Antibiotic Pharmacodynamics

Edited by

John C. Rotschafer

Department of Experimental and Clinical Pharmacology, College of Pharmacy, University of Minnesota, Minneapolis, MN, USA

David R. Andes

Division of Infectious Diseases, University of Wisconsin, Madison, WI, USA

Keith A. Rodvold

Colleges of Pharmacy and Medicine, University of Illinois at Chicago, Chicago, IL, USA

Humana Press

Editors
John C. Rotschafer
Department of Experimental and Clinical Pharmacology
College of Pharmacy
University of Minnesota
Minneapolis, MN, USA

David R. Andes
Division of Infectious Diseases
University of Wisconsin
Madison, WI, USA

Keith A. Rodvold
Colleges of Pharmacy and Medicine
University of Illinois at Chicago
Chicago, IL, USA

ISSN 1557-2153 ISSN 1940-6053 (electronic)
Methods in Pharmacology and Toxicology
ISBN 978-1-4939-3321-1 ISBN 978-1-4939-3323-5 (eBook)
DOI 10.1007/978-1-4939-3323-5

Library of Congress Control Number: 2016930313

Springer New York Heidelberg Dordrecht London

Printed on acid-free paper

Humana Press is a brand of Springer
Springer Science+Business Media LLC New York is part of Springer Science+Business Media (www.springer.com)

Preface

The discovery of antibiotics is often considered one of man's greatest achievements, but often the clinical and microbiologic outcome depends upon the skill of the clinician directing therapy. Over the last 30 years, two new sciences, pharmacokinetics and pharmacodynamics, have increased our understanding of antibiotic behavior in the human host and how these agents interact with bacteria.

In vitro and In vivo pharmacodynamic modeling characterizes antibiotic performance against specific bacterial pathogens as concentration dependent (time independent) or concentration independent (time dependent). Such knowledge can influence antibiotic delivery methods and determine whether desired pharmacodynamic outcome parameter values will be achieved. As a result, continuous infusion or extended infusions of beta-lactam antibiotics or a single daily dose of aminoglycosides are now commonplace strategies used to optimize antibiotic presentation.

Linking bacterial antibiotic susceptibility in the form of a minimum inhibiting concentration (MIC) with antibiotic pharmacokinetic parameters generates pharmacodynamic outcome parameters. Depending upon the antibiotic and pathogen, the peak antibiotic concentration (Cp-max) to MIC ratio (Cp-max/MIC), the area-under-the-serum-concentration-time-curve (AUC) to MIC ratio (AUC/MIC), and the percent of time that antibiotic concentration remains above MIC (%T> MIC) have all been reported to be useful predictors of antibiotic performance.

These data combined with Monte Carlo modeling strategies can predict the probability of achieving the desired therapeutic goal based on the specific pathogen, bacterial MIC, dose, dosage interval, and method of antibiotic delivery. The advances in antibiotic pharmacodynamics have now found their way into the antibiotic development process used for licensing new antibiotics.

This text offers state-of-the-art contributions written by world renowned experts which provide an extensive background on specific classes of antibiotics summarizing our understanding as to how these antibiotics might be optimally used in a clinical situation.

Minneapolis, MN, USA — *John C. Rotschafer*
Madison, WI, USA — *David R. Andes*
Chicago, IL, USA — *Keith A. Rodvold*

Contents

Preface . . . . *v*
Contributors . . . . *ix*

PART I PHARMACODYNAMICS METHODS FOR ANTI-INFECTIVE AGENTS

1 General Concepts of Pharmacodynamics for Anti-infective Agents 3
Johan W. Mouton

2 In Vitro Pharmacodynamic Models to Evaluate Anti-infective Pharmacodynamics 29
Warren Rose

3 Animal Models to Evaluate Anti-infective Pharmacodynamics 59
Alexander J. Lepak and David R. Andes

4 Pharmacodynamic Issues in Antibiotic Combinations 89
Zackery P. Bulman, Ryan C. Dillon, and Brian T. Tsuji

5 Methodologies for Protein Binding Determination in Anti-infective Agents 109
Jatinder Kaur Mukker, Ravi Shankar Prasad Singh, and Hartmut Derendorf

6 Evaluation of Exposure-Response Relationships Using Clinical Data: Basic Concepts and Applications 127
Sujata M. Bhavnani, Christopher M. Rubino, and Paul G. Ambrose

7 Toxicokinetics and Toxicodynamics of Anti-infective Agents 159
David E. Nix

PART II PHARMACODYNAMICS OF ANTIBACTERIAL AGENTS

8 Pharmacodynamics of Fluoroquinolones 177
Ramy H. Elshaboury, Thomas J. Dilworth, and John C. Rotschafer

9 Aminoglycoside Pharmacodynamics 199
Dana R. Bowers, Amy N. Schilling, and Vincent H. Tam

10 Polymyxin Pharmacokinetics and Pharmacodynamics 221
Soon-Ee Cheah, Jian Li, Phillip J. Bergen, and Roger L. Nation

11 Vancomycin Pharmacodynamics: Optimal vs. Controversial 261
Ben M. Lomaestro

12 Pharmacodynamics of Lipoglycopeptides 285
Eric Wenzler, Siyun Liao, and Keith A. Rodvold

13 Pharmacodynamics of Daptomycin 317
Eric Wenzler, Siyun Liao, and Keith A. Rodvold

14 Pharmacodynamics of Macrolides, Azalides, and Ketolides 345
Wonhee So and David P. Nicolau

PART III PHARMACODYNAMICS OF NON-ANTIBACTERIAL AGENTS

15 Antifungal Pharmacokinetics and Pharmacodynamics 369
William Hope and David R. Andes

16 Pharmacokinetics and Pharmacodynamics of the Tuberculosis Drugs. 385
Aline B. Barth, Eric F. Egelund, and Charles A. Peloquin

17 Pharmacodynamics of Antimalarial Agents. 415
Rahul P. Bakshi and Theresa A. Shapiro

18 Pharmacodynamics of Antiviral Agents 441
Renee-Claude Mercier, Bernadette Jakeman, and Larry Pineda

19 Pharmacodynamics of Antiretroviral Agents. 469
Kajal B. Larson and Edward P. Acosta

PART IV PHARMACODYNAMIC CONSIDERATIONS AND SPECIAL POPULATIONS

20 Implementing a Continuous or Prolonged Infusion Beta-Lactam Program in the Hospital Setting 507
Shawn H. MacVane, Nathaniel J. Rhodes, Marc H. Scheetz, and Joseph L. Kuti

21 Pharmacodynamic Considerations in Critically Ill Patients 537
Mahipal G. Sinnollareddy and Jason A. Roberts

22 Pharmacodynamic Considerations and Special Populations: Pediatrics 561
Jennifer Le and John S. Bradley

23 Pharmacodynamics and Obesity 599
Manjunath P. Pai

24 Drug Development Process and Regulatory Science 621
Evelyn J. Ellis-Grosse and Jogarao Gobburu

25 Antibiotic Stewardship and Applications of Pharmacodynamics 633
Elizabeth D. Hermsen and Lynne Fehrenbacher

Index *649*

Contributors

EDWARD P. ACOSTA • *Division of Pharmacology and Toxicology, School of Medicine, University of Alabama at Birmingham, Birmingham, AL, USA*

PAUL G. AMBROSE • *Institute for Clinical Pharmacodynamics, Latham, NY, USA*

DAVID R. ANDES • *Division of Infectious Diseases, University of Wisconsin, Madison, WI, USA*

RAHUL P. BAKSHI • *Division of Clinical Pharmacology and Malaria Research Institute, The Johns Hopkins University School of Medicine, Baltimore, MD, USA*

ALINE B. BARTH • *College of Pharmacy and Emerging Pathogens Institute, University of Florida, Gainesville, FL, USA*

PHILLIP J. BERGEN • *Centre for Medicine Use and Safety, Monash University, Parkville, VIC, Australia*

SUJATA M. BHAVNANI • *Institute for Clinical Pharmacodynamics, Latham, NY, USA*

DANA R. BOWERS • *Department of Pharmacy, Kingman Regional Medical Center, Kingman, AZ, USA*

JOHN S. BRADLEY • *Skaggs School of Pharmacy and Department of Pediatrics, University of California, San Diego, La Jolla, CA, USA; Rady Children's Hospital of San Diego, San Diego, CA, USA*

ZACKERY P. BULMAN • *The New York State Center of Excellence in Bioinformatics & Life Sciences, University at Buffalo, SUNY, Buffalo, NY, USA; Laboratory for Antimicrobial Pharmacodynamics, School of Pharmacy and Pharmaceutical Sciences, University at Buffalo, SUNY, Buffalo, NY, USA*

SOON-EE CHEAH • *Drug Delivery, Disposition and Dynamics, Monash Institute of Pharmaceutical Sciences, Monash University, Melbourne, VIC, Australia*

HARTMUT DERENDORF • *Department of Pharmaceutics, College of Pharmacy, University of Florida, Gainesville, FL, USA*

RYAN C. DILLON • *Laboratory for Antimicrobial Pharmacodynamics, School of Pharmacy and Pharmaceutical Sciences, University at Buffalo, SUNY, Buffalo, NY, USA*

THOMAS J. DILWORTH • *Department of Pharmacy, Wheaton Franciscan Healthcare – Saint Francis, Milwaukee, WI, USA*

ERIC F. EGELUND • *College of Pharmacy and Emerging Pathogens Institute, University of Florida, Gainesville, FL, USA*

EVELYN J. ELLIS-GROSSE • *e2g Biopharmaceutical Consulting, Marietta, GA, USA*

RAMY H. ELSHABOURY • *Department of Pharmacy, Wheaton Franciscan Healthcare, Milwaukee, WI, USA*

LYNNE FEHRENBACHER • *School of Pharmacy, Concordia University, Mequon, WI, USA*

JOGARAO GOBBURU • *University of Maryland, Baltimore, MA, USA*

ELIZABETH D. HERMSEN • *Merck & Co., Kenilworth, NJ, USA; College of Pharmacy, University of Nebraska Medical Center, Omaha, NE, USA*

WILLIAM HOPE • *Antimicrobial Pharmacodynamics and Therapeutics, Institute of Translational Medicine, University of Liverpool, Liverpool, UK*

BERNADETTE JAKEMAN • *College of Pharmacy, University of New Mexico, Albuquerque, NM, USA*

JOSEPH L. KUTI • *Center for Anti-Infective Research and Development, Hartford Hospital, Hartford, CT, USA*
KAJAL B. LARSON • *Merck Sharp and Dohme Corp., Kenilworth, NJ, USA*
JENNIFER LE • *Skaggs School of Pharmacy and Department of Pediatrics, University of California, San Diego, La Jolla, CA, USA; Miller Children's Hospital of Long Beach, Long Beach, CA, USA*
ALEXANDER J. LEPAK • *Division of Infectious Diseases, University of Wisconsin, Madison, WI, USA*
JIAN LI • *Drug Delivery, Disposition and Dynamics, Monash Institute of Pharmaceutical Sciences, Monash University, Melbourne, VIC, Australia*
SIYUN LIAO • *Department of Pharmacy, University of Cincinnati Medical Center, Cincinnati, OH, USA*
BEN M. LOMAESTRO • *Department of Pharmacy (MC85), Albany Medical Center Hospital, Albany, NY, USA*
SHAWN H. MACVANE • *Center for Anti-Infective Research and Development, Hartford Hospital, Hartford, CT, USA*
RENEE-CLAUDE MERCIER • *College of Pharmacy, University of New Mexico, Albuquerque, NM, USA*
JOHAN W. MOUTON • *Department of Medical Microbiology, Radboudumc, Nijmegen, The Netherlands; Department of Medical Microbiology and Infectious Diseases, Erasmus MC, Rotterdam, The Netherlands*
JATINDER KAUR MUKKER • *Department of Pharmaceutics, College of Pharmacy, University of Florida, Gainesville, FL, USA*
ROGER L. NATION • *Drug Delivery, Disposition and Dynamics, Monash Institute of Pharmaceutical Sciences, Monash University, Melbourne, VIC, Australia; Faculty of Pharmacy and Pharmaceutical Sciences, Monash Institute of Pharmaceutical Sciences, Monash University, Parkville, VIC, Australia*
DAVID P. NICOLAU • *Center for Anti-Infective Research and Development, Hartford Hospital, Hartford, CT, USA; Division of Infectious Diseases, Hartford Hospital, Hartford, CT, USA*
DAVID E. NIX • *Pharmacy Practice & Science, and Medicine, University of Arizona, Tucson, AZ, USA*
MANJUNATH P. PAI • *Albany College of Pharmacy and Health Sciences, Albany, NY, USA*
CHARLES A. PELOQUIN • *Emerging Pathogens Institute, College of Pharmacy, University of Florida, Gainesville, FL, USA*
LARRY PINEDA • *College of Pharmacy, University of New Mexico, Albuquerque, NM, USA*
NATHANIEL J. RHODES • *Midwestern University, Downers Grove, IL, USA; Northwestern Memorial Hospital, Chicago, IL, USA*
JASON A. ROBERTS • *Pharmacy Department, Royal Brisbane and Women's Hospital, Herston, QLD, Australia*
KEITH A. RODVOLD • *Colleges of Pharmacy and Medicine, University of Illinois at Chicago, Chicago, IL, USA*
WARREN ROSE • *Pharmacy Practice Division, School of Pharmacy, University of Wisconsin-Madison, Madison, WI, USA*
JOHN C. ROTSCHAFER • *Department of Experimental and Clinical Pharmacology, College of Pharmacy, University of Minnesota, Minneapolis, MN, USA*
CHRISTOPHER M. RUBINO • *Institute for Clinical Pharmacodynamics, Latham, NY, USA*

MARC H. SCHEETZ • *Midwestern University, Downers Grove, IL, USA; Northwestern Memorial Hospital, Chicago, IL, USA*
AMY N. SCHILLING • *Department of Pharmacy, Memorial Hermann The Woodlands Hospital, The Woodlands, TX, USA*
THERESA A. SHAPIRO • *Division of Clinical Pharmacology and Malaria Research Institute, The Johns Hopkins University School of Medicine, Baltimore, MD, USA*
RAVI SHANKAR PRASAD SINGH • *Department of Pharmaceutics, College of Pharmacy, University of Florida, Gainesville, FL, USA*
MAHIPAL G. SINNOLLAREDDY • *Therapeutics Research Centre, Basil Hetzel Institute for Translational Health Research, The Queen Elizabeth Hospital, Adelaide, SA, Australia*
WONHEE SO • *Center for Anti-Infective Research and Development, Hartford Hospital, Hartford, CT, USA*
VINCENT H. TAM • *Department of Pharmacy Practice and Translational Research, University of Houston College of Pharmacy, Houston, TX, USA*
BRIAN T. TSUJI • *Laboratory for Antimicrobial Pharmacodynamics, School of Pharmacy and Pharmaceutical Sciences, University at Buffalo, SUNY, Buffalo, NY, USA; The New York State Center of Excellence in Bioinformatics & Life Sciences, University at Buffalo, SUNY, Buffalo, NY, USA*
ERIC WENZLER • *College of Pharmacy, University of Illinois at Chicago, Chicago, IL, USA*

Part I

Pharmacodynamics Methods for Anti-Infective Agents

Chapter 1

General Concepts of Pharmacodynamics for Anti-infective Agents

Johan W. Mouton

Abstract

Pharmacokinetics (PK) and pharmacodynamics (PD) have become an important field in the evaluation and application of antimicrobials in all its aspects. PK/PD is used in developing drugs, optimizing therapy, setting clinical breakpoints, and preventing emergence of resistance. This chapter provides a general overview of PK/PD, the major factors that play a role, in vitro–in vivo relationships, pitfalls, and the application to clinical practice.

Key words Pharmacodynamic indices, E_{max} models, Exposure-response relationships

1 Introduction

Pharmacokinetics (PK) and pharmacodynamics (PD) have become an important field in the evaluation and application of antimicrobials in all its aspects. It is now almost unconceivable that the development of antimicrobials would take place without a thorough understanding of PK/PD relationships. But what then is exactly PK/PD? And why is it so important? In this chapter we provide a general overview of the emergence of PK/PD as a separate discipline and highlight important aspects of the field. It should be borne in mind, however, that the field is still evolving and that nothing is set in stone—yet there are certain principles that will not change. Indeed, some dogmas—if ever there were—have been shown to fail under certain circumstances. On the other hand, trying to understand what is going on between antibiotic and microorganism has led to some general principles that are now widely accepted, and exceptions to certain behavior in the past can now readily be explained with new understanding.

Pharmacokinetics and pharmacodynamics link the exposure of an antimicrobial in the host—e.g., the human—to its effect on microbes, and this marks the exposure–effect relationships different from other drugs. Whereas for other drugs, such as a

John C. Rotschafer et al. (eds.), *Antibiotic Pharmacodynamics*, Methods in Pharmacology and Toxicology,
DOI 10.1007/978-1-4939-3323-5_1, © Springer Science+Business Media New York 2016

beta-receptor agonist or aspirin, the drug interacts and exerts its effect directly on a receptor in the human body, antimicrobials interact with receptors on the microorganism with the purpose of inflicting damage in such a way that the microbe cannot survive. It easily follows that the number of different receptors to potentially interact with is much larger for an antimicrobial and a microbe than another drug in the human body. Every species of microorganisms is characterized by its own set of receptors, and the way antimicrobials interact with these receptors is therefore also species specific. Moreover, due to the rapid multiplication of microorganisms and selection of mutants in specific environmental conditions, new populations of the same species with other receptor characteristics may emerge fast—resulting in what is generally known as reduced susceptibility or resistance. The field of antimicrobial pharmacodynamics endeavors to describe this interaction by several methods with the overall purpose to be able to predict the efficacy of antimicrobials in the treatment of infectious diseases. Most of these methods were rather crude in the past, but increasing refinement has led to a growing insight into exactly how antimicrobials can be used more successfully, by optimizing both the dosing for cure and the usage and dosing to reduce or prevent emergence of resistance. Importantly, it was realized that pharmacokinetics play an important role in the overall effect of an antimicrobial, and that the concentrations in different compartments of the host as well as the time course of those concentrations had a marked impact on the overall effect of the antimicrobial. Hence the aggregated term PK/PD emerged to incorporate the impact of pharmacokinetic profiling in the overall outcome of antimicrobial treatment.

PK/PD then describes the effect of the concentration-time course of an antimicrobial on the microbe as well as the longer term outcome thereof including the overall purpose of antimicrobial treatment, that is, cure of the patient, prevention of infection, or prevention of emergence of resistance, as illustrated in Fig. 1.

From the diagram in Fig. 1, it is obvious that there are many factors that play a role from dosing regimen to clinical cure of the patient. In the following, the major components that constitute PK/PD relationships and/or have a significant impact are discussed, but are intended to serve as a general overview. In each of the following chapters much is covered in much more detail. In the first part, pharmacodynamic relationships and parameters are discussed, the interaction of the drug with the microorganism, and methods to describe those. The second part introduces pharmacokinetic profiling and the effect thereof in exposure-response relationships. Although the text and examples primarily concern antibacterials, the principles of PK/PD are similar for antifungal and antiviral drugs. Finally, in the last section a number of applications and considerations are provided.

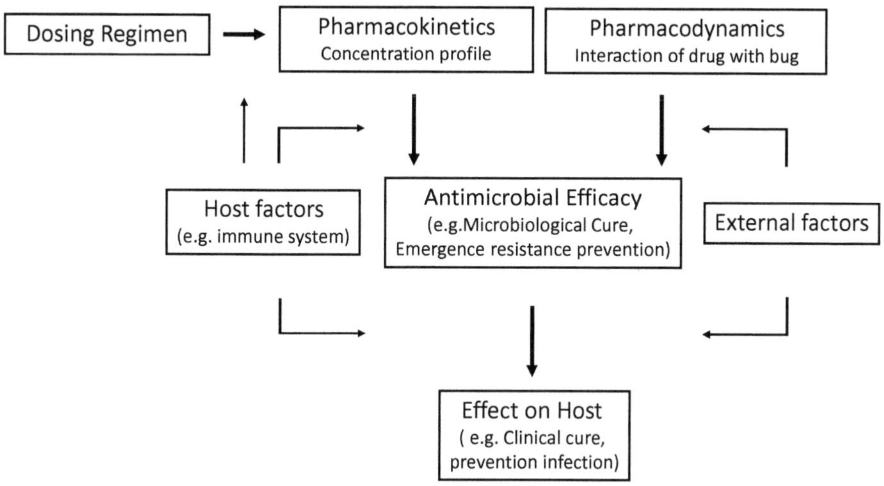

Fig. 1 The interrelationships between dosing, pharmacokinetics, pharmacodynamics, and treatment outcome

2 Concentration-Effect Relationships: Pharmacodynamics

Microorganisms contain many receptors that antimicrobials interact with, some more important than others and in most cases one or two that the antimicrobial agent specifically was developed for. However, it is practically impossible—or has been until now—to define specific drug-receptor interactions; rather an overall measure of activity of an antimicrobial agent against a microorganism is used. The pharmacodynamic parameter most often used to that purpose is the minimum inhibitory concentration (MIC). The MIC is defined as the lowest concentration with no visible growth after (in most cases) 16–20 h of incubation under specifically prescribed conditions [1]. Alternatively, the minimum bactericidal concentration (MBC) is the concentration with no (or few - see below) surviving bacteria in the MIC test and therefore is generally higher than the MIC. Both the MIC and the MBC strive to capture the overall effect of an antimicrobial over a certain period of time: the parameter value of the MIC (or MBC) is the end result of growth and/or kill of bacteria by the antimicrobial over time. It should be noted that "MIC testing" and "susceptibility testing using the MIC test" are often interchangeable but strictly speaking are two separate procedures. The MIC test provides a measure of activity, whereas susceptibility testing also includes an interpretation of the parameter value in the test.

2.1 MIC

The MIC was first described in some way in the report by Ericsson and Sherris, when microbiologists were looking for a method to characterize the activity of an antimicrobial agent and using a measure of activity to distinguish resistant populations from susceptible populations [2]. In the report, twofold dilutions are mentioned as well as the inclusion of 1 mg/L in the dilution series. However, the MIC is dependent on many factors that all represent their effect on the growth rate and kill rate of the bacterial population during the time of incubation. These factors include incubation temperature, atmosphere (CO_2), pH, inoculum, and, importantly, composition of the medium including Mueller-Hinton, the medium often used today. However, Mueller-Hinton is not a very-well-defined medium, and certainly at the time there were significant batch-to-batch and producer-to-producer variations that resulted in a reproducibility of the MIC that was not satisfactory to many. For the disk-diffusion susceptibility testing method this effect was even far more pronounced. It was not possible to reach a consensus in the years following the publication of the report, and many different methods were developed at the time. In Europe, a significant number of countries adopted the ISO sensitest medium instead of Mueller-Hinton, since ISO sensitest was a much better defined medium than Mueller-Hinton and reproducibility—in particular for disk-diffusion—considered superior. Then, in 2002, an initiative was taken by the European Committee on Standardization (CEN) to reach consensus on a reference method for susceptibility testing culminating in two standards from the International Standards Organization (ISO). ISO 25572-1 [1] describes the standard microdilution method for rapidly growing aerobic bacteria and is based on earlier published methods of CLSI [3] and EUCAST [4]. A separate document, ISO 25572-2, describes the validation procedure for other methods [5]. Finally, very recently an ISO standard for Mueller-Hinton medium was agreed on and is in its final stages before publication [6]. For yeasts and molds there is no worldwide consensus, and the MICs of these should therefore always be looked at with some caution and as will become apparent below, this may have significant impact on the interpretation of PK/PD relationships.

Although the microdilution MIC is considered the gold standard, agar dilution has long been the mainstay of MIC testing for large numbers of strains simultaneously, in particular in drug development and epidemiological studies. In this method a series of agar plates is incubated with inocula of up to 40 strains, each agar plate containing, similar to microdilution assay, a twofold increase in antibiotic concentration. The activity of the antibiotic is read as growth or no growth at a certain concentration. The inoculum for agar diffusion is typically somewhat lower than in microdilution, 10E4 cfu (colony-forming units) vs 5 × 10E5 cfu/ml, and is one of the reasons that the MIC is often somewhat lower. Agar diffusion is still being used for screening large numbers of strains, but the values obtained may differ by one- or twofold dilutions from those obtained by microdilution depending on the antimicrobial and strain tested. Thus, for any interpretation and calculation of pharmacodynamic targets (for the definition see below), this method is less suitable, unless having been validated against the ISO standard microdilution method. Yet, the method does provide an alternative to the microdilution method and has the advantage that the effect of the antibiotic can be measured quantitatively. A more in-depth discussion of susceptibility testing can be found in Chap. 2. A variation of this method, using large inocula, is being used to determine the mutant prevention concentration (MPC; see Sect. 4.5).

The MIC is not an "all or nothing" parameter of activity, although this may seem to be the case. The definition clearly states "non-visible growth" as an end point, and the initial inoculum is clearly defined as 3–7 × 10E5 cfu/ml. Non-visible growth after incubation may represent any number of bacteria between 0 and the number resulting in visible cloudiness—in effect around 10E8 bacteria/ml. Effectively, bacteria may not even have been inhibited in growth, but grown from inoculum size to just under the limit of detection by vision—still more than 2 ^{10}logs! Alternatively, significant killing over the incubation period may have resulted in a decline in 2 ^{10}logs, but the MIC would still not have a different value. The implications hereof are discussed in [7]. This lack of precision of the measurement of antimicrobial activity is one of the explanations that PK/PD relationships found by various investigators may vary significantly.

The pharmacodynamic parameter that is somewhat more precise as an estimate of antimicrobial activity is the minimum bactericidal concentration, the MBC.

2.2 MBC

The MBC has long been used as an indication of bactericidality of a compound, in particular in the previous century when PK/PD relationships were not well established and alternative measures of the activity of an antimicrobial were sought. The MBC is determined by plating the contents of each well in the twofold dilution series and ascertaining growth or nongrowth the following day. The lowest concentration with at least a 99.9 % reduction in cfu compared to the initial inoculum is the MBC. This method is seemingly more precise—bacteria either survive or do not. However, the time course of killing is not taken into account—and the duration of incubation in the MIC test of 16–20 h is therefore one of the major factors that contribute to the MBC and is therefore still an arbitrary measure of activity.

2.3 Time-Kill Curves: Fixed Concentrations

Although the MIC captures the overall activity of an antimicrobial in a single value, which has its practical advantages, there are two important drawbacks that also apply to the MBC. The first is that it does not describe the effect of the antimicrobial over time, only the end result after 16–20 h (or other times in certain cases) of incubation. Thus, as an example, whether bacteria are slowly killed over time or rapidly killed over time these different patterns of kill-

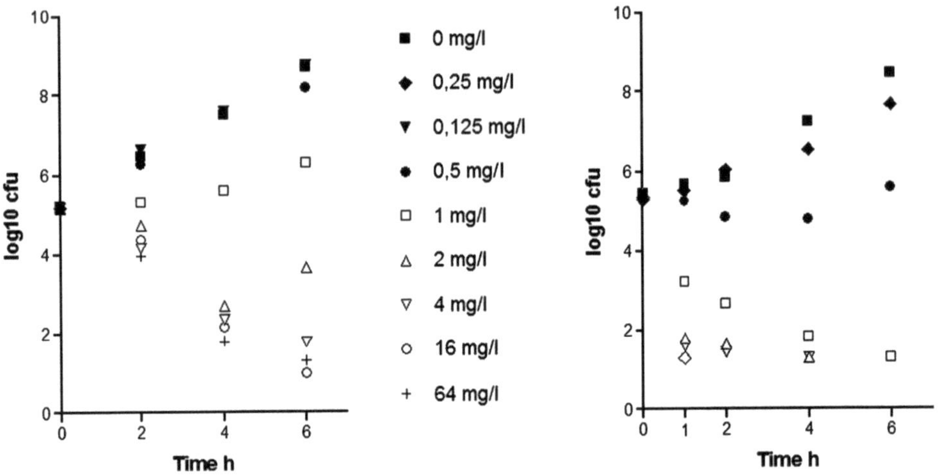

Fig. 2 Timc-kill kinctics of ccftazidimc (*lcft*) and tobramycin (*right*) and *Pscudomonas acruginosa*. Killing by tobramycin at higher concentrations is significantly faster than by ceftazidime

ing all could result in the same MIC and MBC value. Moreover, initial killing after which regrowth occurs is not accounted for either in the MIC test.

Differences in killing behavior of antimicrobials were observed as early as 1948, when Garrod described kill kinetics of streptomycin and penicillin and *Staphylococcus aureus* [8]. Studies over the years by various investigators such as Shah [9], Mattie [10], and the group of Craig [11] have indicated that the behavior and killing characteristics differed between various classes of antimicrobials and ultimately led to the recognition of antimicrobials that show increased killing over a large concentration range and those that do not. In addition, some antimicrobials show relatively fast killing, whereas others show a much slower but persistent killing effect. An example is shown in Fig. 2 for ceftazidime and tobramycin. Killing of ceftazidime is maximized at concentrations of around four times the MIC. Microorganisms exposed to concentrations higher than four times the MIC all show the same rate of decline of cfu. Concentrations lower than the MIC do not have much effect, although there is some growth inhibition at concentrations just below the MIC. In contrast, increasing concentrations of tobramycin result in an increased kill rate, up to the highest concentration measured. The different killing properties of these two classes of agents have led to the terms "concentration-independent" and "concentration-dependent" antimicrobials. The former term is not fully correct of course, since effects are always concentration dependent and only indicate the degree and span of kill rates of the one relative to the other. As discussed later in this chapter, these pharmacodynamic properties of the two classes are associated with their antimicrobial effects in vivo.

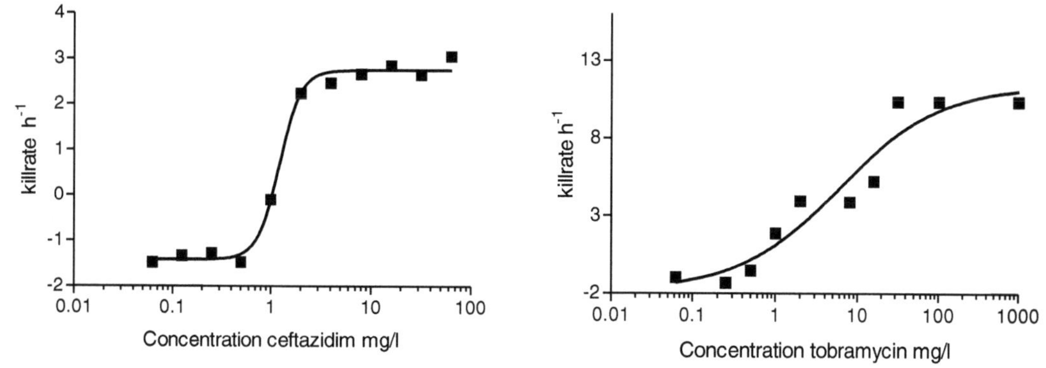

Fig. 3 Kill rates of ceftazidime (*left*) and tobramycin (*right*) against *P. aeruginosa*. Note the different scales used for the *x*-axes and *y*-axes

Another way of expressing the rate of killing of bacteria is plotting the kill rate as a function of concentration, as shown in Fig. 3. At low concentrations the kill rate is negative (because there is growth of the microorganisms) whereas increasing concentrations result in an increased kill rate. The kill rate is maximal at four times the MIC for ceftazidime, and at much higher concentrations for tobramycin. It should be realized that the maximum kill rates are in part dependent on the experimental conditions and the way samples were obtained, in particular for "concentration-dependent" drugs. For instance, some antimicrobials—such as the fluoroquinolones against enterobacteriaceae—kill bacteria at such speed at high concentrations that measurements after even a short period as one-half hour of incubation will underestimate the kill rate, and carryover effects will overestimate it.

2.4 Modeling of Concentration-Time Data

The relationship between concentration and kill rate can be modeled. One of the most often used models to describe the killing of bacteria is the E_{max} model with variable slope, also called the Hill equation:

$$\text{Effect} = E_{max} \times C^{g} / (C^{g} + \text{EC}_{50}{}^{g})$$

where E_{max} is the maximum effect, C the concentration, EC_{50} the concentration where 50 % of the effect is reached, and g the Hill slope. Several variations of the model exist, for instance including a minimum effect (the model shown above assumes the minimum effect to be 0), or including a negative sign. The E_{max} model has shown to be a very useful tool to describe pharmacodynamic relationships and thereby estimate parameter values that can subsequently be used to compare the effects of different drugs or different conditions. It should be borne in mind however that one of the major reasons the model is so effectual is that by the nature of most experiments and the type of observations used, the E_{max}

and E_{min} are predetermined by experimental conditions and not necessarily always represent the "true" effects of a drug. This will be further discussed in Sect. 3.

In Fig. 3, the E_{max} model for the ceftazidime and tobramycin kill rate data indicate that the maximum kill rate of tobramycin is reached at much higher concentrations than for ceftazidime; in addition the Hill slope has a much lower value—represented by the shallower curve for tobramycin. As will be seen later in the chapter, the PK/PD behavior in vivo can be traced directly to these specific attributes.

The effect of an antibiotic on a bacterial population can be described by the natural growth rate of bacteria and the kill rate of the antibiotic, the latter dependent on the antibiotic concentration as described by the E_{max} model. It can be calculated that for every antibiotic there is a certain concentration where the growth rate equals the kill rate and there is no net growth of bacteria, the stationary concentration SC [7, 12, 13]. Above the SC bacteria will outgrow, and below the SC bacteria are killed. The SC is therefore a much more precise estimate of antibacterial effect than the MIC is but arguably much more difficult to measure. The SC is also dependent on experimental and in vivo conditions, whereas the MIC is standardized. In general, the SC is somewhat lower than the MIC. The lower the Hill slope and/or growth rate, the lower the SC is, relative to the MIC. The SC is further discussed in Sect. 3.4.

3 PK/PD

In the section above, the effect of the antimicrobial agent was described at fixed concentrations: the MIC as the lowest concentration with no visible growth, and time-kill curves describing the effect of an antimicrobial agent at various concentrations. Noteworthy, during these tests concentrations during exposure to an inoculum do not change. However, when patients are treated for infections and receive an antibiotic for the treatment of an infection, the concentrations resulting from the dose are not fixed. A dose results in increasing concentrations initially, the speed being dependent on the infusion rate or absorption rate of the drug. After a maximum concentration has been reached, concentrations decline over time due to redistribution and elimination, until the next dose is administered and the cycle starts anew. Thus, the concentration changes over time. Moreover, patients usually receive antibiotics several times a day, the frequency of administration varying depending on the drug. Obviously, the concentration-time profile is much different from that applied in MIC testing and time-kill curve experiments, and it is not possible to use a single concentration to express the activity of the drug in vivo. This was already appreciated in the very early days of antimicrobial chemotherapy. Harry Eagle, in groundbreaking experiments in mice, demonstrated that the frequency of administration of penicillin had a profound effect on its efficacy, even if the total daily dose was the same, indicating that the shape of the concentration profile did have a significant impact on the overall effect of this particular antibiotic [14].

3.1 Pharmacodynamic Indices

Since concentrations change over time during intermittent dosing schedules, other measures of exposure are required to allow expression of exposure of an effect. Over time, three measures have appeared to be particularly useful (Fig. 4). The first is the area under the concentration-time curve (AUC), and it represents the integrated concentration over time. Thus, independent of the shape of the curve, it is a measure for total exposure of the drug to the microorganism. Since most (but not all) of the antimicrobials used today show linear pharmacokinetic behavior after intravenous administration, it follows that there is a linear relationship between dose and AUC. In other words the AUC over a certain time period is, until certain limits, independent of the frequency of administration. The second measure is the peak concentration or maximum concentration Cmax. This is usually defined as the highest concentration in plasma after the distribution phase. The third measure of exposure is the time the concentration remains above the MIC of the microorganism. This is usually expressed as a percentage of the dosing interval (%T > MIC). In contrast to the AUC, the %T > MIC *is* dependent on the shape of the concentration-time curve as illustrated in Fig. 4b. It should be noted that the first two measures, the AUC and the Cmax or peak concentration, can be determined *without* any knowledge of an MIC and are strictly spoken pharmacokinetic parameters, whereas for calculation of the

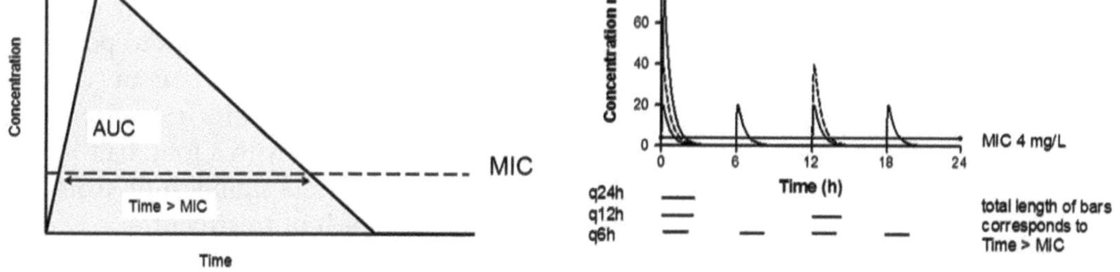

Fig. 4 (**a**) Schematic presentation of the pharmacokinetic parameters Cmax (maximum concentration) and AUC (area under the concentration-time curve; indicated in *light grey*) and the pharmacodynamic index time > MIC. (**b**) Effect of dosing frequency on the %T > MIC: the daily dose is similar for each of the three regimens, the AUC is similar, but the %T > MIC increases if the frequency of administration increases, as indicated by he *horizontal bars* below the figure

%T > MIC the value of the MIC is required. The pharmacodynamic expressions that go together with AUC and peak concentration are the AUC/MIC ratio and the peak/MIC ratio and express the relationship between two independent estimates and are referred to as pharmacodynamic indices rather than pharmacodynamic parameters: a pharmacodynamic index is not a parameter by itself, but the ratio of two independent parameter estimates [15]. Another way of expression is that the exposure of the microorganism to an antibiotic in pharmacokinetic terms is normalized by the potency of the antibiotic and thereby provides a means to establish exposure-response relationships independent of the MIC.

There have been significant discussions as to the dimension and units that should be used for pharmacodynamic indices as they are, in principle, a construct of two independent parameter estimates. This applies in particular to the AUC/MIC. Moreover, the value of the MIC is not an unconditional parameter, but is dependent on certain conditions, such as medium composition, duration of incubation, initial inoculum, atmosphere, and others. In the two papers that defined the use and expressions of pharmacodynamic indices units for AUC/MIC ratio were proposed in the first [16], but in the sequel more expanded paper, units for pharmacodynamic indices were abolished, as there was the general feeling that the use of units was not justified [15] although there is still a debate [17]. Thus, the AUC/MIC ratio is dimensionless, but the two constituent factors AUC and MIC have their own definition. It could also be argued that the MIC is a measure of effect over (the incubation) time rather then a concentration and therefore should have the dimension h.mg/L rendering the ratio dimensionless. For the peak/MIC ratio such a discussion appeared to be meaningless, because even if dimensions would be taken into account, both are expressed similarly (mg/L, although with a total different meaning) and the ratio therefore is dimensionless by default. The %T > MIC is obviously expressed in % of the dosing interval or % of 24 h. However, even with a description of the intended meaning of these expressions, there is still a lot of leeway in the procedures to determine the exact value estimates. There are many different methods to determine an AUC, and the same applies to peak concentration in particular. It is therefore imperative that any description of a pharmacodynamic relationship provides a description of the methods used. In particular, for drugs with a long half-life the estimate of the AUC in steady state differs significantly from that after the first dose, or even the first 24 h of treatment.

3.2 Exposure-Response Relationships

Exposure-response relationships have been established for most antimicrobials, and it has appeared that these differ by class of antibiotic, but are markedly consistent within a class. After Eagle described the dependency of the effect of penicillin on dosing frequency in mice experiments, several decades passed until this was followed up by evaluating the effect of dosing regimens of penicillin by Bakker-Woudenberg in a rat pneumonia model [18] and other antimicrobials in the neutropenic mouse thigh model by Gerber and colleagues [19]. Elaborate studies by the group of Craig showed that for some classes of drugs frequency of administration did matter, while for others it did not [20–22]. The experimental setup that they chose was the mentioned neutropenic mouse thigh model that since has been copied many times and has become some sort of a standard model, if only because virtually every antibiotic has been evaluated in this infection model. Mice are rendered neutropenic and infected with an inoculum typically in the range of 10E6–10E7 per thigh. After 2 h, mice receive dosing regimens varying both in dose and frequency for 24 h. Each mouse receives a different regimen. After 24 h—or in some models 48 or 72 h—the mice are terminated and the number of cfu in each thigh determined by homogenizing the thigh and plating in tenfold dilutions. In the pulmonary model, also often used to determine the efficacy of antimicrobials in lung-infections, the lungs are surgically excised. In separate experiments, the pharmacokinetic characteristics of the drug are determined to establish the exposure for each dosing regimen. By plotting the number of cfu after treatment against the exposure for each mouse an exposure-response curve can then be constructed. An example is provided in Fig. 5, showing the exposure-response relationship of AUC, peak, and %T > MIC for levofloxacin and a strain of *S. pneumoniae* [23]. The data show a clearly better relationship between AUC and response than %T > MIC and response; there is a moderate relationship with the Cmax. As can be observed from the figure, the relationship between exposure and response is of the E_{max} model type and fitting the E_{max} model to the data indeed shows the best relationship with AUC, as inferred from the R^2 of the model fits. The E_{max} model used is similar to that described in the previous section, except that the concentration C and the 50 % effective concentra-

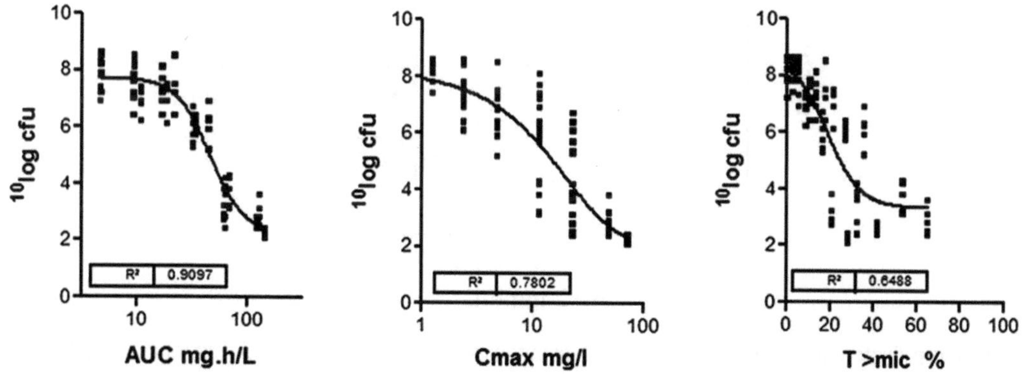

Fig. 5 Relationship between AUC, Cmax, and %T > MIC of levofloxacin and number of cfu of *S. pneumoniae*. Adapted from Scaglione, 2003

tion EC_{50} are substituted by the pharmacokinetic parameter or pharmacodynamic index (PI) values.

The E_{max} model fit allows estimations of the parameters in the model, such as the EI_{50} (the 50 % effective (pharmacodynamic) index). However, another set of parameters has appeared to be very useful over the years. The most important one is the net static effect. This is the dose or exposure resulting in the measure of effect being unchanged from baseline to the time of evaluation (e.g., the number of cfu at $t=0$ h (baseline, start of treatment) and $t=$ time of sampling (usually 24 h)). The use of the term static does not imply that no changes have occurred during the period of reference; indeed kill and regrowth may have repeatedly occurred [15]. Other characteristics include exposures that result in the E_{max}, 90 % of the E_{max}, or a 1 or 2 ^{10}log drop (Fig. 6). The PI value that will result in one of the effects described and is desired is also called the *pharmacodynamic target* (PT). In Fig. 6 the value at "A" is the static effect of pharmacodynamic target and at "B" the 2 ^{10}log drop of pharmacodynamic target. Pharmacodynamic targets have been described for many microorganism–anti-infective combinations and in general show a good concordance with survival and clinical cure (see below), in particular for the free, nonprotein-bound fraction of the drug [24].

As noted in paragraph a, the AUC and the Cmax are pharmacokinetic parameters and effect plots do not necessarily include the MIC, whereas for %T > MIC the MIC is required. Including the MIC in the effect plots such as Fig. 6 by using the AUC/MIC or Cmax/MIC will only have a scalar effect, that is, depending on the MIC, the shape of the curve and the overall relationship do not change. The curve is only shifted to the left (if the MIC is above 1 mg/L) or to the right (if the MIC is below 1 mg/L). In contrast, the overall relationship and shape of the curve between %T > MIC

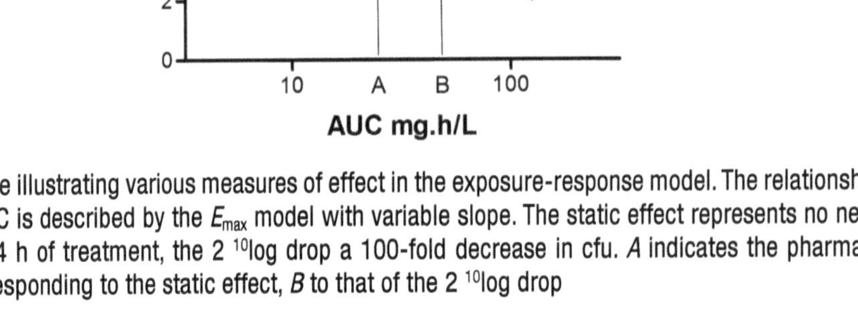

Fig. 6 Figure illustrating various measures of effect in the exposure-response model. The relationship between cfu and AUC is described by the E_{max} model with variable slope. The static effect represents no net change in cfu after 24 h of treatment, the 2 ^{10}log drop a 100-fold decrease in cfu. *A* indicates the pharmacodynamic target corresponding to the static effect, *B* to that of the 2 ^{10}log drop

and effect will change depending on the MIC. Also, given a certain dose and assuming linear pharmacokinetics, the AUC is independent of the shape of the pharmacokinetic curve, whereas %T > MIC can be markedly different for a drug given as a bolus infusion or as extended or continuous infusion. Estimates of %T > MIC are, in general, therefore more difficult and cumbersome to ascertain.

3.3 Protein Binding

One of the issues that has risen to considerable debate in the past is the effect of protein binding and to what extent protein binding plays a role in the outcome of treatment, although it was shown that there was a relationship between the degree of protein binding and the ability of various penicillins to kill *S. aureus* as early as 1947 [25]. The issue has by and large been resolved by elegant analysis of pharmacodynamic results by Craig. By comparing the exposure required for stasis in the infected thigh model for seven different quinolones with different degrees of protein binding properties—varying between less than 20 % to over 80 %—he showed that the AUC/MIC ratio to result in stasis was similar for each of the seven quinolones if only the free fraction of the drug was considered. However, the AUC/MIC of total drug—thus including the protein-bound fraction—was different for each of them, and the AUC/MIC required proportional to the degree of binding (Fig. 7). Likewise, the %T > MIC of cephalosporins required for static effect was comparable if based on unbound antibiotic, but became longer if the unbound fraction was taken into account [26]. In pharmacodynamic expressions, the suffix *f* is often used to indicate that the free fraction of the drug is meant. Thus *f*AUC represents the AUC of the nonprotein-bound fraction, whereas AUC indicates total drug. Methods to establish the degree of pro-

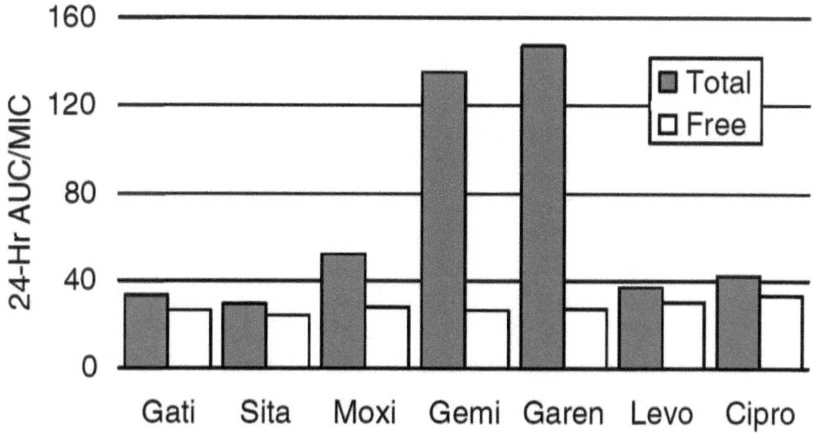

Fig. 7 The 24-AUC/MIC values for total (*grey*) and free drug (*white*) required for a static effect of seven fluoroquinolones. Labels indicate the fluoroquinolone abbreviated by -floxacin. Courtesy of Dr. William A. Craig, MD, 2011

tein binding have evolved over the years, and have helped to interpret the interpretation of protein binding [27].

The degree of protein binding is of considerable importance in the translation and interpretation of pharmacodynamic target values from one setting to the other, such as mice to men, or even in vitro activity to activity in vivo. Protein binding of a number of antibiotics differs considerably across species, and not making allowance for this may result in considerable over- or underestimation of antimicrobial activity. Unfortunately, this was not fully recognized until the last decade of the previous century. Daptomycin most likely failed in initial clinical studies because of its high protein binding not considered [28]; teicoplanin likewise failed initially because of dosing that was too low, and one of the explanations was the relatively high protein binding [29]. The importance of protein binding is further discussed in Chap. 5.

3.4 Exposure-Response Relationships: Differences between Classes

In the section above, exposure-response relationships were demonstrated for levofloxacin, representing the class of the fluoroquinolones. Similar relationships have been determined for other classes of drugs, such as beta-lactams, aminoglycosides, glycopeptides, and many others, and pharmacodynamic targets have been derived from each of these relationships. The one class of antimicrobials that clearly shows a different pharmacodynamic behavior is the beta-lactam class. The beta-lactam class is extensive and many of the drugs that are used belong to this class including the penicillins, cephalosporins, carbapenems, and monobactams. Figure 8 shows the results of dose fractionation studies of levofloxacin and ceftazidime. In contrast to the example of levofloxacin above, the relationship between %T > MIC and effect is clearly superior to that of AUC and effect for ceftazidime. In analogy to deriving pharmacodynamic targets of levofloxacin for AUCs, %T > MIC targets can be determined for beta-lactams. Experimental work shows that the static effect is reached at around 40 %*f*T > MIC for cephalosporins, but may be higher or lower for other subclasses.

3.5 The Relationship between In Vitro and In Vivo Pharmacodynamics

A certain relationship exists between the pharmacodynamic properties of antimicrobials in vitro and in vivo. In general, time-kill kinetics showing an antimicrobial to be "concentration dependent" will show a good relationship with total AUC in vivo, provided that the Hill coefficient does not deviate too much from 1. For most drugs this is the case. In the E_{max} model, the killing effect over time dN/dt is then described by $(E_{max} \times (C/C + EC_{50})) \times N$ where N is the number of bacteria and C is the concentration (static in time-kill curves but changing over time depending on the pharmacokinetic profile). For $C \ll EC_{50}$, and taking the integral over time, this resolves to the integration over C, and the change in bacteria over time thus being linearly related to AUC (E_{max} and EC_{50} being regarded constants). For antimicrobials that show a

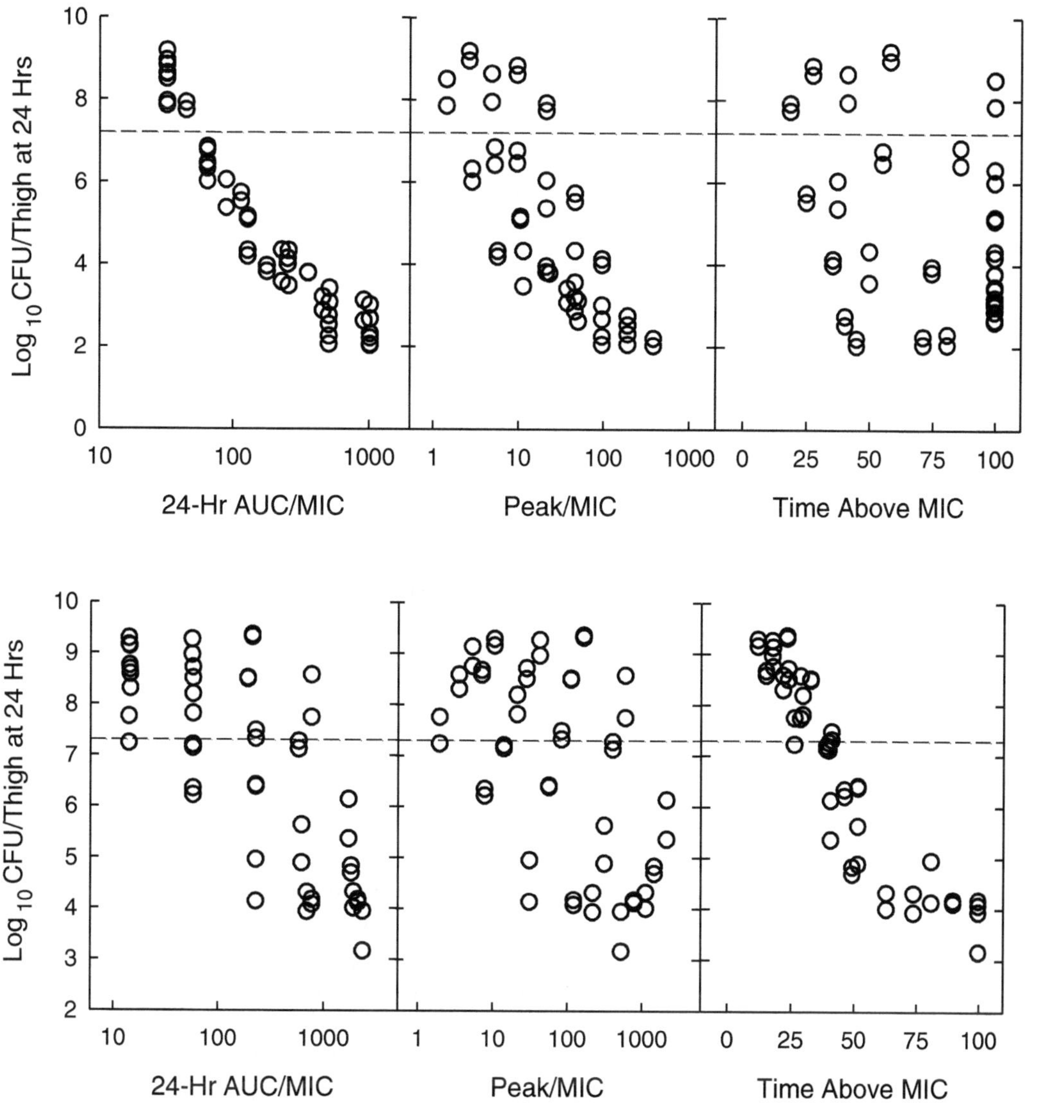

Fig. 8 PK/PD relationships of the fluoroquinolone levofloxacin (upper panel) and the beta-lactam ceftazidime (lower panel). With permission from [38]

"concentration-independent" killing, characterized by a Hill coefficient well above 1, the degree of killing can be described by some sort of a step function, with killing of bacteria above a certain concentration and outgrowth of bacteria if the concentration falls below a certain value. It should be noted that the concentration where there is no growth and no kill of bacteria—the stationary concentration SC as discussed in Sect. 2.4—is not equal to the MIC and may be well below the MIC, in particular if growth is relatively slow compared to in vitro conditions. The difference in SC and MIC may explain some antibacterial effects observed in vivo, such as the post-antibiotic in vivo effect [13]. This is the time lag between concentrations of an antibiotic declining below the MIC in vivo and observed regrowth of bacteria. The lower the SC compared to the MIC, and the longer the half-life of the antibiotic, the longer the post-antibiotic effect. Conversely, a long post-antibiotic effect can also be caused by other persistent effects. Post-exposure and sub-MIC effects have also been described [30].

In a slightly different approach, Tam and colleagues endeavored to distinguish between peak, AUC, and %*f*T > MIC antimicrobials by defining three-dimensional planes separating the effects of in vitro PK/PD characteristics in three categories correlating with in vivo effects with major dependencies on dosing frequency and dose [31]. In their proposal and subsequent simulations, they found that the PI is at least in part, depending on dosing intensity, a combination of average killing characteristics and dosing regimen.

3.6 PK/PD in Patient Populations

Whereas experimental conditions can be controlled in the research setting and PK/PD relationships therefore relatively easy to establish, this is much more difficult in the clinical setting. Moreover, for many drugs fixed dosing regimens have been established—typically found in the hospital formularium—and therefore the variation in pharmacokinetic profiles is relatively low. MICs of microorganisms are not always available, and the definition of treatment success in terms of cure or failure is not always clear either. As a consequence, it took much longer to ascertain exposure-response relationships in patients. Most of the early studies were focused on quinolones and aminoglycosides. One of the first studies to show the relationship between AUC/MIC and microbiological and clinical cure was by Forrest and colleagues in patients with a pseudomonas infection treated with ciprofloxacin [32]. They showed that patients with an AUC/MIC ratio below 125 did significantly worse than patients with an AUC/MIC ratio of 125 or higher. Increasing the ratio up to 250 and beyond resulted in an even better outcome. Subsequent studies by Preston and colleagues [33] and Ambrose and colleagues [34] found similar relationships for quinolones. Relationships for other antimicrobials have also been established, many of these discussed in specific chapters in this book, including antifungal agents [35]. In principle, these studies, and all subsequent ones, follow the same study design as depicted in Fig. 9: estimate the exposure in individual patients using population pharmacokinetic models and/or sampling in individual patients, determine the MIC of the infectious microorganisms, and define microbiological and clinical cure at relevant moments in time. Figure 10 shows an example of such an approach for ceftazidime in the treatment of nosocomial pneumonia [36]. The figure shows the relationship between %*f*T > MIC and clinical efficacy. Logistic regression was used because of the binomial outcome cure versus no cure. Classification and regression

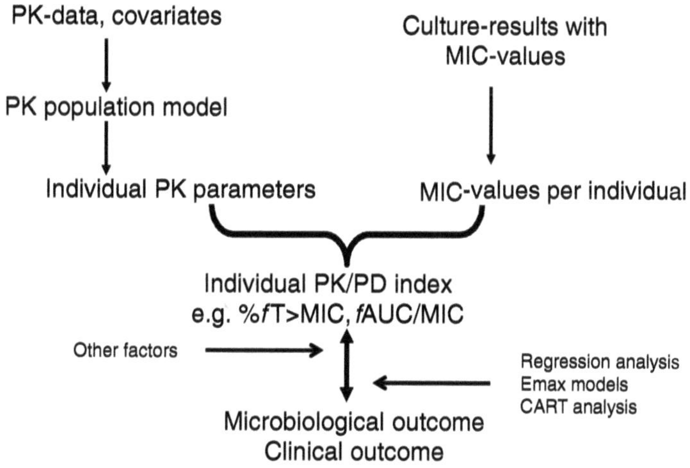

Fig. 9 Diagram showing the general setup of PK/PD analyses in patients. Note the resemblance with Fig. 1

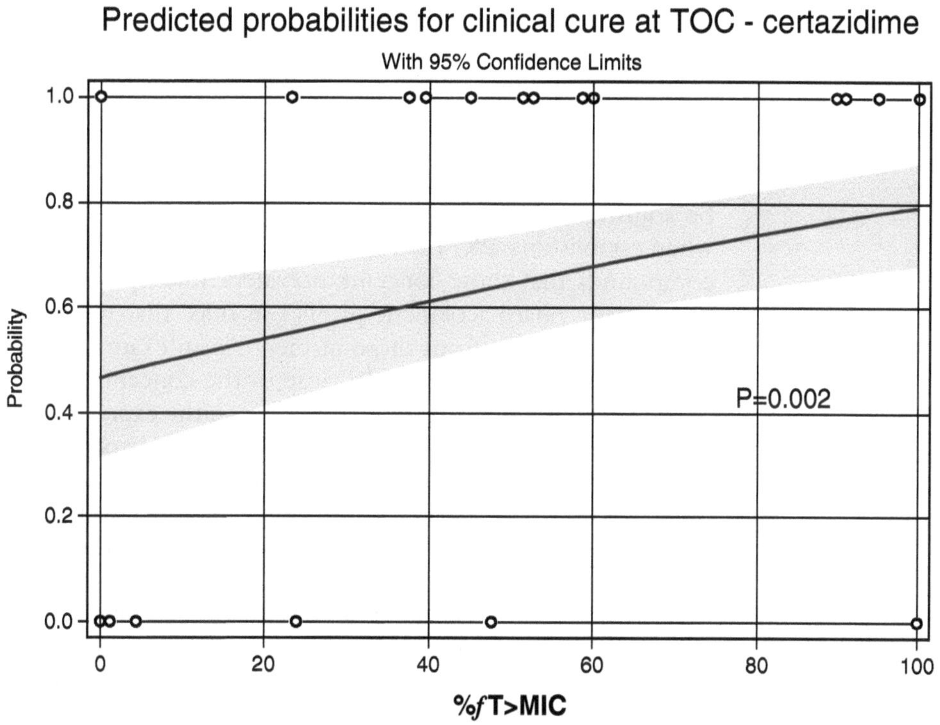

Fig. 10 Logistic regression showing the relationship between %fT > MIC and clinical cure at test of cure (TOC) for ceftazidime against Gram-negative bacteria

tree analysis was performed to determine the value that best distinguishes between a high and a low probability of cure. This was 45 % in this study, and is in the same range as that found in animal models.

4 Some Considerations

It should be clear from the discussions above that there are many factors that have an impact on the parameter estimates that are required to determine pharmacodynamic indices, and that with any interpretation of data the methods used to determine these parameter estimates should be borne in mind. In addition, the experimental or clinical circumstances under which pharmacodynamic relationships are established may bear no predictive value for every situation. One of the issues that is a matter of elaborate discussions is the generability of pharmacodynamic target estimates and exactly which targets should be used to adequately predict treatment success. Here some of these issues are discussed a little more in depth.

4.1 Translation from Mice to Men

Although it has been clearly established that exposure-response relationships found in mice—or other animal species—concur with those in men, as has been shown by Ambrose and colleagues [24], there are a few issues that should be borne in mind. The first is, as discussed above, the degree of protein binding. Although this can be adjusted for by using the free fraction of the compound only when establishing PK/PD relationships, this is not satisfactory for compounds that show concentration-dependent protein binding, because the pharmacokinetic profiles in mice that will result in a certain AUC differ from those in men. As an example, Scaglione and colleagues showed that, because of the concentration dependence of the protein binding of quinolones, the exposure-response relationships of free drug were different from those of total drug in mice, and therefore the pharmacodynamic behavior was to be reinterpreted [23]. A similar situation exists for ceftriaxone and some other drugs. It should be stressed again however that there is a difference in pharmacodynamic behavior of the drug and pharmacodynamic target. The latter is dependent on the compartment where the drug is measured, and the matrix that was used to determine the target. Thus, a pharmacodynamic target derived from concentrations measured in plasma should not be used as a target in epithelial lining fluid (ELF) or other tissue compartment. Similarly, the pharmacodynamic index relationships of free drug are not necessarily the same as for total drug.

The second issue is which pharmacodynamic target derived from the experiment in mice is to be used—the exposure resulting in a static effect, the one-log drop in cfu, or the two-log drop in cfu? Of course, the duration of the experiment has to be considered here as well: 24 h or longer? In general however, the static effect dose is considered to be adequate for non-severe, non-life-threatening infections, whereas the one or two log drop is considered necessary for severe infections, in particular patients with ventilator-associated pneumonia (VAP). Finally, a distinction should be made between targets obtained in neutropenic versus non-neutropenic mice. Many of the species and strains of interest are not virulent in mice, and exposure-response relationships obtained in non-neutropenic mice may overestimate the antibacterial effect of the compound. On the other hand, neutrophils do contribute to the overall effect of an antimicrobial [37] but the overall contribution of neutrophils is also dependent on the class of drugs and infection type [38].

4.2 Exposures in Men

Even if the pharmacodynamic targets are considered valid, there still remains the challenge to estimate the exposure of the antimicrobial in the clinical conditions of interest. For instance, in drug development estimates of pharmacokinetic parameters are derived from studies in human volunteers initially, and exposures are then translated to the use in clinical practice. The variation in individual exposures is accounted for by using Monte Carlo simulations (MCS), a technique that was initially applied by Drusano [39, 40], but now generally applied throughout the drug development process and breakpoint setting. However, although individual variation is accounted for by MCS, the premise is that the variation- and indeed the estimates proper in some cases- reflects the clinical situation. However, the variation observed in ICU patients extends that in volunteers; moreover, hyperclearance in part of this population will most certainly result in underexposure if doses are used that are derived from human volunteer data [41].

4.3 Clinical Breakpoints and Drug Development

Clinical breakpoints are used to distinguish between strains that are clinically resistant or susceptible with the overall purpose to provide an advice to the clinician whether or not the drug could be used for the treatment of infections. Over the years PK/PD has gained a strong influence over the rationale and setting of breakpoints. One of the major reasons is the relationship between PK, MIC, PD, and overall outcome of treatment. Identification of pharmacodynamic targets, the dosing regimens used, and the application of Monte Carlo simulations will result in a clinical breakpoint value that is, by the nature of the process, dependent on the dosing regimens used [42]. Many of the breakpoints of older drugs have been revised to more rational values, initially by the EUCAST [43, 44], but over the last years also by the CLSI and, in a new initiative, the USCAST (www.uscast.org). The USCAST is a breakpoint committee recently established and currently establishing and revising breakpoints in a similar fashion to

EUCAST. Unfortunately, for many older drugs, there is not the information required to go through the whole process of breakpoint setting, in particular pharmacodynamic targets are often missing by the lack of appropriate preclinical studies, but even pharmacokinetic data are sometimes lacking. Currently, there is much interest in rationalizing the use of older drugs.

In the development of new drugs, the application of PK/PD plays a major role in first determining the pharmacodynamic target and the pharmacokinetic profile of the new drug in humans. The indications of the drug and the MIC distributions of the potential causing microorganisms (in particular the ECOFF, the epidemiological cutoff MIC value that distinguishes wild-type from non-wild-type strains, see Chap. 2) will then allow a rational dosing regimen to be established. Thus, for many of the new antimicrobials the clinical breakpoint is similar or very close to the ECOFF. A further discussion can be found in Chap. 30.

4.4 Antiviral and Antifungal Drugs

As noted in the introduction, the principles of pharmacodynamics are not restricted to antibacterials, but also apply to antifungals and antivirals. The pharmacodynamics of most of the antifungals drugs against nonfilamentous fungi has now been reasonably well established. Many of the principles described above have been shown to apply here [45]. Exposure-response relationships have been shown for most antifungals in the clinical setting as well. For antifungal drugs against filamentous fungi exposure-response relationships have been established sparingly. Infections are relatively rare and only for *Aspergillus fumigatus* significant data have been collected. Relationships have been established for azoles in various animal models, but it remains difficult to show these in the clinical setting. There is increasing evidence that PK/PD relationships apply here and dosing can be optimized [46].

Likewise, PK/PD relationships have been established for many antiviral drugs. Although antiviral drugs lagged behind in development compared to antimicrobials, PK/PD relationships were established early on [47] and are used in a similar manner as for antibacterials [48].

4.5 Emergence of Resistance

The major part in this chapter was devoted to the effect of an antimicrobial on microorganisms by describing exposure-response relationships. However, there is another important effect of antimicrobials on bacterial populations. This is the evolution of bacteria as a result of selection pressure in the environment, the selection pressure in this case being exposure to antimicrobial agents. Over the years, it has been shown that PK/PD can explain some of the effects observed. For instance, Firsov showed in a hollow fiber infection model (HFIM) that the increase in MIC of quinolones of *S. aureus* was dependent on the AUC. The relationship could be described by an inverted U shape, indicating that there is an optimal concentration for resistance selection [49]. At very low exposures no increase was found, nor at very high AUCs. The optimum value for resistance selection in that experiment was 43. This is value close to that required for treatment effects. Tam and colleagues used a similar approach to define regimens that would have a lower probability of resistance emergence [50, 51].

Strain-specific parameters have been sought that identify the ease with which resistant mutants can be selected. The parameter that has been used over the last decades is the mutant prevention concentration (MPC) [52]. The MPC is determined using agar dilution methodology (see Sect. 2.1) but with a much higher inoculum, up to 10^{10}. The higher the MPC, the more probable it is that resistance is selected. The MPC was subsequently used to propose and define the mutant selection window (the MPC-MIC) and the tMSW, the time within the mutant selection window [53]. This is the time that, during fluctuating antimicrobial concentrations, the concentration is between the MIC and the MPC and thus dependent on the dosing frequency and the half-life of the antimicrobial (Fig. 11). The reasoning was that concentrations above the MIC do not inhibit growth whereas concentrations below the MPC do not result in kill of the entire bacterial population, and mutants with elevated MICs will be selected—with as a consequence emergence of resistance. This concept was initially applicated to quinolone resistance in an HFIM [49]. In a rat model of infection, Goessens and colleagues showed the concept to be applicable to ceftazidime [54]. In both studies, several dosing frequencies were applied to allow changes in the tMSW. The conclusion here is that the longer the concentration falls within the MSW

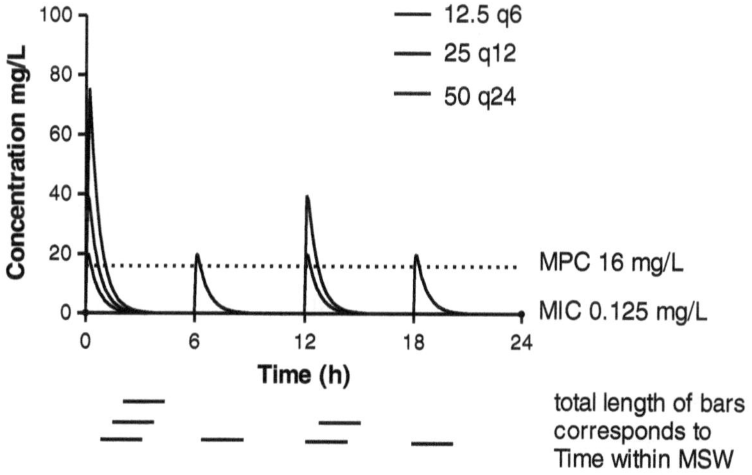

Fig. 11 Diagram showing the tMSW and effect of dosing frequency on the tMSW: the daily dose (mg/kg) is similar for each of the three regimens, but the tMSW increases if the frequency of administration increases, as indicated by the horizontal bars below the figure. Note the differences with Fig. 4b

the higher the probability resistance emerges. Resistance emergence is therefore dependent on both the strain characteristics (as defined by the MSW) as well as the pharmacokinetic characteristics and dosing regimen of the antimicrobial. Optimizing the dosing regimen to reduce resistance emergence would therefore be a potential strategy.

The role of PK/PD in the emergence of resistance has likewise been studied in antivirals [48, 55] and is a major focus in establishing optimal dosing regimens for these drugs.

4.6 PK/PD of Combinations

Pharmacodynamic relationships have been studied in vitro and in vivo for antimicrobial combinations. In vitro, pharmacodynamic models have been developed to describe interaction in checkerboard-type experiments [56] and time-kill curves [57]. Few studies have examined the relationship between pharmacodynamic index and effect. However, similar to the activity-effect relationships for single drugs, pharmacodynamic principles have been shown to be applicable in combinations [58].

5 Concluding Remarks

Over the course of time, the importance and the impact of pharmacokinetics and pharmacodynamics on the optimal use of antimicrobials are increasingly appreciated. It has become recognized that there is no such thing as "one size fits all" and that each drug class has its own specific properties. Time-kill characteristics of antimicrobial agents in vitro have been shown to be related to their effect in vivo, and pharmacodynamic indices have been identified that correlated with microbiological and clinical cure. The PK/PD relationships established allow optimization of therapy not only in the general sense, but also for individual patients. Therapeutic drug monitoring and patient-specific dosing are becoming increasingly used, in particular for drugs with a narrow therapeutic window. However, therapeutic drug monitoring is also used increasingly to ensure that concentrations in individual patients are above the pharmacodynamic target, in particular in patients with unpredictable pharmacokinetics. PK/PD has shifted from explanatory to predictive and guidance of optimal dosing for the population in general to individualized patient care.

References

1. ISO (2006) ISO 20776-1. Clinical Laboratory Testing and in vitro diagnostic test systems - susceptibility testing of infectious agents and evaluation of performance of antimicrobial susceptibility testing devices- Part 1. International Standards Organisation
2. Ericsson HM, Sherris JC (1971) Antibiotic sensitivity testing. Report of an international collaborative study. Acta Pathol Microbiol Scand B: Microbiol Immunol 217(Suppl B):1–90
3. NCCLS (2001) Development of in vitro susceptibility testing criteria and quality control

parameters; approved guideline-Second Edition. NCCLS document M23-A2. NCCLS, Wayne
4. EUCAST (2003) Determination of minimum Inhibitory concentrations (MICs) of antibacterial agents by broth dilution. DISCUSSION DOCUMENT E.Dis 5.1. European Society Clinical Microbiology and Infectious Diseases, Munich, Germany
5. ISO (2008) ISO 20776-2. Clinical Laboratory Testing and in vitro diagnostic test systems - susceptibility testing of infectious agents and evaluation of performance of antimicrobial susceptibility testing devices- Part 2. International Standards Organisation
6. ISO (2014) ISO 16782. Criteria for acceptable lots of dehydrated Mueller-Hinton Agar and Broth for Antimicrobial Susceptibility Testing. International Standards Organisation
7. Mouton JW, Vinks AA (2005) Relationship between minimum inhibitory concentration and stationary concentration revisited: growth rates and minimum bactericidal concentrations. Clin Pharmacokinet 44(7):767–768
8. Garrod LP (1948) The bactericidal action of streptomycin. Br Med J 1(4547):382–386
9. Shah PM, Junghanns SW (1976) Bactericidal dosie-activity relationships with *E. coli*, K. pneumoniae and Staph. aureus (author's transl). Dtsch Med Wochenschr 101(9):325–328
10. Mattie H (1981) Kinetics of antimicrobial action. Rev Infect Dis 3(1):19–27
11. Vogelman B, Craig WA (1986) Kinetics of antimicrobial activity. J Pediatr 108(5 Pt 2):835–840
12. Bouvier d'Yvoire MJY, Maire PH (1996) Dosageregimens of antibacterials. Implications of a pharmacokinetic/pharmacodynamic model. Clin Drug Invest 11:229–239
13. Mouton JW, Vinks AA (2005) Pharmacokinetic/pharmacodynamic modelling of antibacterials in vitro and in vivo using bacterial growth and kill kinetics: the minimum inhibitory concentration versus stationary concentration. Clin Pharmacokinet 44(2):201–210
14. Eagle H, Fleischman R, Levy M (1953) "Continuous" vs. "discontinuous" therapy with penicillin; the effect of the interval between injections on therapeutic efficacy. N Engl J Med 248(12):481–488
15. Mouton JW, Dudley MN, Cars O, Derendorf H, Drusano GL (2005) Standardization of pharmacokinetic/pharmacodynamic (PK/PD) terminology for anti-infective drugs: an update. J Antimicrob Chemother 55(5):601–607
16. Mouton JW, Dudley MN, Cars O, Derendorf H, Drusano GL (2002) Standardization of pharmacokinetic/pharmacodynamic (PK/PD) terminology for anti-infective drugs. Int J Antimicrob Agents 19(4):355–358
17. Toutain PL, Bousquet-Melou A, Martinez M (2007) AUC/MIC: a PK/PD index for antibiotics with a time dimension or simply a dimensionless scoring factor? J Antimicrob Chemother 60(6):1185–1188. doi:10.1093/jac/dkm360
18. Bakker-Woudenberg IA, van Gerwen AL, Michel MF (1979) Efficacy of antimicrobial therapy in experimental rat pneumonia: antibiotic treatment schedules in rats with impaired phagocytosis. Infect Immun 25(1):376–387
19. Gerber AU, Craig WA, Brugger HP, Feller C, Vastola AP, Brandel J (1983) Impact of dosing intervals on activity of gentamicin and ticarcillin against Pseudomonas aeruginosa in granulocytopenic mice. J Infect Dis 147(5):910–917
20. Vogelman B, Gudmundsson S, Leggett J, Turnidge J, Ebert S, Craig WA (1988) Correlation of antimicrobial pharmacokinetic parameters with therapeutic efficacy in an animal model. J Infect Dis 158(4):831–847
21. Leggett JE, Fantin B, Ebert S, Totsuka K, Vogelman B, Calame W, Mattie H, Craig WA (1989) Comparative antibiotic dose-effect relations at several dosing intervals in murine pneumonitis and thigh-infection models. J Infect Dis 159(2):281–292
22. Leggett JE, Ebert S, Fantin B, Craig WA (1990) Comparative dose-effect relations at several dosing intervals for beta- lactam, aminoglycoside and quinolone antibiotics against gram-negative bacilli in murine thigh-infection and pneumonitis models. Scand J Infect Dis Suppl 74:179–184
23. Scaglione F, Mouton JW, Mattina R, Fraschini F (2003) Pharmacodynamics of levofloxacin and ciprofloxacin in a murine pneumonia model: peak concentration/MIC versus area under the curve/MIC ratios. Antimicrob Agents Chemother 47(9):2749–2755
24. Ambrose PG, Bhavnani SM, Rubino CM, Louie A, Gumbo T, Forrest A, Drusano GL (2007) Pharmacokinetics-pharmacodynamics of antimicrobial therapy: it's not just for mice anymore. Clin Infect Dis 44(1):79–86
25. Tompsett R, Shultz S, McDermott W (1947) The relation of protein binding to the pharmacology and antibacterial activity of penicillins X, G, dhydro F, and K. J Bacteriol 53:581–595
26. Craig WA (1995) Interrelationship between pharmacokinetics and pharmacodynamics in determining dosage regimens for broad-spectrum cephalosporins. Diagn Microbiol Infect Dis 22(1-2):89–96

27. Zeitlinger MA, Derendorf H, Mouton JW, Cars O, Craig WA, Andes D, Theuretzbacher U (2011) Protein binding: do we ever learn? Antimicrob Agents Chemother 55(7):3067–3074. doi:10.1128/AAC.01433-10
28. Garrison MW, Vance-Bryan K, Larson TA, Toscano JP, Rotschafer JC (1990) Assessment of effects of protein binding on daptomycin and vancomycin killing of *Staphylococcus aureus* by using an in vitro pharmacodynamic model. Antimicrob Agents Chemother 34(10):1925–1931
29. Calain P, Krause KH, Vaudaux P, Auckenthaler R, Lew D, Waldvogel F, Hirschel B (1987) Early termination of a prospective, randomized trial comparing teicoplanin and flucloxacillin for treating severe staphylococcal infections. J Infect Dis 155(2):187–191
30. Lowdin E, Odenholt-Tornqvist I, Bengtsson S, Cars O (1993) A new method to determine postantibiotic effect and effects of subinhibitory antibiotic concentrations. Antimicrob Agents Chemother 37(10):2200–2205
31. Tam VH, Nikolaou M (2011) A novel approach to pharmacodynamic assessment of antimicrobial agents: new insights to dosing regimen design. PLoS Comput Biol 7(1):e1001043
32. Forrest A, Nix DE, Ballow CH, Goss TF, Birmingham MC, Schentag JJ (1993) Pharmacodynamics of intravenous ciprofloxacin in seriously ill patients. Antimicrob Agents Chemother 37(5):1073–1081
33. Preston SL, Drusano GL, Berman AL, Fowler CL, Chow AT, Dornseif B, Reichl V, Natarajan J, Corrado M (1998) Pharmacodynamics of levofloxacin: a new paradigm for early clinical trials [see comments]. JAMA 279(2):125–129
34. Ambrose PG, Grasela DM, Grasela TH, Passarell J, Mayer HB, Pierce PF (2001) Pharmacodynamics of fluoroquinolones against Streptococcus pneumoniae in patients with community-acquired respiratory tract infections. Antimicrob Agents Chemother 45(10):2793–2797
35. Rodriguez-Tudela JL, Almirante B, Rodriguez-Pardo D, Laguna F, Donnelly JP, Mouton JW, Pahissa A, Estrella MC (2007) Correlation of the MIC and Dose/MIC ratio of fluconazole to the therapeutic response of patients with mucosal candidiasis and candidaemia. Antimicrob Agents Chemother 51(10):3599–3604
36. Muller AE, Punt N, Mouton JW (2013) Optimal exposures of ceftazidime predict the probability of microbiological and clinical outcome in the treatment of nosocomial pneumonia. J Antimicrob Chemother 68(4):900–906. doi:10.1093/jac/dks468, dks468 [pii]
37. Drusano GL, Fregeau C, Liu W, Brown DL, Louie A (2010) Impact of burden on granulocyte clearance of bacteria in a mouse thigh infection model. Antimicrob Agents Chemother 54(10):4368–4372. doi:10.1128/AAC.00133-10, AAC.00133-10 [pii]
38. Andes D, Craig WA (2002) Animal model pharmacokinetics and pharmacodynamics: a critical review. Int J Antimicrob Agents 19(4):261–268
39. Drusano GL, D'Argenio DZ, Preston SL, Barone C, Symonds W, LaFon S, Rogers M, Prince W, Bye A, Bilello JA (2000) Use of drug effect interaction modeling with Monte Carlo simulation to examine the impact of dosing interval on the projected antiviral activity of the combination of abacavir and amprenavir. Antimicrob Agents Chemother 44(6):1655–1659
40. Drusano GL, Preston SL, Hardalo C, Hare R, Banfield C, Andes D, Vesga O, Craig WA (2001) Use of preclinical data for selection of a phase II/III dose for evernimicin and identification of a preclinical MIC breakpoint. Antimicrob Agents Chemother 45(1):13–22
41. Roberts JA, Abdul-Aziz MH, Lipman J, Mouton JW, Vinks AA, Felton TW, Hope WW, Farkas A, Neely MN, Schentag JJ, Drusano G, Frey OR, Theuretzbacher U, Kuti JL, on behalf of The International Society of Anti-Infective P, the P, Pharmacodynamics Study Group of the European Society of Clinical M, Infectious D (2014) Individualised antibiotic dosing for patients who are critically ill: challenges and potential solutions. Lancet Infect Dis 14(6):498–509. doi:10.1016/S1473-3099(14)70036-2
42. Mouton JW, Brown DF, Apfalter P, Canton R, Giske CG, Ivanova M, Macgowan AP, Rodloff A, Soussy CJ, Steinbakk M, Kahlmeter G (2012) The role of pharmacokinetics/pharmacodynamics in setting clinical MIC breakpoints: the EUCAST approach. Clin Microbiol Infect 18(3):E37–E45. doi:10.1111/j.1469-0691.2011.03752.x
43. Kahlmeter G, Brown DF, Goldstein FW, MacGowan AP, Mouton JW, Osterlund A, Rodloff A, Steinbakk M, Urbaskova P, Vatopoulos A (2003) European harmonization of MIC breakpoints for antimicrobial susceptibility testing of bacteria. J Antimicrob Chemother 52(2):145–148
44. Kahlmeter G, Brown DF, Goldstein FW, MacGowan AP, Mouton JW, Odenholt I, Rodloff A, Soussy CJ, Steinbakk M, Soriano F, Stetsiouk O (2006) European Committee on Antimicrobial Susceptibility Testing (EUCAST) Technical Notes on antimicrobial susceptibility testing. Clin Microbiol Infect 12(6):501–503
45. Andes D (2006) Pharmacokinetics and pharmacodynamics of antifungals. Infect Dis Clin North Am 20(3):679–697

46. Seyedmousavi S, Mouton JW, Melchers WJ, Bruggemann RJ, Verweij PE (2014) The role of azoles in the management of azole-resistant aspergillosis: from the bench to the bedside. Drug Resist Updat 17(3):37–50. doi:10.1016/j.drup.2014.06.001
47. Drusano GL (1993) Pharmacodynamics of antiretroviral chemotherapy. Infect Control Hosp Epidemiol 14(9):530–536
48. McSharry JJ, Drusano GL (2011) Antiviral pharmacodynamics in hollow fibre bioreactors. Antivir Chem Chemother 21(5):183–192. doi:10.3851/IMP1770
49. Firsov AA, Vostrov SN, Lubenko IY, Drlica K, Portnoy YA, Zinner SH (2003) In vitro pharmacodynamic evaluation of the mutant selection window hypothesis using four fluoroquinolones against *Staphylococcus aureus*. Antimicrob Agents Chemother 47(5):1604–1613
50. Tam VH, Louie A, Deziel MR, Liu W, Leary R, Drusano GL (2005) Bacterial-population responses to drug-selective pressure: examination of garenoxacin's effect on *Pseudomonas aeruginosa*. J Infect Dis 192(3):420–428
51. Tam VH, Louie A, Fritsche TR, Deziel M, Liu W, Brown DL, Deshpande L, Leary R, Jones RN, Drusano GL (2007) Impact of drug-exposure intensity and duration of therapy on the emergence of *Staphylococcus aureus* resistance to a quinolone antimicrobial. J Infect Dis 195(12):1818–1827. doi:10.1086/518003, JID37660 [pii]
52. Blondeau JM, Zhao X, Hansen G, Drlica K (2001) Mutant prevention concentrations of fluoroquinolones for clinical isolates of *Streptococcus pneumoniae*. Antimicrob Agents Chemother 45(2):433–438. doi:10.1128/AAC.45.2.433-438.2001
53. Zhao X, Drlica K (2002) Restricting the selection of antibiotic-resistant mutant bacteria: measurement and potential use of the mutant selection window. J Infect Dis 185(4):561–565
54. Goessens WH, Mouton JW, Ten Kate MT, Bijl AJ, Ott A, Bakker-Woudenberg IA (2007) Role of ceftazidime dose regimen on the selection of resistant Enterobacter cloacae in the intestinal flora of rats treated for an experimental pulmonary infection. J Antimicrob Chemother 59(3):507–516
55. Drusano GL, Bilello JA, Stein DS, Nessly M, Meibohm A, Emini EA, Deutsch P, Condra J, Chodakewitz J, Holder DJ (1998) Factors influencing the emergence of resistance to indinavir: role of virologic, immunologic, and pharmacologic variables. J Infect Dis 178(2):360–367
56. Meletiadis J, Verweij PE, TeDorsthorst DT, Meis JF, Mouton JW (2005) Assessing in vitro combinations of antifungal drugs against yeasts and filamentous fungi: comparison of different drug interaction models. Med Mycol 43(2):133–152
57. Yuan Z, Ledesma KR, Singh R, Hou J, Prince RA, Tam VH (2010) Quantitative assessment of combination antimicrobial therapy against multidrug-resistant bacteria in a murine pneumonia model. J Infect Dis 201(6):889–897. doi:10.1086/651024
58. Mouton JW, van Ogtrop ML, Andes D, Craig WA (1999) Use of pharmacodynamic indices to predict efficacy of combination therapy in vivo. Antimicrob Agents Chemother 43(10):2473–2478

Chapter 2

In Vitro Pharmacodynamic Models to Evaluate Anti-infective Pharmacodynamics

Warren Rose

Abstract

In vitro models have provided valuable insight into the pharmacodynamics of antimicrobials and have improved treatment approaches for patients. The use of in vitro models continues to help guide dosing decision for new antimicrobials and reevaluate those used already in clinical practice as resistance emerges. The design of in vitro PD models has not changed significantly since their introduction, but historically the models have been unique to individual laboratories with different methods scattered throughout the literature. The basic principle of the in vitro PK/PD model is to allow for assessment of antimicrobial activity under dynamic exposure conditions. This chapter presents the materials and methods for four different in vitro model types that have been used consistently in the literature to assess antimicrobial PK/PD for a given scenario: one-compartment model, hollow fiber model, biofilm model, and combination therapy model. In addition, this information is supplemented with information to design dosing schemes for the models as well as assess the PD outcomes of the antibiotic simulation. This information provides the basics for in vitro dynamic assessment, and the models can be customized from the presented method to address a specific research question or clinical situation.

Key words Pharmacokinetics, Pharmacodynamics, One-compartment model, Area under the curve, Hollow fiber, Combination model, Killing curve

1 Introduction

The in vitro pharmacokinetic/pharmacodynamic model remains a highly useful tool to evaluate both new antimicrobials in development as well as reassess available antimicrobials for dosing scheme optimization and mitigate resistance development. The basic principle of the in vitro PK/PD model is to allow for assessment of antimicrobial activity under dynamic exposure conditions. This provides a significant advantage for assessment of antimicrobial effectiveness over static assays that include susceptibility testing and in vitro time-kill curve methods, which fail to represent the clinical scenario where antibiotic distribution, metabolism, and elimination alter the antibiotic exposure. To understand how antimicrobials interact with organisms under dynamic antimicrobial

John C. Rotschafer et al. (eds.), *Antibiotic Pharmacodynamics*, Methods in Pharmacology and Toxicology, DOI 10.1007/978-1-4939-3323-5_2,

Table 1
Classification and application characteristics of in vitro PD models: adapted from [8]

Type	Application
Static models	Kill curves, basic PD assessment
Intracellular models	PK/PD of intracellular bacteria different from extracellular
One-compartment PK/PD models	Direct PK/PD relationships for given simulation
Multi-compartment PK/PD models	Different PK profiles or bacterial growing conditions. Simulate PK of antibiotic with numerous theoretical compartments
Models of combination therapy	PK/PD synergy with two or more antimicrobials
PK/PD biofilm models	Bacteria in biofilms: properties distinct from single organisms, e.g., increased antimicrobial resistance

conditions, a number of in vitro pharmacokinetic/pharmacodynamic (PK/PD) models have been developed by various investigators over the last few decades and are classified in Table 1. These models have been valuable in understanding the dynamic drug exposures and dose–response relationships that are needed for continued drug development and optimization.

In order to determine the pharmacodynamics of an antibiotic, the impact of the antimicrobial on organism growth must be directly assessed, and for this, in vitro PK/PD models have many advantages. The antimicrobial effects from the in vitro model have translated well to the animal PD model and the patient setting [1–5]. However unlike the animal model, which necessitates human-scaled antimicrobial exposure due to altered animal metabolism [6], the in vitro PD model can simulate exact human PK exposures [7]. Also, the in vitro PD model is highly flexible to measure multiple time points throughout the treatment simulation, microbial resistance development and mutation frequencies (mutant selection window), combinations of antibiotics, and prolonged treatment courses [4, 8–10]. The models can also be easily adjusted to accurately simulate a range of altered clearance environments that are commonly found in patients with renal or hepatic dysfunction [11, 12]. There are some inherent limitations of in vitro PD models that should also be discussed. Primarily, these are simply models of simulated exposures and do not simulate all in vivo conditions, host factors, tissue dynamics, and concentrations at the site of infection. However, when drug clearance from a site such as epithelial lining fluid in the lung is known, these exposures have been simulated separately [13]. Also, these models often determine PK/PD endpoint with *free* drug simulations, not total drug that would be administered in patients. However, free drug only has been shown to account for the in vivo antibiotic activity [6]. In vitro PD models should be used as guidance for antimicrobial effectiveness and are not intended to replace the in vivo model or patient condition.

Although a large number of in vitro PD models have been developed, the overall concept of providing dynamic antibiotic exposures over time remains fairly consistent. The historical development of in vitro PD model is beyond the scope of this chapter and has been reviewed by Grasso et al. [14], Li and Zhu [15], as well as two quality book chapters on in vitro dynamic models with the technical aspects of modeling and the methodology of pharmacodynamic studies [4, 5]. A more recent review of in vitro PD models provides a comprehensive discussion of basic designs for dynamic models with either bacterial loss or no bacterial loss and the advantages and disadvantages of these different model types [8]. However, the protocol method and design of available in vitro PD models and interpretation of results have not been presented for investigators to establish models for PK/PD analysis in their own laboratory. This chapter presents the materials and methods for four different in vitro model types that have been used consistently in the literature to assess antimicrobial PK/PD for a given scenario. This information provides the basics for in vitro dynamic assessment, and the models can be customized from the presented method to address a specific research question (e.g., inoculum effect or altered clearance simulations).

2 Materials

2.1 One-Compartment PK/PD Models

The one-compartment in vitro PK/PD model is perhaps the most widely used and versatile model available. While it is relatively simplistic in its design, this allows for a variety of applications for antibiotic PK/PD assessment. The design of the one-compartment model is depicted in Fig. 1 and consists of central compartment flask containing growth media and bacteria. Fresh media is pumped into the central compartment via a peristaltic pump and the waste media is eliminated from the model by pressure of the inflow media or removed by a second pump. Antibiotics can be administered and samples taken through a sample port throughout the model duration. A magnetic stir bar provides continuous mixing of media, organism, and antibiotic. One limitation of this model is the loss of bacteria by the flow removal of waste media from the central compartment. However, this is usually not a significant factor for overall bacterial quantification if the clearance from the model is lower than the doubling rate of bacteria. Concerns may arise with excess bacterial clearance from the model when quantifying the emergence of resistance in a bacterial population during drug exposure. Some investigators have used filters in the waste flow to capture bacteria at this step [16, 17], but this will not be presented in the one-compartment method for this chapter.

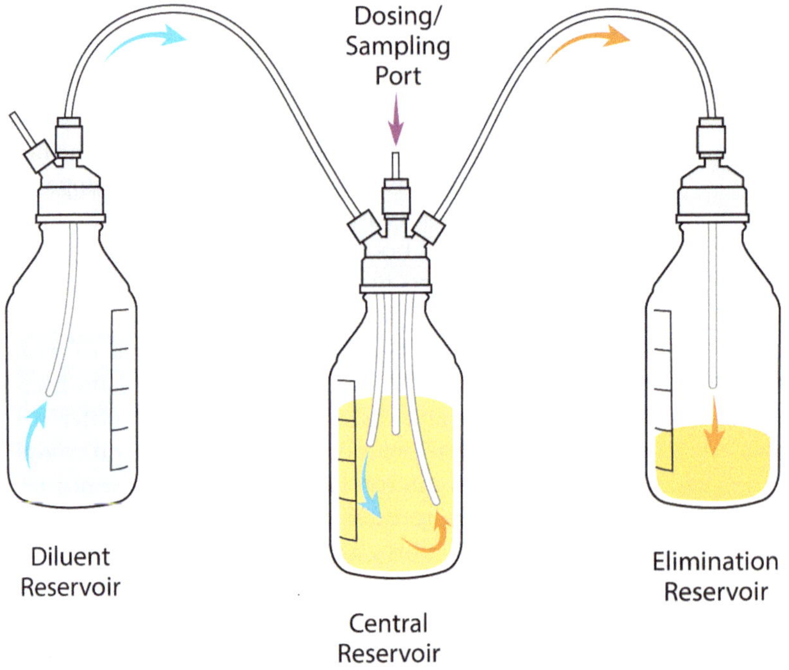

Fig. 1 One-compartment PD model depiction of the central reservoir system. Supplemental diluent media is supplied to the model and waste is removed at an equivalent rate. Antibiotic doses can be administered and samples removed from the central reservoir

There are a variety of ways to create one-compartment in vitro models for PK/PD assessment. The simplistic design of the model requires a culture flask and a sealed cap with ports to allow delivery and removal of media, administration of antibiotic, and collection of samples. Some researchers in this field have customized glass flasks for these requirements, but the models themselves still maintain the same principles. This method provides materials that can be readily purchased for this purpose, but culture reservoirs with different volumes and accessories are available to fit specific research needs.

1. Growth media: Mueller-Hinton broth supplemented with 25 mg/L calcium and 12.5 mg/L magnesium as recommended by Clinical and Laboratory Standards Institute (CLSI) for Antimicrobial testing (*see* **Note 1**) [18] (#275710; BD Biosciences)
2. Reservoir for one-compartment in vitro model (Kimax GL 45 500 mL; #02-542C: Fisher Scientific)
3. Four-port model cap (#OF945T4F; Fisher Scientific)
4. Magnetic stir bar (#14-513-60; Fisher)
5. Peristaltic pump (Masterflex L/S Digital Drive: #EW-07551-30; Cole-Parmer)

6. Peristaltic pump head (Masterflex L/S Easy-Load pump head for precision tubing; #EW-07516-00; Cole-Parmer)
7. Silicone tubing (*see* **Note 2**); (Masterfex L/S 14: #EW-96410-14; Cole-Parmer)
8. Silicone tubing (Masterflex L/S 16; #EW-96410-16; Cole-Parmer)
9. Straight Tubing connector (Masterflex: #EW-30612-47; Cole-Parmer)
10. Male Luer lock connector (#T-45504-04; Cole-Parmer)
11. Stirring hotplate (Corning; #S50446HP; Fisher)
12. Flask for fresh media supplementation and waste media (*see* **Note 3**) (#4980; Fisher)
13. Rubber stopper, two hole, Size No. 10 (*see* **Notes 4** and **5**) (#14-140M; Fisher)
14. Syringe Filter (GE SPARTAN: #09-302-152; Fisher)
15. Syringe 3 ml Luer-Lok™ (#309657; BD)

2.2 Two-Compartment Models: Hollow Fiber Multi-compartment PK/PD Model

Two-compartment models offer the advantages of a simulated second compartment for drug distribution as well as maintaining bacteria in the secondary space for a more accurate assessment of resistance development and other microbe-related assessments. Unlike the one-compartment models, bacterial growth in the two-compartment model is maintained in the second compartment and therefore no loss of organism occurs via the clearance flow from the model. Many investigators have customized multi-compartment models using a variety of methods that permit antibiotics and nutrient media to freely distribute from the central compartment into the peripheral compartment but maintain bacteria within the peripheral compartment. A common method established bacteria in artificial membranes as the second compartment and attached tubing for access for bacterial sampling. The types of artificial membranes that have been used for this modeling include cellulose acetate, dialysis membranes, polycarbonate, polysulfone, and regenerated cellulose [19–23]. The drug is administered into the central compartment and allowed to diffuse into the peripheral compartment at the simulated infection site [21, 24]. Other types of two-compartment models have modified the one-compartment model to include introducing custom-made infected tissue in the model as a second peripheral compartment. Some examples of these pharmacodynamic models include the simulated endocardial vegetation model developed and extensively used by Rybak [25] and simulated tissue cage model [26] among other similar types. These models are highly customized two-compartment models that have been described in detail in the literature, and their development is beyond the scope of this chapter.

The hollow fiber model system was first utilized by Zinner et al. in 1981 [21] through the use of an artificial capillary membrane system to provide a separation between the central and peripheral compartments. The polysulfone fibers allow diffusion of media and antibiotics to the peripheral compartment. This design was further developed into a multi-compartmental model by Blaser et al. [27, 28]. A significant advance in the increased utilization of multi-compartmental modeling was made by developing hollow fiber bioreactors for two-compartment PK/PD assessments. FiberCell Systems has developed a variety of hollow fiber bioreactors for commercial purchase and use. The reactor itself consists of small tubular filters approximately 200 μm in diameter and sealed at the end of the chamber. Media and antibiotics circulating through the central system flow through the filter into the secondary space where it interacts with the microorganism. The microorganism resides in the extracapillary space for convenient sampling and quantification. The hollow fiber model can also be used for other PK/PD applications beyond antimicrobial killing. The extracapillary space within the cartridge can trap extracellular proteins produced by bacteria, such as toxins and virulence factors, and allows for dual assessment of antimicrobial killing and toxin production/suppression from simulated PK/PD exposures. The antimicrobial/antitoxin effects of select antimicrobials have been evaluated in two separate studies in this model for *Bacillus anthracis* and *Staphylococcus aureus* [29, 30].

A schematic representation of the cartridge and fiber filter system is displayed in Fig. 2. A central media compartment that is dosed with the antimicrobial supplies the cartridge with the supplemented media. Dilution media is supplied to the central compartment and removed at an equivalent rate by peristaltic pumps to provide the dynamic antibiotic concentrations in the model. The clearance of antibiotic from the model is determined based on the antibiotic half-life and follows the principles outlined in Sect. 3.5. Hollow fiber models have been used in applications for cell culture growth and antimicrobial PK/PD studies in a variety of microorganisms including bacteria, viruses, and parasites [31, 32]. Although a variety of two-compartment models have been explored and are in use as described in this section, the hollow fiber system will be the representative two-compartment model for this method.

1. Growth media: Mueller-Hinton broth supplemented with 25 mg/L calcium and 12.5 mg/L magnesium as recommended by Clinical and Laboratory Standards Institute for Antimicrobial testing [18] (*see* **Note 1**) (#275710; BD Biosciences).
2. Duet Pump (# P3202; FiberCell Systems).

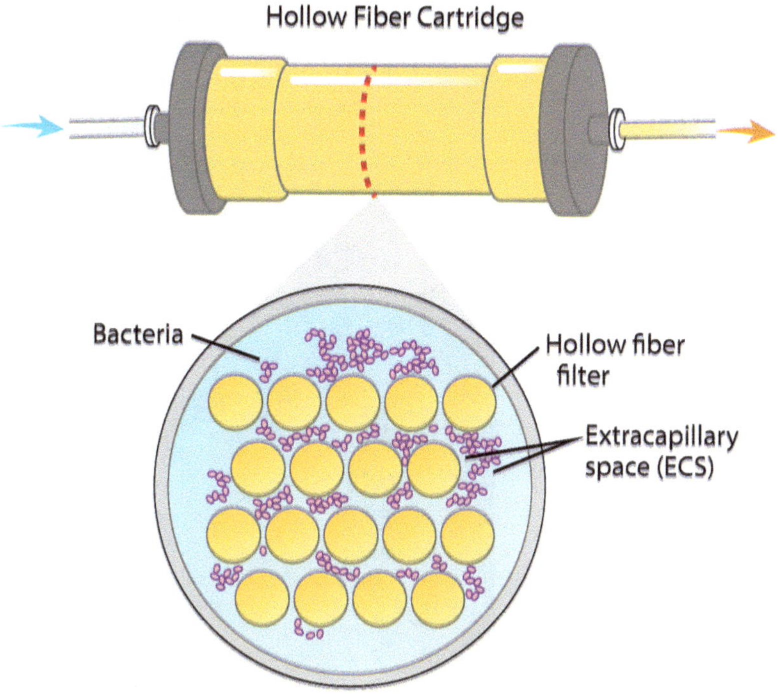

Fig. 2 Two-compartment hollow fiber model depiction. The cross section of the hollow fiber cartridge displays the separation of organism in the extracapillary space while allowing media and antibiotics to freely diffuse in the model

3. Hollow-Fiber cartridge (#C2011; Fiber Cell Systems): A variety of cartridges are available for commercial use and have different volumes and molecular weight cutoffs that can be selected for the intended application. Antimicrobial pharmacodynamic assessments are usually performed in the C2011 cartridge. The methods for this model will use this cartridge.
4. Central compartment reservoir (Nalgene; #03-311-1C: Fisher).
5. Central compartment reservoir cap (#A1007; FiberCell Systems): The reservoir cap is designed to deliver antibiotics and media to the central reservoir while maintaining a constant volume. There are five tubes with luer connectors on the cap as displayed in Fig. 3. Two connectors are for the recirculation circuit through the hollow fiber cartridge, one is for diluent into the central reservoir, one is for diluent out of the central reservoir, and one is for a vent filter to maintain constant pressure within the central reservoir.
6. Peristaltic pump (Masterflex L/S Digital Drive: #EW-07551-30; Cole-Parmer).
7. Peristaltic pump head (Masterflex L/S Easy-Load pump head for precision tubing: #EW-07516-00; Cole-Parmer).

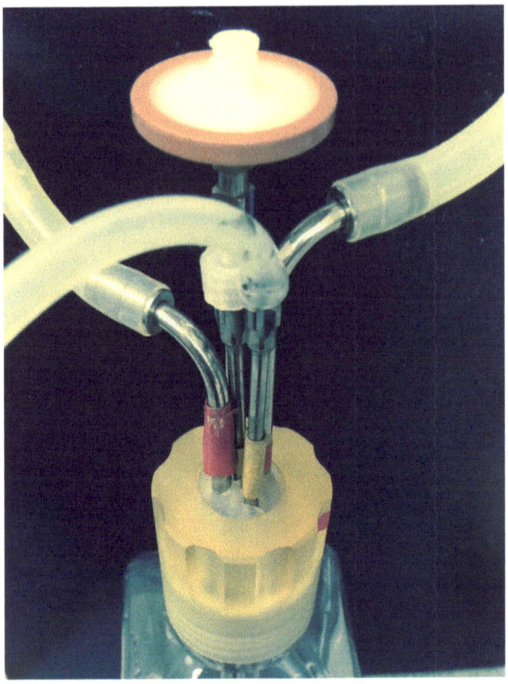

Fig. 3 Image of the hollow fiber model reservoir cap with five tube connections. Two connectors are for the recirculation circuit through the hollow fiber cartridge, one is for diluent into the central reservoir, one is for diluent out of the central reservoir, and one is for a vent filter to maintain constant pressure within the central reservoir

8. Silicone tubing (*see* **Note 2**) (Masterflex L/S 14: #EW-96410-14; Cole-Parmer).
9. 3-Way Stopcock with Luer Connections (#EW-30600-07; Cole-Parmer): This item is made of polycarbonate, which is autoclavable. The item must be completely rinsed with distilled water prior to autoclave sterilization to remove detergent residues that may lead to crazing and spotting.
10. Male Luer lock connector (#T-45504-04; Cole-Parmer).
11. Injection Site with Male Luer Lock (#MX492; Smiths Medical).
12. Syringe Filter (GE SPARTAN: #09-302-152; Fisher).
13. Syringe 3 ml Luer-Lok™ (#309657; BD).
14. Syringe 20 ml Luer-Lok™ (#302830; BD).
15. Tabletop incubator (*see* **Note 6**).
16. Flask for fresh media supplementation and waste media (*see* **Note 3**); #4980; Fisher).
17. Rubber stopper, two hole, Size No. 10 (*see* **Notes 4** and **5**) (#14-140M; Fisher).

2.3 PK/PD Biofilm Models

A variety of models have been proposed to evaluate antimicrobial efficacy against mature biofilms. However, few of these have the ability to incorporate PK/PD simulations of antibiotics against both bacteria in the planktonic and biofilm cell state. Some models have introduced second compartments into the one-compartment model that contain biofilm in a tissue cage, membrane, or catheter-related bacteremia model [33, 34]. In these models, artificially induced biofilm is developed in a secondary compartment [35] consisting of a small-diameter plastic chamber with a cellulose membrane or a glass microfiber filter inside or developed in catheters available for clinical use that have been artificially colonized with biofilm-embedded bacteria [33]. These PK/PD models use the sample principles as other pharmacokinetic models, but the development of biofilm can be cumbersome, the techniques being unique to each investigator, and has not been protocolized for routine use outside of the published literature. The Center for Biofilm Engineering at Montana State University has developed commercial assays for biofilm development and analysis, including a model that can be adapted for use in PK/PD simulations. The system has been used to assess biofilm and antibiotic activity for a variety of aerobic bacteria including *Pseudomonas aeruginosa* and *Staphylococcus aureus* [36–38]. The CDC Biofilm Reactor is reviewed in this section as a reproducible and reusable commercial model for PK/PD biofilm assessment.

1. Conditioning media: Tryptic soy broth (#211822; BD Biosciences): Broth can be supplemented with 1–10 % glucose to facilitate biofilm development.
2. Growth media: Mueller-Hinton broth supplemented with 25 mg/L calcium and 12.5 mg/L magnesium as recommended by Clinical and Laboratory Standards Institute for Antimicrobial testing [18] (*see* **Note 1**) (#275710; BD Biosciences).
3. CDC Biofilm reactor model (#CBR 90-2; BioSurface Technologies Corporation).
4. Digital stirring hotplate (Corning; #11-500-150; Fisher).
5. Large volume carboy (Nalgene 20L; #02-960-20A; Fisher) with 2 port cap accessory (Nalgene; #02-923-15M; Fisher).
6. Reservoirs for fresh media supplementation (*see* **Note 3**) (#4980; Fisher).
7. Rubber stopper, two hole, Size No. 10 (*see* **Notes 4** and **5**) (#14-140M; Fisher).
8. Silicone tubing (Masterflex L/S 16: #EW-96410-16; Cole-Parmer).
9. Straight Tubing connector (Masterflex: #EW-30612-47; Cole-Parmer).
10. Female Luer lock connector (#EW-45501-04; Cole-Parmer).

2.4 Combination Therapy Models

Combination therapy modeling employs the basic principle of adding a second drug in the simulation. For antibiotics with different half-lives this requires a supplement chamber to replace antibiotic that is removed by the faster clearance. Therefore, the materials required for this supplemental chamber are provided in this section and can be combined with the other models presented to achieve a combination simulation.

1. Supplemental dose reservoir (Kimax GL 45 500 mL; #02-542C: Fisher Scientific)
2. Four-port model cap for supplemental dose reservoir (#OF945T4F; Fisher Scientific)
3. Flask for fresh media supplementation to dose reservoir (Pyrex Flask; #4980; Fisher)
4. Magnetic stir bar (#14-513-60; Fisher)
5. Y-connector (Masterflex L/S 13-14; #EW-30614-43; Cole-Parmer)

3 Methods

3.1 Pharmacokinetic Principles for In Vitro PK/PD Modeling

The one-compartment model system uses the principles of central compartment dilution effects for a simplistic yet powerful tool for pharmacodynamic analysis. The system follows first-order kinetic parameters that allow for central compartment clearance of a drug's specific half-life. This principle is possible when the volume of the drug in the central compartment is kept the same from a similar rate of volume supplementation to elimination. The first-order kinetic equation is used for this effect in which the time-dependent rate of change in the amount of drug is proportional to the drug concentration:

$$C = C_0 e^{-k_e t}$$

where

C = concentration of antibiotic

C_0 = concentration of antibiotic following drug administration

t = time

k_e = elimination rate constant defined as

$k_e = \frac{\mathrm{Cl}}{V_c}$ and $k_e = \frac{\ln 2}{t_{1/2}}$.

Using the transitive property of equality

$$\frac{\mathrm{Cl}}{V_c} = \frac{\ln 2}{t_{1/2}}$$

And solving for Cl

$$\mathrm{Cl} = (\ln 2)\left(\frac{V_c}{t_{1/2}}\right)$$

where

Cl = clearance

V_c = volume of central compartment

$t_{1/2}$ = half-life of antibiotic

The dose of antibiotic is supplied to the central compartment at each scheduled interval according to the regimen simulation (e.g., a dose of amoxicillin is administered every 8 h to the model). The amount of drug to administer to provide each desired concentration can be calculated by

$$\mathrm{Dose} = V_c\,(C_0)$$

The target concentration C_0 can be obtained from healthy volunteer data or from Phase III or Phase IV studies in specific populations with infections. Often the steady state C_0 in serum is targeted from these studies. While it is possible that drug accumulation may occur with subsequent antibiotic doses, it often does not result in substantial accumulation that would affect the PK/PD assessment. For example, Fig. 4 displays limited drug accumulation, represented by no change in maximum or minimum concentration with repeated dosing, with a beta-lactam antibiotic given frequently in a one-compartment model over several days. Therefore an adjustment for residual antibiotic in the model prior to the next dose is often not necessary. However, this could be accounted for by subtracting the estimated residual concentration from the C_0 used in the next dose.

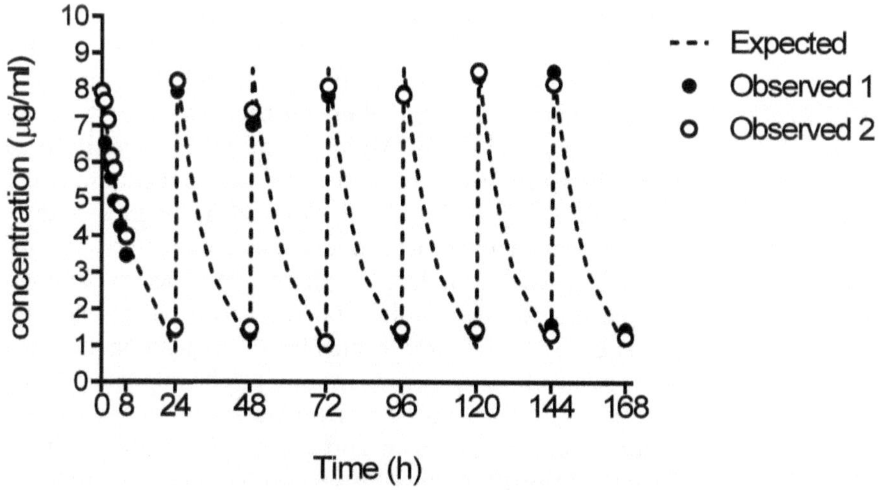

Fig. 4 Concentration-time curve of ceftaroline with repeated dosing in a one-compartment in vitro PD model. The observed pharmacokinetics in the model closely matched the expected values. Adapted from [2]

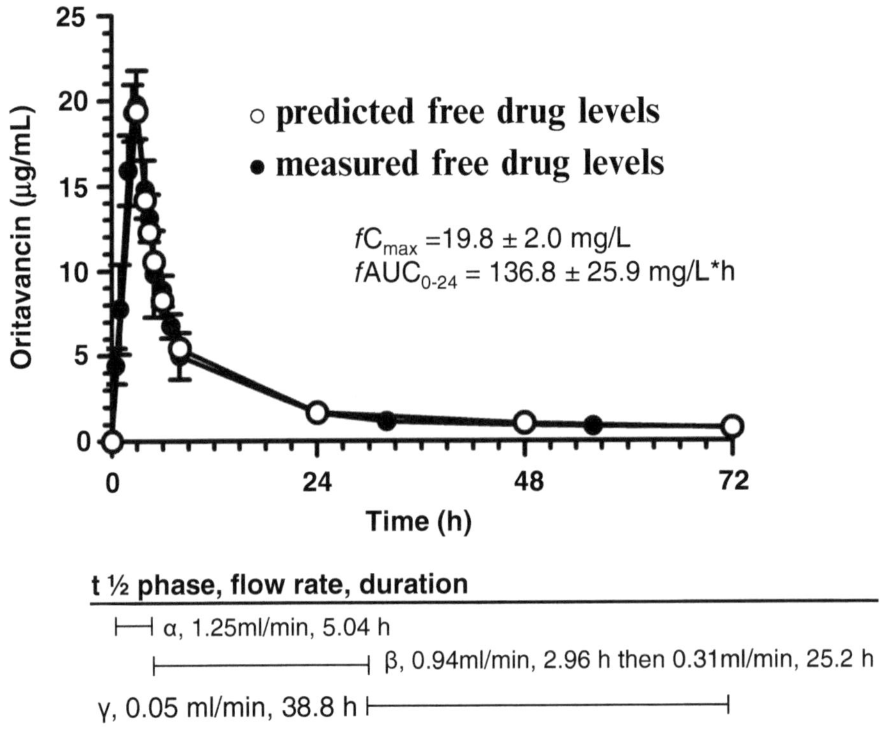

Fig. 5 Concentration-time curve profile of oritavancin using a single 3-h infusion dose in a one-compartment in vitro model. The antibiotic displays a three-phase half-life, which was able to be simulated in the model and was comparable to predicted values from prior pharmacokinetic studies. Adapted from [39]

The clearance of the model, or flow rate (*F*) of the media into and out of the central compartment, is synonymous. Therefore in the one-compartment system, antibiotic pharmacokinetics can be accurately determined using these equations. While this equation is commonly used to simulate a monoexponential decay of drug, these principles can be used to simulate an approximated multi-exponential decay. This can be accomplished through calculating the elimination rate and adjusting the clearance of the model for each exponential decay. Multiple antibiotics have been simulated using this multi-exponential decay function including levofloxacin, amoxicillin, cefuroxime, and oritavancin. Figure 5 displays the one-compartment in vitro model time concentration profile of oritavancin, which simulated a three-phase decay elimination and demonstrated comparable expected and predicted concentrations [39]. Using these same principles of changes in drug clearance, these relatively basic in vitro models can be important tools to evaluate PK/PD relationship in simulations of renal dysfunction and other altered metabolism and clearance situations. Investigators have used these models with success for these PK/PD assessments of altered clearance [11, 12].

3.2 One-Compartment PK/PD Models

The one-compartment model can be used for a variety of applications and simulations. The method described in this section uses a standard inoculum and growth condition, but some of these variables can be altered to evaluate other effects on pharmacodynamics such as inoculum, stationary versus static phase growth, and mixed infection models among others [40–42]. Although this model has been used for a variety of microorganisms, this method will use aerobic bacteria as the model organism type.

3.2.1 Media and Organism Preparation

1. It is preferred that bacteria are in exponential growth phase for the initiation of the model simulation. Inoculate 10 ml of media with a single colony of bacteria from overnight growth on a solid agar. Incubate at 35 °C a rotating shaking platform until media turbidity is present. Dilute culture to a McFarland turbidity standard of 0.5 (10^8 cfu/ml). This is the inoculum that is introduced into the model.
2. Autoclave sterilize dilution media used for PK/PD simulation (*see* **Note 7**).
3. Autoclave sterilize tubing to connect inflow (supplement) and outflow (waste).

3.2.2 Model Preparation

1. Prepare the model top by connecting the four top ports with tubing. Attach the syringe filter to the one port that is used as an air vent. Another port is used to receive dilution medium. The dilution port should have a straight tubing connector to facilitate attachment of dilution tubing to the port. A third port is for waste removal and should also contain a straight connector. The last port is for dosing/sampling the model. The dosing/sampling port should have a female luer connector to facilitate attachment of syringe at the time of dose or sample. Connect tubing to the opposite end of the dose/sample port (i.e., interior of the model) to a length that extends into the media. This allows withdrawal of media from the model during sampling time points. Screw the cap onto the model. Wrap the exposed exterior and sample/dose port with foil. Add magnetic stir bar and non-sterile Mueller-Hinton broth to a target volume for the model, and autoclave sterilize the model for 20 min.
2. Place the model on the stir hotplate. Connect inflow and outflow tubing to the model and attach tubing the peristaltic pumps. Start the model flow for the target antibiotic simulation. After verifying that media is supplementing and exiting the model, inject 1 % v/v of the prepared inoculum into the model so that the starting standard inoculum is 1×10^6 cfu/ml. Flush the port with a small amount of sterile media to ensure that the inoculation reaches the model. Take the first time point from the sample port with a syringe prior to administering antibiotics. Reattach the flush syringe to the sample port and ensure

that the luer port remains closed to the environment outside the model. Administer antibiotic dose to the model through the dosing port on the model cap. This is the starting time point for the antibiotic simulation. The number and frequency of samples depend on the experimental hypothesis, but many take frequent samples in the first few hours to assess PK/PD with initial exposure. There are no limitations to the number of samples that can be obtained for each model during the simulated exposure (*see* **Note 9**).

3.2.3 Analysis

1. Serially dilute each sample as needed and plate on growth agar using standard microbiology techniques or an automated serial dilution plating machine. Incubate the plates for 18–24 h at 35 °C and then count bacterial colonies by manual recording or use colony detection software supplied with the automated method. The bacterial density in the chamber is calculated by the manual method with the equation

$$\log_{10}\left(\frac{\text{cfu}}{\text{ml}}\right)=\log_{10}\left[\left(\frac{\text{Mean}\,\dfrac{\text{cfu}}{\text{plate}}}{\text{Volume of plated sample}}\right)(\text{Dilution of plated sample})\right]$$

3.3 Hollow Fiber Multi-compartment PK/PD Model

The hollow fiber unit consists of the cartridge represented in Fig. 2 and the circulatory tubing that attaches to the duet pump. This set comes pre-sterilized by ethylene oxide from the manufacturer for a one-time-use application. The central compartment reservoir and reservoir cap that attach to the hollow fiber unit to supply media and antibiotics to the system can be autoclave sterilized and reused. This method describes the hollow fiber setup and use for aerobic bacteria.

3.3.1 Model Preparation

1. The central reservoir and cap require sterilization prior to connecting to the hollow fiber model. Prepare the ports on the cap (Fig. 3) by connecting tubing with male luer connectors for the inflow supplement and outflow waste use. The ports used to circulate media and antibiotics from the central compartment to the hollow fiber model should be attached with tubing containing a female luer connection. For the two ports that are used for withdrawal of media from the central compartment, attach tubing on the underside of the cap port to reach the media in the reservoir for withdrawal. Attach the vent filter to the final port. Fill the central reservoir with unsterilized media and note the volume used as it is representative of the V_c for dosing and clearance calculations described in the PD principles

method. Cover all exposed luer connections with foil and autoclave.

2. Autoclave sterilize dilution media used for PK/PD simulation.
3. Connect the 3-way stopcock valve to tubing that is designated for removing media from the central compartment model to waste. Autoclave sterilize this tubing-stopcock as well as tubing to deliver fresh media to the central compartment (inflow supplement).
4. The hollow fiber model requires that the hydrophilic polysulfone fibers are saturated with media prior to introduction of organism into the extracapillary space. It is ideal to prepare the hollow fiber model in a laminar flow hood to minimize contamination risk. Unwrap the model from the sterile package. The model contains four luer ports, two on the cartridge for sample access of bacteria in the extracapillary space, one for delivery of antibiotic from the central compartment, and one for media return to central compartment. These are covered with male luer caps to maintain sterility of the ports outside of the package. Do not remove these caps at this time. Connect the tubing that delivers media to the hollow fiber model to the appropriate port on the central reservoir cap. Connect the tubing that returns media back to the central compartment from the hollow fiber model to the appropriate port on the central reservoir cap. Place the hollow model and central reservoir on the Duet Pump, ensuring that the model latches to the base and the vertical circulatory tubing on the top of the model is secured in the pump slot on the Duet (Fig. 6).

The extracapillary space in the cartridge has a holder volume of 20 ml. Withdraw 10 ml of Mueller-Hinton broth into two 20 ml syringes. Attach syringes onto each port on the cartridge and slowly deliver the 20 ml total volume to the extracapillary space. Leave the syringes on these ports throughout the duration of the experiment to maintain sterility. They are removed only at the time of sampling and immediately reattached. Place the Duet Pump with hollow fiber model in a tabletop incubator or warm room. Start the Duet Pump to begin media circulation throughout the model. The C2011 cartridge and supplied tubing have a volume space of approximately 50 ml. So this volume will be removed from the central reservoir but should be accounted for as the model volume when using V_C in calculations. Allow the pump to circulate media overnight to adequately soak the fibers, but an 18–24-h soak period is preferred.

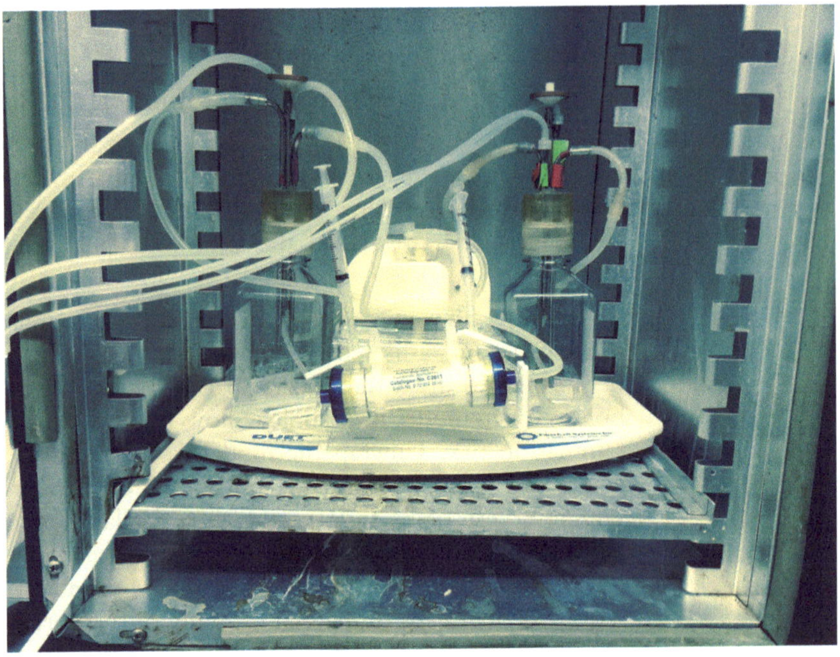

Fig. 6 Image of the hollow fiber model Duet Pump system and connected tubing. The hollow fiber cartridge and central reservoir are held on the Duet Pump system and circulated throughout the model, while pumps provide supplemental media and remove waste (not pictured)

3.3.2 Organism Preparation

It is preferred that bacteria are in exponential growth phase for the initiation of the model simulation. Inoculate 10 ml of media with a single colony of bacteria from overnight growth on a solid agar. Incubate at 35 °C a rotating shaking platform until media turbidity is present. Dilute culture to a McFarland turbidity standard of 0.5 (10^8 cfu/ml). This is the stock inoculum that is introduced into the model.

3.3.3 PK/PD Simulation

1. Connect sterile inflow tubing to the central reservoir inflow port and attach tubing to the peristaltic pump. Connect the sterile 3-way stopcock and tubing to the female luer exit port on the central reservoir and attach tubing to the peristaltic pump. Attach the injection site septum with the male luer to the open female luer on the 3-way stopcock. Start the model flow for the target antibiotic simulation, and ensure that both inflow and outflow rates on the pumps are the same. After verifying that media is supplementing and exiting the model, inject 0.2 ml (1 % v/v) of the prepared inoculum into the model using a 1 ml luer syringe so that the starting standard inoculum is 1×10^6 cfu/ml in the extracapillary space.
2. For sample collection, mix the media and organism in the extracapillary space by withdrawing and reinserting the extracapillary fluid culture using the 20 ml syringes on the cartridge ports for

several cycles. Withdraw 0.5–1 ml from each port using the 20 ml syringes and place each sample in a separate Eppendorf tube for analysis. Return syringes to the ports on the cartridge. The initial sample should be done prior to introducing antibiotic to the model.

3. Administer antibiotic dose to the central model through the dosing port on the central reservoir cap. This is the starting time point for the antibiotic simulation. Continue to administer antibiotic doses at the indicated dosing period for each antibiotic during the entire simulation period. The number and frequency of samples depend on the experimental hypothesis, but many take frequent samples in the first few hours to assess PK/PD with initial exposure. There are no limitations to the number of samples that can be obtained for each model during the simulated exposure (*see* **Note 9**).
4. Pharmacokinetic samples from the central compartment are obtained from the injection site on the 3-way stopcock as the medium is leaving the central compartment. Ideally the time of the PK sample collection should coincide with at least the PK/PD samples taken from the hollow fiber model cartridge. PK can also be obtained from the extracapillary space in the cartridge from the sample collection described in the step above. The PK in the two compartments can be compared.

3.3.4 Analysis

Bacterial quantification from the samples is determined using the same method described for the one-compartment models. Since the hollow fiber model is ideal for quantification of resistance development, susceptibility testing can also be done using standard techniques described in a separate chapter. Another advantage of this model is the ability to quantify toxins and assess virulence factors resulting from antibiotic exposure. Example protocols for these methods are described in the literature with the hollow fiber model and other applications [29, 30].

3.4 PK/PD Biofilm Models

The protocol for CDC model is available upon purchase of the reactor model (http://www.biofilms.biz/biofilm-reactors) and is presented here. All components are autoclavable and reusable for repeat model experiments. The reactor consists of a 1 l beaker with an effluent spout at the 400 ml mark for media elimination (Fig. 7). The unsealed removable top contains eight vertical rods that each houses three coupons that support biofilm growth and are used for assessment of antibiotic activity (Fig. 8). The model top also has three ports for administration of dilution media into the model, sample collection and dose administration, and sterile air ventilation. A variety of coupon materials are available to use in the model including those with clinical applications such as polycarbonate, stainless steel, titanium, polyurethane, and Teflon among

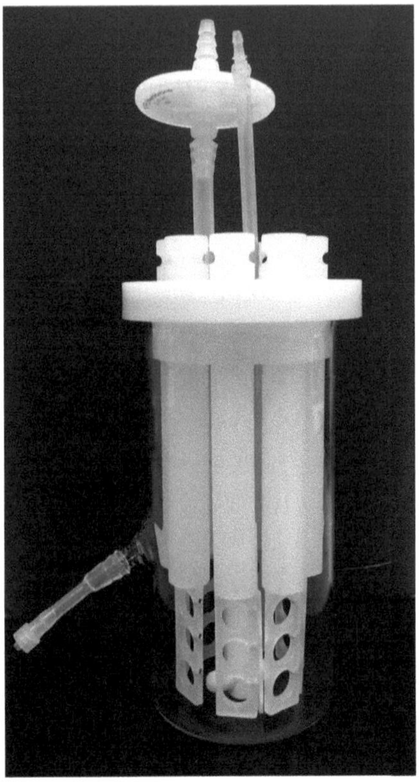

Fig. 7 Image of the CDC biofilm PD model with eight removable rods

Fig. 8 Image of an individual rod with three biofilm coupons from the CDC biofilm model

others. A stir bar/vane supplies continuous consistent high sheer against the coupons and mixing of growth media and antibiotics via a magnetic stir plate. Antimicrobial activity can be assessed from the residual organism on the coupons (biofilm) and in the growth medium (planktonic). The protocol for the model and PK/PD assessment are presented.

3.4.1 Media and Organism Preparation

1. Inoculate 100 ml of growth media (tryptic soy broth) with a single colony of bacteria from overnight growth on a solid agar. Incubate at 35 ± 2 °C overnight on a rotating shaking platform (120 rpm).

2. Sterilize the continuous flow media (20 L of 100 mg/L TSB). It is recommended to first sterilize 20 L of distilled water and aseptically add concentrated TSB (2.0 g TSB/500 mL) to equal the final concentration of 100 mg/L TSB.
3. Sterilize Mueller-Hinton broth to a volume required for the duration of antibiotic therapy (volume = flow rate × duration of simulation). This medium will be used for the assessment of antibiotic PK/PD simulation.

3.4.2 CDC Model Preparation

1. The model rods, beaker, and top can be cleaned with general laboratory soap prior to each use. It is important to vigorously clean the coupons between uses to eliminate attached bacteria and biofilm. The recommended cleaning procedure is two series of immersing the coupons in laboratory soap and sonicating for 3–5 min and rinsing. Finally the coupons should be soaked in 2 M HCl, rinsed with sterile water, and let to air-dry. Place the coupons in the model rod so they are flush with each coupon slot ($n = 3$ coupons/rod, 24 per model) and tighten.
2. Prepare the model top by inserting the coupon rods, attaching the stir bar/vane, and connecting the three top ports with tubing. One port is used as an air vent (PFTE filter provided with model purchase), another for receiving supplemental dilution medium, and the third for dosing/sampling the model. The supplemental dilution port should have a straight tubing connector to facilitate attachment of influent tubing to the port. The dosing/sampling port should have a female luer connector to facilitate attachment of syringe at the time of dose or sample. Connect tubing to the opposite end of the dose/sample port (i.e., interior of the model) to a length below the 400 ml effluent port level. This allows withdrawal of media from the model during sampling time points. Wrap the exposed exterior influent and sample/dose port with foil and place top with rods, coupons, and stir bar/vane into the effluent beaker. Attach tubing to the effluent port on the beaker, insert a straight connector to the opposite end, and wrap with foil. Clamp the effluent tubing with clamp scissors to hold media in the reaction chamber during the batch phase. Add 500 ml of non-sterile TSB batch media (300 mg/L TSB) and autoclave sterilize the model for 20 min.
3. The batch phase of the model allows for initial bacterial growth and attachment on coupons in the model. Place the reactor on the digital stir hotplate and inject 1 ml of the 100 ml overnight culture into the batch media through the injection port with a luer syringe. Flush the port with 5 ml TSB to ensure that the inoculation reaches the batch media. Do not remove the flush syringe to ensure that the luer port remains closed to the environment outside the model. The inoculum in the batch is

approximately 10^8 cfu/ml. Start the stir bar/vane rotating at 125 rpm and confirm that this rotation is maintained throughout the batch phase of 24 h (*see* **Note 8**).

4. The continuous flow phase is designed to further facilitate biofilm development on the coupons. Prior to beginning the continuous flow phase autoclave sterilize tubing to connect to the supplemental and waste carboys. Aseptically connect the tubing to the model and carboys, attach the supplemental tubing to the peristaltic pump, and unclamp the waste port. The rods and stir bar/vane should displace approximately 150 ml media which should exit the effluent port once unclamped, so that 350 ml is maintained as the reactor working volume. A continuous flow rate should be used so that the residence time of the media in the model is less than the doubling time of the bacteria to ensure that non-adhered bacteria are cleared from the model and only biofilm-attached cells remain. In the case of *Pseudomonas aeruginosa* (ATCC 700888), a residence time of 30 min can be used. With a model volume of 350 ml, the flow rate for the continuous flow phase should be set at 11.67 ml/min (350 ml/30 min). The continuous flow phase is operated for 24 h.
5. The antibiotic PK/PD simulation begins following the continuous flow phase. The dilution media for supplementation during the antibiotic simulation is Mueller-Hinton broth, so the dilution supplement should be exchanged for this medium and new tubing connected to the model and peristaltic pump. This new medium should maintain the same flow rate as the continuous flow phase (e.g., from above 11.67 ml/min) for the first 30 min prior to antibiotic dose to introduce appropriate media to the model for antibiotic activity. After 30 min, reduce the clearance to that of the modeled antibiotic (see Subheading 3.1). Dosing to the model and sampling of the media for bacterial enumeration can follow the procedures outlined in the other in vitro PK/PD models.

3.4.3 Analysis

1. The CDC model contains a maximum of 24 coupons for analysis, so therefore the model is limited in duration of antimicrobial simulation to the number of time points (coupons) selected for analysis. The biofilms are formed on the coupon side facing the stir bar/vane, so take note of the coupon side for analysis of anti-biofilm activity. Remove a single rod and rest the bottom on a sterile petri dish while removing the coupon with a flame-sterilized hemostat taking caution not to disturb the biofilm side of the coupon. Place the rod back into the model to continue simulation for the remaining coupons in the rod.

2. The biofilm is scraped from the coupon using sterile supplies. Although many different types of supplies could be used for this, a sterile wooden stick is sufficient to ensure that all biofilm is removed. The scraped biofilm is placed in sterile water and the coupon is rinsed with sterile water to remove any remaining, which is added to the biofilm suspension. The total biofilm suspension volume of 10 ml is important in this step to calculate the bacterial burden in biofilm.
3. Homogenize the sample at 20,500 rpm for 30 s to disaggregate the biofilm and universally disperse the cells in suspension prior to plating. Serially dilute the sample on growth agar using standard microbiology techniques or an automated serial dilution plating machine. Incubate the plates for 18–24 h at 35 °C and then count bacterial colonies by manual recording or use colony detection software supplied with the automated method. The bacterial density on the coupon is calculated by the equation:

$$\log_{10}\left(\frac{\text{cfu}}{\text{cm}^2}\right)=\log_{10}\left[\frac{\left(\dfrac{\text{Mean}\,\dfrac{\text{cfu}}{\text{plate}}}{\text{Volume of plated sample}}\right)(\text{Dilution of plated sample})}{\left(\dfrac{\text{Volume scraped into}}{\text{Surface area scraped}}\right)}\right]$$

The diameter of the coupons supplied for this model is 1.27 cm; therefore the surface area scraped is 5.06 cm^2.

4. The samples taken from the sample port for planktonic bacterial growth in the media should be taken at the same time points as the coupon samples for direct comparison. These samples are plated using standard microbiology techniques described in earlier sections.

3.5 Combination Therapy Models

The development of antimicrobial resistance combined with relatively few new treatment options has increased the interest for combination therapy for situations where monotherapy was traditionally considered adequate. The models described so far have all been used in both single- and combination-therapy experiments. A separate chapter discusses the pharmacodynamic issues of combination therapy, so this section presents the basic design of the combination model that can be incorporated in the methods described for the presented models.

The concept of combination antibacterial modeling in the in vitro dynamic systems allows two antibiotics to be administered simultaneously. For antibacterials with the same half-life, this is easily done in any of the models described so far since both antibiotics will be cleared from the dosing compartment at the same rate. However, when two drugs with different half-lives are studied, one of the antibiotics will be cleared at an inappropriately faster rate. Therefore, this requires a supplement chamber to replace the antibiotic that is removed at the faster rate. This method describes modeling with two antibiotics, but the sample principles can be used to model three or more antibiotics with different half-lives.

3.5.1 Overall Model Design

The combination model was originally described by Blaser et al. [43], and it remains mostly unchanged from the original design [2, 44, 45]). A representative diagram of the design of the two-antimicrobial combination model is provided in Fig. 9. The models described in earlier sections will serve as the central reaction model (M_1) in this method. The supplemental chamber model (M_2) provides supplemental drug to M_1 due to the more rapid clearance of the overall model. The inflow and clearance of the M_2 supplement chamber should be set for the antimicrobial with the lower half-life (slower clearance, C_S). The M_1 inflow rate is set at clearance of the faster drug (C_F) minus C_S ($C_F - C_S$). Therefore the clearance of drug from M_1 is set at the clearance of the drug with the faster half-life. Both antibiotics are dosed into the M_1 chamber at the targeted interval simulation. At the same time, an equivalent dose of the antibiotic with the slower half-life is administered into the M_2 chamber. This allows the antibiotic with the slower half-life to be supplemented back into M_1 to account for the drug lost due

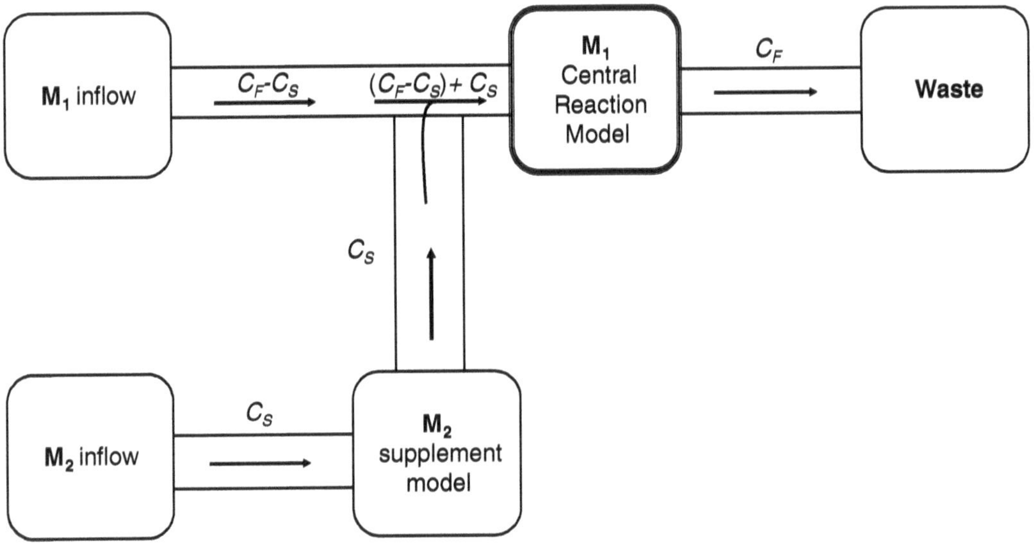

Fig. 9 Schematic diagram of the in vitro combination PD model

to C_F. The total inflow and outflow clearance for M_1 will be equivalent $[(C_F - C_S) + C_S = C_F]$.

An example of this diagram using a 250 ml model simulation is Drug A (half-life of 12 h and a dose given once daily) in combination with Drug B (half-life of 1 h and a dose given every 6 h). Based on the calculating model clearance rates provided in the PK/PD principles section of this chapter, the clearance rates of Drug A = 14.4 ml/h and Drug B = 173.3 ml/h. Therefore $C_F = 173.3$ ml/h, $C_S = 14.4$ ml/h, and $C_F - C_S = 158.9$ ml/h. Drug A is administered into M_1 and M_2 once daily while Drug B is administered into M_1 every 6 h. The preparation, sampling, and PK/PD analysis of the combination model are similar to the methods presented for the other single-drug models in this chapter (*see* **Note 9**). The inflow tubing for M_1 and M_2 should be connected with a y-site so that the flow rates entering M_1 are equivalent to the clearance (C_F).

3.6 Antimicrobial Effect Endpoint Analysis

The classification of the antimicrobial effect can be obtained from the killing curves for a given antibiotic and reflect the entire antimicrobial activity over the duration of exposure. While a general comparison between two antibiotics or among multiple antibiotics for a particular organism can be obtained by visual interpretation of the killing curves, a more intricate approach is needed for a mathematical and statistical comparison of the activities. The primary objective of this analysis is to provide an interpretation of the relationship between antibiotic and organism effect. To further justify the model as a clinically translatable tool, the analysis and interpretation should ideally be able to predict clinical outcomes of antibiotic treatment.

The initial analysis of the antimicrobial effect compares the antimicrobial killing curve to the antibiotic-free growth curve over time. As depicted in Fig. 10, a number of relevant endpoints have been utilized from these comparative curves to indicate the antimicrobial effect [46]. The initial and most widely used indices are T_{90}, T_{99}, and $T_{99.9}$ indicating the time to achieve a 1-log, 2-log, and 3-log reduction from the initial starting inoculum, respectively. For this reason many in vitro PD model studies sample frequently from the model after the initial dose to determine this parameter. While it is possible to determine the time to achieve the defined reduction by visual estimation, it is more accurate to use logarithmic extrapolation of the killing curve data points from the starting inoculum for each experiment to find the rate of bacterial elimination.

Defining the initial killing with an antimicrobial is an important component of PD determination; however additional indices can be measured to determine the effect of the antimicrobial over the duration of the antimicrobial exposure (Fig. 10). These include the area between control growth and bacterial killing curves

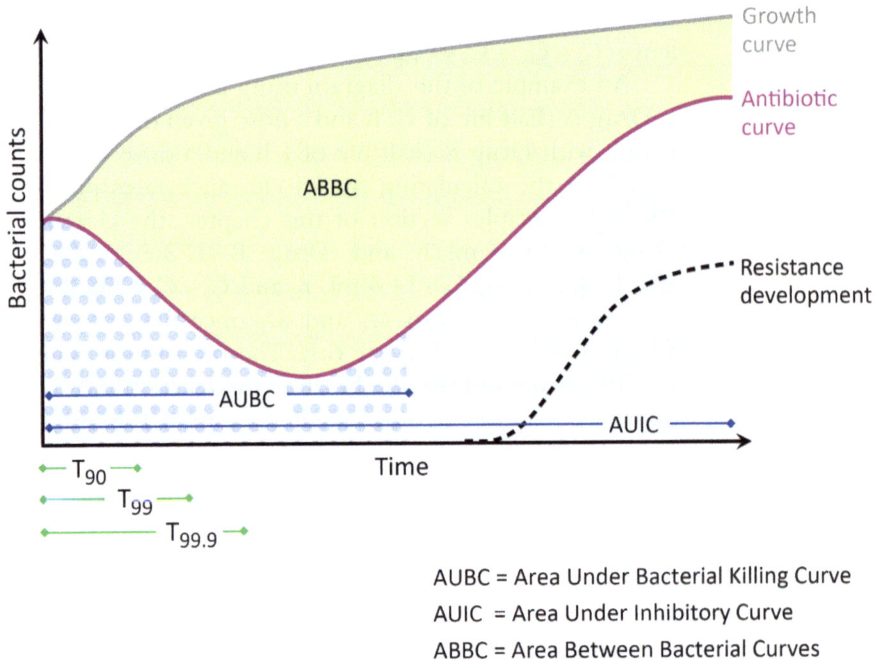

Fig. 10 Antimicrobial effect endpoints. Adapted from [46]

(ABBC), area under the bacterial killing curve (AUBC or AUBKC), and the area under the inhibitory curve (AUIC). These indices can be calculated by the AUC trapezoidal method of the bacterial counts from the initial starting time (T_0) until the cessation of bacterial killing for AUBC or end of antimicrobial exposure for AUIC. The ABBC is calculated by simply subtracting the trapezoidal AUC of the entire experiment duration for the antibiotic curve from the AUC of the growth curve. The AUBC and AUIC are inversely related to bacterial killing: as killing increases, AUBC and AUIC decrease [47].

The pharmacodynamic parameter that predicts the clinical effectiveness of most antimicrobials is the AUC relative to the MIC of the organism (AUC/MIC). The above three indices are relatively accurate in predicting the AUC/MIC response; however some limitations exist and require cautious interpretation. All three endpoints may underestimate the effect at high AUC/MIC, while AUBC may underestimate the true effect at small AUC/MIC [48]. In these situations, other indices of the total antimicrobial effect can be utilized to predict the PD response that have described in more detailed modeling [5]. Resistance development, as depicted in Fig. 10, has become an increasingly important index in the current era of multi-drug resistance, so this is now often screened as part of the analysis, which is a particular advantage of the prolonged duration simulations and continuous sampling supported with the in vitro PD model [49–51]. In addition to these endpoints, detailed mathematical modeling provides robust interpretation of PK/PD effects of antimicrobials from these models and computer simulations [52–54].

4 Notes

1. The recommended media for use in the in vitro PD model is recommended by CLSI for antibiotic testing against most bacteria. Some bacteria may require different media for optimal growth conditions. Similarly, some antibiotics may require different chemical supplementation in order to demonstrate appropriate activity.
2. The Masterflex size 14 tubing is used with the peristaltic pump to provide a flow rate range of 0.21–130 ml/min. This is well within the range of flow rates for most antimicrobials. Those with prolonged half-lives may require smaller bore tubing that can accommodate slower flow rates, such as Masterflex size 13 tubing.
3. The size of the inflow flask should depend on the volume needed for supplementation throughout the simulated exposures. Ideally the size and volume should accommodate the entire experiment without the need for additional media supplementation. This reduces the potential for environmental contamination.
4. No. 10 stoppers are designed for use with 2, 4, and 6 L flasks. Stoppers are available in other sizes to accommodate other flasks.
5. The No. 10 rubber stopper has two predrilled holes. To set up the system, thread 16 size tubing through one hole to a length that can reach the bottom of the flask to remove the entire media contents during the simulation. Thread 16 size tubing through the second hole at a length to just inside the flask. Connect the air filter to the tube in the second hole and allow sterile air diffusion within the flask.
6. A standard tabletop incubator can house the hollow fiber model system. The model with the hollow fiber cartridge and central compartment on the Duet Pump are placed inside the incubator. The connected supplemental inflow and waste tubing remain outside the incubator (room air) with the peristaltic pump to supply/remove media from the model. To prevent the supplement/waste tubing from pinching when closing the autoclave door, cutting the door seal to allow enough room to place the tubes is recommended. This prevents the tubes from pinching but also does not interfere with the integrity of the seal that may lead to heat loss. Alternatively, if a warm room is

available for use, this would be a more optimal setup for the entire system.

7. The dilution media should be autoclaved with the rubber stopper system in place to ensure sterility after the autoclave cycle.
8. As provided in the materials, a digital stir hotplate provides accurate measurement of the rotation needed to create the biofilm in this phase.
9. Removal of large volumes of media during the sampling points may alter the pharmacokinetics of the model due to increased elimination. It is recommended to sample only volumes required for analysis.

References

1. LaPlante KL, Leonard SN, Andes DR, Craig WA, Rybak MJ (2008) Activities of clindamycin, daptomycin, doxycycline, linezolid, trimethoprim-sulfamethoxazole, and vancomycin against community-associated methicillin-resistant *Staphylococcus aureus* with inducible clindamycin resistance in murine thigh infection and in vitro pharmacodynamic models. Antimicrob Agents Chemother 52(6):2156–2162. doi:10.1128/AAC.01046-07, AAC.01046-07 [pii]
2. Rose WE, Schulz LT, Andes D, Striker R, Berti AD, Hutson PR, Shukla SK (2012) Addition of ceftaroline to daptomycin after emergence of daptomycin-nonsusceptible *Staphylococcus aureus* during therapy improves antibacterial activity. Antimicrob Agents Chemother 56(10):5296–5302. doi:10.1128/AAC.00797-12, AAC.00797-12 [pii]
3. Vidaillac C, Gardete S, Tewhey R, Sakoulas G, Kaatz GW, Rose WE, Tomasz A, Rybak MJ (2013) Alternative mutational pathways to intermediate resistance to vancomycin in methicillin-resistant *Staphylococcus aureus*. J Infect Dis 208(1):67–74. doi:10.1093/infdis/jit127
4. Rybak MJ, Allen GP, Hershberger E (2001) In vitro antibiotic pharmacodynamic models. In: Nightingale CH, Murakawa T, Ambrose PG (eds) Antimicrobial pharmacodynamics in theory and clinical practice. Marcell Dekker, New York, pp 41–65
5. Firsov AA, Zinner SH, Lubenko IY (2007) In vitro dynamic models as tools to predict antibiotic pharmacodynamics. In: Nightingale CH, Ambrose PG, Drusano GL, Murakawa T (eds) Antimicrobial pharmacodynamics in theory and clinical practice, 2nd edn. CRC Press, New York, pp 45–78
6. Craig WA (1998) Pharmacokinetic/pharmacodynamic parameters: rationale for antibacterial dosing of mice and men. Clin Infect Dis 26(1):1–10, quiz 11–12
7. White RL (2001) What in vitro models of infection can and cannot do. Pharmacotherapy 21(11 Pt 2):292S–301S
8. Gloede J, Scheerans C, Derendorf H, Kloft C (2010) In vitro pharmacodynamic models to determine the effect of antibacterial drugs. J Antimicrob Chemother 65(2):186–201. doi:10.1093/jac/dkp434
9. Firsov AA, Portnoy YA, Strukova EN, Shlykova DS, Zinner SH (2014) Predicting bacterial resistance using the time inside the mutant selection window: possibilities and limitations. Int J Antimicrob Agents 44(4):301–305. doi:10.1016/j.ijantimicag.2014.06.013
10. Leonard SN, Rolek KM (2013) Evaluation of the combination of daptomycin and nafcillin against vancomycin-intermediate *Staphylococcus aureus*. J Antimicrob Chemother 68(3):644–647. doi:10.1093/jac/dks453, dks453 [pii]
11. Cappelletty DM (1999) Evaluation of several dosing regimens of cefepime, with various simulations of renal function, against clinical isolates of *Pseudomonas aeruginosa* in a pharmacodynamic infection model. Antimicrob Agents Chemother 43(1):129–133
12. Rao GG, Ly NS, Haas CE, Garonzik S, Forrest A, Bulitta JB, Kelchlin PA, Holden PN, Nation RL, Li J, Tsuji BT (2014) New dosing strategies for an old antibiotic: pharmacodynamics of front-loaded regimens of colistin at simulated pharmacokinetics in patients with kidney or liver disease. Antimicrob Agents Chemother 58(3):1381–1388. doi:10.1128/AAC.00327-13
13. MacVane SH, So W, Nicolau DP, Kuti JL (2014) In vitro activity of human-simulated epithelial lining fluid exposures of ceftaroline, ceftriaxone, and vancomycin against methicillin-susceptible and -resistant

Staphylococcus aureus. Antimicrob Agents Chemother 58(12):7520–7526. doi:10.1128/AAC.03742-14
14. Grasso S (1985) Historical review of in-vitro models. J Antimicrob Chemother 15(Suppl A):99–102
15. Li RC, Zhu ZY (1997) In vitro models for prediction of antimicrobial activity: a pharmacokinetic and pharmacodynamic perspective. J Chemother 9(Suppl 1):55–63
16. Nolting A, Dalla Costa T, Rand KH, Derendorf H (1996) Pharmacokinetic-pharmacodynamic modeling of the antibiotic effect of piperacillin in vitro. Pharm Res 13(1):91–96
17. Dalla Costa T, Nolting A, Rand K, Derendorf H (1997) Pharmacokinetic-pharmacodynamic modelling of the in vitro antiinfective effect of piperacillin-tazobactam combinations. Int J Clin Pharmacol Ther 35(10):426–433
18. Clinical (2010) Clinical and Laboratory Standards Institute, C. L. S. I., Performance standards for antimicrobial susceptibility testing, vol 20th informational supplement M100-S20. CLSI, Wayne, PA
19. Al-Asadi MJ, Greenwood D, O'Grady F (1979) In vitro model simulating the form of exposure of bacteria to antimicrobial drugs encountered in infection. Antimicrob Agents Chemother 16(1):77–80
20. Toothaker RD, Welling PG, Craig WA (1982) An in vitro model for the study of antibacterial dosage regimen design. J Pharm Sci 71(8):861–864
21. Zinner SH, Husson M, Klastersky J (1981) An artificial capillary in vitro kinetic model of antibiotic bactericidal activity. J Infect Dis 144(6):583–587
22. Guggenbichler JP, Semenitz E, Konig P (1985) Kill kinetics and regrowth pattern of bacteria exposed to antibiotic concentrations simulating those observed in vivo. J Antimicrob Chemother 15(Suppl A):139–146
23. Bonapace CR, Friedrich LV, Bosso JA, White RL (2002) Determination of antibiotic effect in an in vitro pharmacodynamic model: comparison with an established animal model of infection. Antimicrob Agents Chemother 46(11):3574–3579
24. Renkin EM (1985) Capillary transport of macromolecules: pores and other endothelial pathways. J Appl Physiol 58(2):315–325
25. Aeschlimann JR, Zervos MJ, Rybak MJ (1998) Treatment of vancomycin-resistant Enterococcus faecium with RP 59500 (quinupristin-dalfopristin) administered by intermittent or continuous infusion, alone or in combination with doxycycline, in an in vitro pharmacodynamic infection model with simulated endocardial vegetations. Antimicrob Agents Chemother 42(10):2710–2717
26. Haller I (1985) Penetration of antibiotics through cell culture monolayers. J Antimicrob Chemother 15(Suppl A):197–199
27. Blaser J, Stone BB, Zinner SH (1985) Two compartment kinetic model with multiple artificial capillary units. J Antimicrob Chemother 15(Suppl A):131–137
28. Blaser J, Stone BB, Groner MC, Zinner SH (1985) Impact of netilmicin regimens on the activities of ceftazidime-netilmicin combinations against Pseudomonas aeruginosa in an in vitro pharmacokinetic model. Antimicrob Agents Chemother 28(1):64–68
29. Louie A, Vanscoy BD, Heine HS 3rd, Liu W, Abshire T, Holman K, Kulawy R, Brown DL, Drusano GL (2012) Differential effects of linezolid and ciprofloxacin on toxin production by *Bacillus anthracis* in an in vitro pharmacodynamic system. Antimicrob Agents Chemother 56(1):513–517. doi:10.1128/AAC.05724-11
30. Pichereau S, Pantrangi M, Couet W, Badiou C, Lina G, Shukla SK, Rose WE (2012) Simulated antibiotic exposures in an in vitro hollow-fiber infection model influence toxin gene expression and production in community-associated methicillin-resistant *Staphylococcus aureus* strain MW2. Antimicrob Agents Chemother 56(1):140–147. doi:10.1128/AAC.05113-11, AAC.05113-11 [pii]
31. Brown AN, McSharry JJ, Weng Q, Adams JR, Kulawy R, Drusano GL (2011) Zanamivir, at 600 milligrams twice daily, inhibits oseltamivir-resistant 2009 pandemic H1N1 influenza virus in an in vitro hollow-fiber infection model system. Antimicrob Agents Chemother 55(4):1740–1746. doi:10.1128/AAC.01628-10
32. Louie A, Grasso C, Bahniuk N, Van Scoy B, Brown DL, Kulawy R, Drusano GL (2010) The combination of meropenem and levofloxacin is synergistic with respect to both Pseudomonas aeruginosa kill rate and resistance suppression. Antimicrob Agents Chemother 54(6):2646–2654. doi:10.1128/AAC.00065-10
33. Wiederhold NP, Coyle EA, Raad II, Prince RA, Lewis RE (2005) Antibacterial activity of linezolid and vancomycin in an in vitro pharmacodynamic model of gram-positive catheter-related bacteraemia. J Antimicrob Chemother 55(5):792–795. doi:10.1093/jac/dki106
34. Tang HJ, Chen CC, Ko WC, Yu WL, Chiang SR, Chuang YC (2011) In vitro efficacy of antimicrobial agents against high-inoculum or biofilm-embedded meticillin-resistant *Staphylococcus aureus* with vancomycin minimal inhibitory concentrations equal to 2 mug/mL (VA2-MRSA). Int J Antimicrob Agents 38(1):46–51. doi:10.1016/j.ijantimicag.2011.02.013

35. Yasuda H, Koga T, Fukuoka T (1999) In vitro and in vivo models of bacterial biofilms. Methods Enzymol 310:577–595
36. Parra-Ruiz J, Vidaillac C, Rose WE, Rybak MJ (2010) Activities of high-dose daptomycin, vancomycin, and moxifloxacin alone or in combination with clarithromycin or rifampin in a novel in vitro model of *Staphylococcus aureus* biofilm. Antimicrob Agents Chemother 54(10):4329–4334. doi:10.1128/AAC.00455-10, AAC.00455-10 [pii]
37. Hall Snyder AD, Vidaillac C, Rose W, McRoberts JP, Rybak MJ (2014) Evaluation of high-dose daptomycin versus vancomycin alone or combined with clarithromycin or rifampin against *Staphylococcus aureus* and *S. epidermidis* in a novel in vitro PK/PD model of bacterial biofilm. Infect Dis Ther. doi:10.1007/s40121-014-0055-5
38. Lora-Tamayo J, Murillo O, Bergen PJ, Nation RL, Poudyal A, Luo X, Yu HY, Ariza J, Li J (2014) Activity of colistin combined with doripenem at clinically relevant concentrations against multidrug-resistant *Pseudomonas aeruginosa* in an in vitro dynamic biofilm model. J Antimicrob Chemother 69(9):2434–2442. doi:10.1093/jac/dku151
39. Belley A, Arhin FF, Sarmiento I, Deng H, Rose W, Moeck G (2013) Pharmacodynamics of a simulated single 1,200-milligram dose of oritavancin in an in vitro pharmacokinetic/pharmacodynamic model of methicillin-resistant *Staphylococcus aureus* infection. Antimicrob Agents Chemother 57(1):205–211. doi:10.1128/AAC.01428-12, AAC.01428-12 [pii]
40. LaPlante KL, Rybak MJ, Leuthner KD, Chin JN (2006) Impact of Enterococcus faecalis on the bactericidal activities of arbekacin, daptomycin, linezolid, and tigecycline against methicillin-resistant Staphylococcus aureus in a mixed-pathogen pharmacodynamic model. Antimicrob Agents Chemother 50(4):1298–1303. doi:10.1128/AAC.50.4.1298-1303.2006, 50/4/1298 [pii]
41. Bowker KE, Garvey MI, Noel AR, Tomaselli SG, Macgowan AP (2013) Comparative antibacterial effects of moxifloxacin and levofloxacin on *Streptococcus pneumoniae* strains with defined mechanisms of resistance: impact of bacterial inoculum. J Antimicrob Chemother 68(5):1130–1138. doi:10.1093/jac/dks537
42. Cremades R, Rodriguez JC, Garcia-Pachon E, Galiana A, Ruiz-Garcia M, Lopez P, Royo G (2011) Comparison of the bactericidal activity of various fluoroquinolones against *Mycobacterium tuberculosis* in an in vitro experimental model. J Antimicrob Chemother 66(10):2281–2283. doi:10.1093/jac/dkr281
43. Blaser J (1985) In-vitro model for simultaneous simulation of the serum kinetics of two drugs with different half-lives. J Antimicrob Chemother 15(Suppl A):125–130
44. Deris ZZ, Yu HH, Davis K, Soon RL, Jacob J, Ku CK, Poudyal A, Bergen PJ, Tsuji BT, Bulitta JB, Forrest A, Paterson DL, Velkov T, Li J, Nation RL (2012) The combination of colistin and doripenem is synergistic against *Klebsiella pneumoniae* at multiple inocula and suppresses colistin resistance in an in vitro pharmacokinetic/pharmacodynamic model. Antimicrob Agents Chemother 56(10):5103–5112. doi:10.1128/AAC.01064-12
45. Oku T, Imanishi J, Kishida T (1986) Antiviral effect of two aryl-oligopeptides, FR41565 and FR48217. Antivir Res 6(4):233–239
46. Firsov AA, Vostrov SN, Shevchenko AA, Cornaglia G (1997) Parameters of bacterial killing and regrowth kinetics and antimicrobial effect examined in terms of area under the concentration-time curve relationships: action of ciprofloxacin against *Escherichia coli* in an in vitro dynamic model. Antimicrob Agents Chemother 41(6):1281–1287
47. MacGowan A, Rogers C, Bowker K (2000) The use of in vitro pharmacodynamic models of infection to optimize fluoroquinolone dosing regimens. J Antimicrob Chemother 46(2):163–170
48. Firsov AA, Lubenko IY, Portnoy YA, Zinner SH, Vostrov SN (2001) Relationships of the area under the curve/MIC ratio to different integral endpoints of the antimicrobial effect: gemifloxacin pharmacodynamics in an in vitro dynamic model. Antimicrob Agents Chemother 45(3):927–931. doi:10.1128/AAC.45.3.927-931.2001
49. Zhanel GG, Denisuik A, Vashisht S, Yachison C, Adam HJ, Hoban DJ (2014) Pharmacodynamic activity of ertapenem versus genotypically characterized extended-spectrum beta-lactamase (ESBL)-, KPC- or NDM-producing *Escherichia coli* with reduced susceptibility or resistance to ertapenem using an in vitro model. J Antimicrob Chemother 69(9):2448–2452. doi:10.1093/jac/dku149
50. Hagihara M, Housman ST, Nicolau DP, Kuti JL (2014) In vitro pharmacodynamics of polymyxin B and tigecycline alone and in combination against carbapenem-resistant *Acinetobacter baumannii*. Antimicrob Agents Chemother 58(2):874–879. doi:10.1128/AAC.01624-13
51. Werth BJ, Steed ME, Ireland CE, Tran TT, Nonejuie P, Murray BE, Rose WE, Sakoulas G, Pogliano J, Arias CA, Rybak MJ (2014) Defining daptomycin resistance prevention exposures in vancomycin-resistant *Enterococcus faecium* and *E. faecalis*. Antimicrob Agents

Chemother 58(9):5253–5261. doi:10.1128/AAC.00098-14
52. Landersdorfer CB, Ly NS, Xu H, Tsuji BT, Bulitta JB (2013) Quantifying subpopulation synergy for antibiotic combinations via mechanism-based modeling and a sequential dosing design. Antimicrob Agents Chemother 57(5):2343–2351. doi:10.1128/AAC.00092-13
53. Venisse N, Gregoire N, Marliat M, Couet W (2008) Mechanism-based pharmacokinetic-pharmacodynamic models of in vitro fungistatic and fungicidal effects against *Candida albicans*. Antimicrob Agents Chemother 52(3):937–943. doi:10.1128/AAC.01030-07
54. Bhagunde P, Chang KT, Singh R, Singh V, Garey KW, Nikolaou M, Tam VH (2010) Mathematical modeling to characterize the inoculum effect. Antimicrob Agents Chemother 54(11):4739–4743. doi:10.1128/AAC.01831-09

Chapter 3

Animal Models to Evaluate Anti-infective Pharmacodynamics

Alexander J. Lepak and David R. Andes

Abstract

Animal models in the PK/PD evaluation of antimicrobial therapy have proven to be a critical element in drug development and dosing refinement for numerous infectious diseases. There are several variables that are taken into consideration when animal models are utilized. These can include host-specific variables such as the animal species, route of infection, infection site, immune status, end organ/tissue sampling and optimal endpoint measure. Pathogen-specific variables include the genus/species, inoculum size, virulence, and drug susceptibility. Finally, therapeutic variables include route of drug administration, timing of therapy, dose level and frequency, metabolism and elimination, and duration of therapy. This list of variables may seem challenging; however, carefully controlled animal model studies are the cornerstone of PK/PD therapeutic evaluations that lead to dosing regimen optimization, limiting drug-related toxicity, guiding therapeutic drug monitoring, and setting of drug susceptibility breakpoints.

Key words In vivo, Animal, Pharmacodynamics, PK/PD

1 Pharmacokinetics in Animal Models

Pharmacokinetic (PK) measurements are necessary to ensure that an anti-infective agent will be present at sufficient concentrations and microbiologically active at a given site of infection in a mammalian host. PK, as it relates to pharmacodynamic (PD) studies, is primarily measured in terms of elimination half-life ($T_{1/2}$), area under the drug concentration curve (AUC), and maximal concentrations achieved (Cmax). The design of PK studies incorporates the number of animals necessary to achieve statistically reproducible PK measures and the number of time points necessary for optimal PK estimates. Many of these studies are performed in rodent models; however other mammals such as hamsters, rabbits, and guinea pigs are utilized. Drug concentration measurements are most commonly performed using HPLC or mass spectroscopy (i.e., LC/MS-MS) methods; however bioassays perform very well and are still utilized.

John C. Rotschafer et al. (eds.), *Antibiotic Pharmacodynamics*, Methods in Pharmacology and Toxicology,
DOI 10.1007/978-1-4939-3323-5_3, © Springer Science+Business Media New York 2016

1.1 Tissue Site

An important consideration in PK studies is which compartment or tissue site is relevant for drug concentration and PK parameter determination. Traditionally, bloodstream (i.e., whole blood, serum, or plasma) measurements of drug concentration have been utilized; however, there are situations in which tissue-specific or target-organ drug concentration measurement is necessary and potentially more informative. This is especially true for sites of infection that are considered sequestered (e.g., brain, CSF, urine, eye, placenta) or for pathogens that are primarily intracellular in nature. For example, many PK/PD investigations now include measurement of drug concentration in the epithelial lining fluid (ELF) compartment for drugs that are being considered for the treatment of pulmonary infections. The lack of efficacy of daptomycin in pulmonary infections, due to inactivation of drug by surfactant, is a prime example of the need to consider site-specific animal infection models and drug PK [1]. Additionally, penetration to sites of infection can be preferentially different leading to lower PD targets based on the specific site of infection. An example of this important finding is the revelation of PD targets that are approximately one-half in lung versus thigh infection models for an investigational oxazolidinone based on preferential penetration into ELF [2, 3].

An additional concern is in the processing of tissue samples for PK measurement. The most common method of processing tissue samples for drug concentration measurement is tissue homogenization [4, 5]. However, tissues have two distinct fluid components consisting of the interstitial and intracellular compartments. When homogenized, these two compartments are irrevocably mixed. Since the intracellular compartment is usually of larger volume, drugs that concentrate more in the interstitial compartment will appear to be much lower in total concentration than drugs that accumulate in the intracellular compartment (e.g., beta-lactams versus fluoroquinolones). More recently a technique to determine interstitial tissue-specific drug concentrations via microdialysis has been applied [6, 7].

1.2 Effect of Animal Species on Antibiotic Pharmacokinetics

The host animal species can have dramatic effects on the PK of a drug. Smaller mammals often exhibit more rapid metabolism and elimination, and therefore half-lives in these models can be considerably shorter than in larger mammals such as humans [8]. The route of administration can also affect drug PK in a host-specific manner, as demonstrated by rifampicin where the $t_{1/2}$ in rats was 4.7 h following intravenous administration, but increased to 9.3 h following oral administration [9]. Interestingly, this same increase in half-life was not evident in mice. Finally, even the strain of animal can affect the PK. For example, BALB/c mice and DBA/2 mice display markedly different serum drug concentrations of itraconazole over time [10].

1.3 Effect of Infection on Antibiotic Pharmacokinetics

The infection process can have a dramatic effect on the PK of a drug. Perhaps the most well-known scenario that has long been recognized to demonstrate this effect is bacterial meningitis, where bacterial and host inflammatory-induced damage to the blood–brain barrier produces profound changes in the penetration of antibiotics [11–13]. For example, vancomycin penetrates poorly through an intact blood–brain barrier due to the presence of intact tight junctions [12, 14]. However, significant damage occurs to these tight junctions during bacterial meningitis leading to increased permeability. In a study utilizing rabbits, there was a near-fourfold increase in CSF vancomycin levels in animals with meningitis versus healthy controls [12]. Sepsis can also impact drug pharmacokinetics via a variety of mechanisms including increased volume of distribution and organ dysfunction leading to altered metabolism and elimination [15–17]. The translatability of preclinical animal model PK to patients therefore usually includes both uninfected and infected animal PK to determine if the disease state significantly alters drug PK.

1.4 Effect of Animal Age

Age can have a profound effect on drug PK in many mammalian species. However, the clinical applicability of using age-related PK in an animal model and correlating it to age-related PK in a human is limited. For example, plasma PKs of five beta-lactam antibiotics are markedly different in neonatal versus adult mice [18]. However, there is no corollary study in humans (i.e., neonates) to determine if these differences are applicable. When differences do occur in the animal model, it can provide the stimulus to study the PK in the age groups the antibiotic is being developed for in humans. However, when age-related differences do not occur in the animal model, it does not necessarily indicate that there are no significant clinical differences in drug PK in different aged humans. With this caveat aside, there are examples of age-related changes in antimicrobial PK in animal models [19, 20]. In general, drug concentrations are higher in aged animals compared to young animals for a given dose. Differential rates of metabolism and elimination most likely account for these differences, which are often clinically relevant in humans as well. For example, aged rats (22–24 months) had higher concentrations (Cmax and AUC) and prolonged elimination rates ($T_{1/2}$) compared to young rats (2–3 months) [19].

1.5 Strategies to Mimic Human PK in Animal Models

The two most common strategies to attempt to mimic human PK in an animal model where there is rapid metabolism or clearance of the drug are to either directly alter the clearance/metabolism or provide a means of very rapid drug replenishment by frequent or continuous dosing systems. Impairment in renal clearance of a drug can result in slower elimination, which is relevant if this is the major clearance organ (e.g., cephalexin [21]). In mice, this has been accomplished by a single subcutaneous injection of uranyl nitrate (10 mg/kg) 3 days prior to animal infection [22]. Uranyl nitrate produces acute tubular necrosis and subsequent stable but decreased renal glomerulofiltration for a maximal duration of 7 days [23, 24]. For example, Craig and colleagues administered uranyl nitrate to mice receiving amikacin and demonstrated an increased half-life, peak concentration, and AUC for each dose when compared to non-renally impaired mice [24]. The resultant PK parameters and concentration-time curves more appropriately simulated human amikacin PK. Antimicrobial agents actively secreted by renal tubular cells can be competitively blocked by other compounds that utilize the same excretion process. An example of this is probenecid, a weak organic acid which blocks the secretion of penicillin and other cephalosporins [25]. A variety of renal impairment mechanisms have also been reported for rats [21]. This includes proximal tubular necrosis induced by cisplatin (one dose at 5 mg/kg IP), papillary necrosis induced by 2-bromoethylamine hydrobromide (one dose at 75 mg/kg IV), glomerulonephritis induced by sodium aurothiomalate (6 weekly injections of 0.05 mg/kg IV), and anti-rabbit antibodies to rat glomerular basement membrane (single IV injection).

Continuous dosing of antimicrobials has been utilized to counteract the effect of rapid antimicrobial clearance in small rodents. There are a number of systems that have been utilized including tissue cage infusion [26], infusion pumps [27–31], and more recently sophisticated computer programmable pumps [32]. These systems work best from an efficacy standpoint for time-dependent drugs in which the time above MIC is the driving pharmacodynamic index.

2 Host Susceptibility to Infection

2.1 Immune Suppression

Animal models of anti-infective therapy often utilize immune suppression. There are several reasons for this model design. First, an unconfounded evaluation of antimicrobial effect can be performed if the immune system is removed or significantly inhibited from affecting the outcome. Therefore, one will get a more robust drug-effect evaluation by removing confounders that will artificially enhance antimicrobial efficacy. Secondly, many animals are inherently resistant to microbes that are pathogens in humans and immune suppression is required to mimic disease in patients. The effects of immune suppression have been explored in a number of studies. As might be expected, in general there is a reduction in the amount of drug, and thus PK/PD target, necessary to achieve similar microbiological outcome (i.e., net stasis or 1-log kill) in non-neutropenic compared to neutropenic antibacterial models [33]. This reduction can be as much as two- to fourfold lower but appears to vary dependent upon the drug class and microorganism.

The influence of immune suppression has also been demonstrated for fungal infections, although with varied impact when one compares *Aspergillus* and *Candida*. For example, transiently neutropenic mice infected with *Aspergillus* had dramatically higher survival rates with treatment (amphotericin B or echinocandin) than would be expected based on clinical outcome in patients [34]. This discrepancy is likely linked to immune system recovery. This hypothesis was supported by use of the same animal model but producing persistent neutropenia over the study period [35]. In this experiment, persistent neutropenic animals treated with both compounds at the doses studied had 100 % mortality with only a differential effect noted based on the number of days the animals survived until death between the two drug groups. Therefore, immune suppression has a notable effect on antimicrobial efficacy in filamentous fungal models. Conversely, the effects of neutropenia appear to be less impactful in disseminated *Candida* infection models as similar PK/PD targets have been found in neutropenic and non-neutropenic animals [36, 37].

2.2 Effect of Age on Susceptibility to Infection

Host susceptibility and response to infection can change dramatically in very young or advanced age animal models, as in humans. It has been well established that very young (i.e., neonates) and elderly humans are more susceptible to certain infectious diseases, and this can often be attributed to differences in immune function at these age extremes. Neonatal animal models have been established to study common infectious diseases noted in this group including group B streptococcal infection [38, 39], staphylococcal infection including late-onset sepsis with CONs [40–43], and invasive candidiasis [43, 44]. Unfortunately, only a limited number of these studies have also included an evaluation of antimicrobial therapy. Conversely, aged animal models have focused primarily on specific immune function such as studying innate immune responses (e.g., cytokine response and neutrophil function) as well as adaptive immune responses (e.g., T- and B-cell-specific responses). Common infections noted in elderly humans have been modeled in aged animals including bacterial peritonitis, intra-abdominal abscess and sepsis via cecal ligation, invasive candidiasis, and *Clostridium difficile* [45–49]. Unfortunately, while susceptibility to infection has been examined in aged animal models, antimicrobial efficacy in these models is also limited.

3 Common Animal Infection Models for Antimicrobial PK/PD Study

3.1 Animal Models of Bacterial Thigh Infection (Selbie)

The rodent thigh lesion model was originally described by Selbie and Simon in 1952 [50] and continues to be the workhorse for animal model PK/PD antimicrobial efficacy studies. This model is commonly employed in the development of new antimicrobial agents and has been shown to be helpful for predicting efficacy for a number of human applications (e.g., skin and soft tissue infection, intra-abdominal infections, and septicemia). The model is also attractive as use of two thighs per animal (two biological replicates) limits the total needed for each experiment. Briefly, the model involves intramuscular injection of an inoculum into the dorsal thighs. Mice are then treated with an antimicrobial agent for a defined period, euthanized at study endpoint, and CFU enumerated from each thigh. In order to make the data most meaningful, zero hour control mice are optimal to determine the viable burden at the start of therapy. This allows one to determine whether infectious burden increased, decreased, or remained stable over time. Untreated controls are also necessary to assess fitness of each bacterial strain in the animal model. Most studies utilize a neutropenic mouse model. While CFU determination of pathogen abundance is most commonly performed, novel techniques such as fluorescent protein markers, serum biomarkers of infection, image scoring, quantitative PCR, and antigen/antibody testing have been developed for certain pathogens as a means to monitor infectious burden in animals.

3.2 Animal Models of Acute Bacterial Pneumonia

Murine models of acute pneumonia are increasingly incorporated into drug development and PK/PD studies for drugs intended for this infection site. The reliance upon these lung infection models has stemmed from the recognition of differential penetration of antimicrobials to the site of bronchopneumonia, the epithelial lining fluid, ELF. Many contemporary lung infection models have been described, including a recent thorough review of murine models to mimic human pneumonia [51]. The models include infection with common community pulmonary pathogens including *S. pneumoniae*, *H. influenzae*, *C. pneumoniae*, and *M. pneumoniae*. Important considerations in the models include host immune dysfunction, organism pathogenicity in mice, route of infection, inoculum size, experimental duration, and endpoint (e.g., mortality, organism burden). Similar to the thigh model, mice are commonly rendered neutropenic. For a few organisms, immune suppression alone is insufficient to yield highly reproducible results in biological replicates. One strategy to overcome this has been to utilize a chemical irritant (1 % formalin) just prior to inoculation [52]. Decreased fitness has also been noted in drug-resistant isolates where presumably the loss of fitness is secondary to genetic changes in the isolate [53]. Therefore, it is important at the outset to ensure that all organisms utilized have relatively similar degrees of pathogenesis in the animal model.

The route of infection for production of pneumonia includes aerosolization of the inoculum with subsequent inhalation, intranasal instillation with ensuing aspiration, injection into the trachea via percutaneous puncture with a fine needle, or direct instillation into the lungs by tracheal intubation. One advantage of aerosolized inoculation is the ability to infect large numbers of animals in a chamber at the same time with similar inoculum burden. For example, nebulization of 10^8 CFU/mL of *K. pneumoniae* via a Collison nebulizer for 45 min produces a similar degree of pneumonia in up to 100 mice at the same time [54]. Experiment duration can vary depending on pathogenicity of the infecting organism, but usually does not need to be prolonged more than 24–48 h for bacterial pathogens to produce death in untreated control mice. Finally, determination of organism burden is most commonly performed by quantitative culture techniques (CFU determination). The aforementioned pneumonia model techniques are now increasingly utilized for hospital/health care-acquired pneumonia. Representative examples include *Acinetobacter* [55–64], MRSA [3, 65–72], *Pseudomonas aeruginosa* [73–81], and *Klebsiella pneumoniae* [82–89]. Additionally, anthrax models have been developed in recent years given the continued threat of bioterrorism [90–97].

3.3 Animal Models of Chronic Bacterial Pneumonia

Chronic pneumonia usually occurs in the setting of preexisting lung conditions such as chronic obstructive pulmonary disease (COPD) and cystic fibrosis (CF). These lung diseases produce intermittent obstruction and variable loss of immune function with subsequent risk for chronic or recurrent infection. These preexisting conditions do not exist in rodents and bacteria commonly involved in these infections are rapidly cleared from the airways in rodents [98–100]. Therefore, strategies to mimic periodic obstruction and prevent bacterial clearance have been developed. To date the most common method used to achieve airway obstruction is the preparation of the bacterial inoculum in agarose or alginate beads [99, 101]. This method has been employed successfully to yield a persistent *P. aeruginosa* infection in rats for up to 35 days [99].

The pathogen of choice for most chronic pneumonia studies is *P. aeruginosa*. This is clinically applicable as it is not only the most common isolate found in colonization and infection in COPD and CF patients, but is also particularly difficult to treat and has high propensity of acquiring drug resistance. A representative example includes the guinea pig model of chronic *P. aeruginosa* pneumonia [102]. Infection was established using agar bead-encased bacteria and the compounds tested included ticarcillin (120 mg/kg), ciprofloxacin (10 mg/kg), and tobramycin (1.7 mg/kg). Ciprofloxacin was judged to be most efficacious, followed by tobramycin and ticarcillin, which was ineffective (based on CFU counts). Notably, no single-drug treatment was able to completely eradicate the infecting organism in this chronic model. Murine models have also been adapted to investigate the impact of antimicrobial therapy in chronic *P. aeruginosa* pneumonia [103–107]. For example, Macia and colleagues examined ciprofloxacin and tobramycin monotherapy and combination therapy in a murine model of chronic pneumonia using a reference strain and its hypermutable derivative [104]. After exposure to ciprofloxacin, infection with the hypermutable isolate of *P. aeruginosa* resulted in a rapid increase in drug-resistant subpopulations. This effect was not observed with tobramycin monotherapy. Finally, the combination of the two drugs appeared synergistic against the hypermutable isolate. Thus this study design appears useful for investigation of PK/PD dosing strategies to prevent the emergence of resistance. Inhalational drug administration is an additional area of investigation garnering more interest for chronic pneumonia [103, 108–112]. The advantage of this route of administration method is directly targeting antimicrobial therapy to the site of infection as well as limiting systemic toxicity that can be problematic for certain antimicrobial agents.

3.4 Animal Models of Fungal Infections

Fungal pathogens have the capability to cause localized infection (e.g., esophageal candidiasis or skin), pneumonia (pulmonary aspergillosis), disseminated infection (e.g., invasive candidiasis), or a combination of the two (e.g., invasive aspergillosis or cryptococcosis). Therefore, models have been developed to study site-specific infections as well as disseminated infection [113–116]. There are important differences from bacterial animal models that require additional consideration. Examples include the inoculum size and type of immune suppression. Many fungal pathogens require a high inoculum to produce disease, most commonly on the order of 7–9 $\log_{10}$. This very high inoculum though can lead to relatively small growth in end-organ burden prior to study endpoint or animal death (i.e., 1 $\log_{10}$ or less) [117]. Additionally, while many bacterial studies utilize a neutropenic host animal, it is almost universally employed for fungal studies. This is required as most fungal pathogens fail to establish an infection in specific sites (e.g., lung) in the animal host without significant immune suppression. This factor may be intuitive as it is well documented that immune suppression is often a necessary risk factor for human disease for many opportunistic fungal pathogens. A common additional step in immune suppression in pulmonary mold infection models is the utilization of high doses of corticosteroids [118–123]. An alternative strategy is to use a rodent model with specific immune deficiencies bread into their background [124, 125]. For example, SCID mice devoid of B- or T-cell immunity have been used for a mucosal candidiasis model to mimic infection in patients with HIV [125]. Additional host factor modifications have also been incorporated to mimic human disease. For example, a murine model of diabetic ketoacidosis, a major risk factor for disseminated and cerebral zygomycosis, has been successfully described and utilized to examine antifungal therapy in this setting [126, 127].

Use of animal models for investigation for antifungal therapy is most common for *Candida* species, and includes oropharyngeal and esophageal candidiasis [128, 129], vaginitis [130], and invasive candidiasis [10, 36, 37, 115, 119, 131–169]. Disseminated infection induced via tail vein injection of the inoculum is the most commonly utilized model. Quantitation of infectious burden at the end of therapy is assessed in tissue homogenate, frequently the kidneys. Additionally, fungal burdens and treatment effect noted in the kidneys of mice have correlated very closely with other, more difficult-to-sample tissue compartments such as the brain [170]. In a neutropenic murine model of invasive candidiasis, an inoculum of 6–7 $\log_{10}$ *C. albicans* will progress to death in 24–72 h in untreated animals [37]. However, study of organism growth or decline over longer treatment periods can be accomplished utilizing a lower starting inoculum [138]. For other *Candida* spp. (such as *C. glabrata*), severe infection is more difficult to establish, and it often does not result in appreciable animal mortality [133, 134, 144, 171].

A well-recognized clinical complication of invasive candidiasis is dissemination to the eye with subsequent endophthalmitis. Animal models examining drug therapeutic efficacy in animal models of endophthalmitis have also been developed [172–180]. These models have provided important guidance on therapeutic options for this relatively pharmacologically protected body site. Models mimicking human fungal keratitis have also been described [181–192].

Filamentous fungal pathogen models (most commonly *Aspergillus*) have also undergone significant experimental refinement over the past decade. Many of these pathogens are acquired via the respiratory tract and therefore pulmonary inoculation models with dissemination most closely mimic human disease [123]. However, disseminated models via intravenous injection of the organism inoculum have also been utilized [193]. These models often employ significant immune suppression in the form of a combination of chemotherapy-induced neutropenia and corticosteroid treatment. Durations of 7 days or longer are often utilized as in general, despite the immunosuppression, filamentous fungi require longer incubation periods to grow to significant levels and/or disseminate via a pulmonary infection route. One challenge of filamentous fungal PK/PD investigation has been reproducible quantitation of organism burden. Filamentous fungi do not grow in discrete colonies on an agar plate as do bacteria and yeast. Additionally, concern has been raised that homogenization can fracture a filament into multiple pieces leading to overestimation of organism burden. Current molecular assessments of organism burden have largely alleviated this limitation. The most common surrogate methods of organism burden include galactomannan measurement [122] or real-time quantitative PCR (qPCR) [121, 194, 195]. For example, a recent study evaluated the utility of qPCR to assess disease progression, treatment outcome, and animal mortality in a 7-day study of invasive pulmonary aspergillosis (IPA) in a murine model [121]. The study found a strong relationship between qPCR result and treatment efficacy. For every 1-log increased growth of organism based on qPCR, a 17 % increase in mortality was observed. Additionally, the increase in survival was most profound at the dose exposure that was associated with net stasis (static dose) of organism burden. Thus, stasis or net cidal drug activity based on qPCR was a very strong predictor of clinical survival in this model. Other measures of organism viability and abundance have also been utilized such as XTT, DiBAC staining, chitin measurement, histopathology grading, lung weights, pulmonary infarct scoring, and galactomannan measurement [196, 197]. These types of models have also been recently expanded to examine less common filamentous fungal pathogens including *Zygomycetes* [126, 198–201].

Models mimicking fungal meningitis for pathogens that commonly cause primary CNS infection, or have a high likelihood of dissemination to the CNS, have been developed for a number of pathogens (e.g., *Cryptococcus*, *Aspergillus*, and dimorphic pathogens *Blastomyces*, *Histoplasma*, and *Coccidioides*). Infection is induced by either intravenous or intracisternal injection of a defined inoculum and organism burden is quantified in the cerebrospinal fluid and brain parenchyma as a measure of outcome. One of the more common pathogens examined in these animal is *Cryptococcus* sp. [202–211], including the emerging species *Cryptococcus gattii* [208]. Animal models of CNS aspergillosis, many developed and perfected by Clemons and Stevens, have been described and utilized with success to determine therapeutic efficacy of various antifungal agents [212–219]. Additionally, CNS models of invasive candidiasis have been developed to better understand treatment strategies for this rare pediatric complication [44, 220, 221]. Dimorphic fungal pathogens are often acquired via the pulmonary route but can disseminate to involve the CNS. A number of animal model investigations have examined antifungal therapy in animal models of CNS coccidioidomycosis and other dimorphic fungi [222]. Finally, animal models of CNS phaeohyphomycosis have been described for this rare but severe infectious entity [223–225]. PK/PD studies using animal models are very limited though for animal models examining CNS fungal infections.

The efficacy of agents directed at dermatophytes has been evaluated in animal models with cutaneous infection [226–230]. Most commonly, the site of infection (skin, foot pad, or nail) is mechanically abraded prior to topical inoculation to predispose the tissue to infection. The infection often takes several days or weeks to establish and therefore initiation of systemic or local topical therapy is delayed. After therapy, which may also require a prolonged period of time, tissue samples are cultured and examined by histopathology to determine drug efficacy. Rare fungal infections that can occur in patients with severe or prolonged immunosuppression have also been studied to a limited extent. Some examples include blastoschizomycosis [231–233], fusariosis [234–237], scedosporiosis [238–240], and trichosporonosis [241, 242]. PK/PD evaluation in these models is in general lacking.

3.5 Animal Models of Sexually Transmitted Infections

Animal models of human sexually transmitted infections (STIs) can be problematic owing to the high-level specificity many of the STI pathogens display for a human host. Despite this, a number of models (in some cases utilizing a different infecting species that is specific for the urogenital tract of the animal) have been successfully developed. Unfortunately, robust PK/PD studies do not exist in STI models. However, the continued epidemiological burden of STIs throughout the world and increasing rates of drug resistance (i.e., *Neisseria gonorrhea*) make PK/PD study an important area for future investigation.

Mice were traditionally considered resistant to disseminated gonococcal infection [243] despite some early successful studies [244]. A recent advance in the field is the successful development of a reproducible murine model [245, 246]. Mice are made susceptible to colonization and infection with *N. gonorrhea* via the combination of pretreatment with antibiotics (e.g., vancomycin and TMP-sulfa) and estradiol [245, 247]. The model has also been used recently to examine the effects of fluoroquinolone resistance mutation development and associated compensatory mutations to restore wild-type fitness [248].

Animal models examining antimicrobial efficacy in syphilis have been developed for localized disease (i.e., dermal), genitourinary tract disease, CNS/disseminated disease, and congenital disease. Most models utilize rabbits as the animal host; however a model in the hamster has also been well described [249]. Localized infection is induced by intradermal injection of live spirochetes. Antimicrobial therapy is usually withheld until signs of an active syphilitic lesion are present and confirmed by dark-field microscopic analysis of a skin scraping. Once active infection is confirmed, antimicrobial therapy is administered. Representative examples of the use of this protocol to show antimicrobial efficacy for localized disease include penicillin g [250], aztreonam [251], cefetamet [252], cefmetazole [253], an investigational penem [250], ceftriaxone [254], and azithromycin [255]. A hamster model of intradermal infection demonstrating efficacy of clarithromycin has also been described [256]. Genitourinary tract disease models have primarily been limited to orchitis infection models. In this model, animals receive an inoculum of syphilis spirochetes directly into the testes. It has been utilized on a limited basis to determine drug efficacy, with encouraging results from a study of ceftriaxone, ceftizoxime, and penicillin g [257, 258]. Central nervous system infection with syphilis can be achieved by direct intracisternal injection of *T. pallidum*. Marra and colleagues utilized this procedure to develop a rabbit model of CNS syphilis that very closely mimicked human disease including a 6 % rate of uveitis in the animal model [259]. A year later the same group demonstrated potentially improved results for penicillin g versus ceftriaxone in the rabbit model, although it lacked power to definitively show a statistical difference between the two drugs [260]. Finally, congenital syphilis has been described in a rabbit and hamster model [261–263]; however, antimicrobial therapy in congenital syphilis models has not been well explored.

Chlamydia trachomatis is a major cause of STI worldwide and remains the most common STI in the USA. Attempts at developing an animal model have, however, proven challenging [264]. Reproducible establishment of infection of the upper genital tract in female mice with human isolates of *C. trachomatis* requires hormonal manipulation, inbred animals, and surgical intervention to place the organisms directly into the site (i.e., salpingitis) [265]. However, in 1994 Beale and Upshon developed a novel upper genital tract infection model in mice [265]. They utilized *C. trachomatis* MoPN (primarily a mouse respiratory pathogen) and were able to demonstrate upper genital track disease in progesterone-treated mice administered the inoculum by intravaginal injection. Additionally, minocycline, doxycycline, amoxicillin-clavulanate, and azithromycin were all effective when initiated 1 or 7 days post-infection. Both doxycycline and azithromycin were highly effective in restoring animal fertility. A study of azithromycin efficacy in female mice demonstrated that the antimicrobial agent could reverse chlamydial-induced damage and restore fertility if administered within 2 or 7 days of infection [266]. Conversely, if administered 12 or more days after infection, even at very high doses, it failed to prevent infertility. A male murine model of genital tract disease caused by *C. trachomatis* MoPN has also been described [267] that similarly mimics disease in human males. However, evaluation of antimicrobial therapy in this model has not been performed. Another strategy to circumvent problems with establishing genital tract disease with human isolates of *C. trachomatis* is to utilize a species that does cause intrinsic genital tract infection in the animal host. This has been accomplished using the isolate *C. muridarum* to infect the urogenital tract of mice [268–273] and *C. caviae* in guinea pigs [274–276].

3.6 Animal Models of Urinary Tract Infections

Models of urinary tract infections (UTI) are commonly used to assess antimicrobial efficacy given it is one of the most common infectious diseases of humans. Rodents (i.e., mice and rats) are the most common animal model utilized and there are few important factors one needs to consider. First, not all bacteria are inherently pathogenic in the rodent urinary system and therefore in some studies manipulation (i.e., obstruction or direct instillation into renal parenchyma) is necessary. Secondly, vesicoureteral reflux is a naturally occurring phenomenon in rodents due to the lack of ureterovesical valves [277]. In its simplest form, UTI can be induced in rodents by instillation of normally pathogenic microorganisms, such as *E. coli*, into the bladder by urethral catheterization and clamping the catheter or urethra for a short period of time to prevent immediate inoculation expulsion and promote infection [278–281]. As long as the bacterial strain has necessary virulence factors (i.e., type 1 or type P fimbriae), a UTI with high bacterial counts in the bladder and kidney will ensue over a period of 1–8 days. This model has been successfully employed to study antimicrobial efficacy and PK/PD relationships of antimicrobial therapy [279, 282–284]. Urinary obstruction models provide a framework to study pyelonephritis and UTI with organisms that are not intrinsically pathogenic to the rodent urinary system [285, 286]. This model is more technically demanding as it usually requires animal surgery to directly inoculate the bladder with the pathogen and then ligate one ureter to cause an obstructed infection. Antimicrobial therapy has also been examined using this model although given the complexity there is less robust pharmacodynamic analyses than the unobstructed model [287–289]. Direct instillation of organism into the parenchyma (i.e., poles) of one or both kidneys has also been demonstrated as a means to study antimicrobial efficacy in the urinary system but is also technically demanding [290–292]. A final mechanism that has been utilized is hematogenous seeding of the urinary system to produce UTI [293, 294]. This model has been particularly useful to examine antimicrobial therapy for other common bacterial pathogens of the urinary system including *Enterococcus*, *Staphylococcus*, and *Klebsiella* [295–298].

3.7 Animal Models of Infectious Endocarditis

Animal models of endocarditis have been utilized for decades to examine optimal antimicrobial therapy for this common life-threatening infection. Additionally, they are perhaps the area of animal model evaluation that has garnered the most translatable clinical applicability [299–305]. The most common animal species utilized are rabbits, although rodent models have also been developed. The infection model itself usually consists of canalization of the right carotid artery with a polyethylene intravenous catheter and advancing it across the aortic valve. This results in the development of sterile vegetations on the aortic valve which can then be colonized/infected with a bacterial inoculum through the catheter. This model remains a very important tool in optimizing antimicrobial therapy for endocarditis, especially combination therapy with aminoglycosides and novel combinations for aminoglycoside-resistant Enterococcal endocarditis and methicillin-resistant *Staphylococcus aureus* endocarditis [306–315].

3.8 Animal Models of Intraperitoneal Infection

Peritoneal infections can be produced by one of the two mechanisms: direct inoculation of organism into the peritoneal cavity or cecal perforation as the result of ligation and puncture (CLP). The former mechanism was initially performed by surgically placing a gelatin-incased inoculum into the peritoneal cavity [316–318]. However, more recently this has been simplified by direct inoculation of the inoculum by syringe into the peritoneal cavity to produce an infectious peritonitis [317–326]. To enhance pathogenicity talcum (magnesium hydropolysilicate) is often utilized in inoculum preparation and serves as a foreign body irritant to promote infection while having no effect on antimicrobial therapy. The CLP model is another surgical technique to mimic secondary bacterial peritonitis [327, 328]. In this model, the animal is anesthetized and the abdominal cavity is aseptically entered whereby the cecum is identified, ligated, and perforated with a needle before closing the abdomen.

References

1. Silverman JA, Mortin LI, Vanpraagh AD, Li T, Alder J (2005) Inhibition of daptomycin by pulmonary surfactant: in vitro modeling and clinical impact. J Infect Dis 191:2149–2152
2. Louie A, Liu W, Kulawy R, Drusano GL (2011) In vivo pharmacodynamics of torezolid phosphate (TR-701), a new oxazolidinone antibiotic, against methicillin-susceptible and methicillin-resistant Staphylococcus aureus strains in a mouse thigh infection model. Antimicrob Agents Chemother 55:3453–3460
3. Lepak AJ, Marchillo K, Pichereau S, Craig WA, Andes DR (2012) Comparative pharmacodynamics of the new oxazolidinone tedizolid phosphate and linezolid in a neutropenic murine Staphylococcus aureus pneumonia model. Antimicrob Agents Chemother 56:5916–5922
4. Mouton JW, Theuretzbacher U, Craig WA, Tulkens PM, Derendorf H, Cars O (2008) Tissue concentrations: do we ever learn? J Antimicrob Chemother 61:235–237
5. Redington J, Ebert SC, Craig WA (1991) Role of antimicrobial pharmacokinetics and pharmacodynamics in surgical prophylaxis. Rev Infect Dis 13(Suppl 10):S790–799
6. Liu P, Muller M, Derendorf H (2002) Rational dosing of antibiotics: the use of plasma concentrations versus tissue concentrations. Int J Antimicrob Agents 19:285–290
7. Brunner M, Derendorf H, Muller M (2005) Microdialysis for in vivo pharmacokinetic/pharmacodynamic characterization of anti-infective drugs. Curr Opin Pharmacol 5:495–499
8. Andes D, Craig WA (2002) Animal model pharmacokinetics and pharmacodynamics: a critical review. Int J Antimicrob Agents 19:261–268
9. Bruzzese T, Rimaroli C, Bonabello A, Mozzi G, Ajay S, Cooverj ND (2000) Pharmacokinetics and tissue distribution of rifametane, a new 3-azinomethyl-rifamycin derivative, in several animal species. Arzneimittelforschung 50: 60–71
10. MacCallum DM, Odds FC (2002) Influence of grapefruit juice on itraconazole plasma levels in mice and guinea pigs. J Antimicrob Chemother 50:219–224
11. Andes DR, Craig WA (1999) Pharmacokinetics and pharmacodynamics of antibiotics in meningitis. Infect Dis Clin N Am 13:595–618
12. Krontz DP, Strausbaugh LJ (1980) Effect of meningitis and probenecid on the penetration of vancomycin into cerebrospinal fluid in rabbits. Antimicrob Agents Chemother 18:882–886
13. Scheld WM (1989) Drug delivery to the central nervous system: general principles and relevance to therapy for infections of the central nervous system. Rev Infect Dis 11(Suppl 7):S1669–1690
14. Levy RM, Gutin PH, Baskin DS, Pons VG (1986) Vancomycin penetration of a brain abscess: case report and review of the literature. Neurosurgery 18:632–636
15. Ngeleka M, Auclair P, Tardif D, Beauchamp D, Bergeron MG (1989) Intrarenal distribution of vancomycin in endotoxemic rats. Antimicrob Agents Chemother 33: 1575–1579

16. Ganzinger U, Haslberger A (1985) Pharmacokinetics of cephalosporins in normal and septicemic rabbits. Antimicrob Agents Chemother 28:473–477
17. Mimoz O, Jacolot A, Padoin C, Quillard J, Tod M, Louchahi K, Samii K, Petitjean O (1996) Influence of experimental rat model of multiple organ dysfunction on cefepime and amikacin pharmacokinetics. Antimicrob Agents Chemother 40:819–821
18. Morita E, Mizuno N, Nishikata M, Miyake K (1990) Comparison of the pharmacokinetics of five beta-lactam antibiotics between neonatal and adult rats. Dev Pharmacol Ther 14:223–230
19. Tanira MO, Ali BH, Bashir AK (1997) Effect of endotoxin on gentamicin pharmacokinetics in old and young adult rats. Life Sci 60:413–424
20. Thadepalli H, Chuah SK, Reddy U, Hanna N, Clark R, Polzer RJ, Gollapudi S (1997) Efficacy of trovafloxacin for treatment of experimental Bacteroides infection in young and senescent mice. Antimicrob Agents Chemother 41:1933–1936
21. Maiza A, Daley-Yates PT (1993) Variability in the renal clearance of cephalexin in experimental renal failure. J Pharmacokinet Biopharm 21:19–30
22. Giacomini KM, Roberts SM, Levy G (1981) Evaluation of methods for producing renal dysfunction in rats. J Pharm Sci 70:117–121
23. Andes D, Craig WA (1998) In vivo activities of amoxicillin and amoxicillin-clavulanate against *Streptococcus pneumoniae*: application to breakpoint determinations. Antimicrob Agents Chemother 42:2375–2379
24. Craig WA, Redington J, Ebert SC (1991) Pharmacodynamics of amikacin in vitro and in mouse thigh and lung infections. J Antimicrob Chemother 27(Suppl C):29–40
25. Nierenberg DW (1987) Drug inhibition of penicillin tubular secretion: concordance between in vitro and clinical findings. J Pharmacol Exp Ther 240:712–716
26. Thonus I, de Lange-Macdaniel A, Otte C, Michel M (1979) Tissue cage infusion: a technique for the achievement of prolonged steady state in experimental animals. J Pharmacol Methods 2:63–69
27. Astry CL, Nelson S, Karam GH, Summer WR (1987) Interactions of clindamycin with antibacterial defenses of the lung. Am Rev Respir Dis 135:1015–1019
28. Naziri W, Cheadle WG, Trachtenberg LS, Montgomery WD, Polk HC Jr (1995) Second place winner of the Conrad Jobst Award in the gold medal paper competition. Increased antibiotic effectiveness in a model of surgical infection through continuous infusion. Am Surg 61:11–15
29. Thauvin C, Eliopoulos GM, Willey S, Wennersten C, Moellering RC Jr (1987) Continuous-infusion ampicillin therapy of enterococcal endocarditis in rats. Antimicrob Agents Chemother 31:139–143
30. Tran Ba Huy P, Meulemans A, Wassef M, Manuel C, Sterkers O, Amiel C (1983) Gentamicin persistence in rat endolymph and perilymph after a two-day constant infusion. Antimicrob Agents Chemother 23:344–346
31. Roosendaal R, Bakker-Woudenberg IA, van den Berghe-van Raffe M, Vink-van den Berg JC, Michel BM (1989) Impact of the dosage schedule on the efficacy of ceftazidime, gentamicin and ciprofloxacin in Klebsiella pneumoniae pneumonia and septicemia in leukopenic rats. Eur J Clin Microbiol Infect Dis 8:878–887
32. Robaux MA, Dube L, Caillon J, Bugnon D, Kergueris MF, Navas D, Le Conte P, Baron D, Potel G (2001) In vivo efficacy of continuous infusion versus intermittent dosing of ceftazidime alone or in combination with amikacin relative to human kinetic profiles in a *Pseudomonas aeruginosa* rabbit endocarditis model. J Antimicrob Chemother 47:617–622
33. Craig WA, Andes DR, Stamstad T (2010) In vivo pharmacodynamics of new lipopeptide MX-2401. Antimicrob Agents Chemother 54:5092–5098
34. Verweij PE, Oakley KL, Morrissey J, Morrissey G, Denning DW (1998) Efficacy of LY303366 against amphotericin B-susceptible and -resistant Aspergillus fumigatus in a murine model of invasive aspergillosis. Antimicrob Agents Chemother 42:873–878
35. Petraitis V, Petraitiene R, Groll AH, Bell A, Callender DP, Sein T, Schaufele RL, McMillian CL, Bacher J, Walsh TJ (1998) Antifungal efficacy, safety, and single-dose pharmacokinetics of LY303366, a novel echinocandin B, in experimental pulmonary aspergillosis in persistently neutropenic rabbits. Antimicrob Agents Chemother 42:2898–2905
36. Louie A, Drusano GL, Banerjee P, Liu QF, Liu W, Kaw P, Shayegani M, Taber H, Miller MH (1998) Pharmacodynamics of fluconazole in a murine model of systemic candidiasis. Antimicrob Agents Chemother 42:1105–1109
37. Andes D, van Ogtrop M (1999) Characterization and quantitation of the pharmacodynamics of fluconazole in a neutropenic murine disseminated candidiasis infection model. Antimicrob Agents Chemother 43:2116–2120

38. Madoff LC, Michel JL, Gong EW, Rodewald AK, Kasper DL (1992) Protection of neonatal mice from group B streptococcal infection by maternal immunization with beta C protein. Infect Immun 60:4989–4994
39. Rodewald AK, Onderdonk AB, Warren HB, Kasper DL (1992) Neonatal mouse model of group B streptococcal infection. J Infect Dis 166:635–639
40. Kronforst KD, Mancuso CJ, Pettengill M, Ninkovic J, Power Coombs MR, Stevens C, Otto M, Mallard C, Wang X, Goldmann D, Levy O (2012) A neonatal model of intravenous Staphylococcus epidermidis infection in mice <24 h old enables characterization of early innate immune responses. PLoS One 7:e43897
41. Oluola O, Kong L, Fein M, Weisman LE (2007) Lysostaphin in treatment of neonatal *Staphylococcus aureus* infection. Antimicrob Agents Chemother 51:2198–2200
42. Placencia FX, Kong L, Weisman LE (2009) Treatment of methicillin-resistant *Staphylococcus aureus* in neonatal mice: lysostaphin versus vancomycin. Pediatr Res 65:420–424
43. Venkatesh MP, Pham D, Fein M, Kong L, Weisman LE (2007) Neonatal coinfection model of coagulase-negative Staphylococcus (Staphylococcus epidermidis) and Candida albicans: fluconazole prophylaxis enhances survival and growth. Antimicrob Agents Chemother 51:1240–1245
44. Flattery AM, Hickey E, Gill CJ, Powles MA, Misura AS, Galgoci AM, Ellis JD, Zhang R, Sandhu P, Ronan J, Abruzzo GK (2011) Efficacy of caspofungin in a juvenile mouse model of central nervous system candidiasis. Antimicrob Agents Chemother 55:3491–3497
45. Ashman RB, Papadimitriou JM, Fulurija A (1999) Acute susceptibility of aged mice to infection with Candida albicans. J Med Microbiol 48:1095–1102
46. Hyde SR, Stith RD, McCallum RE (1990) Mortality and bacteriology of sepsis following cecal ligation and puncture in aged mice. Infect Immun 58:619–624
47. Murciano C, Villamon E, Yanez A, O'Connor JE, Gozalbo D, Gil ML (2006) Impaired immune response to *Candida albicans* in aged mice. J Med Microbiol 55:1649–1656
48. Pawlowski SW, Calabrese G, Kolling GL, Platts-Mills J, Freire R, AlcantaraWarren C, Liu B, Sartor RB, Guerrant RL (2010) Murine model of Clostridium difficile infection with aged gnotobiotic C57BL/6 mice and a BI/NAP1 strain. J Infect Dis 202:1708–1712
49. Turnbull IR, Wlzorek JJ, Osborne D, Hotchkiss RS, Coopersmith CM, Buchman TG (2003) Effects of age on mortality and antibiotic efficacy in cecal ligation and puncture. Shock 19:310–313
50. Selbie FR, Simon RD (1952) Virulence to mice of Staphylococcus pyogenes: its measurement and its relation to certain in vitro properties. Br J Exp Pathol 33:315–326
51. Mizgerd JP, Skerrett SJ (2008) Animal models of human pneumonia. Am J Physiol Lung Cell Mol Physiol 294:L387–398
52. Miyazaki S, Nunoya T, Matsumoto T, Tateda K, Yamaguchi K (1997) New murine model of bronchopneumonia due to cell-bound Haemophilus influenzae. J Infect Dis 175: 205–209
53. Fukuoka T, Kawada H, Kitayama A, Koga T, Kubota M, Harasaki T, Kamai Y, Ohya S, Yasuda H, Iwata M, Kuwahara S (1998) Efficacy of CS-834 against experimental pneumonia caused by penicillin-susceptible and -resistant Streptococcus pneumoniae in mice. Antimicrob Agents Chemother 42:23–27
54. Leggett J (1999) Murine models of pneumonia using aerosol infection. Academic, San Diego
55. Mutlu Yilmaz E, Sunbul M, Aksoy A, Yilmaz H, Guney AK, Guvenc T (2012) Efficacy of tigecycline/colistin combination in a pneumonia model caused by extensively drug-resistant *Acinetobacter baumannii*. Int J Antimicrob Agents 40:332–336
56. Song JY, Cheong HJ, Lee J, Sung AK, Kim WJ (2009) Efficacy of monotherapy and combined antibiotic therapy for carbapenem-resistant *Acinetobacter baumannii* pneumonia in an immunosuppressed mouse model. Int J Antimicrob Agents 33:33–39
57. Dudhani RV, Turnidge JD, Nation RL, Li J (2010) fAUC/MIC is the most predictive pharmacokinetic/pharmacodynamic index of colistin against *Acinetobacter baumannii* in murine thigh and lung infection models. J Antimicrob Chemother 65:1984–1990
58. Harris G, Kuo Lee R, Lam CK, Kanzaki G, Patel GB, Xu HH, Chen W (2013) A Mouse model of *Acinetobacter baumannii*-associated pneumonia using a clinically isolated hypervirulent strain. Antimicrob Agents Chemother 57:3601–3613
59. Koomanachai P, Kim A, Nicolau DP (2009) Pharmacodynamic evaluation of tigecycline against *Acinetobacter baumannii* in a murine pneumonia model. J Antimicrob Chemother 63:982–987

60. Pachon-Ibanez ME, Docobo-Perez F, Jimenez-Mejias ME, Ibanez-Martinez J, Garcia-Curiel A, Pichardo C, Pachon J (2011) Efficacy of rifampin, in monotherapy and in combinations, in an experimental murine pneumonia model caused by panresistant *Acinetobacter baumannii* strains. Eur J Clin Microbiol Infect Dis 30:895–901
61. Pachon-Ibanez ME, Docobo-Perez F, Lopez-Rojas R, Dominguez-Herrera J, Jimenez-Mejias ME, Garcia-Curiel A, Pichardo C, Jimenez L, Pachon J (2010) Efficacy of rifampin and its combinations with imipenem, sulbactam, and colistin in experimental models of infection caused by imipenem-resistant *Acinetobacter baumannii*. Antimicrob Agents Chemother 54:1165–1172
62. Pichardo C, Pachon-Ibanez ME, Docobo-Perez F, Lopez-Rojas R, Jimenez-Mejias ME, Garcia-Curiel A, Pachon J (2010) Efficacy of tigecycline vs. imipenem in the treatment of experimental *Acinetobacter baumannii* murine pneumonia. Eur J Clin Microbiol Infect Dis 29:527–531
63. Tang HJ, Chuang YC, Ko WC, Chen CC, Shieh JM, Chen CH, Lee NY, Chiang SR (2012) Comparative evaluation of intratracheal colistimethate sodium, imipenem, and meropenem in BALB/c mice with carbapenem-resistant *Acinetobacter baumannii* pneumonia. Int J Infect Dis 16:e34–40
64. Yuan Z, Ledesma KR, Singh R, Hou J, Prince RA, Tam VH (2010) Quantitative assessment of combination antimicrobial therapy against multidrug-resistant bacteria in a murine pneumonia model. J Infect Dis 201:889–897
65. Bhalodi AA, Crandon JL, Biek D, Nicolau DP (2012) Efficacy of ceftaroline fosamil in a staphylococcal murine pneumonia model. Antimicrob Agents Chemother 56:6160–6165
66. Crandon JL, Kuti JL, Nicolau DP (2010) Comparative efficacies of human simulated exposures of telavancin and vancomycin against methicillin-resistant *Staphylococcus aureus* with a range of vancomycin MICs in a murine pneumonia model. Antimicrob Agents Chemother 54:5115–5119
67. Docobo-Perez F, Lopez-Rojas R, Dominguez-Herrera J, Jimenez-Mejias ME, Pichardo C, Ibanez-Martinez J, Pachon J (2012) Efficacy of linezolid versus a pharmacodynamically optimized vancomycin therapy in an experimental pneumonia model caused by methicillin-resistant *Staphylococcus aureus*. J Antimicrob Chemother 67:1961–1967
68. Karau MJ, Tilahun AY, Schmidt SM, Clark CR, Patel R, Rajagopalan G (2012) Linezolid is superior to vancomycin in experimental pneumonia caused by superantigen-producing *Staphylococcus aureus* in HLA class II transgenic mice. Antimicrob Agents Chemother 56:5401–5405
69. Koomanachai P, Crandon JL, Banevicius MA, Peng L, Nicolau DP (2009) Pharmacodynamic profile of tigecycline against methicillin-resistant *Staphylococcus aureus* in an experimental pneumonia model. Antimicrob Agents Chemother 53:5060–5063
70. Laohavaleeson S, Tessier PR, Nicolau DP (2008) Pharmacodynamic characterization of ceftobiprole in experimental pneumonia caused by phenotypically diverse *Staphylococcus aureus* strains. Antimicrob Agents Chemother 52: 2389–2394
71. Reyes N, Skinner R, Kaniga K, Krause KM, Shelton J, Obedencio GP, Gough A, Conner M, Hegde SS (2005) Efficacy of telavancin (TD-6424), a rapidly bactericidal lipoglycopeptide with multiple mechanisms of action, in a murine model of pneumonia induced by methicillin-resistant *Staphylococcus aureus*. Antimicrob Agents Chemother 49:4344–4346
72. Tessier PR, Keel RA, Hagihara M, Crandon JL, Nicolau DP (2012) Comparative in vivo efficacies of epithelial lining fluid exposures of tedizolid, linezolid, and vancomycin for methicillin-resistant *Staphylococcus aureus* in a mouse pneumonia model. Antimicrob Agents Chemother 56:2342–2346
73. Aoki N, Tateda K, Kikuchi Y, Kimura S, Miyazaki C, Ishii Y, Tanabe Y, Gejyo F, Yamaguchi K (2009) Efficacy of colistin combination therapy in a mouse model of pneumonia caused by multidrug-resistant *Pseudomonas aeruginosa*. J Antimicrob Chemother 63: 534–542
74. Bretonniere C, Jacqueline C, Caillon J, Guitton C, Le Mabecque V, Miegeville AF, Villers D, Potel G, Boutoille D (2010) Efficacy of doripenem in the treatment of *Pseudomonas aeruginosa* experimental pneumonia versus imipenem and meropenem. J Antimicrob Chemother 65:2423–2427
75. Crandon JL, Nicolau DP (2013) Human simulated studies of aztreonam and aztreonam-avibactam to evaluate activity against challenging gram-negative organisms, including metallo-beta-lactamase producers. Antimicrob Agents Chemother 57:3299–3306
76. Crandon JL, Schuck VJ, Banevicius MA, Beaudoin ME, Nichols WW, Tanudra MA, Nicolau DP (2012) Comparative in vitro and in vivo efficacies of human simulated doses of ceftazidime and ceftazidime-avibactam against *Pseudomonas aeruginosa*. Antimicrob Agents Chemother 56:6137–6146

77. Hagihara M, Crandon JL, Urban CM, Nicolau DP (2013) KPC presence in *Pseudomonas aeruginosa* has minimal impact on the in vivo efficacy of carbapenem therapy. Antimicrob Agents Chemother 57:1086–1088
78. Jacqueline C, Roquilly A, Desessard C, Boutoille D, Broquet A, Le Mabecque V, Amador G, Potel G, Caillon J, Asehnoune K (2013) Efficacy of ceftolozane in a murine model of *Pseudomonas aeruginosa* acute pneumonia: in vivo antimicrobial activity and impact on host inflammatory response. J Antimicrob Chemother 68:177–183
79. Louie A, Fregeau C, Liu W, Kulawy R, Drusano GL (2009) Pharmacodynamics of levofloxacin in a murine pneumonia model of *Pseudomonas aeruginosa* infection: determination of epithelial lining fluid targets. Antimicrob Agents Chemother 53:3325–3330
80. Morinaga Y, Yanagihara K, Nakamura S, Yamamoto K, Izumikawa K, Seki M, Kakeya H, Yamamoto Y, Yamada Y, Kohno S, Kamihira S (2008) In vivo efficacy and pharmacokinetics of tomopenem (CS-023), a novel carbapenem, against *Pseudomonas aeruginosa* in a murine chronic respiratory tract infection model. J Antimicrob Chemother 62:1326–1331
81. Sabet M, Miller CE, Nolan TG, Senekeo-Effenberger K, Dudley MN, Griffith DC (2009) Efficacy of aerosol MP-376, a levofloxacin inhalation solution, in models of mouse lung infection due to *Pseudomonas aeruginosa*. Antimicrob Agents Chemother 53:3923–3928
82. Bakker-Woudenberg IA, ten Kate MT, Goessens WH, Mouton JW (2006) Effect of treatment duration on pharmacokinetic/pharmacodynamic indices correlating with therapeutic efficacy of ceftazidime in experimental *Klebsiella pneumoniae* lung infection. Antimicrob Agents Chemother 50:2919–2925
83. Docobo-Perez F, Nordmann P, Dominguez-Herrera J, Lopez-Rojas R, Smani Y, Poirel L, Pachon J (2012) Efficacies of colistin and tigecycline in mice with experimental pneumonia due to NDM-1-producing strains of *Klebsiella pneumoniae* and *Escherichia coli*. Int J Antimicrob Agents 39:251–254
84. Goessens WH, Mouton JW, Ten Kate MT, Sorgel F, Kinzig M, Bakker-Woudenberg IA (2013) The therapeutic effect of tigecycline, unlike that of Ceftazidime, is not influenced by whether the *Klebsiella pneumoniae* strain produces extended-spectrum beta-lactamases in experimental pneumonia in rats. Antimicrob Agents Chemother 57:643–646
85. Hilliard JJ, Melton JL, Hall L, Abbanat D, Fernandez J, Ward CK, Bunting RA, Barron A, Lynch AS, Flamm RK (2011) Comparative effects of carbapenems on bacterial load and host immune response in a *Klebsiella pneumoniae* murine pneumonia model. Antimicrob Agents Chemother 55:836–844
86. Hirsch EB, Guo B, Chang KT, Cao H, Ledesma KR, Singh M, Tam VH (2013) Assessment of antimicrobial combinations for *Klebsiella pneumoniae* carbapenemase-producing *K. pneumoniae*. J Infect Dis 207:786–793
87. Padilla E, Alonso D, Domenech-Sanchez A, Gomez C, Perez JL, Alberti S, Borrell N (2006) Effect of porins and plasmid-mediated AmpC beta-lactamases on the efficacy of beta-lactams in rat pneumonia caused by *Klebsiella pneumoniae*. Antimicrob Agents Chemother 50:2258–2260
88. Pichardo C, del Carmen CM, Bernabeu-Wittel M, Pascual A, Jimenez-Mejias ME, de Cueto M, Pachon-Ibanez ME, Garcia I, Pachon J, Martinez-Martinez L (2005) Activity of cefepime and carbapenems in experimental pneumonia caused by porin-deficient *Klebsiella pneumoniae* producing FOX-5 beta-lactamase. Clin Microbiol Infect 11:31–38
89. Pichardo C, Rodriguez-Martinez JM, Pachon-Ibanez ME, Conejo C, Ibanez-Martinez J, Martinez-Martinez L, Pachon J, Pascual A (2005) Efficacy of cefepime and imipenem in experimental murine pneumonia caused by porin-deficient *Klebsiella pneumoniae* producing CMY-2 beta-lactamase. Antimicrob Agents Chemother 49:3311–3316
90. Ambrose PG, Forrest A, Craig WA, Rubino CM, Bhavnani SM, Drusano GL, Heine HS (2007) Pharmacokinetics-pharmacodynamics of gatifloxacin in a lethal murine *Bacillus anthracis* inhalation infection model. Antimicrob Agents Chemother 51:4351–4355
91. Deziel MR, Heine H, Louie A, Kao M, Byrne WR, Basset J, Miller L, Bush K, Kelly M, Drusano GL (2005) Effective antimicrobial regimens for use in humans for therapy of *Bacillus anthracis* infections and postexposure prophylaxis. Antimicrob Agents Chemother 49:5099–5106
92. Gill SC, Rubino CM, Bassett J, Miller L, Ambrose PG, Bhavnani SM, Beaudry A, Li J, Stone KC, Critchley I, Janjic N, Heine HS (2010) Pharmacokinetic-pharmacodynamic assessment of faropenem in a lethal murine *Bacillus anthracis* inhalation postexposure prophylaxis model. Antimicrob Agents Chemother 54:1678–1683

93. Heine HS, Bassett J, Miller L, Bassett A, Ivins BE, Lehoux D, Arhin FF, Parr TR Jr, Moeck G (2008) Efficacy of oritavancin in a murine model of *Bacillus anthracis* spore inhalation anthrax. Antimicrob Agents Chemother 52:3350–3357
94. Heine HS, Bassett J, Miller L, Hartings JM, Ivins BE, Pitt ML, Fritz D, Norris SL, Byrne WR (2007) Determination of antibiotic efficacy against *Bacillus anthracis* in a mouse aerosol challenge model. Antimicrob Agents Chemother 51:1373–1379
95. Heine HS, Bassett J, Miller L, Purcell BK, Byrne WR (2010) Efficacy of Daptomycin against *Bacillus anthracis* in a murine model of anthrax spore inhalation. Antimicrob Agents Chemother 54:4471–4473
96. Heine HS, Purcell BK, Bassett J, Miller L, Goldstein BP (2010) Activity of dalbavancin against *Bacillus anthracis* in vitro and in a mouse inhalation anthrax model. Antimicrob Agents Chemother 54:991–996
97. Kao LM, Bush K, Barnewall R, Estep J, Thalacker FW, Olson PH, Drusano GL, Minton N, Chien S, Hemeryck A, Kelley MF (2006) Pharmacokinetic considerations and efficacy of levofloxacin in an inhalational anthrax (postexposure) rhesus monkey model. Antimicrob Agents Chemother 50:3535–3542
98. Hansen EJ, Toews GB (1992) Animal models for the study of noninvasive *Haemophilus influenzae* disease: pulmonary clearance systems. J Infect Dis 165(Suppl 1):S185–187
99. O'Reilly T (1995) Relevance of animal models for chronic bacterial airway infections in humans. Am J Respir Crit Care Med 151:2101–2107, discussion 2107–2108
100. Toews GB, Gross GN, Pierce AK (1979) The relationship of inoculum size to lung bacterial clearance and phagocytic cell response in mice. Am Rev Respir Dis 120:559–566
101. Johansen HK, Hoiby N (1999) Rat model of chronic *Pseudomonas aeruginosa*. Academic, San Diego
102. Schiff JB, Small GJ, Pennington JE (1984) Comparative activities of ciprofloxacin, ticarcillin, and tobramycin against experimental *Pseudomonas aeruginosa* pneumonia. Antimicrob Agents Chemother 26:1–4
103. Hraiech S, Bregeon F, Brunel JM, Rolain JM, Lepidi H, Andrieu V, Raoult D, Papazian L, Roch A (2012) Antibacterial efficacy of inhaled squalamine in a rat model of chronic *Pseudomonas aeruginosa* pneumonia. J Antimicrob Chemother 67:2452–2458
104. Macia MD, Borrell N, Segura M, Gomez C, Perez JL, Oliver A (2006) Efficacy and potential for resistance selection of antipseudomonal treatments in a mouse model of lung infection by hypermutable *Pseudomonas aeruginosa*. Antimicrob Agents Chemother 50:975–983
105. Moser C, Van Gennip M, Bjarnsholt T, Jensen PO, Lee B, Hougen HP, Calum H, Ciofu O, Givskov M, Molin S, Hoiby N (2009) Novel experimental *Pseudomonas aeruginosa* lung infection model mimicking long-term host-pathogen interactions in cystic fibrosis. APMIS 117:95–107
106. Song Z, Wu H, Mygind P, Raventos D, Sonksen C, Kristensen HH, Hoiby N (2005) Effects of intratracheal administration of novispirin G10 on a rat model of mucoid *Pseudomonas aeruginosa* lung infection. Antimicrob Agents Chemother 49:3868–3874
107. van Gennip M, Moser C, Christensen LD, Bjarnsholt T, Calum H, Jensen PO, Christophersen L, Hougen HP, Ciofu O, Molin S, Givskov M, Hoiby N (2009) Augmented effect of early antibiotic treatment in mice with experimental lung infections due to sequentially adapted mucoid strains of *Pseudomonas aeruginosa*. J Antimicrob Chemother 64:1241–1250
108. Beaulac C, Sachetelli S, Lagace J (1999) Aerosolization of low phase transition temperature liposomal tobramycin as a dry powder in an animal model of chronic pulmonary infection caused by *Pseudomonas aeruginosa*. J Drug Target 7:33–41
109. Cannon CL, Hogue LA, Vajravelu RK, Capps GH, Ibricevic A, Hindi KM, Kascatan-Nebioglu A, Walter MJ, Brody SL, Youngs WJ (2009) In vitro and murine efficacy and toxicity studies of nebulized SCC1, a methylated caffeine-silver(I) complex, for treatment of pulmonary infections. Antimicrob Agents Chemother 53:3285–3293
110. Ferrari F, Lu Q, Girardi C, Petitjean O, Marquette CH, Wallet F, Rouby JJ (2009) Nebulized ceftazidime in experimental pneumonia caused by partially resistant *Pseudomonas aeruginosa*. Intensive Care Med 35:1792–1800
111. Goldstein I, Wallet F, Nicolas-Robin A, Ferrari F, Marquette CH, Rouby JJ (2002) Lung deposition and efficiency of nebulized amikacin during *Escherichia coli* pneumonia in ventilated piglets. Am J Respir Crit Care Med 166:1375–1381
112. Lu Q, Girardi C, Zhang M, Bouhemad B, Louchahi K, Petitjean O, Wallet F, Becquemin MH, Le Naour G, Marquette CH, Rouby JJ (2010) Nebulized and intravenous colistin in experimental pneumonia caused by *Pseudomonas aeruginosa*. Intensive Care Med 36:1147–1155
113. Zak O, Sande MA (1982) Correlation of in vitro antimicrobial activity of antibiotics

with results of treatment in experimental animal models and human infection. Hans Huber Publishers, Bern

114. Zak O, Sande MA (1999) Handbook of animal models of infection. Academic, San Diego, CA
115. Capilla J, Clemons KV, Stevens DA (2007) Animal models: an important tool in mycology. Med Mycol 45:657–684
116. Guarro J (2011) Lessons from animal studies for the treatment of invasive human infections due to uncommon fungi. J Antimicrob Chemother 66:1447–1466
117. Dannaoui E, Mouton JW, Meis JF, Verweij PE (2002) Efficacy of antifungal therapy in a nonneutropenic murine model of zygomycosis. Antimicrob Agents Chemother 46:1953–1959
118. Lewis RE, Prince RA, Chi J, Kontoyiannis DP (2002) Itraconazole preexposure attenuates the efficacy of subsequent amphotericin B therapy in a murine model of acute invasive pulmonary aspergillosis. Antimicrob Agents Chemother 46:3208–3214
119. Wiederhold NP, Kontoyiannis DP, Chi J, Prince RA, Tam VH, Lewis RE (2004) Pharmacodynamics of caspofungin in a murine model of invasive pulmonary aspergillosis: evidence of concentration-dependent activity. J Infect Dis 190:1464–1471
120. Patterson TF, George D, Ingersoll R, Miniter P, Andriole VT (1991) Efficacy of SCH 39304 in treatment of experimental invasive aspergillosis. Antimicrob Agents Chemother 35:1985–1988
121. Lepak AJ, Marchillo K, Vanhecker J, Andes DR (2013) Posaconazole pharmacodynamic target determination against wild-type and Cyp51 mutant isolates of *Aspergillus fumigatus* in an in vivo model of invasive pulmonary aspergillosis. Antimicrob Agents Chemother 57:579–585
122. Howard SJ, Lestner JM, Sharp A, Gregson L, Goodwin J, Slater J, Majithiya JB, Warn PA, Hope WW (2011) Pharmacokinetics and pharmacodynamics of posaconazole for invasive pulmonary aspergillosis: clinical implications for antifungal therapy. J Infect Dis 203:1324–1332
123. Sheppard DC, Rieg G, Chiang LY, Filler SG, Edwards JE Jr, Ibrahim AS (2004) Novel inhalational murine model of invasive pulmonary aspergillosis. Antimicrob Agents Chemother 48:1908–1911
124. Clemons KV, Stevens DA (2001) Efficacy of ravuconazole in treatment of mucosal candidosis in SCID mice. Antimicrob Agents Chemother 45:3433–3436
125. Ju JY, Polhamus C, Marr KA, Holland SM, Bennett JE (2002) Efficacies of fluconazole, caspofungin, and amphotericin B in Candida glabrata-infected p47phox-/- knockout mice. Antimicrob Agents Chemother 46:1240–1245
126. Luo G, Gebremariam T, Lee H, French SW, Wiederhold NP, Patterson TF, Filler SG, Ibrahim AS (2013) Efficacy of liposomal amphotericin B and posaconazole in intratracheal models of murine mucormycosis. Antimicrob Agents Chemother 57:3340–3347
127. Ibrahim AS, Avanessian V, Spellberg B, Edwards JE Jr (2003) Liposomal amphotericin B, and not amphotericin B deoxycholate, improves survival of diabetic mice infected with *Rhizopus oryzae*. Antimicrob Agents Chemother 47:3343–3344
128. Foldvari M, Jaafari MR, Radhi J, Segal D (2005) Efficacy of the antiadhesin octyl O-(2-acetamido-2-deoxy-beta-D-galactopyranosyl)-(1-4)-2-O-propyl-beta-D-galactopy ranoside (Fimbrigal-P) in a rat oral candidiasis model. Antimicrob Agents Chemother 49:2887–2894
129. Takakura N, Sato Y, Ishibashi H, Oshima H, Uchida K, Yamaguchi H, Abe S (2003) A novel murine model of oral candidiasis with local symptoms characteristic of oral thrush. Microbiol Immunol 47:321–326
130. Calderon L, Williams R, Martinez M, Clemons KV, Stevens DA (2003) Genetic susceptibility to vaginal candidiasis. Med Mycol 41:143–147
131. Andes D (2005) Use of an animal model of disseminated candidiasis in the evaluation of antifungal therapy. Methods Mol Med 118: 111–128
132. Andes D, Ambrose PG, Hammel JP, Van Wart SA, Iyer V, Reynolds DK, Buell DN, Kovanda LL, Bhavnani SM (2011) Use of pharmacokinetic-pharmacodynamic analyses to optimize therapy with the systemic antifungal micafungin for invasive candidiasis or candidemia. Antimicrob Agents Chemother 55:2113–2121
133. Andes D, Diekema DJ, Pfaller MA, Bohrmuller J, Marchillo K, Lepak A (2010) In vivo comparison of the pharmacodynamic targets for echinocandin drugs against Candida species. Antimicrob Agents Chemother 54:2497–2506
134. Andes D, Diekema DJ, Pfaller MA, Prince RA, Marchillo K, Ashbeck J, Hou J (2008) In vivo pharmacodynamic characterization of anidulafungin in a neutropenic murine candidiasis model. Antimicrob Agents Chemother 52:539–550
135. Andes D, Forrest A, Lepak A, Nett J, Marchillo K, Lincoln L (2006) Impact of antimicrobial dosing regimen on evolution of drug resistance in vivo: fluconazole and *Candida albicans*. Antimicrob Agents Chemother 50:2374–2383

136. Andes D, Lepak A, Nett J, Lincoln L, Marchillo K (2006) In vivo fluconazole pharmacodynamics and resistance development in a previously susceptible *Candida albicans* population examined by microbiologic and transcriptional profiling. Antimicrob Agents Chemother 50:2384–2394
137. Andes D, Marchillo K, Conklin R, Krishna G, Ezzet F, Cacciapuoti A, Loebenberg D (2004) Pharmacodynamics of a new triazole, posaconazole, in a murine model of disseminated candidiasis. Antimicrob Agents Chemother 48:137–142
138. Andes D, Marchillo K, Lowther J, Bryskier A, Stamstad T, Conklin R (2003) In vivo pharmacodynamics of HMR 3270, a glucan synthase inhibitor, in a murine candidiasis model. Antimicrob Agents Chemother 47:1187–1192
139. Andes D, Marchillo K, Stamstad T, Conklin R (2003) In vivo pharmacokinetics and pharmacodynamics of a new triazole, voriconazole, in a murine candidiasis model. Antimicrob Agents Chemother 47:3165–3169
140. Andes D, Marchillo K, Stamstad T, Conklin R (2003) In vivo pharmacodynamics of a new triazole, ravuconazole, in a murine candidiasis model. Antimicrob Agents Chemother 47:1193–1199
141. Andes D, Safdar N, Marchillo K, Conklin R (2006) Pharmacokinetic-pharmacodynamic comparison of amphotericin B (AMB) and two lipid-associated AMB preparations, liposomal AMB and AMB lipid complex, in murine candidiasis models. Antimicrob Agents Chemother 50:674–684
142. Andes D, Stamsted T, Conklin R (2001) Pharmacodynamics of amphotericin B in a neutropenic-mouse disseminated-candidiasis model. Antimicrob Agents Chemother 45:922–926
143. Andes D, van Ogtrop M (2000) In vivo characterization of the pharmacodynamics of flucytosine in a neutropenic murine disseminated candidiasis model. Antimicrob Agents Chemother 44:938–942
144. Andes DR, Diekema DJ, Pfaller MA, Marchillo K, Bohrmueller J (2008) In vivo pharmacodynamic target investigation for micafungin against *Candida albicans* and *C. glabrata* in a neutropenic murine candidiasis model. Antimicrob Agents Chemother 52:3497–3503
145. Arendrup MC, Perlin DS, Jensen RH, Howard SJ, Goodwin J, Hope W (2012) Differential in vivo activities of anidulafungin, caspofungin, and micafungin against *Candida glabrata* isolates with and without FKS resistance mutations. Antimicrob Agents Chemother 56:2435–2442
146. Sugar AM (1991) Interactions of amphotericin B and SCH 39304 in the treatment of experimental murine candidiasis: lack of antagonism of a polyene-azole combination. Antimicrob Agents Chemother 35:1669–1671
147. Sugar AM, Goldani LZ, Picard M (1991) Treatment of murine invasive candidiasis with amphotericin B and cilofungin: evidence for enhanced activity with combination therapy. Antimicrob Agents Chemother 35:2128–2130
148. Sugar AM, Hitchcock CA, Troke PF, Picard M (1995) Combination therapy of murine invasive candidiasis with fluconazole and amphotericin B. Antimicrob Agents Chemother 39:598–601
149. Sugar AM, Liu XP (1998) Interactions of itraconazole with amphotericin B in the treatment of murine invasive candidiasis. J Infect Dis 177:1660–1663
150. Wiederhold NP, Najvar LK, Bocanegra R, Kirkpatrick WR, Patterson TF (2012) Comparison of anidulafungin's and fluconazole's in vivo activity in neutropenic and non-neutropenic models of invasive candidiasis. Clin Microbiol Infect 18:E20–23
151. Wiederhold NP, Najvar LK, Bocanegra R, Molina D, Olivo M, Graybill JR (2007) In vivo efficacy of anidulafungin and caspofungin against *Candida glabrata* and association with in vitro potency in the presence of sera. Antimicrob Agents Chemother 51:1616–1620
152. Wiederhold NP, Najvar LK, Bocanegra RA, Kirkpatrick WR, Patterson TF (2011) Caspofungin dose escalation for invasive candidiasis due to resistant *Candida albicans*. Antimicrob Agents Chemother 55:3254–3260
153. Sanati H, Ramos CF, Bayer AS, Ghannoum MA (1997) Combination therapy with amphotericin B and fluconazole against invasive candidiasis in neutropenic-mouse and infective-endocarditis rabbit models. Antimicrob Agents Chemother 41:1345–1348
154. Rex JH, Nelson PW, Paetznick VL, Lozano-Chiu M, Espinel-Ingroff A, Anaissie EJ (1998) Optimizing the correlation between results of testing in vitro and therapeutic outcome in vivo for fluconazole by testing critical isolates in a murine model of invasive candidiasis. Antimicrob Agents Chemother 42: 129–134
155. Spellberg B, Fu Y, Edwards JE Jr, Ibrahim AS (2005) Combination therapy with amphotericin B lipid complex and caspofungin acetate of disseminated zygomycosis in diabetic ketoacidotic mice. Antimicrob Agents Chemother 49:830–832

156. Spellberg B, Ibrahim AS, Edwards JE Jr, Filler SG (2005) Mice with disseminated candidiasis die of progressive sepsis. J Infect Dis 192:336–343
157. Marine M, Pastor FJ, Guarro J (2010) Efficacy of posaconazole in a murine disseminated infection by *Candida tropicalis*. Antimicrob Agents Chemother 54:530–532
158. Howard SJ, Livermore J, Sharp A, Goodwin J, Gregson L, Alastruey-Izquierdo A, Perlin DS, Warn PA, Hope WW (2011) Pharmacodynamics of echinocandins against *Candida glabrata*: requirement for dosage escalation to achieve maximal antifungal activity in neutropenic hosts. Antimicrob Agents Chemother 55:4880–4887
159. Hope WW, Drusano GL, Moore CB, Sharp A, Louie A, Walsh TJ, Denning DW, Warn PA (2007) Effect of neutropenia and treatment delay on the response to antifungal agents in experimental disseminated candidiasis. Antimicrob Agents Chemother 51:285–295
160. Hope WW, Mickiene D, Petraitis V, Petraitiene R, Kelaher AM, Hughes JE, Cotton MP, Bacher J, Keirns JJ, Buell D, Heresi G, Benjamin DK Jr, Groll AH, Drusano GL, Walsh TJ (2008) The pharmacokinetics and pharmacodynamics of micafungin in experimental hematogenous *Candida meningoencephalitis*: implications for echinocandin therapy in neonates. J Infect Dis 197:163–171
161. Hope WW, Warn PA, Sharp A, Howard S, Kasai M, Louie A, Walsh TJ, Drusano GL, Denning DW (2006) Derivation of an in vivo drug exposure breakpoint for flucytosine against *Candida albicans* and Impact of the MIC, growth rate, and resistance genotype on the antifungal effect. Antimicrob Agents Chemother 50:3680–3688
162. Clancy CJ, Cheng S, Nguyen MH (2009) Animal models of candidiasis. Methods Mol Biol 499:65–76
163. Lepak A, Castanheira M, Diekema D, Pfaller M, Andes D (2012) Optimizing Echinocandin dosing and susceptibility breakpoint determination via in vivo pharmacodynamic evaluation against *Candida glabrata* with and without fks mutations. Antimicrob Agents Chemother 56:5875–5882
164. Lepak A, Nett J, Lincoln L, Marchillo K, Andes D (2006) Time course of microbiologic outcome and gene expression in *Candida albicans* during and following in vitro and in vivo exposure to fluconazole. Antimicrob Agents Chemother 50:1311–1319
165. Gumbo T, Drusano GL, Liu W, Kulawy RW, Fregeau C, Hsu V, Louie A (2007) Once-weekly micafungin therapy is as effective as daily therapy for disseminated candidiasis in mice with persistent neutropenia. Antimicrob Agents Chemother 51:968–974
166. Gumbo T, Drusano GL, Liu W, Ma L, Deziel MR, Drusano MF, Louie A (2006) Anidulafungin pharmacokinetics and microbial response in neutropenic mice with disseminated candidiasis. Antimicrob Agents Chemother 50:3695–3700
167. Louie A, Banerjee P, Drusano GL, Shayegani M, Miller MH (1999) Interaction between fluconazole and amphotericin B in mice with systemic infection due to fluconazole-susceptible or -resistant strains of *Candida albicans*. Antimicrob Agents Chemother 43:2841–2847
168. Louie A, Deziel M, Liu W, Drusano MF, Gumbo T, Drusano GL (2005) Pharmacodynamics of caspofungin in a murine model of systemic candidiasis: importance of persistence of caspofungin in tissues to understanding drug activity. Antimicrob Agents Chemother 49:5058–5068
169. MacCallum DM, Coste A, Ischer F, Jacobsen MD, Odds FC, Sanglard D (2010) Genetic dissection of azole resistance mechanisms in *Candida albicans* and their validation in a mouse model of disseminated infection. Antimicrob Agents Chemother 54:1476–1483
170. MacCallum DM, Odds FC (2004) Need for early antifungal treatment confirmed in experimental disseminated *Candida albicans* infection. Antimicrob Agents Chemother 48:4911–4914
171. Brieland J, Essig D, Jackson C, Frank D, Loebenberg D, Menzel F, Arnold B, DiDomenico B, Hare R (2001) Comparison of pathogenesis and host immune responses to *Candida glabrata* and *Candida albicans* in systemically infected immunocompetent mice. Infect Immun 69:5046–5055
172. Livermore JL, Felton TW, Abbott J, Sharp A, Goodwin J, Gregson L, Warn PA, Howard SJ, Hope WW (2013) Pharmacokinetics and pharmacodynamics of anidulafungin for experimental *Candida endophthalmitis*: insights into the utility of echinocandins for treatment of a potentially sight-threatening infection. Antimicrob Agents Chemother 57:281–288
173. Deren YT, Ozdek S, Kalkanci A, Akyurek N, Hasanreisoglu B (2010) Comparison of antifungal efficacies of moxifloxacin, liposomal amphotericin B, and combination treatment in experimental *Candida albicans* endophthalmitis in rabbits. Can J Microbiol 56:1–7
174. Demant E, Easterbrook M (1977) An experimental model of candida endophthalmitis. Can J Ophthalmol 12:304–307
175. Edwards JE Jr, Montgomerie JZ, Foos RY, Shaw VK, Guze LB (1975) Experimental

hematogenous endophthalmitis caused by *Candida albicans*. J Infect Dis 131:649–657
176. Gupta SK, Dhingra N, Velpandian T, Jaiswal J (2000) Efficacy of fluconazole and liposome entrapped fluconazole for *C. albicans* induced experimental mycotic endophthalmitis in rabbit eyes. Acta Ophthalmol Scand 78:448–450
177. Kusbeci T, Avci B, Cetinkaya Z, Ozturk F, Yavas G, Ermis SS, Inan UU (2007) The effects of caspofungin and voriconazole in experimental *Candida endophthalmitis*. Curr Eye Res 32:57–64
178. Louie A, Liu W, Miller DA, Sucke AC, Liu QF, Drusano GL, Mayers M, Miller MH (1999) Efficacies of high-dose fluconazole plus amphotericin B and high-dose fluconazole plus 5-fluorocytosine versus amphotericin B, fluconazole, and 5-fluorocytosine monotherapies in treatment of experimental endocarditis, endophthalmitis, and pyelonephritis due to *Candida albicans*. Antimicrob Agents Chemother 43:2831–2840
179. Omuta J, Uchida K, Yamaguchi H, Shibuya K (2007) Histopathological study on experimental endophthalmitis induced by bloodstream infection with *Candida albicans*. Jpn J Infect Dis 60:33–39
180. Savani DV, Perfect JR, Cobo LM, Durack DT (1987) Penetration of new azole compounds into the eye and efficacy in experimental *Candida endophthalmitis*. Antimicrob Agents Chemother 31:6–10
181. Yuan X, Hua X, Wilhelmus KR (2010) The corneal expression of antimicrobial peptides during experimental fungal keratitis. Curr Eye Res 35:872–879
182. Yuan X, Mitchell BM, Wilhelmus KR (2008) Gene profiling and signaling pathways of *Candida albicans* keratitis. Mol Vis 14: 1792–1798
183. Zhong W, Yin H, Xie L (2009) Expression and potential role of major inflammatory cytokines in experimental keratomycosis. Mol Vis 15:1303–1311
184. Wu TG, Wilhelmus KR, Mitchell BM (2003) Experimental keratomycosis in a mouse model. Invest Ophthalmol Vis Sci 44:210–216
185. Hu J, Wang Y, Xie L (2009) Potential role of macrophages in experimental keratomycosis. Invest Ophthalmol Vis Sci 50:2087–2094
186. O'Day DM, Head WS, Csank C, Shetlar DJ, Robinson RD, McCollum GW, Yang R, Zhu TL, Wang MX (2000) Differences in virulence between two *Candida albicans* strains in experimental keratitis. Invest Ophthalmol Vis Sci 41:1116–1121
187. Ohno S, Fuerst DJ, Okumoto M, Grabner G, Smolin G (1983) The effect of K-582, a new antifungal agent, on experimental *Candida keratitis*. Invest Ophthalmol Vis Sci 24:1626–1629
188. Pleyer U, Legmann A, Mondino BJ, Lee DA (1992) Use of collagen shields containing amphotericin B in the treatment of experimental *Candida albicans*-induced keratomycosis in rabbits. Am J Ophthalmol 113:303–308
189. Ray WA, O'Day DM, Head WS, Robinson RD (1984) Variability in isolate recovery rates from multiple and single breeds of outbred pigmented rabbits in an experimental model of Candida keratitis. Curr Eye Res 3:949–953
190. Ishibashi Y, Kaufman HE (1986) Topical ketoconazole for experimental Candida keratitis in rabbits. Am J Ophthalmol 102:522–526
191. Goldblum D, Frueh BE, Sarra GM, Katsoulis K, Zimmerli S (2005) Topical caspofungin for treatment of keratitis caused by *Candida albicans* in a rabbit model. Antimicrob Agents Chemother 49:1359–1363
192. Mitchell BM, Wu TG, Jackson BE, Wilhelmus KR (2007) *Candida albicans* strain-dependent virulence and Rim13p-mediated filamentation in experimental keratomycosis. Invest Ophthalmol Vis Sci 48:774–780
193. Mavridou E, Bruggemann RJ, Melchers WJ, Mouton JW, Verweij PE (2010) Efficacy of posaconazole against three clinical *Aspergillus fumigatus* isolates with mutations in the cyp51A gene. Antimicrob Agents Chemother 54:860–865
194. Vallor AC, Kirkpatrick WR, Najvar LK, Bocanegra R, Kinney MC, Fothergill AW, Herrera ML, Wickes BL, Graybill JR, Patterson TF (2008) Assessment of *Aspergillus fumigatus* burden in pulmonary tissue of guinea pigs by quantitative PCR, galactomannan enzyme immunoassay, and quantitative culture. Antimicrob Agents Chemother 52:2593–2598
195. Bowman JC, Abruzzo GK, Anderson JW, Flattery AM, Gill CJ, Pikounis VB, Schmatz DM, Liberator PA, Douglas CM (2001) Quantitative PCR assay to measure *Aspergillus fumigatus* burden in a murine model of disseminated aspergillosis: demonstration of efficacy of caspofungin acetate. Antimicrob Agents Chemother 45:3474–3481
196. Lewis RE, Ben-Ami R, Best L, Albert N, Walsh TJ, Kontoyiannis DP (2013) Tacrolimus enhances the potency of posaconazole against *Rhizopus oryzae* in vitro and in an experimental model of mucormycosis. J Infect Dis 207:834–841
197. Hope WW, Petraitis V, Petraitiene R, Aghamolla T, Bacher J, Walsh TJ (2010) The initial 96 hours of invasive pulmonary aspergillosis: histopathology, comparative kinetics of galactomannan and (1->3) beta-d-glucan and consequences of delayed antifungal therapy. Antimicrob Agents Chemother 54:4879–4886
198. Ibrahim AS, Bowman JC, Avanessian V, Brown K, Spellberg B, Edwards JE Jr, Douglas

CM (2005) Caspofungin inhibits *Rhizopus oryzae* 1,3-beta-D-glucan synthase, lowers burden in brain measured by quantitative PCR, and improves survival at a low but not a high dose during murine disseminated zygomycosis. Antimicrob Agents Chemother 49:721–727

199. Lewis RE, Albert ND, Liao G, Hou J, Prince RA, Kontoyiannis DP (2010) Comparative pharmacodynamics of amphotericin B lipid complex and liposomal amphotericin B in a murine model of pulmonary mucormycosis. Antimicrob Agents Chemother 54:1298–1304
200. Lamaris GA, Ben-Ami R, Lewis RE, Chamilos G, Samonis G, Kontoyiannis DP (2009) Increased virulence of Zygomycetes organisms following exposure to voriconazole: a study involving fly and murine models of zygomycosis. J Infect Dis 199:1399–1406
201. Rodriguez MM, Serena C, Marine M, Pastor FJ, Guarro J (2008) Posaconazole combined with amphotericin B, an effective therapy for a murine disseminated infection caused by *Rhizopus oryzae*. Antimicrob Agents Chemother 52:3786–3788
202. Clemons KV, Stevens DA (1998) Comparison of fungizone, Amphotec, Am Bisome, and Abelcet for treatment of systemic murine cryptococcosis. Antimicrob Agents Chemother 42:899–902
203. Calvo E, Pastor FJ, Rodriguez MM, Pujol I, Guarro J (2010) Antifungal therapy in a murine model of disseminated infection by *Cryptococcus gattii*. Antimicrob Agents Chemother 54:4074–4077
204. Lengerova M, Kocmanova I, Racil Z, Hrncirova K, Pospisilova S, Mayer J, Najvar LK, Wiederhold NP, Kirkpatrick WR, Patterson TF (2012) Detection and measurement of fungal burden in a guinea pig model of invasive pulmonary aspergillosis by novel quantitative nested real-time PCR compared with galactomannan and (1,3)-beta-D-glucan detection. J Clin Microbiol 50:602–608
205. Larsen RA, Bauer M, Thomas AM, Sanchez A, Citron D, Rathbun M, Harrison TS (2005) Correspondence of in vitro and in vivo fluconazole dose-response curves for *Cryptococcus neoformans*. Antimicrob Agents Chemother 49:3297–3301
206. Schwarz P, Dromer F, Lortholary O, Dannaoui E (2006) Efficacy of amphotericin B in combination with flucytosine against flucytosine-susceptible or flucytosine-resistant isolates of *Cryptococcus neoformans* during disseminated murine cryptococcosis. Antimicrob Agents Chemother 50:113–120
207. Serena C, Pastor FJ, Marine M, Rodriguez MM, Guarro J (2007) Efficacy of voriconazole in a murine model of cryptococcal central nervous system infection. J Antimicrob Chemother 60:162–165
208. Thompson GR III, Wiederhold NP, Najvar LK, Bocanegra R, Kirkpatrick WR, Graybill JR, Patterson TF (2012) A murine model of *Cryptococcus gattii* meningoencephalitis. J Antimicrob Chemother 67:1432–1438
209. Widmer F, Wright LC, Obando D, Handke R, Ganendren R, Ellis DH, Sorrell TC (2006) Hexadecylphosphocholine (miltefosine) has broad-spectrum fungicidal activity and is efficacious in a mouse model of cryptococcosis. Antimicrob Agents Chemother 50:414–421
210. Wiederhold NP, Najvar LK, Bocanegra R, Kirkpatrick WR, Sorrell TC, Patterson TF (2013) Limited activity of miltefosine in murine models of cryptococcal meningoencephalitis and disseminated cryptococcosis. Antimicrob Agents Chemother 57:745–750
211. Zaragoza O, Mihu C, Casadevall A, Nosanchuk JD (2005) Effect of amphotericin B on capsule and cell size in *Cryptococcus neoformans* during murine infection. Antimicrob Agents Chemother 49:4358–4361
212. Chiller TM, Sobel RA, Luque JC, Clemons KV, Stevens DA (2003) Efficacy of amphotericin B or itraconazole in a murine model of central nervous system Aspergillus infection. Antimicrob Agents Chemother 47:813–815
213. Clemons KV, Espiritu M, Parmar R, Stevens DA (2005) Comparative efficacies of conventional amphotericin b, liposomal amphotericin B (AmBisome), caspofungin, micafungin, and voriconazole alone and in combination against experimental murine central nervous system aspergillosis. Antimicrob Agents Chemother 49:4867–4875
214. Clemons KV, Parmar R, Martinez M, Stevens DA (2006) Efficacy of Abelcet alone, or in combination therapy, against experimental central nervous system aspergillosis. J Antimicrob Chemother 58:466–469
215. Clemons KV, Schwartz JA, Stevens DA (2012) Experimental central nervous system aspergillosis therapy: efficacy, drug levels and localization, immunohistopathology, and toxicity. Antimicrob Agents Chemother 56:4439–4449
216. Clemons KV, Stevens DA (2005) The contribution of animal models of aspergillosis to understanding pathogenesis, therapy and virulence. Med Mycol 43(Suppl 1):S101–110
217. Imai J, Singh G, Fernandez B, Clemons KV, Stevens DA (2005) Efficacy of Abelcet and caspofungin, alone or in combination, against CNS aspergillosis in a murine model. J Antimicrob Chemother 56:166–171

218. Imai JK, Singh G, Clemons KV, Stevens DA (2004) Efficacy of posaconazole in a murine model of central nervous system aspergillosis. Antimicrob Agents Chemother 48:4063–4066
219. Singh G, Imai J, Clemons KV, Stevens DA (2005) Efficacy of caspofungin against central nervous system *Aspergillus fumigatus* infection in mice determined by TaqMan PCR and CFU methods. Antimicrob Agents Chemother 49: 1369–1376
220. Warn PA, Livermore J, Howard S, Felton TW, Sharp A, Gregson L, Goodwin J, Petraitiene R, Petraitis V, Cohen-Wolkowiez M, Walsh TJ, Benjamin DK Jr, Hope WW (2012) Anidulafungin for neonatal hematogenous *Candida meningoencephalitis*: identification of candidate regimens for humans using a translational pharmacological approach. Antimicrob Agents Chemother 56:708–714
221. Kang CI, Rouse MS, Mandrekar JN, Steckelberg JM, Patel R (2009) Anidulafungin treatment of candidal central nervous system infection in a murine model. Antimicrob Agents Chemother 53:3576–3578
222. Sorensen KN, Clemons KV, Stevens DA (1999) Murine models of blastomycosis, coccidioidomycosis, and histoplasmosis. Mycopathologia 146:53–65
223. Calvo E, Pastor FJ, Guarro J (2010) Antifungal therapies in murine disseminated phaeohyphomycoses caused by Exophiala species. J Antimicrob Chemother 65:1455–1459
224. Calvo E, Pastor FJ, Rodriguez MM, Mayayo E, Salas V, Guarro J (2010) Murine model of a disseminated infection by the novel fungus Fonsecaea monophora and successful treatment with posaconazole. Antimicrob Agents Chemother 54:919–923
225. Al-Abdely HM, Najvar LK, Bocanegra R, Graybill JR (2005) Antifungal therapy of experimental cerebral phaeohyphomycosis due to *Cladophialophora bantiana*. Antimicrob Agents Chemother 49:1701–1707
226. Itoyama T, Uchida K, Yamaguchi H (1997) Therapeutic effects of omoconazole nitrate on guinea-pigs experimentally infected with Trichophyton mentagrophytes. J Antimicrob Chemother 39:825–827
227. Itoyama T, Uchida K, Yamaguchi H, Fujita S (1997) Therapeutic effects of omoconazole nitrate on experimental tinea pedis, an intractable dermatophytosis, in guinea-pigs. J Antimicrob Chemother 40:441–444
228. Koga H, Nanjoh Y, Kaneda H, Yamaguchi H, Tsuboi R (2012) Short-term therapy with luliconazole, a novel topical antifungal imidazole, in guinea pig models of tinea corporis and tinea pedis. Antimicrob Agents Chemother 56:3138–3143
229. Saunte DM, Simmel F, Frimodt-Moller N, Stolle LB, Svejgaard EL, Haedersdal M, Kloft C, Arendrup MC (2007) In vivo efficacy and pharmacokinetics of voriconazole in an animal model of dermatophytosis. Antimicrob Agents Chemother 51:3317–3321
230. Shimamura T, Kubota N, Nagasaka S, Suzuki T, Mukai H, Shibuya K (2011) Establishment of a novel model of onychomycosis in rabbits for evaluation of antifungal agents. Antimicrob Agents Chemother 55: 3150–3155
231. Serena C, Marine M, Marimon R, Pastor FJ, Guarro J (2007) Effect of antifungal treatment in a murine model of blastoschizomycosis. Int J Antimicrob Agents 29:79–83
232. Serena C, Rodriguez MM, Marine M, Pastor FJ, Guarro J (2007) Combined therapies in a murine model of blastoschizomycosis. Antimicrob Agents Chemother 51:2608–2610
233. Serena C, Rodriguez MM, Marine M, Pastor FJ, Guarro J (2008) Micafungin combined with fluconazole, an effective therapy for murine blastoschizomycosis. J Antimicrob Chemother 61:877–879
234. Wiederhold NP, Najvar LK, Bocanegra R, Graybill JR, Patterson TF (2010) Efficacy of posaconazole as treatment and prophylaxis against *Fusarium solani*. Antimicrob Agents Chemother 54:1055–1059
235. Ruiz-Cendoya M, Marine M, Guarro J (2008) Combined therapy in treatment of murine infection by *Fusarium solani*. J Antimicrob Chemother 62:543–546
236. Ruiz-Cendoya M, Marine M, Rodriguez MM, Guarro J (2009) Interactions between triazoles and amphotericin B in treatment of disseminated murine infection by *Fusarium oxysporum*. Antimicrob Agents Chemother 53:1705–1708
237. Lionakis MS, Chamilos G, Lewis RE, Wiederhold NP, Raad II, Samonis G, Kontoyiannis DP (2006) Pentamidine is active in a neutropenic murine model of acute invasive pulmonary fusariosis. Antimicrob Agents Chemother 50:294–297
238. Rodriguez MM, Calvo E, Serena C, Marine M, Pastor FJ, Guarro J (2009) Effects of double and triple combinations of antifungal drugs in a murine model of disseminated infection by *Scedosporium prolificans*. Antimicrob Agents Chemother 53:2153–2155
239. Rodriguez MM, Pastor FJ, Salas V, Calvo E, Mayayo E, Guarro J (2010) Experimental murine scedosporiosis: histopathology and azole treatment. Antimicrob Agents Chemother 54:3980–3984
240. Bocanegra R, Najvar LK, Hernandez S, McCarthy DI, Graybill JR (2005) Caspofungin

and liposomal amphotericin B therapy of experimental murine scedosporiosis. Antimicrob Agents Chemother 49:5139–5141

241. Serena C, Gilgado F, Marine M, Pastor FJ, Guarro J (2006) Efficacy of voriconazole in a guinea pig model of invasive trichosporonosis. Antimicrob Agents Chemother 50:2240–2243
242. Serena C, Pastor FJ, Gilgado F, Mayayo E, Guarro J (2005) Efficacy of micafungin in combination with other drugs in a murine model of disseminated trichosporonosis. Antimicrob Agents Chemother 49:497–502
243. Johnson AP, Tuffrey M, Taylor-Robinson D (1989) Resistance of mice to genital infection with *Neisseria gonorrhoeae*. J Med Microbiol 30:33–36
244. Corbeil LB, Wunderlich AC, Corbeil RR, McCutchan JA, Ito JI Jr, Braude AI (1979) Disseminated gonococcal infection in mice. Infect Immun 26:984–990
245. Jerse AE (1999) Experimental gonococcal genital tract infection and opacity protein expression in estradiol-treated mice. Infect Immun 67:5699–5708
246. Kita E, Katsui N, Emoto M, Sawaki M, Oku D, Nishikawa F, Hamuro A, Kashiba S (1991) Virulence of transparent and opaque colony types of *Neisseria gonorrhoeae* for the genital tract of mice. J Med Microbiol 34:355–362
247. Song W, Condron S, Mocca BT, Veit SJ, Hill D, Abbas A, Jerse AE (2008) Local and humoral immune responses against primary and repeat *Neisseria gonorrhoeae* genital tract infections of 17beta-estradiol-treated mice. Vaccine 26:5741–5751
248. Kunz AN, Begum AA, Wu H, D'Ambrozio JA, Robinson JM, Shafer WM, Bash MC, Jerse AE (2012) Impact of fluoroquinolone resistance mutations on gonococcal fitness and in vivo selection for compensatory mutations. J Infect Dis 205:1821–1829
249. Alder JD (1999) The hamster model of syphilis. Academic, San Diego
250. Baughn RE, Adams C, Musher DM (1984) Evaluation of Sch 29482 in experimental syphilis and comparison with penicillin G benzathine in disseminated disease and localized infection. Antimicrob Agents Chemother 26:401–404
251. Lukehart SA, Baker-Zander SA, Holmes KK (1984) Efficacy of aztreonam in treatment of experimental syphilis in rabbits. Antimicrob Agents Chemother 25:390–391
252. Fitzgerald TJ (1992) Effects of cefetamet (Ro 15-8074) on *Treponema pallidum* and experimental syphilis. Antimicrob Agents Chemother 36:598–602
253. Baker-Zander SA, Lukehart SA (1989) Efficacy of cefmetazole in the treatment of active syphilis in the rabbit model. Antimicrob Agents Chemother 33:1465–1469
254. Johnson RC, Bey RF, Wolgamot SJ (1982) Comparison of the activities of ceftriaxone and penicillin G against experimentally induced syphilis in rabbits. Antimicrob Agents Chemother 21:984–989
255. Lukehart SA, Fohn MJ, Baker-Zander SA (1990) Efficacy of azithromycin for therapy of active syphilis in the rabbit model. J Antimicrob Chemother 25(Suppl A):91–99
256. Alder J, Jarvis K, Mitten M, Shipkowitz NL, Gupta P, Clement J (1993) Clarithromycin therapy of experimental *Treponema pallidum* infections in hamsters. Antimicrob Agents Chemother 37:864–867
257. Korting HC, Haag R, Walter D, Riethmuller U, Meurer M (1993) Efficacy of ceftizoxime in the treatment of incubating syphilis in rabbits. Chemotherapy 39:331–335
258. Korting HC, Walther D, Riethmuller U, Meurer M (1987) Ceftriaxone given repeatedly cures manifest syphilis in the rabbit. Chemotherapy 33:376–380
259. Marra C, Baker-Zander SA, Hook EW III, Lukehart SA (1991) An experimental model of early central nervous system syphilis. J Infect Dis 163:825–829
260. Marra CM, Slatter V, Tartaglione TA, Baker-Zander SA, Lukehart SA (1992) Evaluation of aqueous penicillin G and ceftriaxone for experimental neurosyphilis. J Infect Dis 165: 396–397
261. Kajdacsy-Balla A, Howeedy A, Bagasra O (1987) Syphilis in the Syrian hamster. A model of human venereal and congenital syphilis. Am J Pathol 126:599–601
262. Kajdacsy-Balla A, Howeedy A, Bagasra O (1993) Experimental model of congenital syphilis. Infect Immun 61:3559–3561
263. Wicher V, Wicher K (1999) Guinea-pig model of acquired and congenital syphilis. Academic, San Diego
264. Moller BR, Mardh PA (1982) Animal models for the study of Chlamydial infections of the urogenital tract. Scand J Infect Dis Suppl 32:103–108
265. Beale AS, Upshon PA (1994) Characteristics of murine model of genital infection with *Chlamydia trachomatis* and effects of therapy with tetracyclines, amoxicillin-clavulanic acid, or azithromycin. Antimicrob Agents Chemother 38:1937–1943
266. Tuffrey M, Woods C, Inman C, Ward M (1994) The effect of a single oral dose of

azithromycin on chlamydial infertility and oviduct ultrastructure in mice. J Antimicrob Chemother 34:989–999

267. Pal S, Sarcon AK, de la Maza LM (2010) A new murine model for testing vaccines against genital *Chlamydia trachomatis* infections in males. Vaccine 28:7606–7612
268. Carey A, Cunningham K, Andrew D, Hafner L, Timms P, Beagley K (2011) A comparison of the effects of a chlamydial vaccine administered during or after a C. muridarum urogenital infection of female mice. Vaccine 29:6505–6513
269. Imtiaz MT, Schripsema JH, Sigar IM, Kasimos JN, Ramsey KH (2006) Inhibition of matrix metalloproteinases protects mice from ascending infection and chronic disease manifestations resulting from urogenital *Chlamydia muridarum* infection. Infect Immun 74:5513–5521
270. Imtiaz MT, Schripsema JH, Sigar IM, Ramsey KH (2006) Outcome of urogenital infection with *Chlamydia muridarum* in CD14 gene knockout mice. BMC Infect Dis 6:144
271. Johnson RM, Kerr MS, Slaven JE (2012) Plac8-dependent and inducible NO synthase-dependent mechanisms clear *Chlamydia muridarum* infections from the genital tract. J Immunol 188:1896–1904
272. Johnson RM, Yu H, Kerr MS, Slaven JE, Karunakaran KP, Brunham RC (2012) PmpG303-311, a protective vaccine epitope that elicits persistent cellular immune responses in *Chlamydia muridarum*-immune mice. Infect Immun 80:2204–2211
273. Reeves DM, Nagarajan U, O'Connell C, Andrews CW Jr, Darville T (2007) Lack of an effect of antibiotic treatment on prolonged detection of chlamydial DNA in murine genital tract infection. Antimicrob Agents Chemother 51:2646–2648
274. Binet R, Bowlin AK, Maurelli AT, Rank RG (2010) Impact of azithromycin resistance mutations on the virulence and fitness of *Chlamydia caviae* in guinea pigs. Antimicrob Agents Chemother 54:1094–1101
275. Frazer LC, Darville T, Chandra-Kuntal K, Andrews CW Jr, Zurenski M, Mintus M, AbdelRahman YM, Belland RJ, Ingalls RR, O'Connell CM (2012) Plasmid-cured *Chlamydia caviae* activates TLR2-dependent signaling and retains virulence in the guinea pig model of genital tract infection. PLoS One 7:e30747
276. Wang Y, Nagarajan U, Hennings L, Bowlin AK, Rank RG (2010) Local host response to chlamydial urethral infection in male guinea pigs. Infect Immun 78:1670–1681
277. Roberts JA (1992) Vesicoureteral reflux and pyelonephritis in the monkey: a review. J Urol 148:1721–1725
278. Hagberg L, Engberg I, Freter R, Lam J, Olling S, Svanborg EC (1983) Ascending, unobstructed urinary tract infection in mice caused by pyelonephritogenic *Escherichia coli* of human origin. Infect Immun 40:273–283
279. Hvidberg H, Struve C, Krogfelt KA, Christensen N, Rasmussen SN, Frimodt-Moller N (2000) Development of a long-term ascending urinary tract infection mouse model for antibiotic treatment studies. Antimicrob Agents Chemother 44:156–163
280. Johnson JR, Berggren T, Manivel JC (1992) Histopathologic-microbiologic correlates of invasiveness in a mouse model of ascending unobstructed urinary tract infection. J Infect Dis 165:299–305
281. Johnson JR, Brown JJ (1996) Defining inoculation conditions for the mouse model of ascending urinary tract infection that avoid immediate vesicoureteral reflux yet produce renal and bladder infection. J Infect Dis 173:746–749
282. Kerrn MB, Frimodt-Moller N, Espersen F (2003) Effects of sulfamethizole and amdinocillin against *Escherichia coli* strains (with various susceptibilities) in an ascending urinary tract infection mouse model. Antimicrob Agents Chemother 47:1002–1009
283. Frimodt-Moller N (2002) Correlation between pharmacokinetic/pharmacodynamic parameters and efficacy for antibiotics in the treatment of urinary tract infection. Int J Antimicrob Agents 19:546–553
284. Tsuchimori N, Yamazaki T, Okonogi K (1997) Therapeutic effects of cefozopran against experimental mixed urinary tract infection with *Enterococcus faecalis* and *Pseudomonas aeruginosa* in mice. J Antimicrob Chemother 39:423–425
285. Glauser MP, Ransley P, Bille J (1986) Urinary tract infections, pyelonephritic scars, and chemotherapy, experimental models in antimicrobial chemotherapy, vol 1. Academic, London
286. Brooks SJ, Lyons JM, Braude AI (1974) Immunization against retrograde pyelonephritis. I. Production of an experimental model of severe ascending *Escherichia coli* pyelonephritis without bacteremia in rats. Am J Pathol 74:345–358
287. Glauser MP, Bonard M (1982) Treatment of experimental ascending *Escherichia coli* pyelonephritis with ceftriaxone alone and in combination with gentamicin. Chemotherapy 28: 410–416

288. Glauser MP, Lyons JM, Braude AI (1979) Prevention of pyelonephritis due to *Escherichia coli* in rats with gentamicin stored in kidney tissue. J Infect Dis 139:172–177
289. Glauser MP, Lyons JM, Braude AI (1979) Synergism of ampicillin and gentamicin against obstructive pyelonephritis due to *Escherichia coli* in rats. J Infect Dis 139:133–140
290. Bergeron MG, Marois Y (1986) Benefit from high intrarenal levels of gentamicin in the treatment of *E. coli* pyelonephritis. Kidney Int 30:481–487
291. LeBrun M, Grenier L, Gourde P, Bergeron MG, Labrecque G, Beauchamp D (1999) Effectiveness and toxicity of gentamicin in an experimental model of pyelonephritis: effect of the time of administration. Antimicrob Agents Chemother 43:1020–1026
292. Miller TE, Findon G, Rainer SP, Gavin JB (1992) The pathobiology of subclinical pyelonephritis--an experimental evaluation. Kidney Int 41:1356–1365
293. Frosco MB, Melton JL, Stewart FP, Kulwich BA, Licata L, Barrett JF (1996) In vivo efficacies of levofloxacin and ciprofloxacin in acute murine hematogenous pyelonephritis induced by methicillin-susceptible and-resistant *Staphylococcus aureus* strains. Antimicrob Agents Chemother 40:2529–2534
294. Kaijser B, Larsson P (1982) Experimental acute pyelonephritis caused by enterobacteria in animals. A review. J Urol 127:786–790
295. Fu KP, Foleno BD, Lafredo SC, LoCoco JM, Isaacson DM (1993) In vitro and in vivo antibacterial activities of FK037, a novel parenteral broad-spectrum cephalosporin. Antimicrob Agents Chemother 37:301–307
296. Griffith DC, Harford L, Williams R, Lee VJ, Dudley MN (2003) In vivo antibacterial activity of RWJ-54428, a new cephalosporin with activity against gram-positive bacteria. Antimicrob Agents Chemother 47:43–47
297. Montgomerie JZ, Schick DG (1998) Treatment of enterococcal pyelonephritis with trovafloxacin and rifampin: in vitro-in vivo contrast. Antimicrob Agents Chemother 42:188–189
298. Sapico FL, Ginunas VJ, Montgomerie JZ, Canawati HN (1991) Cefpirome, alone and in combination with gentamicin for enterococcal pyelonephritis in the rodent model. Diagn Microbiol Infect Dis 14:297–300
299. Bayer AS, Greenberg DP, Yih J (1988) Correlates of therapeutic efficacy in experimental methicillin-resistant *Staphylococcus aureus* endocarditis. Chemotherapy 34:46–55
300. Baddour LM (1994) Virulence factors among gram-positive bacteria in experimental endocarditis. Infect Immun 62:2143–2148
301. Carbon C (1993) Experimental endocarditis: a review of its relevance to human endocarditis. J Antimicrob Chemother 31(Suppl D):71–85
302. Eliopoulos GM, Thauvin-Eliopoulos C, Moellering RC Jr (1992) Contribution of animal models in the search for effective therapy for endocarditis due to enterococci with high-level resistance to gentamicin. Clin Infect Dis 15:58–62
303. Gutschik E (1993) The Enterococcus endocarditis model in experimental animals and its relevance to human infection. J Antimicrob Chemother 31(Suppl D):87–95
304. Lefort A, Fantin B (1999) Rabbit model of bacterial endocarditis. In: Zak O, Sande MA (eds) Handbook of animal models of infection. Academic, San Diego, pp 611–618
305. Santoro J, Levison ME (1978) Rat model of experimental endocarditis. Infect Immun 19:915–918
306. Dube L, Caillon J, Jacqueline C, Bugnon D, Potel G, Asseray N (2012) The optimal aminoglycoside and its dosage for the treatment of severe *Enterococcus faecalis* infection. An experimental study in the rabbit endocarditis model. Eur J Clin Microbiol Infect Dis 31:2545–2547
307. Batard E, Jacqueline C, Boutoille D, Hamel A, Drugeon HB, Asseray N, Leclercq R, Caillon J, Potel G, Bugnon D (2002) Combination of quinupristin-dalfopristin and gentamicin against methicillin-resistant *Staphylococcus aureus*: experimental rabbit endocarditis study. Antimicrob Agents Chemother 46:2174–2178
308. Jacqueline C, Asseray N, Batard E, Le Mabecque V, Kergueris MF, Dube L, Bugnon D, Potel G, Caillon J (2004) In vivo efficacy of linezolid in combination with gentamicin for the treatment of experimental endocarditis due to methicillin-resistant *Staphylococcus aureus*. Int J Antimicrob Agents 24: 393–396
309. Miro JM, Garcia-de-la-Maria C, Armero Y, Soy D, Moreno A, del Rio A, Almela M, Sarasa M, Mestres CA, Gatell JM, Jimenez de Anta MT, Marco F, Hospital Clinic Experimental Endocarditis Study G (2009) Addition of gentamicin or rifampin does not enhance the effectiveness of daptomycin in treatment of experimental endocarditis due to methicillin-resistant *Staphylococcus aureus*. Antimicrob Agents Chemother 53: 172–4177

310. Navas D, Caillon J, Gras-Le Guen C, Jacqueline C, Kergueris MF, Bugnon D, Potel G (2004) Comparison of in vivo intrinsic activity of cefepime and imipenem in a *Pseudomonas aeruginosa* rabbit endocarditis model: effect of combination with tobramycin simulating human serum pharmacokinetics. J Antimicrob Chemother 54:767–771
311. Gavalda J, Torres C, Tenorio C, Lopez P, Zaragoza M, Capdevila JA, Almirante B, Ruiz F, Borrell N, Gomis X, Pigrau C, Baquero F, Pahissa A (1999) Efficacy of ampicillin plus ceftriaxone in treatment of experimental endocarditis due to *Enterococcus faecalis* strains highly resistant to aminoglycosides. Antimicrob Agents Chemother 43:639–646
312. Gavalda J, Onrubia PL, Gomez MT, Gomis X, Ramirez JL, Len O, Rodriguez D, Crespo M, Ruiz I, Pahissa A (2003) Efficacy of ampicillin combined with ceftriaxone and gentamicin in the treatment of experimental endocarditis due to *Enterococcus faecalis* with no high-level resistance to aminoglycosides. J Antimicrob Chemother 52:514–517
313. Yang SJ, Xiong YQ, Boyle-Vavra S, Daum R, Jones T, Bayer AS (2010) Daptomycin-oxacillin combinations in treatment of experimental endocarditis caused by daptomycin-nonsusceptible strains of methicillin-resistant *Staphylococcus aureus* with evolving oxacillin susceptibility (the "seesaw effect"). Antimicrob Agents Chemother 54:3161–3169
314. Tsaganos T, Skiadas I, Koutoukas P, Adamis T, Baxevanos N, Tzepi I, Pelekanou A, Giamarellos-Bourboulis EJ, Giamarellou H, Kanellakopoulou K (2008) Efficacy and pharmacodynamics of linezolid, alone and in combination with rifampicin, in an experimental model of methicillin-resistant *Staphylococcus aureus* endocarditis. J Antimicrob Chemother 62:381–383
315. Jacqueline C, Caillon J, Grossi O, Le Mabecque V, Miegeville AF, Bugnon D, Batard E, Potel G (2006) In vitro and in vivo assessment of linezolid combined with ertapenem: a highly synergistic combination against methicillin-resistant *Staphylococcus aureus*. Antimicrob Agents Chemother 50:2547–2549
316. Weinstein WM, Onderdonk AB, Bartlett JG, Louie TJ, Gorbach SL (1975) Antimicrobial therapy of experimental intraabdominal sepsis. J Infect Dis 132:282–286
317. Frimodt-Moller N, Knudsen JD (1999) The mouse peritonitis/sepsis model. In: Zak O, Sande MA (eds) Handbook of animal models of infection. Academic, San Diego, pp 127–136
318. Frimodt-Moller N (1993) The mouse peritonitis model: present and future use. J Antimicrob Chemother 31(Suppl D):55–60
319. Michea-Hamzehpour M, Pechere JC, Marchou B, Auckenthaler R (1986) Combination therapy: a way to limit emergence of resistance? Am J Med 80:138–142
320. Michea-Hamzehpour M, Auckenthaler R, Regamey P, Pechere JC (1987) Resistance occurring after fluoroquinolone therapy of experimental *Pseudomonas aeruginosa* peritonitis. Antimicrob Agents Chemother 31: 1803–1808
321. Pechere JC, Marchou B, Michea-Hamzehpour M, Auckenthaler R (1986) Emergence of resistance after therapy with antibiotics used alone or combined in a murine model. J Antimicrob Chemother 17(Suppl A): 11–18
322. Pechere JC, Vladoianu IR (1992) Development of resistance during ceftazidime and cefepime therapy in a murine peritonitis model. J Antimicrob Chemother 29:563–573
323. Marchou B, Michea-Hamzehpour M, Lucain C, Pechere JC (1987) Development of beta-lactam-resistant *Enterobacter cloacae* in mice. J Infect Dis 156:369–373
324. Lucain C, Regamey P, Bellido F, Pechere JC (1989) Resistance emerging after pefloxacin therapy of experimental *Enterobacter cloacae* peritonitis. Antimicrob Agents Chemother 33:937–943
325. Mimoz O, Gregoire N, Poirel L, Marliat M, Couet W, Nordmann P (2012) Broad-spectrum beta-lactam antibiotics for treating experimental peritonitis in mice due to *Klebsiella pneumoniae* producing the carbapenemase OXA-48. Antimicrob Agents Chemother 56:2759–2760
326. Vimont S, Aubert D, Mazoit JX, Poirel L, Nordmann P (2007) Broad-spectrum beta-lactams for treating experimental peritonitis in mice due to *Escherichia coli* producing plas mid-encoded cephalosporinases. J Antimicrob Chemother 60:1045–1050
327. Shrotri M, Peyton JC, Cheadle WG (1999) Mouse peritonitis using ceccal ligation and puncture. In: Zak O, Sande MA (eds) Handbook of animal models of infection. Academic, San Diego, pp 173–181
328. Dupont H, Montravers P (1999) Rat polymicrobial peritonitis infection model. In: Zak O, Sande MA (eds) Handbook of animal models of infection. Academic, San Diego, pp 189–194

Chapter 4

Pharmacodynamic Issues in Antibiotic Combinations

Zackery P. Bulman, Ryan C. Dillon, and Brian T. Tsuji

Abstract

For over decades, antibiotics have been used in various combinations to treat infections. From a clinical perspective a number of studies have shown that combination treatments can significantly reduce mortality in certain subsets of patients including those who are both bacteremic and severely ill. However, there is significant controversy over their current role and definitions of appropriate applications of antibiotic combinations, particularly as it to relates to pharmacodynamics and measurements of effect. The emerging health care crisis surrounding multidrug-resistant bacteria and the lack of novel antibiotics highlight the importance of optimizing these combinations. The fundamental principles of effective combination regimens are increased bactericidal activity with decreased potential for resistance selection upon treatment and to minimize exposure-associated toxicity. Furthermore, quantification of two drug's combined effect is of major importance when weighing the benefits and disadvantages of their use compared to monotherapy. Qualitative terms like synergy, additivity, or antagonism all help to categorize the nature of the interaction between two antibiotics. There has been much debate as to which definitions of drug interactions are most appropriate but the two main metrics used to help qualify the nature of the combination (or interactions between any two drugs) are Loewe additivity and Bliss independence. Overall, despite the apparent benefits of combination therapy, pharmacodynamic concerns exist about these regimens including: definitions of synergy, indifference, and antagonism; duration of studies; bacterial inoculum; model systems utilized; and a number of other issues exist. The primary objective of the chapter is to review the state of the art pharmacodynamic issues regarding antibiotic combinations.

Key words Antibiotic combinations, Pharmacokinetics, Pharmacodynamics, Synergy, Interaction

1 Introduction

Clinically, antibiotics have been used in various combinations for many years to treat infections but with mixed results when compared to monotherapy. There is conflict over their current role and a trend toward defining appropriate applications of antibiotic combinations, particularly as it relates to pharmacodynamics and measurements of effect. The emerging health care crisis surrounding multidrug-resistant bacteria and the lack of novel antibiotics highlight the importance of optimizing these combinations [1, 2].

John C. Rotschafer et al. (eds.), *Antibiotic Pharmacodynamics*, Methods in Pharmacology and Toxicology,
DOI 10.1007/978-1-4939-3323-5_4, © Springer Science+Business Media New York 2016

The fundamental principles of effective combination regimens are increased bactericidal activity (synergy or additive) with decreased potential for resistance selection upon treatment [3, 4]. Of additional benefit is decreased dose-associated toxicity of drugs. Overall, despite these apparent benefits, concerns exist about these regimens, including increased costs, more drug-related adverse events, and potential selection for superinfections [3, 5]. The primary objective of the current chapter is to review the state of the art pharmacodynamic issues of antibiotic combinations.

2 Defining the Rationale for Combination Therapy: What Is the Mortality Benefit?

Before one analyzes the rationale for utilizing a combination therapy from a pharmacodynamics perspective, it is critical to understand the original tenants of combination therapy from a mortality benefit perspective. Such an understanding is important to assess the effectiveness and importance of combination regimens in clinical practice through a review of studies that have assessed the mortality benefit of multiple antibiotics vs. monotherapy. Analysis of published literature allows us the greatest insight into when antibiotic combinations can have the maximum impact on survival in addition to the pharmacodynamics issues. Generally, these studies have shown that combination treatments can significantly reduce mortality in certain subsets of patients including those who are both bacteremic and severely ill [6–9]. Meta-analyses investigating antibiotic combinations have consistently shown that antibiotic combinations generally do not demonstrate a mortality benefit in comparison to monotherapy in infectious processes such as ventilator-associated pneumonia (VAP) and gram-negative bacteremia [5, 10]. However, early combination therapy has been shown to significantly reduce mortality in critically ill patients with bacterial pathogens with the potential to display multidrug resistance [5, 7–9, 11].

Safdar et al. conducted a meta-analysis investigating combination antimicrobial therapy in reduction of mortality during gram-negative bacteremia [5]. The authors examined 17 studies including 3077 patients that met their inclusion criteria of documented gram-negative bacteremia and single or multiple antibiotics with mortality as a primary outcome. The summary odds ratio (OR) was calculated to be 0.96 (95 % CI 0.70–1.32), which established their conclusion that there is no overall mortality benefit of combination antibiotics vs. monotherapy in documented gram-negative bacteremia. The authors challenged their results by exploring specific subgroups to determine the authenticity of their conclusion. They questioned whether the design of the studies and those published before 1990, where less potent gram-negative antibiotics were available, would change the outcome of their study. The investigators found no significant difference in these subgroups. Interestingly, when only looking at the five studies that examined specifically *Pseudomonas* spp. bacteremia, there was a significant reduction in mortality when the patient was started on combination antibiotics vs. monotherapy [OR 0.50 (95 % CI 0.2–0.79)], with an approximate 50 % reduction in mortality observed. The authors concluded that there may not be mortality benefit when using combination antibiotics in suspected gram-negative bacteremia except in the case of documented or presumed *Pseudomonas* spp. infection. This could possibly be attributed to the resilience of *Pseudomonas* spp. and its characteristic multidrug-resistant strains [12]. Therefore, it may be of benefit to start combination antibiotics on patients with previously documented or suspected bacteremia with *Pseudomonas* spp.

Baddour et al. conducted a prospective, observational study assessing 592 patients 15 years or older with bacteremia due to *Streptococcus pneumoniae*, where the primary outcome was mortality at 14 days [6]. Monotherapy was compared to combination therapy and there was no significant difference in mortality (10.4 % vs. 11.5 %, p=NS). When the investigators looked at the patients who presented with a Pitt bacteremia score >4 there was a significant reduction in mortality at 14 days for the patients treated with combination antibiotics (23.4 % vs. 55.3 %, p=0.0015) (Fig. 1).

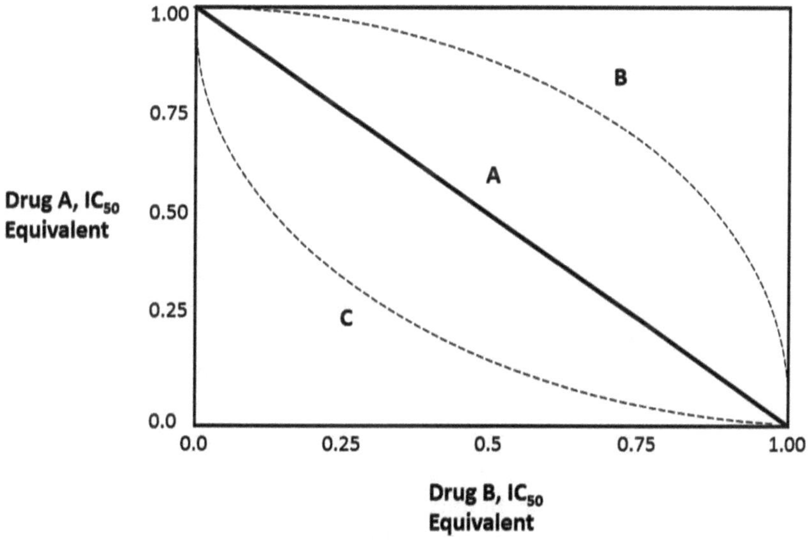

Fig. 1 Isobologram analysis. *Line A* is the line of additivity which connects the independent concentrations of drug A and drug B that are required to generate the designated effect (IC_{50}). *Lines B* and *C* represent experimental data points which indicate antagonism and synergism of the drug combination, respectively. Experimental data points falling on *line A* would indicate additivity

This study concludes that patients with *Streptococcus pneumoniae* bacteremia may not benefit from combination antimicrobials in terms of mortality. However, the patients included who were deemed critically ill with this bacteremia as described by a Pitt bacteremia score greater than 4 had a significant mortality benefit when treated with a combination of antibiotics vs. monotherapy. This is consistent with the general conclusion that critically ill patients see more benefit when combination antibiotics are started empirically.

Correlating to the previous conclusions, two other studies evaluated the mortality advantage of early combination antimicrobials in septic shock patients as defined as systemic inflammatory response syndrome (SIRS) criteria with a source of infection and hypotension despite adequate fluid resuscitation [8, 13, 14]. Kumar et al. designed a retrospective, propensity-matched cohort study with 4662 eligible cases and 1223 propensity-matched pairs generated [8]. The primary outcome was 28-day mortality. The study was restricted to antibiotic combinations that included beta-lactams with aminoglycosides, fluoroquinolones, or macrolides/clindamycin. There was a significant reduction in hospital mortality related to combination antibiotics vs. monotherapy [47.8 % vs. 37.4 %, OR 0.69 (95 % CI 0.59–0.81, $p < 0.0001$)]. Of note the trial was limited by the nature of the retrospective design and the inability to account for unknown confounders. The study does however raise the possibility of antibiotic combinations being superior to monotherapy in critically ill patients and acknowledges the need for randomized controlled trials. Their conclusion does concur with other publications regarding its benefit in the severely ill population we have visited.

Rodriguez et al. designed a prospective obervational cohort study in 529 patients who required ICU admission for community-acquired pneumonia with the primary outcome of 28-day mortality [13]. They found that mortality was similar for patients receiving combination antimicrobials vs. monotherapy. When the authors analyzed the subgroup of patients who presented with clinically defined septic shock they found a significant reduction in 28-day mortality when combination antimicrobials were used [hazard ratio (HR), 1.69 (95 % CI 1.09–2.60, $p = 0.01$)]. This again adds to the evidence of the mortality benefit in the critically ill.

At this point we have examined some of the published literature surrounding the use of combination antimicrobials vs. monotherapy and have seen that the mortality benefit seems to lie within the severely ill and critically unstable patient populations. Most of the current studies that have examined the non-critically ill patients with community-acquired infections find that monotherapy can be sufficient in comparison to combination therapy. There is insufficient evidence to broadly determine that combination is superior in community-acquired infections [5, 15, 16]. We can extrapolate that concept to the theory that community-acquired pathogens are generally more susceptible to current antimicrobials. When evaluating critically ill patients with the possibility of multidrug-resistant pathogens, the need for adequate coverage utilizing combination antimicrobials that attack the pathogen at multiple sites appears to be increased [5, 11].

Determining whether to empirically start a combination of antibiotics requires individual assessment of the clinical picture. Some risk factors will encourage the use of multidrug regimens in order to ensure proper spectrum coverage of the infectious process. Additionally, patient characteristics such as host defenses, site of infection, perceived inoculum, and clinical presentation (e.g., age, vital signs, mental status) should be evaluated during the decision-making process. Antimicrobial properties should also be carefully considered, such as the pharmacokinetics (PK)/pharmacodynamics (PD) of the individual drugs as well as how these can fluctuate when combination regimens are utilized. There is satisfactory data to support the mortality benefit of empiric antibiotic combinations in severe infections especially when resilient pathogens are suspected.

Highlighting the effectiveness and importance of combination regimens in clinical practice are recent studies that have assessed the mortality benefit of multiple antibiotics vs. monotherapy. Generally, these studies have shown that combination treatments can significantly reduce mortality in certain subsets of patients including those who are both bacteremic and severely ill [6, 7]. Early combination therapy has also been shown to reduce mortality in patients with suspected *P. aeruginosa* infections or sepsis [5, 8, 9]. Collectively, these studies are critical to appreciate the pharmacodynamic issues of combination therapy.

3 General Principles of Antibiotic Combination Therapy Considering Pharmacodynamics

Clinically, antibiotics have been utilized in various combinations for many years to treat infections, but with mixed results when compared to monotherapy. Consequently, there is much debate concerning their role in therapy and a trend toward defining appropriate applications of antibiotic combinations. As the crisis involving multidrug-resistant bacteria escalates and the deficit of novel antibiotic agents persists, the significance of optimizing combination therapy becomes evident [1, 2]. The effectiveness of combination regimens is based on the fundamental principles of increased bactericidal activity (either synergistic or additive) and the decreased potential for resistance [3, 4]. Additionally, we see the benefit of decreased dose-associated toxicity, as observed with nephrotoxic drugs such as vancomycin and aminoglycosides as a result of lowered doses when used in combination. Regardless of these apparent benefits, concerns still exist surrounding the higher costs, increased drug-related adverse events, and potential selection for superinfection [3, 5].

Synergistic activity, a quality that is determined in vitro, results in the concurrent use of two antimicrobial agents having a greater collective effect than the sum of their respective activity measured independently [17]. A hallmark example of a combination that exhibits synergy is the use of β-lactams with aminoglycosides, which has been proven to be effective against various gram-positive and gram-negative organisms [18]. These two drug classes in particular have found great utility in the treatment of serious infections such as endocarditis where rapid killing of the invading organism is imperative. The mechanism behind the concerted activity of β-lactams and aminoglycosides is inherently complex as a direct result of the complicated mechanisms of action of the individual drugs. Simply put, β-lactams are able to make the bacterial cell wall permeable enough for the aminoglycosides to penetrate them and inhibit protein synthesis. This relationship is critical when the β-lactams may not be sufficient to exclusively kill the organisms and can only cause nonlethal damage and/or if the aminoglycosides are unable to independently permeate the cell wall to carry out its desired effect. Even in cases where both agents demonstrate individual efficacy, synergy is still observable since the drugs work through different pathways and are able to attack the organism from different angles. It is important to note that both of these drugs are considered to be bactericidal agents rather than bacteriostatic, a factor which is postulated to play a role in whether a combination will be synergistic, antagonistic, or additive [19]. These assumptions are also based upon the mechanisms of the agents that fall under those categories. It is proposed that when a bactericidal drug which acts on actively multiplying organisms is combined with a bacteriostatic agent which prevents multiplication, the action of the bactericidal agent becomes nullified. Conversely, two bactericidal agents would destroy multiplying bacteria through different pathways creating a synergistic affect and two bacteriostatic agents would likely result in additive effects. However, we must also consider that this definition is not fixed and can vary for an antibiotic depending on the bacteria as demonstrated in the aforementioned example where the β-lactam was not sufficient to kill the organism and displayed characteristics that were primarily bacteriostatic.

In addition to providing augmented efficacy, combination antibiotic therapy offers the benefit of combatting the emergence of resistance. The rise of antibiotic-resistant bacteria has become a considerable challenge to physicians and pharmacists alike, whom are faced with not only increasingly resistant organisms, but also a lack of new agents to eliminate them [1]. Ironically, antibiotics themselves are primarily responsible for the development of resistance as they created an environment with selective pressures that was conducive to the evolution of these resilient strains [17]. Bearing in mind the complex metabolism of bacteria, it is easy to see how a rapidly dividing, unicellular organism can transform in a manner that makes it elusive to the mechanisms of existing antibiotics [19]. A single change in the metabolic pathway during a course of treatment can result in the depletion of the sensitive strain with continued administration while creating a population of entirely resistant organisms. Combination therapy has the potential to avoid such a situation when using antimicrobials with varied mechanisms of action, thereby restricting the number of pathways through which the organism can evade elimination [17]. This principle is critical in the treatment of chronic diseases such as the human immunodeficiency virus (HIV) where indefinite treatment durations foster an ideal environment for resistance and pharmacologic agents are limited. In such cases, combination therapy has become the standard of treatment. Despite its utility in suppressing the incidence of resistance, we must exercise caution in utilizing combination therapy to avoid the development of increasingly resistant strains. Although some situations call for the empiric use of combination antibiotics, there are instances where there is no proven benefit to using more than one agent [9, 20]. It is pertinent for clinicians to be familiar with antimicrobial susceptibility in their geographic area in order to appropriately implement combination antibiotic therapy.

4 Definitions of Synergy to Evaluate Antibiotic Pharmacodynamics

Quantification of two drug's combined effect is of major importance when weighing the benefits and disadvantages of their use compared to monotherapy. Qualitative terms like synergy, additivity, or antagonism all help to categorize the nature of the interaction between two antibiotics. There has been much debate as to which definitions of drug interactions are most appropriate but the two main metrics used to help qualify the nature of the combination (or interactions between any two drugs) are Loewe additivity and Bliss independence [21].

4.1 Loewe Additivity

Loewe additivity is one of the two main reference models used to analyze drug-drug interactions and is founded on the principle that a drug cannot act synergistically with itself or another drug similar in nature [22, 23]. Loewe additivity is defined as the magnitude of the effect when an agent is added onto itself. For example, if drugs "A" and "B" are the same or close in structure, the activity of "A" when used in combination with "B" at the same concentration will be the same as using twice as much drug "A." In other words, both drugs must have linearly proportional increases in their magnitude of inhibition for increasing doses of the drugs in order to be considered additive. Isoboles, or lines of constant inhibition, are measured by obtaining pharmacodynamic data in a two-dimensional range of dosages for the drugs. Thus, Loewe synergism is defined as a magnitude of effect greater than that expected by the additivity principle when two unique compounds are used in combination. It is this principle that is also the basis of more contemporary methods of analyzing drug interactions including isobologram analysis, combination index analysis, and curve shift analysis. Isobologram analysis (*see* Fig. 2) looks at interactions between two drugs at a fixed effect level (i.e., 50 %) and compares drug concentrations required to achieve that effect level alone and in combination with one another [24]. Combination experiments are run and the concentrations of each drug at which some fixed effect level (i.e., 50 %) is achieved are determined. Experimental data falling above the line of additivity is interpreted as antagonism, data falling on the line is considered additivity, and data below the line is synergism.

The next drug interaction analyzing method is the combination index (CI) which is calculated by the equation below where $C_{A,x}$ and $C_{B,x}$ are the concentrations of drugs A and B used in combination that attain a predetermined effect level ("x"). $IC_{x,A}$ and $IC_{x,B}$ are the concentrations of drug A and B monotherapy, each attained at the same effect level, "x" [25]. A CI value of 1 indicates additivity, CI > 1 indicates antagonism, and a CI < 1 indicates synergism. It has been considered the simplest way of quantifying synergism or antagonism of compounds given the simplicity of its equation, efficient data analysis, and ability to reduce trial size:

$$\mathrm{CI} = \frac{C_{\mathrm{A,x}}}{\mathrm{IC}_{\mathrm{x,A}}} + \frac{C_{\mathrm{B,x}}}{\mathrm{IC}_{\mathrm{x,B}}}$$

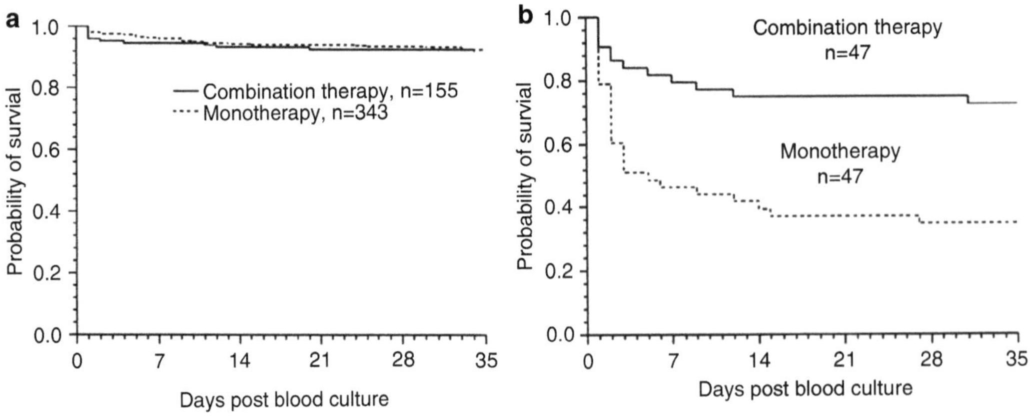

Fig. 2 (**a**) Kaplan-Meier survival plot for patients with pneumococcal bacteremia and a Pitt bacteremia score ≤4. (**b**) Kaplan-Meier survival plot for patients with pneumococcal bacteremia and with a Pitt bacteremia score >4 (Baddour et al. 2014).

Curve shift analysis is another method of evaluating for the presence of Loewe synergy. Two-dimensional graphs are formed which plot the experimental concentration normalized to the IC_{50} value vs. effect of two agents, "A" and "B," alone and in combination at a variety of ratios [23]. The data are then fit to the Hill equation by nonlinear regression. Shift of the curves to the left for the combination of "A" and "B" defines synergy in this analysis model where a shift to the right would be defined as antagonism of two interacting drugs (Fig. 3).

4.2 Bliss Independence

Bliss independence is a second major reference model used to interpret drug combination interactions. Bliss independence is founded on the principle that two drugs will not interact with one another but can each contribute to a common pharmacodynamic endpoint [26]. For antibiotics to be considered Bliss independent, the product of growth inhibition by each drug measured independently should be equal to the effect seen when the two drugs are used together at the same concentrations [27]. For example, Bliss independent drugs "A" and "B" both cause 25 % inhibition of bacterial growth independently and in combination they cause a decrease in growth of $(0.25+0.25)-0.25\times0.25$ which is equal to 43.75 %. If the pharmacodynamic studies show that inhibition is greater than this threshold, it would be considered synergistic, while a value less than 43.75 % would be antagonistic.

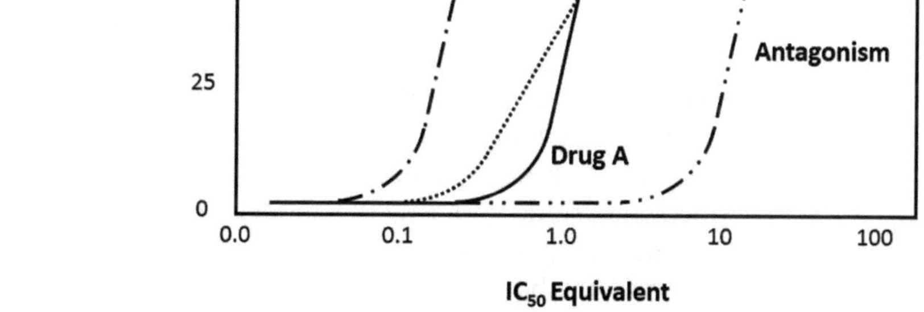

Fig. 3 Analysis synergy. The *solid line* labeled as "Drug A" and *dotted line* labeled "Drug B" show the fitted Hill function for experimental data of each when given as monotherapy. *Dashed lines*, "Synergism" and "Antagonism," represent the interaction of drugs "A" and "B" and their activity relative to the agents acting alone

5 Traditional Methods of Evaluating Synergism in In Vitro Studies: Pharmacodynamic Advantages and Disadvantages

5.1 In Vitro Studies

In vitro studies are often used to study combination therapies with the goal of defining the interaction using either the Loewe additivity or Bliss independence model. Determining the best method to define such interactions depends on the experimental system used [21, 28]. When using the checkerboard method to analyze antibiotic combinations, the fractional inhibitory concentration (FIC) index is used. Briefly, the checkerboard method requires serial dilution of two drugs into every well of a microdilution plate which each contains a specific inoculum of bacterial cells in liquid media. The plates are then incubated and the MIC measured with the naked eye as the first well that completely inhibited bacterial growth. The FIC is calculated as seen below [28]:

$$\text{FIC index} = \frac{\text{MIC of drug A in combination}}{\text{MIC of drug A alone}} + \frac{\text{MIC of drug B in combination}}{\text{MIC of drug B alone}}$$

The literature suggests various definitions for synergy with this method but it has traditionally been defined as an FIC index of ≤0.5. Additivity is described by an FIC index of 1.0, and antagonism as an FIC index of 2.0. However, more recent analysis has shown that an FIC index of >4 should be considered the cutoff of antagonism given imprecision of the technique and because an FIC index of 2.0 is probably more indicative of an indifferent effect [29]. As common as the checkerboard method is, it is still less discriminatory than other more sophisticated in vitro methods (e.g., static or PK/PD time-kill models) for assessing the interactions of antimicrobial agents [30–32]. E-test results are not always concordant with checkerboard or time-kill methods, which are also used to test for synergy [33, 34].

Time-kill methods can have advantages over other methods used to assess synergy such as the checkerboard technique or E-test method. Primarily, the time-kill method measures the bactericidal activity of the combination being tested at many points over time (viable counts; CFU/mL), whereas the checkerboard technique provides only inhibitory data and usually from a single time point (after 16–24 h of incubation) [28]. Time-kill models can be subdivided into static and PK/PD models. In static time-kill models, with the exception of a small degree of loss in drug activity due to bacterial metabolism or inactivation, bacteria are exposed to static (fixed) concentrations of an antibacterial agent over a defined period of time. In PK/PD models [35, 36], the most common of which is the one-compartment model, the test organism is presented with a dynamic concentration of drug designed to mimic in vivo PK. PK/PD models typically consist of a central reservoir containing the organism, a diluent reservoir, and a waste reservoir. Drug is added to the central reservoir to achieve the desired peak concentration and the elimination profile is mimicked by addition of sterile, drug-free media to the central reservoir and removal of an equal volume of drug-containing media into the waste reservoir; various adaptations of this standard model are available to simultaneously mimic the in vivo PK of two or more drugs with differing half-lives [37].

Synergy combinations have traditionally been defined as a 100-fold increase in killing, a ≥2-log_{10} lower CFU/mL, relative to its most active component at 24 h for static and PK/PD time-kill methods [28]. Antagonism is defined by the opposite of the expression for synergism where a 100-fold decrease, a ≥2-log_{10} higher CFU/mL, in killing at 24 h with the combination compared with the most active single drug alone is antagonistic. In theory, these definitions should require that at least one of the drugs being tested produces minimal to no significant inhibition or killing alone so you are basically able to assess the addition of an inactive compound to a more bactericidal antibiotic. Criteria have yet to be created to allow evaluation of interactions when using two or more drugs when each has activity alone. Consequently, these same definitions for synergy are often used for all time-kill experiments given the lack of an appropriate alternative even when there are multiple drugs which display significant bacterial killing. Many variations exist in the literature making comparison between studies difficult. As an example, synergy is sometimes reported as described above, with the added qualification that the number of surviving organisms in the presence of the combination must be ≥2-log_{10} CFU/mL below the starting inoculum which may alter some combinations previously defined as synergistic [38–42]. As such, it is important to pay close attention when interpreting time-kill experiment results and comparing them to other studies. Static and PK/PD time-kill experiments both provide more granular data than either the checkerboard or E-test methods and when analyzed appropriately can help to predict the time course of the combination's pharmacodynamic effect.

6 Pharmacodynamic Analysis and Mathematical Modeling Issues in Antibiotic Combinations

Analysis of combinations using the basic definitions of synergy, additivity, or antagonism is simple and convenient, yet not without significant limitations. A significant drawback of using simple static metrics and definitions of drug combinations is that the labels do not always describe the interactions appropriately and lack the clinical and translational applicability to ensure mortality benefit in critically ill patients with difficult-to-treat infections. For example, a combination that is labeled as synergistic that does not result in a good clinical outcome may not be meaningful. Similarly, antagonistic interactions do not always suggest an unfavorable outcome, and in some instances may be beneficial. The following examples will help illustrate the drawbacks of the basic classification method.

Linezolid is a synthetic antibacterial agent of the oxazolidinone class and inhibits protein synthesis at the 50S ribosome site. Nisin, a rapidly killing peptide antibiotic, works by inducing pore formation in the bacterial membrane and also inhibiting peptidoglycan synthesis. In an in vitro study, linezolid and nisin were dosed simultaneously against a simulated high-inoculum MRSA infection and pharmacodynamic activity based purely on definition suggested little benefit of the combination [43]. Based on the definition of Bliss independence, this combination was considered additive. The combination's classification as additive and not synergistic is misleading though because linezolid may be helpful to prolong bacterial replication time making other antibiotics more effective. It is also important given some of the limitations of spectrum for linezolid against certain gram-negative and anaerobic bacteria that it can work with other antibiotics without antagonizing their effect [44].

Antagonism in drug combinations is usually portrayed negatively but the combination of rifampicin and vancomycin is a perfect example of how it can be useful clinically. Rifampicin is a bactericidal semisynthetic derivative of the rifamycins class of antibiotics that inhibits bacterial RNA polymerase responsible for DNA transcription whereas vancomycin is a glycopeptide antibiotic that primarily inhibits cell-wall biosynthesis. In vitro studies have traditionally defined this combination as antagonistic based on the Bliss independence model but more recent analysis shows that it may actually be an independent combination [45, 46]. Despite its negative classification as either an antagonistic or an independent combination, it is still of clinical utility as adjunctive therapy when treating certain acute *S. aureus* infections as it may help prevent the emergence of resistance or reduce the signs and symptoms of virulence among others.

The presence of synergy is not always the prediction of success just like antagonism, independence, or additivity are not always predictors of combination failure. Two antibiotics with independently low bactericidal capacities could have synergy together as defined by the static models but this would likely not be predictive of a good clinical response. Grouping combinations based on simplified labels like antagonism, synergy, or additivity are often helpful but still may misrepresent the outcome of the interaction between the agents. Being labeled as synergistic or additive is only as valuable as its ability to accurately predict pharmacodynamic activity based on that type of interaction. Part of this failure may be due to the exclusion of mechanistic information which would allow for a fuller understanding of how drugs interact to promote their combined effects. Given the inadequate representation of synergy by these basic models, newer approaches have sought to better define activity of antibiotic combinations.

Traditional methods that look at the 24-h time point to assess the bactericidal activity of the combination fail to take into consideration the entire time course of synergistic killing or of resistance prevention. Qualitative approaches used to describe the time course of antibiotic combinations are scarce [47]. In vitro and mathematical modeling can provide data throughout the time course of treatment allowing for a more accurate description of the interaction between two antibiotics in combination. Analysis of these methods can be done with the log ratio area formula. Assessment of the combination can be made using the living bacterial density measurements (CFU) from throughout the time course for the samples grown with the more active antibiotic (consider drug "A" to be the more active antibiotic) and those grown with both antibiotics in combination (drugs "A" and "B"). These measurements will be used to make the determination of area under the CFU curve for the duration of the experiment (consider the example experimental duration to be 48 h; thus $AUCFU_{0-48}$). This calculation will employ the use of the trapezoidal rule. Comparison of the calculated AUCFU of the combination sample to that of the control (drug "A" monotherapy) will enable us to approximate the effect by using the log ratio area equation below. The log ratio area formula shows the log-transformed decrease in area under the entire time course CFU curve for a specified set of concentrations of antibiotics relative to the absence of one of the antibiotics. The log ratio area formula provides more robust analysis when for example compared to taking the log difference at the 24-h time point as it accounts for the drug's killing effect throughout the entire experiment:

$$\text{Log ratio area} = \log_{10}\left(\frac{\text{AUCFU}_{\text{drug}}}{\text{AUCFU}_{\text{control}}}\right)$$

Antibiotic failure due to evolution and persistence of heterogeneous subpopulations is a major concern. Failing to account for the small subpopulation of bacteria that are not susceptible to a chosen antibiotic therapy can lead to a selective pressure in favor of the resistant strain. For example, the prevalence of heterogeneous VISA (hVISA) in MRSA infections is reported to be 1.67 %, so treatment failure would be anticipated in all of these patients if vancomycin monotherapy is selected [48]. Traditional synergy definitions will not sufficiently account for the additional suppression or killing by an antibiotic whose bacterial target may only comprise <1 % of the overall infection and may classify these combinations as either additive or independent. It is important not to overlook their benefit based simply on these classical, static definitions. Recent analysis has described this type of antibiotic combination, where one agent is added to attack a specific subset of less susceptible organisms, as subpopulation synergy (Fig. 4) [43]. A better understanding of the role of subpopulation synergy in predicting antibiotic pharmacodynamics is required before it can practically be applied in the clinical setting.

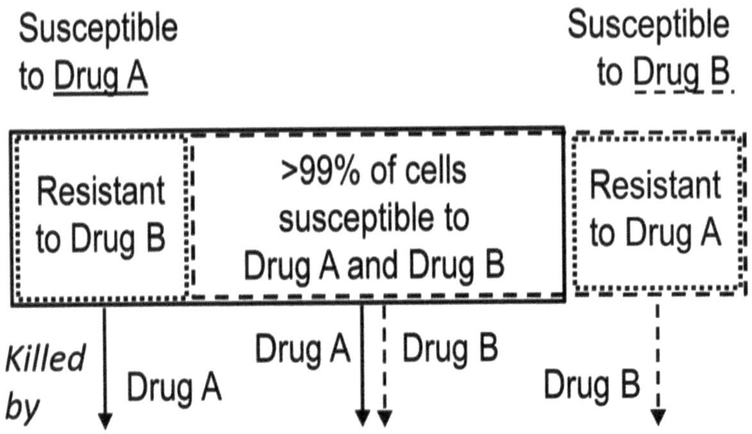

Fig. 4 Subpopulation synergy concept depicting combination treatment with drugs "A" and "B" against a population of bacteria to which there is a subpopulation susceptible to "A" (*inside solid rectangle*) and a second susceptible to "B" (*long dashed lines*). Bacteria in either of the *dotted line boxes* are resistant to either drug "A" or "B." Without drug "B," the subpopulation that is resistant to drug "A" would be selected for and cause a persistent and resistant infection. Adapted with permission from Landersdorfer et al. [43]

7 Innovative Strategies to Combination Treatment

There are many novel approaches to combination regimens that aim to focus the effort of antibiotic killing on the nature of the infection. Of important consideration in these approaches is the severity of the infection, density or starting inoculum, and behavior or communication within the bacterial population. Not all types of infections will warrant or benefit from multiple antibiotic treatment. Therefore, considering the specific infections and their mechanisms of progression and human mortality can help to limit combination use to patients who can most benefit.

Short-course combination therapy using 2 weeks of gentamicin has been successful in severe infections with high density such as with infective endocarditis [49, 50]. The nature of infective endocarditis as a sequestered, high-inoculum infection lends itself well to early antibiotic combination treatment. With focuses to prevent resistance and achieve rapid and sustainable bactericidal activity, these types of infections can particularly benefit from combinations [51]. However, in an attempt to achieve maximal killing while reducing drug-induced nephrotoxicity associated with aminoglycosides and vancomycin, shorter duration regimens would be optimal. Studies have shown that a single high dose of gentamicin (5 mg/kg) on the first day of treatment for simulated *Staphylococcus aureus* infective endocarditis with either daptomycin or vancomycin resulted in early enhanced killing (within 4 h) and may be of benefit to gain synergy while minimizing toxicity [52]. This is an example of a 'pulse' combination regimen, which provides intentionally high doses of one antibiotic agent (ie. gentamicin) in short duration at the start of therapy but ultimately with lower overall exposure than traditional dosing while maintaining normal doses of the second, principal, antibiotic (ie. daptomycin or vancomycin).

Although not fully understood, it is thought that these pulse combinations may act synergistically by killing susceptible organisms within a heterogeneous population immediately reducing the inoculum to a more manageable concentration. Recent criticism of synergistic combination regimens may also support the use of initial brief periods of multiple agents before quickly reducing to monotherapy so as to prevent the evolution of prominently multidrug-resistant populations [53].

Additionally, it may be useful to front-load antibiotic combination regimens, similar in concept to the standard azithromycin dosing, where you can start by treating a patient with higher doses of one or multiple drugs and then subsequently reduce them to lessen exposure and help to prevent toxicity. This differs from 'pulse' dosing in that you do not discontinue either antibiotic immediately after the loading dose. In using a loading dose, you can achieve a high C_{max} for a brief period of time which will help to drive early killing, especially for antibiotics considered to be concentration dependent. Antibiotics which are rapidly bactericidal and have concentration dependent bacterial killing that are active against high bacterial density, such as the polymyxin class, linezolid or daptomycin, make good candidates for front loading regimen exploration.Linezolid frontloaded regimens have shown promise where simulated doses of either 1,200 mg every 12 hours for 5 days or 2,400 mg every 12 hours for 5 days followed by 300 mg every 12 hours for each case sustained bacterial killing against MRSA in vitro [63]. Since overall exposure to linezolid in this example is significantly higher than when it is traditionally dosed, assessment of front-loaded combinations may be useful in an attempt to maintain early killing while reducing risk for dose associated toxicities. Polymyxins, formerly abandoned due to dose limiting toxicity, are now commonly used as salvage regimens of multidrug resistant gram-negative infections. It could be important to start a higher initial dose for drugs like colistin methanesulfonate (polymyxin E) which have relatively low clinically achievable plasma concentrations [64]. Although, using a front-loaded colistin methanesulfonate monotherapy regimen against P. aeruginosa may not be sufficient for complete bacterial reduction in critically ill patients and combination with other antibiotics such as doripenem, which has shown the ability to achieve substantially improved bacterial killing profiles in vitro compared to monotherapy, may be required [65]. In this case, an additional antibiotic with synergistic killing activity is thought to sustain the killing initiated by front-loaded colistin methanesulfonate [66]. Patients with renal or hepatic dysfunction that may have trouble clearing or metabolizing an antibiotic may especially benefit from a front-loaded regimen since the dosing frequency is already likely to be reduced. It is important to consider starting a higher initial dose for drugs like colistin which have relatively low clinically achievable plasma concentrations [54]. Using a front-loaded colistin regimen against *P. aeruginosa* as monotherapy may not be sufficient for complete bacterial reduction in critically ill patients and combination with doripenem achieved substantially improved bacterial killing profiles in vitro [55]. In this case, an additional antibiotic with synergistic killing activity is thought to sustain the killing achieved by front-loaded colistin [56]. In general, front-loaded antibiotic combinations are most likely to be useful for patients that require antibiotics with a poor pharmacokinetic profile and/or have toxic adverse event profiles since you are increasing C_{max} while maintaining similar *f*AUC values [56].

Although synergy in microbiology is traditionally defined by increased bactericidal activity, broadening the interpretation to incorporate other antimicrobial targets of therapy such as bacterial virulence may ultimately allow us to improve treatment outcomes. Virulence is the degree of pathogenicity of a microbe which is determined by its ability to harm the host organism or cause disease. *Pseudomonas aeruginosa* controls many of its virulence factors by the density-dependent cell-cell method of communication known as quorum sensing (QS). The QS system in gram-negative infections employs small, self-generated, diffusible *N*-acyl l-homoserine lactone (AHLs) signaling molecules which activate transcriptional regulators to promote synthesis of virulence factors among others (biofilm formation, cell aggregation, swarming motility, exopolysaccharide formation, etc.). These virulence factors governed by this mechanism include elastase, alkaline protease, phosphatase, exotoxin A, rhamnolipids, pyocyanin, and lactin-binding protein [57, 58]. Deficiency in the QS mechanism and resultant reductions in virulence factor synthesis have been shown to reduce time to mortality and decrease rates of pneumonia and bacteremia in the murine model [58, 59]. Studies have also shown that QS is a realistic target for virulence attenuation adding credence to the argument that it may be appropriate to add synergy to combination antibiotic regimens under a more broad multiple mechanism-based definition [60, 61]. Therefore, adding antibiotics to modulate virulence and not strictly for additive bactericidal activity is of potential value in virulent infections. While the specific mechanism may differ, treatment of *S. aureus* which uses a peptide-based QS system to control virulence and *Acinetobacter baumannii*, whose QS control on virulence has not been well defined, may also benefit from these concepts [60, 62].

Azithromycin has been used for years with success in cystic fibrosis patients that have chronic *P. aeruginosa* colonization in order to reduce inflammation despite its intrinsic lack of bactericidal activity. Although the mechanism of its benefit has never been completely identified it has been suggested that it is likely at least in part due to its ability to inhibit virulence [63]. Here we use azithromycin to exemplify multiple mechanism synergy in the treatment of *P. aeruginosa* infections. Azithromycin is a macrolide antibiotic that inhibits protein synthesis by binding to the 50S subunit of the bacterial ribosome. Traditionally, azithromycin is not used in the treatment of *P. aeruginosa* given its lack of bactericidal or bacteriostatic activity [64]. Its QS-specific inhibition of virulence is likely the result of interference with AHL signal synthesis. Azithromycin has been shown to reduce QS-gene expression in tracheal aspirates of patients colonized by *P. aeruginosa* and although the population analysis of these patients suggests a trend toward the more virulent wild type after treatment, no direct measure of virulence was made [61]. Additionally, if used in the treatment of an acute *P. aeruginosa* infection that is to be completely eradicated, such as in hospital-acquired pneumonia, population evolution will not impact outcomes as they could in persistent colonizations. Since azithromycin lacks bactericidal activity against *P. aeruginosa* alone, it must be used in addition to another antibiotic such as piperacillin-tazobactam, a carbapenem or an anti-pseudomonal cephalosporin which can make up for its lack of killing. The benefit to an azithromycin combination regimen against *P. aeruginosa* has yet to be defined clinically but limited in vitro data suggests that it may add bactericidal activity in addition to the potential for reduced virulence. One in vitro study showed additive effects in combination with colistin, but virulence was not measured [65]. Other studies have shown that azithromycin may have a role in combination therapy for multidrug-resistant *P. aeruginosa* where azithromycin with tobramycin, doxycycline, trimethoprim, polymyxin B, or rifampin has also resulted in increased activity [4, 66, 67]. In order to improve our knowledge regarding combination regimens and their clinical effectiveness moving forward, it will be important to consider multiple mechanism synergy. Looking beyond basic measures and definitions of synergy may lead to novel combination dosing strategies and more studies are warranted.

References

1. Boucher HW, Talbot GH, Bradley JS, Edwards JE, Gilbert D, Rice LB et al (2009) Bad bugs, no drugs: no ESKAPE! An update from the Infectious Diseases Society of America. Clin Infect Dis 48(1):1–12. doi:10.1086/595011, Epub 2008/11/28
2. Payne DJ, Gwynn MN, Holmes DJ, Pompliano DL (2007) Drugs for bad bugs: confronting the challenges of antibacterial discovery. Nat Rev Drug Discov 6(1):29–40. doi:10.1038/nrd2201, Epub 2006/12/13
3. Moore NM, Flaws ML (2011) Treatment strategies and recommendations for Pseudomonas aeruginosa infections. Clin Lab Sci 24(1):52–56, Epub 2011/03/17
4. Rahal JJ (2006) Novel antibiotic combinations against infections with almost completely resistant Pseudomonas aeruginosa and Acinetobacter species. Clin Infect Dis 43(Suppl 2):S95–S99. doi:10.1086/504486, Epub 2006/08/09
5. Safdar N, Handelsman J, Maki DG (2004) Does combination antimicrobial therapy reduce mortality in Gram-negative bacteraemia? A meta-analysis. Lancet Infect Dis 4(8):519–527
6. Baddour LM, Yu VL, Klugman KP, Feldman C, Ortqvist A, Rello J et al (2004) Combination antibiotic therapy lowers mortality among severely ill patients with pneumococcal bacteremia. Am J Respir Crit Care Med 170(4):440–

444. doi:10.1164/rccm.200311-1578OC, Epub 2004/06/09

7. Korvick JA, Bryan CS, Farber B, Beam TR Jr, Schenfeld L, Muder RR et al (1992) Prospective observational study of Klebsiella bacteremia in 230 patients: outcome for antibiotic combinations versus monotherapy. Antimicrob Agents Chemother 36(12):2639–2644, Epub 1992/12/11. PubMed Central PMCID: PMC245520
8. Kumar A, Zarychanski R, Light B, Parrillo J, Maki D, Simon D et al (2010) Early combination antibiotic therapy yields improved survival compared with monotherapy in septic shock: a propensity-matched analysis. Crit Care Med 38(9):1773–1785. doi:10.1097/CCM.0b013e3181eb3ccd, Epub 2010/07/20
9. Micek ST, Welch EC, Khan J, Pervez M, Doherty JA, Reichley RM et al (2010) Empiric combination antibiotic therapy is associated with improved outcome against sepsis due to Gram-negative bacteria: a retrospective analysis. Antimicrob Agents Chemother 54(5): 1742–1748. doi:10.1128/AAC.01365-09, Epub 2010/02/18. PubMed Central PMCID: PMC2863648
10. Aarts MA, Hancock JN, Heyland D, McLeod RS, Marshall JC (2008) Empiric antibiotic therapy for suspected ventilator-associated pneumonia: a systematic review and meta-analysis of randomized trials. Crit Care Med 36(1):108–117. doi:10.1097/01.CCM.0000297956.27474.9D, Epub 2007/11/17
11. Tumbarello M, Viale P, Viscoli C, Trecarichi EM, Tumietto F, Marchese A et al (2012) Predictors of mortality in bloodstream infections caused by Klebsiella pneumoniae carbapenemase-producing K. pneumoniae: importance of combination therapy. Clin Infect Dis 55(7):943–950. doi:10.1093/cid/cis588, Epub 2012/07/04
12. Lister PD, Wolter DJ, Hanson ND (2009) Antibacterial-resistant Pseudomonas aeruginosa: clinical impact and complex regulation of chromosomally encoded resistance mechanisms. Clin Microbiol Rev 22(4):582–610. doi:10.1128/CMR.00040-09, PubMed Central PMCID: PMC2772362
13. Rodriguez A, Mendia A, Sirvent JM, Barcenilla F, de la Torre-Prados MV, Sole-Violan J et al (2007) Combination antibiotic therapy improves survival in patients with community-acquired pneumonia and shock. Crit Care Med 35(6):1493–1498. doi:10.1097/01.CCM.0000266755.75844.05, Epub 2007/04/25
14. Dellinger RP, Levy MM, Rhodes A, Annane D, Gerlach H, Opal SM et al (2013) Surviving Sepsis Campaign: international guidelines for management of severe sepsis and septic shock, 2012. Intensive Care Med 39(2): 165–228. doi:10.1007/s00134-012-2769-8, Epub 2013/01/31
15. Solomkin J, Zhao YP, Ma EL, Chen MJ, Hampel B, Team DS (2009) Moxifloxacin is non-inferior to combination therapy with ceftriaxone plus metronidazole in patients with community-origin complicated intra-abdominal infections. Int J Antimicrob Agents 34(5):439–445. doi:10.1016/j.ijantimicag.2009.06.022, Epub 2009/08/21
16. Torres A, Garau J, Arvis P, Carlet J, Choudhri S, Kureishi A et al (2008) Moxifloxacin monotherapy is effective in hospitalized patients with community-acquired pneumonia: the MOTIV study—a randomized clinical trial. Clin Infect Dis 46(10):1499–1509. doi:10.1086/587519, Epub 2008/04/19
17. Leekha S, Terrell CL, Edson RS (2011) General principles of antimicrobial therapy. Mayo Clin Proc 86(2):156–167. doi:10.4065/mcp.2010.0639, Epub 2011/02/02. PubMed Central PMCID: PMCPmc3031442
18. Davis BD (1982) Bactericidal synergism between β-lactams and aminoglycosides: mechanism and possible therapeutic implications. Rev InfectDis4(2):237–245.doi:10.2307/4452714
19. Gal K (1965) Combined antibiotic therapy. Can Med Assoc J 93(16):844–847, Epub 1965/10/16. PubMed Central PMCID: PMCPmc1928965
20. Zembower TR, Noskin GA, Postelnick MJ, Nguyen C, Peterson LR (1998) The utility of aminoglycosides in an era of emerging drug resistance. Int J Antimicrob Agents 10(2):95–105. doi:10.1016/S0924-8579(98)00033-8
21. Greco WR, Bravo G, Parsons JC (1995) The search for synergy: a critical review from a response surface perspective. Pharmacol Rev 47(2):331–385, Epub 1995/06/01
22. Loewe S (1926) Effect of combinations: mathematical basis of problem. Arch Exp Pathol Pharmakol 114:313–326
23. Zhao L, Au JL, Wientjes MG (2010) Comparison of methods for evaluating drug-drug interaction. Front Biosci (Elite Ed) 2:241–249, PubMed Central PMCID: PMCPmc2885905
24. Fraser TR (1872) Lecture on the antagonism between the actions of active substances. Br Med J 2(617):457–459, Epub 1872/10/26. PubMed Central PMCID: PMCPmc2294062
25. Chou T-C (2010) Drug combination studies and their synergy quantification using the Chou-Talalay method. Cancer Res 70(2): 440–446
26. Bliss C (1939) The toxicity of poisons applied jointly. Ann Appl Biol 26(3):585–615
27. Yeh PJ, Hegreness MJ, Aiden AP, Kishony R (2009) Drug interactions and the evolution of

antibiotic resistance. Nat Rev Microbiol 7(6):460–466

28. Pillai SK, Moellering RC, Eliopoulos GM (2005) Antimicrobial combinations. In: Lorian V (ed) Antibiotics in laboratory medicine, 5th edn. Lippincott Williams & Wilkins, Philadelphia, PA
29. Anonymous (2011) Instructions to authors. Antimicrob Agents Chemother 55(1):1–23
30. Cappelletty DM, Rybak MJ (1996) Comparison of methodologies for synergism testing of drug combinations against resistant strains of Pseudomonas aeruginosa. Antimicrob Agents Chemother 40(3):677–683, Epub 1996/03/01. PubMed Central PMCID: PMC163179
31. Wootton M, Hedges AJ, Bowker KE, Holt HA, Reeves DS, MacGowan AP (1995) A critical assessment of the agar dilution chequerboard technique for studying in-vitro antimicrobial interactions using a representative beta-lactam, aminoglycoside and fluoroquinolone. J Antimicrob Chemother 35(5):569–576
32. Norden CW, Wentzel H, Keleti E (1979) Comparison of techniques for measurement of in vitro antibiotic synergism. J Infect Dis 140(4):629–633, Epub 1979/10/01
33. Tan TY, Ng LS, Tan E, Huang G (2007) In vitro effect of minocycline and colistin combinations on imipenem-resistant Acinetobacter baumannii clinical isolates. J Antimicrob Chemother 60(2):421–423. doi:10.1093/jac/dkm178, Epub 2007/06/02
34. Orhan G, Bayram A, Zer Y, Balci I (2005) Synergy tests by E test and checkerboard methods of antimicrobial combinations against Brucella melitensis. J Clin Microbiol 43(1):140–143
35. Gloede J, Scheerans C, Derendorf H, Kloft C (2010) In vitro pharmacodynamic models to determine the effect of antibacterial drugs. J Antimicrob Chemother 65(2):186–201. doi:10.1093/jac/dkp434, Epub 2009/12/23
36. Velkov T, Bergen PJ, Lora-Tamayo J, Landersdorfer CB, Li J (2013) PK/PD models in antibacterial development. Curr Opin Microbiol. doi:10.1016/j.mib.2013.06.010
37. Blaser J (1985) In-vitro model for simultaneous simulation of the serum kinetics of two drugs with different half-lives. J Antimicrob Chemother 15(Suppl A):125–130, Epub 1985/01/01
38. Souli M, Rekatsina PD, Chryssouli Z, Galani I, Giamarellou H, Kanellakopoulou K (2009) Does the activity of the combination of imipenem and colistin in vitro exceed the problem of resistance in metallo-beta-lactamase-producing Klebsiella pneumoniae isolates? Antimicrob Agents Chemother 53(5):2133–2135. doi:10.1128/AAC.01271-08, Epub 2009/03/05. [pii] AAC.01271-08. PubMed Central PMCID: PMC2681524
39. Entenza JM, Moreillon P (2009) Tigecycline in combination with other antimicrobials: a review of in vitro, animal and case report studies. Int J Antimicrob Agents 34(1):8.e1–8.e9. doi:10.1016/j.ijantimicag.2008.11.006, Epub 2009/01/24. [pii] S0924-8579(08)00598-0
40. Principe L, Capone A, Mazzarelli A, D'Arezzo S, Bordi E, Di Caro A et al (2013) In vitro activity of doripenem in combination with various antimicrobials against multidrug-resistant Acinetobacter baumannii: possible options for the treatment of complicated infection. Microb Drug Resist 19(5):407–414. doi:10.1089/mdr.2012.0250
41. Pankuch GA, Lin G, Seifert H, Appelbaum PC (2008) Activity of meropenem with and without ciprofloxacin and colistin against Pseudomonas aeruginosa and Acinetobacter baumannii. Antimicrob Agents Chemother 52(1):333–336
42. Galani I, Orlandou K, Moraitou H, Petrikkos G, Souli M (2014) Colistin/daptomycin: an unconventional antimicrobial combination synergistic in vitro against multidrug-resistant Acinetobacter baumannii. Int J Antimicrob Agents. doi:10.1016/j.ijantimicag.2013.12.010
43. Landersdorfer CB, Ly NS, Xu H, Tsuji BT, Bulitta JB (2013) Quantifying subpopulation synergy for antibiotic combinations via mechanism-based modeling and a sequential dosing design. Antimicrob Agents Chemother 57(5):2343–2351
44. Sweeney MT, Zurenko GE (2003) In vitro activities of linezolid combined with other antimicrobial agents against staphylococci, enterococci, pneumococci, and selected gram-negative organisms. Antimicrob Agents Chemother 47(6):1902–1906
45. Watanakunakorn C, Guerriero JC (1981) Interaction between vancomycin and rifampin against Staphylococcus aureus. Antimicrob Agents Chemother 19(6):1089–1091
46. Deresinski S (2009) Vancomycin in combination with other antibiotics for the treatment of serious methicillin-resistant Staphylococcus aureus infections. Clin Infect Dis 49(7):1072–1079
47. Bulitta JB, Landersdorfer CB, Forrest A, Brown SV, Neely MN, Tsuji BT et al (2011) Relevance of pharmacokinetic and pharmacodynamic modeling to clinical care of critically ill patients. Curr Pharm Biotechnol 12(12):2044–2061
48. Liu C, Chambers HF (2003) Staphylococcus aureus with heterogeneous resistance to vancomycin: epidemiology, clinical significance, and critical assessment of diagnostic methods. Antimicrob Agents Chemother 47(10):3040–3045

49. Chambers HF, Miller RT, Newman MD (1988) Right-sided Staphylococcus aureus endocarditis in intravenous drug abusers: two-week combination therapy. Ann Intern Med 109(8):619–624
50. Francioli P, Ruch W, Stamboulian D (1995) Treatment of streptococcal endocarditis with a single daily dose of ceftriaxone and netilmicin for 14 days: a prospective multicenter study. Clin Infect Dis 21(6):1406–1410
51. Werth BJ, Barber KE, Ireland CE, Rybak MJ (2014) Evaluation of ceftaroline, vancomycin, daptomycin or ceftaroline plus daptomycin against daptomycin non-susceptible (DNS) methicillin resistant Staphylococcus aureus (MRSA) in an in vitro PK/PD model of simulated endocardial vegetations (SEV). Antimicrob Agents Chemother. doi:10.1128/aac.00088-14, Epub 2014/03/26
52. Tsuji BT, Rybak MJ (2005) Short-course gentamicin in combination with daptomycin or vancomycin against Staphylococcus aureus in an in vitro pharmacodynamic model with simulated endocardial vegetations. Antimicrob Agents Chemother 49(7):2735–2745. doi:10.1128/aac.49.7.2735-2745.2005, Epub 2005/06/28. PubMed Central PMCID: PMCPmc1168654
53. Pena-Miller R, Laehnemann D, Jansen G, Fuentes-Hernandez A, Rosenstiel P, Schulenburg H et al (2013) When the most potent combination of antibiotics selects for the greatest bacterial load: the smile-frown transition. PLoS Biol 11(4):e1001540. doi:10.1371/journal.pbio.1001540, Epub 2013/05/01. PubMed Central PMCID: PMCPmc3635860
54. Plachouras D, Karvanen M, Friberg L, Papadomichelakis E, Antoniadou A, Tsangaris I et al (2009) Population pharmacokinetic analysis of colistin methanesulfonate and colistin after intravenous administration in critically ill patients with infections caused by gram-negative bacteria. Antimicrob Agents Chemother 53(8):3430–3436
55. Bergen PJ, Tsuji BT, Bulitta JB, Forrest A, Jacob J, Sidjabat HE et al (2011) Synergistic killing of multidrug-resistant Pseudomonas aeruginosa at multiple inocula by colistin combined with doripenem in an in vitro pharmacokinetic/pharmacodynamic model. Antimicrob Agents Chemother 55(12):5685–5695
56. Rao GG, Ly NS, Haas CE, Garonzik S, Forrest A, Bulitta JB et al (2014) New dosing strategies for an 'old' antibiotic: pharmacodynamics of front-loaded regimens of colistin at simulated pharmacokinetics of patients with kidney or liver disease. Antimicrob Agents Chemother 58(3):1381–1388
57. Pesci EC, Pearson JP, Seed PC, Iglewski BH (1997) Regulation of las and rhl quorum sensing in Pseudomonas aeruginosa. J Bacteriol 179(10):3127–3132
58. Pearson JP, Feldman M, Iglewski BH, Prince A (2000) Pseudomonas aeruginosa cell-to-cell signaling is required for virulence in a model of acute pulmonary infection. Infect Immun 68(7):4331–4334
59. Ozer EA, Pezzulo A, Shih DM, Chun C, Furlong C, Lusis AJ et al (2005) Human and murine paraoxonase 1 are host modulators of Pseudomonas aeruginosa quorum-sensing. FEMS Microbiol Lett 253(1):29–37
60. Saroj SD, Rather PN (2013) Streptomycin inhibits quorum sensing in Acinetobacter baumannii. Antimicrob Agents Chemother 57(4): 1926–1929
61. Köhler T, Perron GG, Buckling A, Van Delden C (2010) Quorum sensing inhibition selects for virulence and cooperation in Pseudomonas aeruginosa. PLoS Pathog 6(5):e1000883
62. Rutherford ST, Bassler BL (2012) Bacterial quorum sensing: its role in virulence and possibilities for its control. Cold Spring Harb Perspect Med 2(11):a012427
63. Jaffe A, Francis J, Rosenthal M, Bush A (1998) Long-term azithromycin may improve lung function in children with cystic fibrosis. Lancet 351(9100):420. doi:10.1016/s0140-6736(05)78360-4, Epub 1998/03/03
64. Tateda K, Comte R, Pechere J-C, Köhler T, Yamaguchi K, Van Delden C (2001) Azithromycin inhibits quorum sensing in Pseudomonas aeruginosa. Antimicrob Agents Chemother 45(6):1930–1933
65. Timurkaynak F, Can F, Azap ÖK, Demirbilek M, Arslan H, Karaman SÖ (2006) In vitro activities of non-traditional antimicrobials alone or in combination against multidrug-resistant strains of Pseudomonas aeruginosa and Acinetobacter baumannii isolated from intensive care units. Int J Antimicrob Agents 27(3):224–228
66. Landman D, Bratu S, Alam M, Quale J (2005) Citywide emergence of Pseudomonas aeruginosa strains with reduced susceptibility to polymyxin B. J Antimicrob Chemother 55(6): 954–957. doi:10.1093/jac/dki153, Epub 2005/05/11
67. Saiman L, Chen Y, San Gabriel P, Knirsch C (2002) Synergistic activities of macrolide antibiotics against Pseudomonas aeruginosa, Burkholderia cepacia, Stenotrophomonas maltophilia, and Alcaligenes xylosoxidans isolated from patients with cystic fibrosis. Antimicrob Agents Chemother 46(4):1105–1107

Chapter 5

Methodologies for Protein Binding Determination in Anti-infective Agents

Jatinder Kaur Mukker, Ravi Shankar Prasad Singh, and Hartmut Derendorf

Abstract

Most of the drugs bind to different proteins in the body. This binding leads to reduction in the free fraction of the drugs, which is responsible for the pharmacological actions. In case of anti-infective agent, influence of protein binding can be clearly seen by reduction in the anti-infective properties of these molecules. Therefore, evaluation of protein binding is an important aspect in case of anti-infective agents.

Protein binding of a drug molecule can be determined by a number of methods such as microdialysis, equilibrium dialysis (considered as gold standard), and ultrafiltration and ultracentrifugation. In case of anti-infective agents, percent protein binding is always corrected while calculating the minimum inhibitory concentration (MIC) and concentration at half maximum effect (EC_{50}) using time kill curves. However, it is a common practice to use protein binding data from the literature and corrected for MIC and EC_{50} values which may be erroneous due to change in percent protein binding with changes in different protein supplements. Therefore, the focus of this chapter is to describe these techniques in detailed methodological fashion and provide the influence of these protein binding determinations in MIC and EC_{50} by time kill curve determinations.

Key words Protein binding, Anti-infective agents, Microdialysis, Ultrafiltration, Minimum inhibitory concentration, Equilibrium dialysis

1 Introduction

The drugs undergo nonspecific binding with biological proteins [1–5]. Depending upon the physicochemical properties of the drug, it can bind to different proteins including albumin, α-1 acid glycoproteins, lipoproteins, erythrocytes, and various globulins and this binding decreases the free unbound fraction of the drug in the body as the free fraction of the drug is responsible for the pharmacological actions and/or side effects.

In case of anti-infectives as well, efficacy studies show the modulation in pharmacodynamics activity with change in protein binding. The reduction in free fraction of the analyte is clearly reflected

John C. Rotschafer et al. (eds.), *Antibiotic Pharmacodynamics*, Methods in Pharmacology and Toxicology,
DOI 10.1007/978-1-4939-3323-5_5,

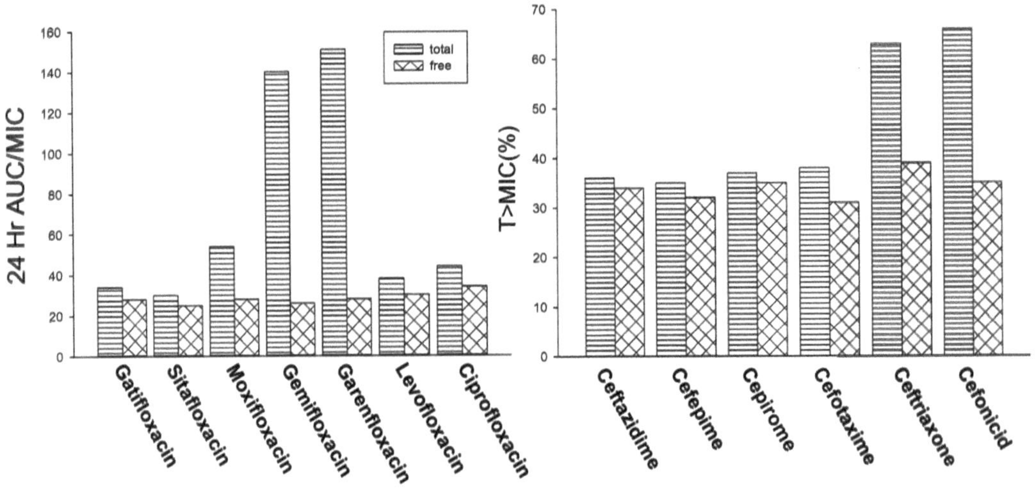

Fig. 1 (*Left*) PK-PD index (area under the concentration time curve over a period of 24 h at a steady state over MIC ratio (AUC/MIC)) of free and total drug concentrations of seven fluoroquinolones (administered as multiple dosing in the thighs of neutropenic mice) as for bacteriostatic actions against *Streptococcus pneumoniae* ATCC 10813 (figure redrawn from ref. 6). (*Right*) PK-PD index (time above MIC (*T*>MIC)) of free and total drug concentrations of six cephalosporin (administered as multiple dosing in the thighs of neutropenic mice) as for bacteriostatic actions against *Klebsiella pneumoniae* ATCC 43615 (figure redrawn from refs. 6, 7)

in the decreased efficacy in case of highly protein-bound anti-infective agents such as ceftriaxone and ertapenem [1]. Similarly, the comparison of pharmacokinetic and pharmacodynamic indices (PK-PD indices) of fluoroquinolones and cephalosporins shows the differential efficacy based on total concentrations but they are equipotent based on their free fractions [6, 7] (Fig. 1). In contrast to the most of the reports, Tsuji et al. reported that daptomycin and telavancin showed efficacy more than predicted based on the free fraction only and thus suggested that bound fraction may also be active [8]. However, this conclusion is based on the use of *in vitro* model of minimum inhibitory concentration (MIC) determination, which is a static model compared to the dynamic nature of *in vivo* system, with analytes being not cleared out of the system and higher concentrations detected compared to the free fraction of these anti-infective agents.

Often the *in vitro* efficacy of anti-infectives is determined based on total concentration despite the knowledge that the unbound fraction is responsible. The potency of anti-infective agent against a specific pathogen is usually reported as changes in the MIC [3, 6]. MIC being a static and variable threshold value against a certain pathogen [9], a more dynamic approach called time kill curves is preferred. Time kill curves evaluate the dynamic growth and antibiotic-induced kill profiles over a time duration which is more detailed evaluation over time [10]. Time kill curve data can be used to calculate the concentration at half maximum effect (EC_{50}) by fitting a simultaneous fit of appropriate mathematical models

[10]. In these pharmacodynamic approaches, protein binding of the anti-infective agents is accounted by the addition of different human serum or protein supplements in the growth media which may only reflect one of the other proteins such as human serum albumin or less expensive animal albumins [5, 11–13]. However, corrections for protein binding are usually done based on literature values, instead of measuring the free fraction of drug in a given experimental condition, which should be done to assess the impact of protein binding on pharmacological actions of anti-infective agents [14, 15]. A number of articles are published on the impact of protein binding on pharmacokinetics and pharmacodynamics of anti-infective agents [16–19]. There are a number of *in vitro* and *in vivo* protein binding determination techniques which can be used in case of anti-infective agent such as microanalysis, equilibrium dialysis, and ultrafiltration and ultracentrifugation. Each technique has its own advantages and disadvantages and is explained in Table 1 [20]. In this chapter we provide protocols of different *in vitro* techniques used in our laboratory for the assessment of the free fraction of the drug. These methods will allow the readers to perform these detailed experiments and to understand the principles and complications behind these techniques.

2 Materials and Methods

Prepare all the solutions using ultrapure water (water prepared by deionization to get a sensitivity of 18 MΩ cm at 25 °C) and HPLC-grade reagents. Prepare and store all the reagents at room temperature (unless indicated specifically). Diligently follow all the waste disposal regulations of the related institute where these experiments will be performed.

2.1 Plasma Protein Binding Determination Using In Vitro Microdialysis (MD)

Microdialysis is a relatively new technique for sampling unbound fraction of the drug (of different molecular sizes) at the site of action (different tissues) and can be used *in vitro*, *in vivo*, and *ex vivo* (Table 1) [20]. It is a nondestructive sampling technique and does not cause any fraction change in unbound concentration while sampling (Fig. 2) [21].

2.1.1 Materials

Materials and reagents required for the free fraction determination by microdialysis are listed below:

1. Unfiltered preclinical/human plasma (*see* **Note 1**).
2. Anti-infective agent (whose protein binding is to be assessed, analyte) (*see* **Note 2**).
3. Microdialysis probe (for example, MD 63 catheter [MDialysis AB, Sweden, P/N: 8010514], polyarylethersulfone (PAES) membrane (20,000 Da cutoff), and polyurethane shaft, inlet and outlet tubes) (*see* **Notes 3, 4,** and **5**).

Table 1
Comparison of different protein binding techniques along with advantages and disadvantages [20]

Technique	Advantages	Problems	Equipment required
Microdialysis	• Can be used *in vitro* and *in vivo* • Free fraction of the drug can be measured at the tissue site	• Need to optimize the flow rate and inlet and outlet tubing • Takes longer time	• Microdialysis probe "with specific molecular weight cutoff" • Peristaltic pump to perfuse the perfusate • HPLC with suitable detector (UV, radiometric, mass spectrometric)
Equilibrium dialysis	• "Gold standard" *in vitro* protein binding • Flexible and automated technique • Percent free fraction can be calculated	• Require longer equilibration duration • Not suitable for unstable drug samples • Not widely available	• 96-Well equilibrium device • HPLC with suitable detector (UV, radiometric, mass spectrometric)
Ultrafiltration	• Percent binding can be calculated • Commercially available cartridges • Available as automated for large number of samples • Comparatively require short duration for the experiment	• Nonspecific binding to the membrane cartridges • Do not represent a true equilibrium • Must correct for the volume shift	• Ultrafiltration device • Fixed-angle centrifuge • HPLC with suitable detector (UV, radiometric, mass spectrometric)

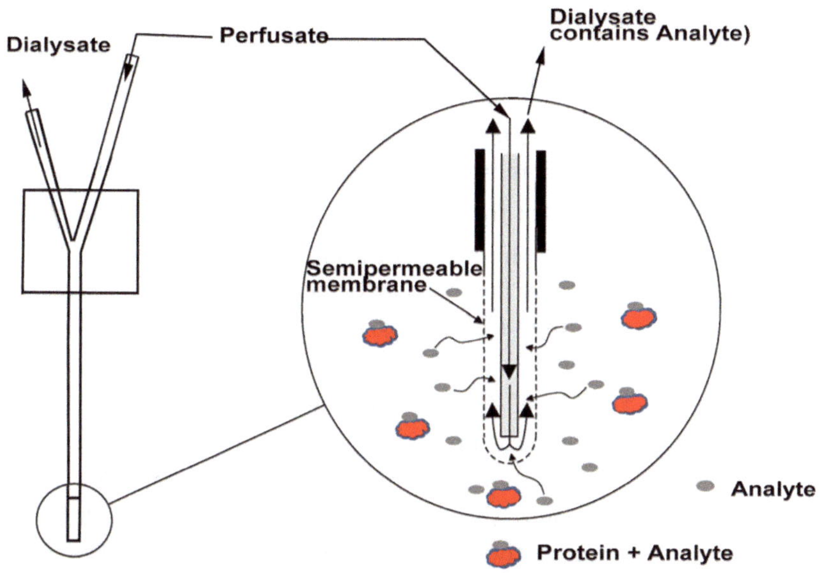

Fig. 2 Diagrammatic representation of microdialysis probe inserted in a tissue containing an analyte of interest. Protein binding of an analyte is taken into consideration in this technique. Flow of the perfusate is shown by the *black arrows* (figure is redrawn from ref. 21)

4. Harvard syringe pump 22 for perfusion.
5. Polypropylene microcentrifuge tubes for sample collection and storage.
6. Analytical equipments: For example, high-performance liquid chromatography (HPLC), LC-MS/MS, and UHPLC-MS/MSPerfusate (required to be optimized for individual compounds) (*see* **Note 6**).

2.1.2 Methods

Detailed methodology to determine the plasma protein binding using *in vitro* microdialysis (MD) is explained below:

MD Setup

1. Place the water reservoir (e.g., a 50 mL beaker) on temperature-controlled heated stir plate to maintain the temperature to 37 °C.
2. Check the integrity of the probe by pumping the perfusate (e.g., saline) and collecting the dialysate while probe was placed in the sample reservoir tube (RT) containing blank saline.
3. Set up Harvard syringe pump 22 to pump the perfusate at a fixed flow rate (0.5–1.5 μL/min) and dialysate samples are collected.

Probe Recovery

The probe recovery is usually determined by extraction efficiency and retrodialysis techniques. The extraction efficiency methodology is explained below:

1. Place the sample reservoir tube (RT) containing analyte in saline in water reservoir maintained at 37 °C.
2. Collect the time zero sample from the RT, immediately.
3. Place the probe in a sample reservoir tube (RT) containing analyte in saline (*see* **Note 7**). Care should be taken that probe does not touch the walls of RT and the membrane should be completely submerged in the sample.
4. Perfuse the perfusate at a fixed flow rate.
5. Allow the probe to equilibrate for 20 min and collect the dialysate samples at 40 and 60 min (*see* **Note 8**).
6. Analyze the samples using developed and validated bioanalytical method as explained in bioanalysis below.
7. Calculate the probe recovery using Eq. (1) (below):

$$\%\ \text{Probe Recovery} = \frac{C_{\text{Dialysate}}}{C_{\text{RT}}} \times 100 \qquad (1)$$

   where $C_{\text{Dialysate}}$ is the dialysate collected between the time interval 40–60 min, and C_{RT} is the concentration of anti-infective drug in the RT (*see* **Note 9**) [17].

8. Repeat the process at least three times and average the probe recoveries to calculate the final percent probe recovery (*see* **Note 10**).

Plasma Protein Binding

1. A syringe containing perfusate is placed on the pump and then fastened.
2. Add an aliquot of the plasma sample previously thawed and incubated at 37 °C for 30 min to RT. The volume of the aliquot should be sufficient to cover the entire length of the membrane (*see* **Notes 11** and 7).
3. The probe should now be placed in plasma samples. The membrane should be completely covered with plasma sample and ideally should not be touching the wall of the RT.
4. The RT should be placed in water reservoir maintained at 37 °C.
5. Firmly attach a collection tube (0.5 mL microcentrifuge tube or microvials) with outlet tube of probe in a rack for sample collection.
6. Turn ON the pump and perfusate is allowed to run through the probe for a period of 20 min (equilibration period). Depending upon the volume of sample, the equilibration period may need

to be increased; higher volume may need longer equilibration period. However, the stability of the compound may be limiting in some cases. Then dialysate samples are collected for a period of 20 min (collection period). The dialysate is collected into collection tube covered. Collect three separate samples, with each 20 min apart (*see* **Notes 12** and **13**).

7. Analyze all the samples using developed and validated bioanalytical method as explained in bioanalysis below (*see* **Note 14**). Usually, the dialysis samples do not need sample cleaning steps; however, sample cleanup may be required in certain cases.
8. Percent free fraction of drug can be calculated by Eq. (2):

$$\%\,\text{Free Fraction} = \frac{C_{\text{Dialysate}(\text{T1},\text{T2})}}{\text{TCRT}} \times \frac{100}{\%\,\text{Probe recovery}} \times 100 \quad (2)$$

where $C_{\text{Dialysate (T1, T2)}}$ is the dialysate collected between the time interval T1 and T2, and TCRT is the total concentration of analyte in reservoir tube.

9. The protein binding should be repeated at least three times and average percent free fraction should be calculated for the anti-infective agent (*see* **Note 15**) [17].

Bioanalysis

1. Analyze all the above-collected samples using a newly developed and validated bioanalytical method using HPLC/LC-MS/MS techniques. Details of method development and validation are out of the scope of this chapter and can be read using UDFDA guidelines (*see* **Note 16**) [22].

2.2 Plasma Protein Binding Determination Using In Vitro Equilibrium Dialysis

Equilibrium dialysis is considered as "gold standard" in determining the protein binding because it represents the true equilibrium before samples are being collected and analyzed for free fraction determination (Fig. 3) (Table 1).

2.2.1 Materials

Materials and reagents required for the *in vitro* equilibrium dialysis are listed below [20]:

1. Dialysis membrane (typical pore sizes for protein binding experiments are between 12,000 and 14,000 kDa mol. Wt. cutoff) (*see* **Note 4**).
2. 96-Well device for equilibrium dialysis.
3. Phosphate buffer saline (PBS), pH 7.4.
4. Unfiltered blank preclinical species/human plasma for analyte samples and control sample preparations (*see* **Notes 11** and **1**).
5. Water bath (at 37 °C) for plasma stability studies.
6. Anti-infective agent (analyte) (*see* **Notes 7** and **17**).
7. Prepare primary and secondary stock solutions of analyte using organic solvents (based on the solubility of the analyte) (*see* **Note 17**).

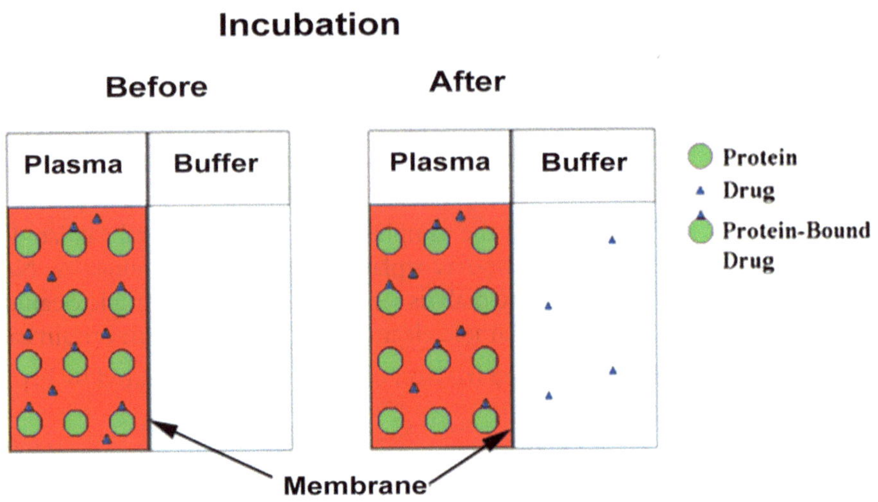

Fig. 3 Basic representation of equilibrium dialysis. Before incubation, protein, drug, and protein-bound drug are in the plasma reservoir. After a fixed incubation period (i.e., true equilibrium), free drug crosses the semi-permeable membrane and can be detected in the buffer reservoir (figure is redrawn from ref. 23 http://www.drumetix.com/php/dmpk-protein-binding.php)

2.2.2 Methods

Detailed methodology to determine the plasma protein binding using *in vitro* equilibrium dialysis is explained below:

1. Soak the equilibrium dialysis membranes in phosphate buffer solution for half an hour before starting the experiment.
2. Add the buffer solution (200 μL) to one side of the 96-well equilibrium dialysis membrane and anti-infective spiked pre-clinical/human plasma (at a required concentration, 200 μL) to the other side of the membrane (*see* **Notes 7** and **11**).
3. Cover the lid of the plate to prevent any evaporation.
4. Incubate the 96-well plate on a horizontally rotating incubator (37 °C) for a specified time (e.g., 2, 4, 6, 8, 24 h can be different based on individual experimental needs) (*see* **Notes 18** and **19**).
5. After incubation, transfer the samples (100 μL) (both buffer and plasma samples) into the sample container (*see* **Notes 2** and **8**).
6. Analyze the samples using appropriate bioanalytical method.
7. Free fraction of the analyte can be calculated using Eq. (3):

$$\%\,\text{Free Fraction} = \frac{C_{\text{buffer}}}{C_{\text{plasma}}} \times 100 \quad (3)$$

where C_{buffer} is the unbound analyte concentration in buffer after dialysis and C_{plasma} is the postdialysis plasma concentration (*see* **Notes 20** and **21**).

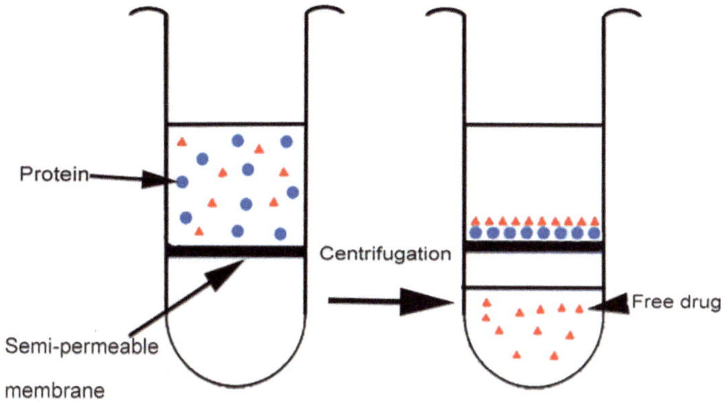

Fig. 4 Diagrammatic representation of ultrafiltration technique to determine plasma protein binding. Centrifugal force allows the free drug to move across the semipermeable membrane and can be detected and analyzed using bioanalytical method (figure redrawn from ref. 24, http://www.cyprotex.com)

2.3 Plasma Protein Binding Determination Using In Vitro Ultrafiltration

It is a rapid and most widely used technique for protein binding determination of the analyte. Centrifugation allows the separation and filter in the cartridge and allows the free analyte to move to the collection vial (Fig. 4).

2.3.1 Materials

Materials and reagents required for the equilibrium dialysis are listed below [20]:

1. Centrifugal filter units with specific molecular weight cutoff (*see* **Note 4**).
2. Centrifuge (at 37 °C) capable of 3000×*g* at fixed-angle rotation.
3. Water bath (at 37 °C) for plasma stability studies.
4. Polypropylene microcentrifuge tubes for sample collection and storage.
5. Unfiltered blank preclinical species/human plasma for samples and control sample preparations (*see* **Notes 1** and **11**).
6. Anti-infective agent (whose protein binding is to be assessed, analyte) (*see* **Note 7**).
7. Prepare primary and secondary stock solutions of anti-infective agent using organic solvents (based on the solubility of the drug) (*see* **Note 17**).

2.3.2 Methods

Detailed methodology to determine the plasma protein binding using *in vitro* ultrafiltration is explained below:

1. Prepare the centrifugal filters for the protein binding experiments by addition of spiked anti-infective solution in preclinical/human plasma/serum (pH 7.4) in the filter. Three replicates of each analyte/plasma type are recommended (*see* **Notes 7** and **11**).

2. Close the centrifugal filter unit tightly by closing its lid.
3. Incubate the samples at 37 °C for 30 min in a temperature-controlled water bath. These samples can be analyzed to determine the plasma stability. Usually not more than 20 % decrease in the concentration (before and after incubation) is considered acceptable for plasma stability (*see* **Note 18**).
4. Centrifuge the samples at 1000 rpm at 37 °C for 30 min.
5. Pipette out the samples from collection cartridges of the ultrafiltration units (post-centrifuged spiked samples (PCSP)) and store in polypropylene microcentrifuge tubes at −80 °C freezer.
6. Collect the plasma sample from the upper part of the cartridge (post-centrifuged ultrafiltrate (PCU)) and store in polypropylene microcentrifuge tubes at −80 °C freezer (*see* **Note 8**).
7. Analyze the samples using appropriate bioanalytical method.
8. Calculate the plasma protein binding using Eq. (4):

$$\% \text{Free Fraction} = \frac{\text{PCSP}}{\text{PCU}} \times 100 \quad (4)$$

2.4 Minimum Inhibitory Concentration and Time Kill Curve Experiments

2.4.1 Materials

Materials and reagents required for the MIC and time kill curve experiments are listed below:

1. Sheep-blood agar plates.
2. Micropipettes.
3. Sterilized pipette tips.
4. Vortexer.
5. Weighing balance for the preparation of broth.
6. CO_2 culture incubator.
7. Autoclave to sterilize different media.
8. McFarland standards.
9. Culture flasks (25 mL, vented caps, canned neck).
10. Glass tubes.
11. Gelman Acrodisc sterile syringe filters.
12. Auto dilution system.
13. Turbidmeter.
14. Turbidity standard.
15. 96-Well and 24-well culture plates.
16. Saline (0.9 % M/V).
17. Lactated Ringer's solution.
18. Mueller-Hinton broth (different types available, based on the specific requirements).
19. Anti-infective agent (analyte) (*see* **Note 7**).

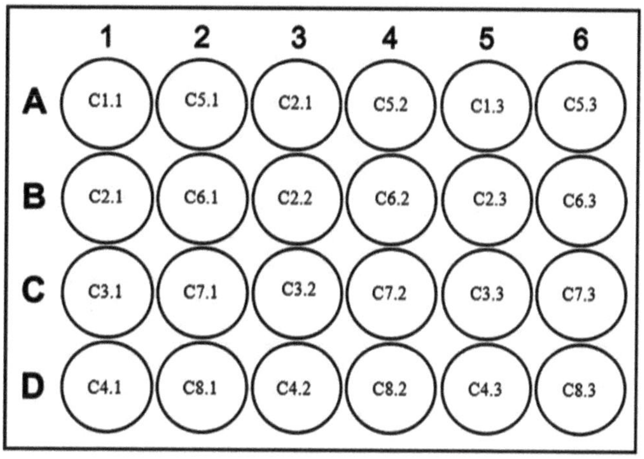

Fig. 5 Schematic representation of the 24-well plate to calculate MIC of an anti-infective agent

2.4.2 Methods

Detailed methodology to determine the MIC and time kill curve is explained below:

Minimum Inhibitory Concentration Determination for Anti-infective Agent by Macrodilution

1. Plate the cryo-preserved bacterial culture and subculture for 3 days on sheep-blood agar plates in order to activate the bacteria.
2. Prepare the broth that will be used in the experiments. Mueller-Hinton broth (440 mg) has to be suspended in purified water (20 mL). Mix thoroughly and heat with frequent agitation. Boil for 1 min to completely dissolve the powder. Autoclave at 121 °C for 15 min. Make sure not to overheat the broth at any time.
3. Prepare five vials containing 15 mL of saline. Autoclave at 121 °C for 15 min.
4. Prepare the primary and secondary stock solutions of anti-infective agent. Filter the secondary stock with a 0.19 μm sterilization filter.
5. Prepare the 24-well plate using the anti-infective secondary stock solution and broth solution (Fig. 5).
6. Perform the turbidmeter calibration using a McFarland standard No. 0.5 and 1.0 (approximately 1.5×10^8 CFU/mL).
7. Prepare a dispersion of bacteria, containing 1.5×10^8 CFU/mL, by picking colonies of specific bacteria from the agar plate. Pick approximately 2–3 colonies and disperse the colonies in the sterilized saline (15 mL vial). Sterilize the picking loop before and after each contact to bacteria or use sterilized disposable loops. Use the turbidmeter to adjust turbidity to the needed CFU/mL.

8. Add the freshly prepared bacterial culture (1.5×10^8 CFU/mL, 10 μL) to each well.
9. Prepare negative control (containing no drug and no bacteria) and positive control (containing no drug but bacteria) samples.
10. Last, incubate the well plates at 37 °C. The wells are read after 20–24 h of incubation, and the MIC is determined as the lowest concentration of the antibiotic allowing no visible growth.

Time Kill Curve Determination

1. Predetermine MIC (μg/mL) (see section "Minimum Inhibitory Concentration Determination for Anti-infective Agent by Macrodilution") for anti-infective agent against a specific bacterial species.
2. Prepare the broth as explained in section "Minimum Inhibitory Concentration Determination for Anti-infective Agent by Macrodilution," step 2.
3. Prepare three vials containing 15 mL of 0.9 % saline. Autoclave at at least 121 °C for at least 15 min. Autoclave 500 mL additional normal saline for dilution.
4. Perform turbidity meter calibration with McFarland standard No. 0.5 and 1.0 (1.5×10^8 CFU/mL and 3.0×10^8 CFU/mL).
5. Prepare bacteria dispersion containing 1.5×10^8 CFU/mL (turbidity meter 0.5) by scratching colonies of bacteria from the agar plate. Pick approximately 2–3 colonies and disperse into sterilized saline. Sterilize the picking loop before and after each contact of bacteria. Use the turbidmeter to adjust turbidity to the needed CFU/mL. Add bacteria or normal saline as needed.
6. Prepare eight culture flasks (50 mL). Out of these eight flasks, six will be C1–C6, seventh is growth control, and eighth is negative control. Dispense Mueller-Hinton broth (20 mL) into each flask. Negative control: no drug and no bacteria; growth control: no drug but bacteria. It is recommended to do the experiment at three concentrations in duplicate.
7. Add the bacteria dispersion (100 μL) containing 1.5×10^8 CFU/mL to each 50 mL culture flasks C1–C6 and to the growth control. Ensure that the organisms are inoculated below the fluid meniscus without touching the flask sides with the pipette and mix gently. Final concentration should be 5×10^5 CFU/mL.
8. Prior to adding the drug, incubate the flasks for 2 h at 37 °C.
9. Add the anti-infective solution to flasks C1–C6, not to the negative and growth control.
10. Remove another 20 μL aliquot from each flask for serial dilution and spot inoculation.

Table 2
Labeling scheme for 8 wells from 1 to 8 (C1–6, growth control, negative control)

Row label	Contents
1	C1
2	C2
3	C3
4	C4
5	C5
6	C6
7	Growth control
8	Negative control

11. Perform a tenfold serial dilution scheme from steps 11a to 11f on the aliquot removed as follows:
    (a) Take a 96-well plate and label 8 wells from 1 to 8 (C1–6, growth control, negative control, as explained in Table 2).
    (b) Add 180 μL of sterile saline to each well.
    (c) Add the removed 20 μL aliquot to the well marked as A.
    (d) Mix using the pipette, and then dispense 20 μL of that well in second column of wells.
    (e) Repeat steps 11c and 11d until reach the 12th column of wells.
    (f) Spot 10 μL of each dilution (dilution pattern will be dependent on the number of bacteria in specific experiment) onto blood agar plates (see Fig. 6).
12. Incubate the inoculated plate at 37 °C for 24 h.
13. Then, repeat sampling (steps 11a–11f) at different time intervals. Time points can be selected based on individual experimental needs.
14. Time kill curves are performed in duplicate.

3 Notes

1. Use of ethylenediaminetetraacetic acid (EDTA) as an anticoagulant is recommended for the plasma harvesting. After harvesting, plasma can be stored at −80 °C and can be reused after thawing it. Heparin interferes with protein binding determination and thus its use is not recommended [20].

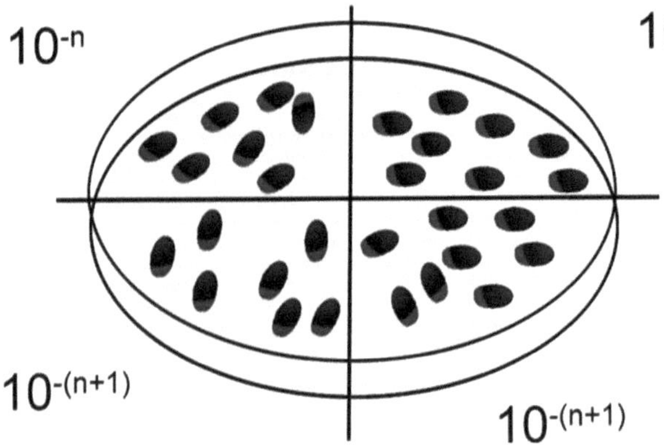

Fig. 6 Spot inoculation of serial dilutions on agar for colony enumeration. Each plate is divided into four parts. Two sectors are used for one dilution step. Each sector is inoculated five times with 10 μL of each dilution (adapted and modified from ref. 25)

However, EDTA also interferes with some antibiotics such as tigecycline.

2. Protein binding techniques can be used to investigate individual protein binding such as human serum albumin, α1-acid glycoprotein, or proteins specific to any preclinical species [20].
3. Recovery of the analyte in microdialysis setup is greatly influenced by length, diameter of the inflow/outflow tubing along with the flow rate of the perfusate. Use of long and narrow tubing with high flow rates results in generating the "back pressure" in the probe and ultrafiltration of the perfusate, which may lead to reduction in relative recovery [26].
4. Selection of a proper probe membrane is critical in microdialysis experiment. The molecular weight cutoff should be considered very carefully. The membrane pore size should be large enough to cross the analyte; however, pore size should be small to maintain the semipermeable nature of the membrane. Different types of membranes are commercially available and some are better suited for the specific analytes than others. Details can be read from the referred articles [26].
5. The length of the microdialysis probe should be long enough to produce the maximum or nearly maximum recovery. Effect of the probe length on microdialysis recovery can be determined very easily using an in vitro microdialysis experiment. Increasing the length of the microdialysis probe is the only way to increase the surface area which will be in contact with the tissue, which is also affected by the size of the tissue [26].

6. Perfusate should be isosmotic and compatible with the organ and analyte to be measured. Flow of the analyte is bidirectional in the microdialysis setup to move the low-molecular-weight solute from and to the tissue and perfusate [26].
7. Most of the protein binding experiments (using microdialysis, equilibrium dialysis, and ultrafiltration) should be designed in such a manner that physiologically feasible concentration/toxicologically relevant concentrations of anti-infective will be used to conduct the experiment [20].
8. Please check for sample storage requirements. Stability of the anti-infective agent at the room temperature should be checked and thus optimal storage conditions should be maintained for the collected samples. Additionally, addition of a protective agent in the collection vial or reducing the temperature will increase the stability of anti-infective agent. For example catecholamines can be protected from oxidative degradation by the addition of ascorbic acid to the perfusate or addition of perchloric acid to the collected samples [26].
9. Always perform a couple of in vitro experiments to optimize the flow rate and detectable volume of the analyte. Series of experiments with one-step variation at a time will help to improve the recovery of the analyte using suitable microdialysis setup.
10. Always check for the loss of the drug molecule due to microdialysis procedure, i.e., binding to the probes, tubing, degradation, or physical interactions such as oxidation. This analysis can be performed by perfusing a known concentration of the anti-infective agent by the inflow and outflow tubing into the collection vials. If significant loss is identified, please identify source of loss by systematically checking all the major components of microdialysis. However, degradation of the compound of interest by certain enzymes or oxidation, binding to the tubing, and probe can be potential source for the loss of the anti-infective agent [26].
11. Preclinical species selection for plasma/serum binding should be based on the purpose/objective of the protein binding experiment which may be allometric scaling or pharmacokinetic studies [20].
12. It is very important to know the "dead volume" of the specific microdialysis setup. This dead volume determination will help to know the lag time between the experiment start-up and collection of the samples. For example, if the capacity of the outflow tubing is 12 μL and perfusion rate is 3.0 μL/min, it will take 4 min as a lag time for collection of samples [26].
13. Collection period should be long enough to get a sufficient volume of analyte for testing. Longer collection period should

be accomplished with slow flow rate which usually increases the relative recovery of the analyte [26].

14. It is always recommended to seal or cover the collected samples from microdialysis experiment. Since the collected samples are usually in small volumes (microliters), evaporation of the samples can be a problem [26].
15. Always conduct a pilot in vivo microdialysis before planning for the full in vivo experiment to test the analyte recovery and bioanalytical detectable ranges [26].
16. Sensitivity of the bioanalytical instrument should be determined using the lowest volume of physiologically relevant anti-infective agent [26].
17. Minimize the use of organic solvents for initial spiking of the anti-infective agent in the plasma (such as dimethylsulfoxide (DMSO)) [20].
18. Stability of the anti-infective agent should always be assessed in all the matrices along with buffer solutions. It should be done over a longer time period for equilibrium dialysis experiment. Stability testing should be performed under same conditions as the equilibrium dialysis apparatus. Samples should be taken at zero and last time point should be assessed to determine percent anti-infective agent [20].
19. Mostly the equilibrium dialysis experiments are performed for the duration of 24 h (due to the efficiency issues). However, this time can be a shorter duration based on the particular experimental conditions [20].
20. One potential issue with equilibrium dialysis is protein breakthrough (i.e., movement of the protein from protein-rich plasma to aqueous side of the dialysis cell). This leads to false evaluation of anti-infective agent in the buffer compartment. This problem can be solved by taking any remaining buffer after the experiment and add acetonitrile to the buffer to precipitate the protein and check for visible particulates. Alternatively, use of the membrane with appropriate molecular weight cutoff can eliminate this problem [20].
21. Loss of anti-infective agent during the experiment by nonspecific binding to the membrane and apparatus and decomposition of the drug due to the stability issue for longer duration can be major issues in case of equilibrium dialysis. This problem can be solved by assessing the pre- and postdialysis plasma and buffer samples and check for the loss of the anti-infective agent during the experiment can be accounted for the calculations [20].

References

1. Schmidt S, Rock K, Sahre M et al (2008) Effect of protein binding on the pharmacological activity of highly bound antibiotics. Antimicrob Agents Chemother 52:3994–4000
2. Zeitlinger MA, Sauermann R, Traunmuller F, Georgopoulos A, Muller M, Joukhadar C (2004) Impact of plasma protein binding on antimicrobial activity using time-killing curves. J Antimicrob Chemother 54:876–880
3. Nix DE, Matthias KR, Ferguson EC (2004) Effect of ertapenem protein binding on killing of bacteria. Antimicrob Agents Chemother 48:3419–3424
4. Popick AC, Crouthamel WG, Bekersky I (1987) Plasma protein binding of ceftriaxone. Xenobiotica 17:1139–1145
5. Svensson CK, Woodruff MN, Baxter JG, Lalka D (1986) Free drug concentration monitoring in clinical practice. Rationale and current status. Clin Pharmacokinet 11:450–469
6. Schmidt S, Gonzalez D, Derendorf H (2010) Significance of protein binding in pharmacokinetics and pharmacodynamics. J Pharm Sci 99:1107–1122
7. Craig WA (2003) Basic pharmacodynamics of antibacterials with clinical applications to the use of beta-lactams, glycopeptides, and linezolid. Infect Dis Clin North Am 17:479–501
8. Tsuji BT, Leonard SN, Rhomberg PR, Jones RN, Rybak MJ (2008) Evaluation of daptomycin, telavancin, teicoplanin, and vancomycin activity in the presence of albumin or serum. Diagn Microbiol Infect Dis 60:441–444
9. Mouton JW, Dudley MN, Cars O, Derendorf H, Drusano GL (2005) Standardization of pharmacokinetic/pharmacodynamic (PK/PD) terminology for anti-infective drugs: an update. J Antimicrob Chemother 55:601–607
10. Schmidt S, Schuck E, Kumar V, Burkhardt O, Derendorf H (2007) Integration of pharmacokinetic/pharmacodynamic modeling and simulation in the development of new anti-infective agents - minimum inhibitory concentration versus time-kill curves. Expert Opin Drug Discov 2:849–860
11. Craig WA, Welling PG (1977) Protein binding of antimicrobials: clinical pharmacokinetic and therapeutic implications. Clin Pharmacokinet 2:252–268
12. Lee BL, Sachdeva M, Chambers HF (1991) Effect of protein binding of daptomycin on MIC and antibacterial activity. Antimicrob Agents Chemother 35:2505–2508
13. Riond JL, Riviere JE (1989) Doxycycline binding to plasma albumin of several species. J Vet Pharmacol Ther 12:253–260
14. Cafini F, Aguilar L, Gonzalez N et al (2007) In vitro effect of the presence of human albumin or human serum on the bactericidal activity of daptomycin against strains with the main resistance phenotypes in Gram-positives. J Antimicrob Chemother 59:1185–1189
15. Laue H, Valensise T, Seguin A, Hawser S, Lociuro S, Islam K (2007) Effect of human plasma on the antimicrobial activity of iclaprim in vitro. J Antimicrob Chemother 60:1388–1390
16. Heuberger J, Schmidt S, Derendorf H (2013) When is protein binding important? J Pharm Sci 102:3458–3467
17. Mukker JK, Singh RP, Derendorf H (2014) Determination of atypical nonlinear plasma-protein-binding behavior of tigecycline using an in vitro microdialysis technique. J Pharm Sci 103:1013–1019
18. Schmidt S, Barbour A, Sahre M, Rand KH, Derendorf H (2008) PK/PD: new insights for antibacterial and antiviral applications. Curr Opin Pharmacol 8:549–556
19. Zeitlinger MA, Derendorf H, Mouton JW et al (2011) Protein binding: do we ever learn? Antimicrob Agents Chemother 55:3067–3074
20. Cohen LH (2004) Plasma protein binding methods in drug discovery. In: Yan Z, Caldwell GW (eds) Optimisation in drug discovery. Humana Press, Totowa, NJ, pp 111–122
21. Azeredo FJ, Dalla Costa T, Derendorf H (2014) Role of microdialysis in pharmacokinetics and pharmacodynamics: current status and future directions. Clin Pharmacokinet 53:205–212
22. Services USDoHaH, Administration FaD (2001) Guidance for industry, bioanalytical method validation. Services USDoHaH, Rockville, MD
23. Equilibrium Dialysis: In Vitro DMPK (ADME). Accessed at http://www.drumetix.com/php/dmpk-protein-binding.php
24. Cyprotex. Ultrafilteration: In Vitro ADME & PK. Accessed at http://www.cyprotex.com/admepk/protein_binding/plasma-protein-binding/
25. Richard Schwalbe LS-M, Avery C. Goodwin (2007) Antimicrobial susceptibility testing protocols. CRC press, Boca Raton, FL, USA
26. Shippenberg TS, Thompson AC (2001) Overview of microdialysis. Curr Protoc Neurosci Chapter 7:Unit7.1

Chapter 6

Evaluation of Exposure-Response Relationships Using Clinical Data: Basic Concepts and Applications

Sujata M. Bhavnani, Christopher M. Rubino, and Paul G. Ambrose

Abstract

An understanding of the relationships between drug exposure and efficacy and/or safety endpoints is useful for optimizing therapy for antimicrobial agents. Such knowledge can help explain why certain patients fail therapy while others are successfully treated and can shed light on whether certain safety endpoints are predictable rather than idiosyncratic. Such exposure-response relationships for efficacy and safety endpoints can together be used to identify both efficacious and safe dosing regimens and thereby balance the competing needs for high efficacy and low toxicity. In order to conduct analyses using clinical data, reliable estimates of drug exposure in individual patients, well-defined and reproducible efficacy and safety endpoints, and appropriate statistical approaches are needed.

Herein, we describe the role of population PK methods to estimate drug exposure in patients and provide examples of exposure-response analyses for efficacy and safety for several antimicrobial agents. The examples described were chosen to illustrate different concepts. Applications of such data to improve patient care are also described.

Key words Exposure-response, Pharmacokinetics, Pharmacodynamics, Pharmacokinetics-pharmacodynamics, Efficacy, Safety

1 Introduction

An understanding of the relationships between drug exposure and response is useful for optimizing patient care. For example, a relationship between drug exposure and an efficacy endpoint can be used to help explain why certain patients fail therapy while others are successfully treated. Similarly, a relationship between drug exposure and a safety endpoint can demonstrate that the event is predictable rather than idiosyncratic. Such exposure-response relationships for efficacy and safety endpoints can together be used to identify both efficacious and safe dosing regimens and thereby balance the competing needs for high efficacy and low toxicity. Three key components are required to conduct robust analyses using clinical data: (1) reliable estimates of drug exposure in individual

John C. Rotschafer et al. (eds.), *Antibiotic Pharmacodynamics*, Methods in Pharmacology and Toxicology,
DOI 10.1007/978-1-4939-3323-5_6,

patients, (2) well-defined and reproducible efficacy and safety endpoints, and (3) appropriate statistical approaches.

The pharmacokinetic (PK) data required to reliably estimate drug exposure in patients are often obtained during the drug development process. Early in drug development, data from healthy volunteers in a highly controlled setting are gathered. In this setting, it is possible to collect numerous blood samples to describe individual subject drug exposure. However, it is challenging to collect enough blood samples to describe individual patient drug exposure in late-stage clinical development, a setting that is generally less well controlled. To overcome this challenge, drug concentration data collected in early- and late-stage drug development are integrated using a process called population PK modeling. The resultant mathematical model allows for the precise and unbiased estimation of drug exposure in individual patients from whom only a limited number of blood samples were collected for drug assay.

Well-defined and reproducible efficacy and safety endpoints along with appropriate statistical approaches to evaluate the relationships between exposure and these endpoints are required. Efficacy and safety endpoints should be defined using objective criteria that are informed by observations collected at meaningful time points so as to capture drug effect. Statistical approaches chosen should consider the study design and nature of the data collected in order to make informative inferences about the data.

Herein, we describe the role of population PK methods to estimate drug exposure in patients and provide examples of exposure-response analyses for efficacy and safety for several antimicrobial agents. The examples described were chosen to illustrate different concepts. Applications of such data to improve patient care are also described. While antimicrobial agents differ in important ways from other classes of drugs, the concepts and approaches described herein apply universally.

2 The Role of Population Pharmacokinetics for Characterizing Drug Exposure

In order to be able to appropriately characterize drug exposure in individual patients and relate exposure to efficacy and/or safety endpoints of interest, sparse samples for PK are required from individual patients. In this section, general PK principles, the basis for developing an understanding of the disposition of the drug through Phase 1 studies, and methodological approaches for quantifying PK properties, including population PK methods, are reviewed. The benefits of population PK methods, including the opportunity to identify sparse but information-rich PK sampling strategies and to use such data to reliably predict drug exposure in individual patients, are described.

Conceptually, PK can be defined as the effect of the human (or animal) body on drugs. A dose of drug is administered, it is then distributed within the body, and clearance organs remove the drug from the system over time. Thus, by defining the PK of a drug, we are quantifying the manner in which drug travels through the body. This is accomplished by observing drug concentrations measured after the administration of a dose or doses of a drug. Most commonly, PK is defined using blood (plasma/serum) concentrations but can also be defined using concentrations collected from so-called effect sites such as tissues, middle ear fluid, or bone. Traditionally, the foundation for our understanding of the PK of drugs comes from Phase 1 studies in normal, healthy volunteers and small populations of diseased patients (e.g., patients with renal or hepatic impairment). The studies have the distinct advantage of being highly controlled and intensive: a relatively homogenous group of subjects are often confined to the study unit for the duration of the study and undergo "dense" PK sampling (over ten blood samples drawn in small time increments often over a long period of time after dosing). These intensive, PK-specific study designs serve to minimize issues relative to unknown variability and provide a reliable definition of the basics of the drug's PK profile. However, their primary advantage (a small, homogenous, captive study population) is also their primary deficiency when considering the clinical use of drugs: healthy people do not usually receive antimicrobial agents. Thus, PK sampling has been incorporated into later stage clinical trials (Phase 2 and 3). This is carried out in an attempt to confirm the PK findings from Phase 1 studies by using data from large populations of patients who will ultimately receive the drug clinically. This strategy allows us to fill the gaps in our PK knowledge by gaining an understanding of the drug's PK in the target population and to further understand factors that contribute to the variability in PK across patients (termed "interindividual variability"). However, conducting PK studies in infected patients presents several potential complicating factors such as a less well-controlled treatment and PK sampling design and the inability to conduct dense PK sampling. As discussed below, these factors can be overcome through a combination of thoughtful study design and innovative data analysis techniques.

Pharmacokinetic properties are quantified using two general methodological approaches: model-independent (also known as non-compartmental or shape, height, area, and moment [SHAM] analyses) and model-dependent. While model-independent approaches have utility, especially when evaluating PK in normal, healthy adults who undergo intensive PK sampling, model-dependent approaches are required when evaluating data obtained from infected patients [1]. Pharmacokinetic models provide several advantages in the context of defining optimal dosing regimens of antibiotics: (1) they allow for a description of the expected time course of drug concentrations (on average and within individuals); (2) they allow for the definition of variability in that time course across and within individuals, which we will call interindividual and intraindividual variability, respectively; (3) when applied appropriately, they allow one to identify those patient-specific factors that minimize the amount of interindividual variability; and (4) they facilitate simulation of the expected time course of drug concentrations following alternative dosing regimens and/or in other populations of interest.

As with the general approach to PK, there are two basic approaches to constructing PK models: models that are fit to data from individual patients and those that are fit to pooled data from a population of patients. Both of these approaches have the advantages described above but each has distinct advantages, depending on the robustness of the available data. When intensive PK data are available, PK modeling of data from individuals can often provide valuable information regarding the structure of the PK model required to define the above-mentioned time course of drug concentrations. However, it is necessary to perform post hoc evaluations in order to quantify the average behavior across individuals and to quantify sources of variability; PK parameters are derived for each individual independently and then pooled in order to use traditional statistics (summary statistics or simple linear regression) to gain insight into the determinants of interindividual variability. This "two-stage" approach, which may be useful when applied to large populations of patients studied intensively, is prone to bias when applied to small populations sampled sparsely [2, 3]. Conversely, population (a.k.a., nonlinear mixed effects) PK models have the advantage of allowing for the identification of both individual and population PK properties [4]. Furthermore, population PK methods have flexibility in that they can be applied to data obtained from heterogeneous sources ranging from tightly controlled, Phase 1 studies through large Phase 3 trials and even to data collected during routine clinical care [5]. In this way, population PK methods allow for the quantification of PK in the target patient population and are highly useful in the process of identifying optimal dosing regimens [6–10].

A second advantage of population PK methods is the ability to quantify the effect of patient-specific factors (covariates) that contribute to the interindividual variability in PK parameters as part of the model (i.e., not as a post hoc analysis in the second stage of the two-stage approach described above). In this way, the interactions between the various PK parameters are taken into consideration during the identification of these factors, resulting in a more reliable quantification of the effects. Although there remains controversy in the optimal means for conducting these covariate analyses [11], the ultimate goal is to identify those factors that result in a meaningful effect from both a statistical and clinical perspective. This is an important consideration given that most approved antimicrobial agents have undergone population PK analyses, the process for which yielded covariate models. However, the dose of very few antimicrobials has required adjustment based upon individual patient factors other than body size. In general, those drugs that require dose adjustment are cleared via the kidneys such that dose amounts or intervals are adjusted secondary to patient renal function [12–14].

Another advantage of population PK methods lies in their ability to inform study design. As described above, it is often not feasible to execute dense PK sampling strategies in Phase 2 or 3 clinical studies. The data needed for PK analyses needs to be collected within the logistical framework of the study, which often necessitates limited PK sampling (e.g., less than five or six samples per patient). It is, therefore, important to maximize the information content of these PK samples to allow for a robust definition of PK in the target population. Optimal sampling theory can be applied to PK models to define the times (both number and timing) that best inform the estimation of parameters for the model [15, 16]. A population PK model can provide the framework for defining these "optimal" PK sampling strategies [16–18].

In summary, population PK methods allow for the opportunity to identify sparse PK sampling strategies. Using sparsely-sampled PK data pooled from many patients, population PK methods also allow for estimation of drug exposure and identification of those patient characteristics which provide clinically relevant insight into the interindividual variability in drug exposure. Such an approach is important in ensuring that drug exposure in individual patients is reliably predicted.

3 Exposure-Response Analyses for Efficacy and Safety

As with all drugs, safety and efficacy are the two components that factor into judging the adequacy of antimicrobial dosing regimens. For well-tolerated agents like meropenem, there are few exposure-related toxicities of clinical consequence [19, 20]. In this best-case scenario, the drug can be dosed in a manner that results in a high percentage of patients with pharmacokinetic-pharmacodynamic (PK-PD) indices that are on the upper plateau of the agent's exposure-response relationship for efficacy with minimal adjustments for patient covariates other than renal dysfunction. For less well-tolerated antibiotics, like aminoglycosides, nephrotoxicity and ototoxicity are clinically relevant exposure-limiting toxicities of concern [21]. In such a circumstance, optimal clinical use must balance the dual requirements of maximizing the probability of efficacy while minimizing the risk of toxicity. Strategies to strike a balance between the competing needs for high efficacy and low toxicity may include limiting the duration of therapy, increasing the interval between exposures, and therapeutic drug monitoring.

Thus, the application of clinically-derived exposure-response relationships for efficacy and safety to evaluate dosing regimens for drug development [22] and use in clinical practice provide the opportunity to balance the competing needs for efficacious and minimally toxic drug exposures. In this section, the certainty that the results of exposure-response analyses for efficacy provide in order to support decisions about dosing regimens and interpretive criteria for in vitro susceptibility testing will be discussed. Later in this section, exposure-response analyses for safety and the integration of relationships for efficacy and safety endpoints to aid in dosing regimen optimization will be discussed.

4 Exposure-Response Analyses for Efficacy

The vast majority of exposure-response analyses for efficacy for antimicrobial agents have been conducted using data collected from adequate and well-controlled clinical studies that were part of a drug development program. From a regulatory perspective, adequate and well-controlled studies have prospectively-defined hypotheses, include a control group, use randomization to ensure group comparability and minimize bias, and use well-defined statistical methods to assess study endpoints. In addition to drug concentration data sufficient to estimate drug exposure, information regarding the infecting pathogen's susceptibility to the study drug is required to conduct exposure-response analyses for efficacy for an antimicrobial agent.

For the evaluation of exposure-response relationships for efficacy, the independent variable represents a measure of drug exposure that is indexed to a measure of susceptibility of the infecting pathogen to the study drug. Although drug dose is a measure of drug exposure, it is not the most informative. This is because for a fixed dose of a drug, there is a resulting range of exposures for a population of patients. Such a distribution of exposures is expected due to random variability and the fact that patients can vary greatly in those covariates known to influence drug exposure, including body size, age, and drug clearing organ function. For antimicrobial agents, preclinical and clinical data have demonstrated the importance of indexing plasma/serum exposures for a drug to a measure of pathogen susceptibility to the same drug, such as the minimum inhibitory concentration (MIC) of the drug to the bacterial isolate of interest [23, 24].

For the majority of antimicrobial agents, preclinical evaluations of exposure-response relationships have demonstrated one or more of the following PK-PD indices to be associated with efficacy: the ratio of the area under the concentration-time curve (AUC) to

MIC (AUC:MIC ratio), the ratio of the maximum concentration (Cmax) to MIC (Cmax:MIC ratio), and the percentage of time during the dosing interval that drug concentrations remain above a threshold concentration (%*T*>threshold) [23, 25]. Alone, each component of the PK-PD index provides important but incomplete information. This principle was effectively demonstrated [24] using clinical trial data evaluating tigecycline for the treatment of patients with complicated intra-abdominal infections (cIAI) [26]. Figure 1 shows the percentage of 71 tigecycline-treated patients with cIAI enrolled in Phase 2 and 3 clinical studies who achieved bacteriologic success by the MIC of the baseline pathogen (the predominant pathogen for which was Enterobacteriaceae from among the 106 baseline pathogens isolated) and by bins of steady-state AUC and AUC:MIC ratio. It is evident from these data that neither pathogen susceptibility, as measured by MIC, nor drug exposure, as measured by AUC, alone provided enough information to explain drug effect. However, when drug exposure was indexed to pathogen susceptibility, as measured by AUC:MIC ratio, response to therapy was reasonably well predicted (i.e., the majority of patients who failed therapy had low AUC:MIC ratio estimates).

The choices for a dependent variable when evaluating exposure-response relationships for efficacy based on clinical data are usually more limited than those for independent variables. Categorical dependent variables, such as clinical or microbiological response to therapy (success or failure) assessed at the test-of-cure visit (i.e., a window of time after the end of study drug) and/or at the end of therapy, have typically been evaluated [27, 28]. Over the years, increasing interest has been placed on efficacy endpoints evaluated earlier in therapy. Updated guidance for the development of antibacterial agents for patients with acute bacterial skin and skin structure infections (ABSSSI) and community-acquired bacterial pneumonia (CABP) that has been issued by the US Food and Drug Administration (US FDA) describes clinical endpoints assessed on days 2–3 and 3–5, respectively [29, 30]. Less experience is available to assess the success of characterizing exposure-response relationships for efficacy using these endpoints. However, given the natural course of infection whereby bacterial eradication is followed by macrophage and inflammatory modulator activity, which is then followed by resolution of signs and symptoms, it may be difficult to identify exposure-response relationships for efficacy using endpoints assessed early after therapy has been initiated. Selecting time points for evaluation at which the difference in treatment effect is expected to be the greatest is optimal not only for clinical trial design but also for the evaluation of exposure-response relationships for efficacy.

Continuous dependent variables, such as change in bacterial density or lesion size, or time-to-event endpoints, such as time to

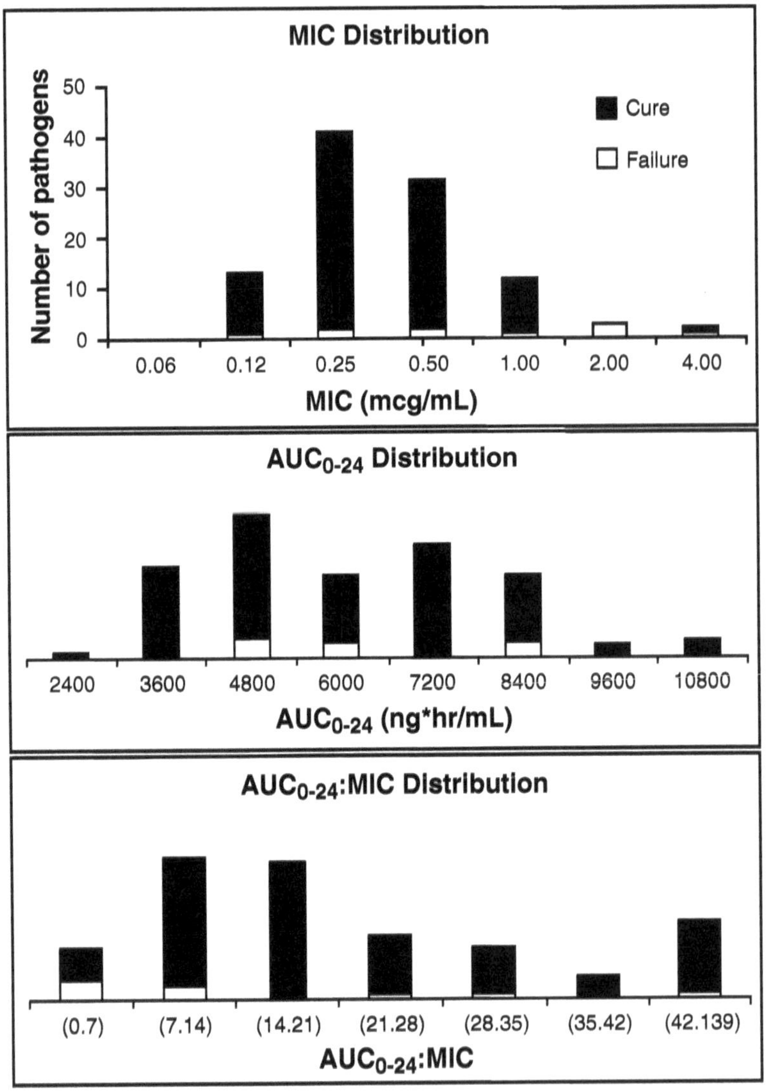

Fig. 1 Bacteriologic response stratified by the MIC of the baseline pathogen, AUC and AUC:MIC ratio for tigecycline-treated patients with cIAI enrolled in Phase 2 and 3 clinical studies. Reproduced from ref. 24 with permission from Oxford University Press

sign and symptom resolution, lesion size reduction, or bacteriologic eradication, may also be evaluated for exposure-response analyses for efficacy. Continuous or time-to-event endpoints are often more sensitive than categorical endpoints for capturing effect when evaluating exposure-response relationships for efficacy. Given the above-described importance of identifying the time point at which treatment effect is greatest, time-to-event analyses provide the advantage of allowing for this objective to be met as well as allowing for the effect of the drug over time to be determined

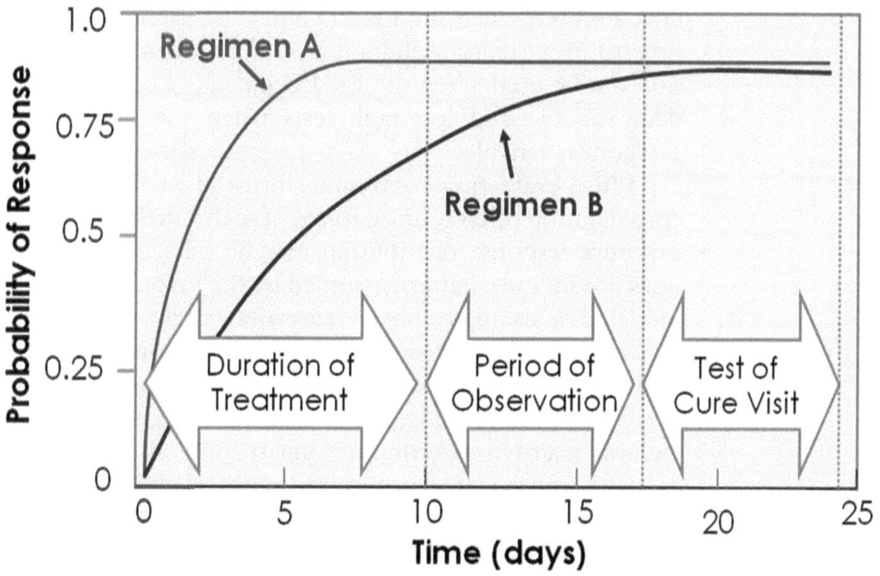

Fig. 2 Schematic for comparing drug regimens using a categorical efficacy endpoint. Reproduced from ref. 31 with permission from Oxford University Press

[31]. Figure 2 illustrates the information lost when one considers only the categorical efficacy endpoint, success or failure, assessed at a fixed time point rather than a time-to-event efficacy endpoint. As seen in this illustration, if the probability of a successful response was only assessed at the test-of-cure visit, Regimens A and B would not appear to be different despite the fact that the probability of a successful response was higher for Regimen A earlier in therapy. Thus, given the above, the evaluation of time-to-event efficacy endpoints is useful for defining the optimal duration of therapy. When used in exposure-response analyses for efficacy, the influence of increasing PK-PD indices on the time to achieving the efficacy endpoint can be assessed, the results of which can be used to inform decisions about dose and duration. An additional benefit for using continuous or time-to-event efficacy endpoints may be the requirement for data from fewer patients to detect differences of clinical interest.

Statistical approaches for characterizing univariable exposure-response relationships for efficacy are determined by the type of efficacy endpoint and the form of the PK-PD index evaluated. For dichotomous efficacy endpoints, logistic regression or Hill-type models can be used when the PK-PD index evaluated is a continuous independent variable; Chi-square or Fisher's exact test may be used for a PK-PD index that is a categorical variable. For continuous efficacy endpoints, linear regression, Spearman correlation, or Hill-type models can be used when the PK-PD index is a continuous independent variable and analysis of variance and Wilcoxon rank-sum test when the PK-PD index is a categorical variable. For time-to-event efficacy endpoints, Cox proportional hazard regression can be used when the PK-PD index is a continuous independent variable and log rank tests when the PK-PD index is a categorical variable.

When evaluating continuous forms of PK-PD indices without consideration of categorical forms of such variables, detection of an exposure-response relationship may be missed if the relationship does not follow a pattern assumed by the underlying mathematical model. For example, linear regression might not be an optimal tool to detect an exposure-response relationship that is not monotonic. By evaluating the PK-PD index in multiple forms, including as a continuous variable, but also divided into groups to characterize nonlinearity or non-monotonicity, one can increase the ability to detect potential exposure-response relationships. Possibilities for group assignments are quartiles, and also two-group and three-group divisions for which thresholds defining categorical independent variables may be optimally determined for the given endpoint of interest. For example, the resulting split of a classification tree for a dichotomous efficacy endpoint can be used to optimally identify a threshold for a two-group categorical independent variable.

Regardless of the type of endpoint, other factors may influence the ability to characterize the nature of the exposure-relationship. Limited sample size, fixed dosing regimens (thus resulting in a relatively more narrow range of exposures), or high efficacy rates can each impede the ability to understand the nature of such relationships. When one or more of these factors are present, identification of a significant relationship in which the PK-PD index is evaluated as a continuous independent variable may be unlikely. It still may be feasible, however, to identify a step function to describe the exposure-response relationship based on a grouped form of the PK-PD index. Such a relationship distinguishes patients with both lower PK-PD indices and percentages of successful response or a longer time to achieve an efficacy endpoint as compared to those with both higher PK-PD indices and percentages of successful response or shorter times to achieve the efficacy endpoint.

When the ability to characterize the nature of the exposure-relationship is limited, another consequence is wide confidence bounds around any mathematical parameters or functions used to describe the exposure-response relationship, thus reflecting inherent uncertainty. However, when inferences about the exposure-response relationships for efficacy based on such clinical data, including the magnitude of PK-PD targets, are consistent with those based on non-clinical data and/or other clinical datasets, the observed uncertainty can be mitigated by other data sources. As discussed later in this section, the application of pre-existing data as an input to conduct Bayesian-based exposure-response analyses represents an informative approach to decrease uncertainty of the findings based on analyses of clinical data.

5 Multivariable Analyses

If significant univariable exposure-response relationships for efficacy are identified or if adjustment for selected variables is deemed necessary to properly understand the relationship between the efficacy endpoint and a PK-PD index, multivariable analyses should be undertaken to evaluate predictors of response in a context in which all potential predictors are taken into account. Potential independent variables that can be considered include demographic characteristics and underlying comorbidities, including previously-defined risk factors. A recent analysis of univariable and multivariable exposure-response analyses for efficacy based on data from 61 tigecycline-treated patients with hospital-acquired or ventilator-associated bacterial pneumonia (HABP and VABP, respectively) [32] is described below. These 61 patients represented a subset of evaluable patients with tigecycline exposure data from among the 474 tigecycline-treated patients enrolled in the randomized, multicenter, double-blind, Phase 3 clinical trial described by Freire et al. [33]. Patients randomized to tigecycline received an intravenous (IV) loading dose of 100 mg of tigecycline followed by 50 mg IV every 12 h infused over 30–60 min for a minimum of 7 days.

In the above-described exposure-response analyses, the independent variable was free-drug AUC:MIC ratio, which was the PK-PD index that was most predictive of efficacy based on nonclinical data [34], and the dependent variables were clinical and microbiological response. As shown in Fig. 3a, b, the fitted functions and associated 95 % pointwise confidence bounds for exposure-response relationships identified using univariable logistic regression are shown overlaid on a histogram describing the observed distribution of free-drug AUC:MIC ratio. The solid box shown on each fitted function represents the threshold for free-drug AUC:MIC ratio when evaluated as a two-group variable as identified using classification tree analysis. A number of useful points were evident based on these results. First, as the free-drug AUC:MIC ratio increased, so too did the probability of clinical and microbiological success. Second, as expected, the 95 % pointwise confidence bounds around the logistic function were tight in the free-drug AUC:MIC ratio range in which the data density was high. Third, a large proportion of patients (31 %) had observed free-drug AUC:MIC ratios associated with a low probability of clinical success, which may indicate suboptimal tigecycline dose selection in this patient population.

In addition to free-drug AUC:MIC ratio, other independent variables were evaluated for associations with clinical and microbiological response in patients with HABP or VABP. Figure 4a shows the relationship between the probability of clinical success and albumin concentration stratified by free-drug AUC:MIC ratio,

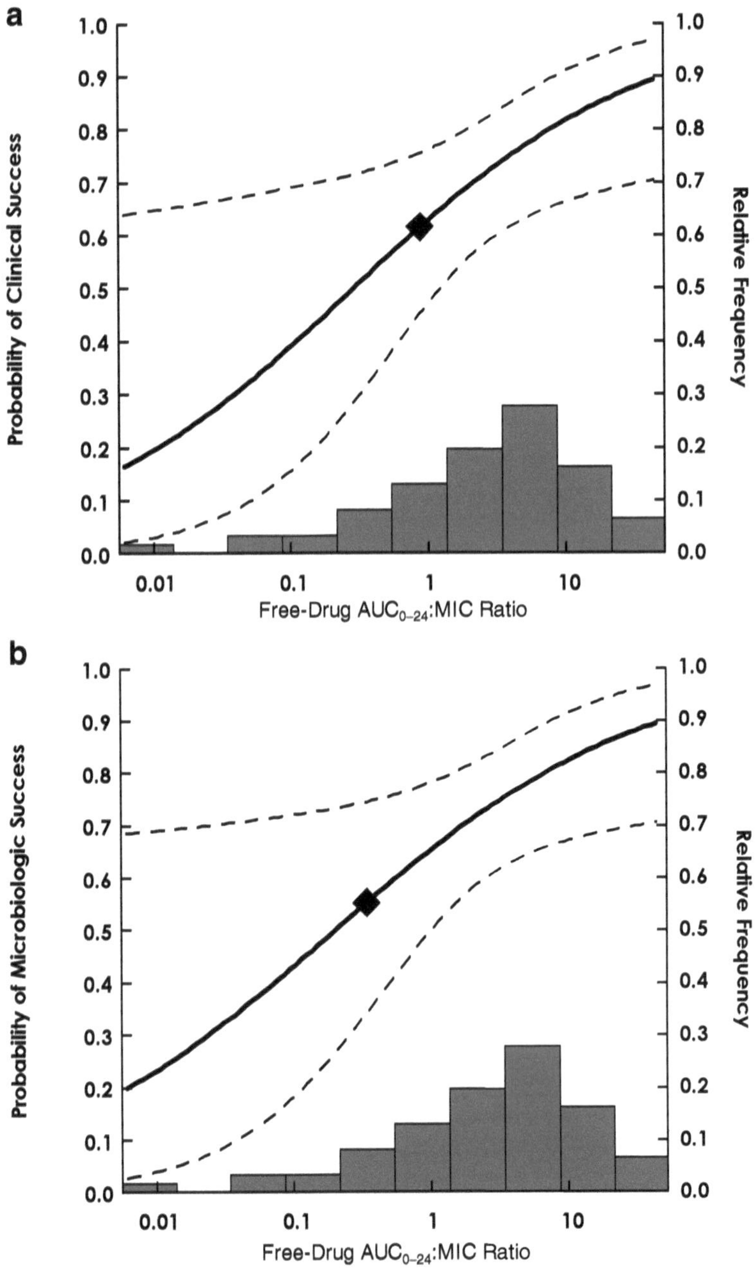

Fig. 3 Fitted functions for the relationship between the probability of clinical (**a**) and microbiological (**b**) success and free-drug AUC_{0-24}:MIC ratio based on univariable logistic regression models ($p=0.023$ and 0.031, respectively) overlaid on a histogram describing the observed free-drug AUC_{0-24}:MIC ratio distribution. The *dashed lines* represent the 95 % pointwise confidence bands derived based on the standard error of the logistic regression model parameters. The *solid box* on each fitted function represents the threshold for free-drug AUC_{0-24}:MIC ratio of 0.9 and 0.35 for the probability of clinical and microbiological success, respectively, derived based on classification tree analysis

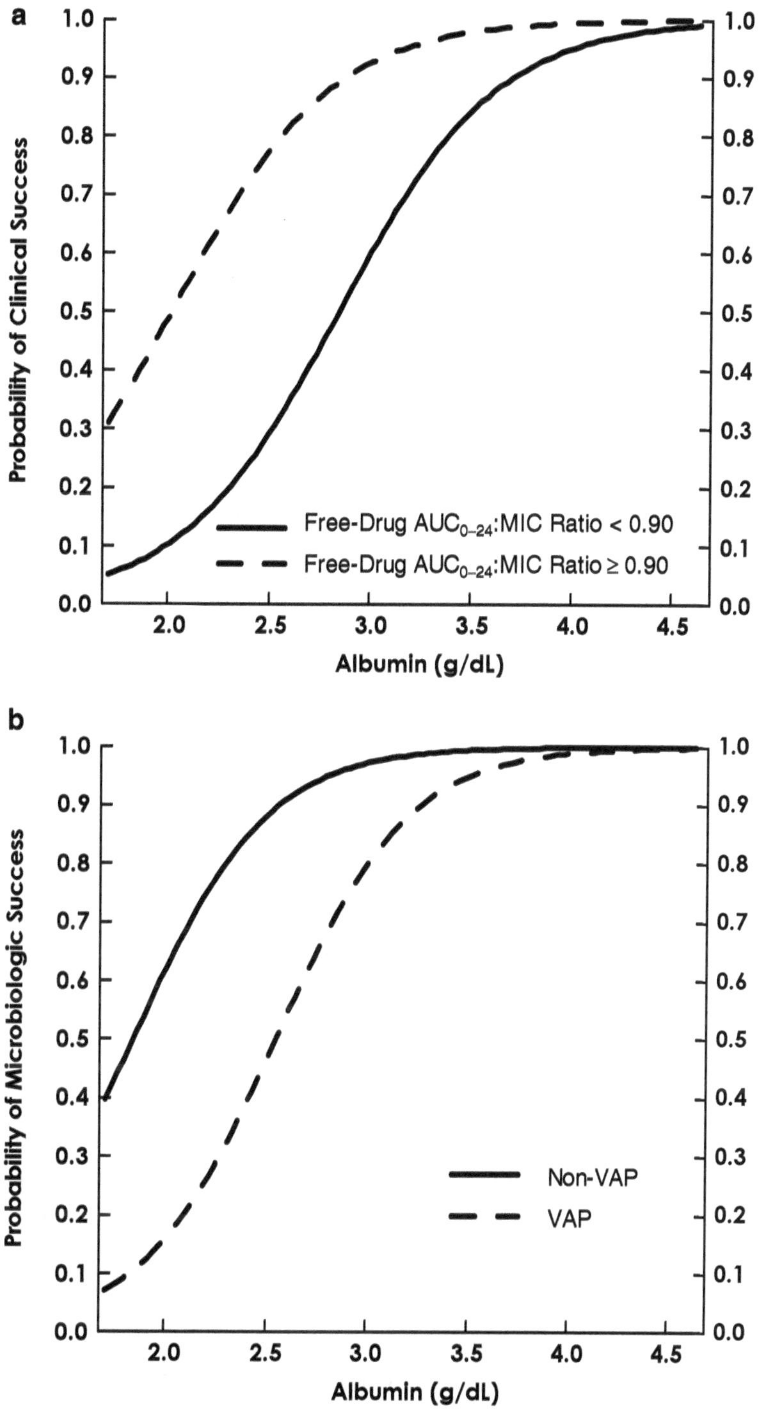

Fig. 4 Fitted functions for the relationship between the probability of clinical or microbiological success and albumin relative to free-drug AUC_{0-24}:MIC ratio evaluated as a two-group categorical variable (**a**) or VABP status (**b**)

evaluated as a two-group variable (as identified using classification tree analysis). As demonstrated by the logistic function shown, the model-predicted probability of clinical success approached one for patients with and without adequate tigecycline exposure and normal baseline albumin concentration (4 g/dL). However, for patients with very low baseline albumin (2.0 g/dL), the influence of inadequate (free-drug AUC:MIC ratio <0.90) versus adequate (free-drug AUC:MIC ratio ≥0.90) tigecycline exposure on the probability of clinical success was greater (0.35 compared to <0.1). In Fig. 4b, the relationship between the probability of microbiological success and albumin concentration stratified by VABP status is shown. Similar to tigecycline exposure, the influence of VABP status on the probability of microbiological success was far greater for patients with very low compared to normal baseline albumin concentrations. Given that MIC distributions for baseline pathogens differed for patients stratified by VABP status, the ability to identify a relationship between the probability of microbiological success and MIC was confounded when evaluated together with VABP status.

Not unexpectedly, the above-described findings demonstrate the ability of independent variables other than tigecycline free-drug AUC:MIC ratio to predict the probability of clinical or microbiological response to therapy in this patient population. While the sample size of this evaluation and the number of independent variables that could be incorporated into a multivariable model were limited, the above-described analysis results illustrate the potential of independent variables other than drug exposure to influence response. The retention of a significant exposure-response relationship in a multivariable model that contains other influential independent variables provides an added degree of certainty about the presence of the relationship.

When evaluating the results of multivariable models, it is useful to assess model-predicted response relative to observed response for cohorts of patients described by independent variables included in the final models. In the above-described analysis of tigecycline-treated patients with HABP or VABP, the performance of each of the logistic regression models presented was assessed by comparing the agreement between the observed proportion of patients with a successful response and the average model-estimated probability of a successful response among cohorts of patients described by combinations of independent variables. The data demonstrated that there was good agreement between observed proportions and average model-estimated probabilities of successful responses, even for those cohorts for which the sample size was limited. While there are a variety of other ways for evaluating the fit of a model resulting from the various statistical approaches described earlier, discussion of these approaches is beyond the scope of this chapter.

6 Application of a Bayesian Approach

Statistical approaches that have historically been used to evaluate data, including exposure-response data, have been based on frequentist inference. Alternative statistical approaches, such as Bayesian inference, have rarely been considered. The two approaches differ with regard to whether or not prior information is used. For frequentist analyses, the quantification of the data does not include consideration of prior data. Inferences based on the results of these analyses may, however, be made in the context of such prior information. In contrast, both prior information and the study data influence the results and conclusions when Bayesian analyses are conducted.

When considering prior information for exposure-response analyses of an antimicrobial agent using clinical data, there is a unique opportunity to consider in vitro and/or in vivo PK-PD findings. Such data, which represents a pre-screen for an antimicrobial agent, is generated before clinical development is initiated. Using the example of the evaluation of tigecycline for patients with HABP or VABP once again, in vitro studies demonstrated tigecycline's activity against target pathogens [35, 36]. In vivo studies conducted using a neutropenic murine-thigh infection model served to characterize the magnitude of the free-drug AUC:MIC ratio associated with efficacy [34]. Subsequent clinical studies of tigecycline-treated patients with cIAI and ABSSSI, indications for which US FDA approval was received [37], demonstrated efficacy. Moreover, exposure-response relationships were also characterized based on these data; results of such analyses confirmed the preclinical observation that increasing AUC:MIC ratio was associated with improved response [26, 38, 39]. Thus, for antimicrobial agents that enter late-stage clinical development, valuable preclinical and clinical priors are available for use when conducting exposure-response analyses for efficacy. To demonstrate the utility of Bayesian principles applied to such analyses, the above-described dataset of 61 patients with HABP or VABP [32] was evaluated using frequentist and Bayesian logistic regression analyses [40]. Specific objectives of the analyses were to determine and compare the magnitude of treatment effect and the ability of clinical trial endpoints to capture drug benefit.

When selecting prior information to be incorporated into a Bayesian analysis, it is important to justify the use of such external data. For tigecycline in the treatment of patients with HABP or VABP, the above-described in vivo data from a neutropenic murine-thigh infection model [34] were selected. These included the slope and the dynamic range based on the exposure-response relationship for *Staphylococcus aureus*, a major target pathogen. The slope was a useful parameter to inform the analysis since, as indicated by the

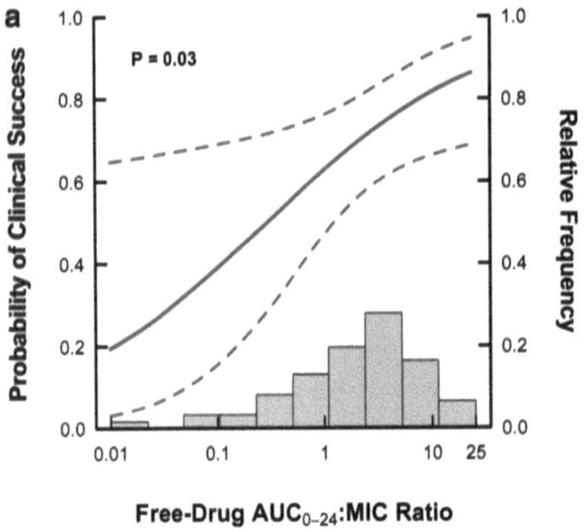

Fig. 5 Frequentist (**a**) and Bayesian (**b**) logistic regression-estimated relationships between the probability of clinical success and the tigecycline free-drug AUC:MIC ratio based on data from 61 patients with HABP. The *solid lines* represent the fitted functions based on logistic regression while the *dashed lines* represent the upper and lower 95 % pointwise confidence and credible bounds, respectively. The *green histogram* represents the distribution of observed values for free-drug AUC:MIC ratio

positive sign for the parameter, higher free-drug AUC:MIC ratios were associated with a greater magnitude of effect. Lower and upper limits of free-drug AUC:MIC ratio of 0.01 and 25, respectively, which represented the range over which the majority of drug effect in animals was observed [34] and which was encompassed in the range observed in HABP/VABP patients [32], were selected.

Figure 5a, b shows fitted functions representing the exposure-response relationships for clinical response based on frequentist and Bayesian logistic regression, respectively. For the frequentist analysis, 95 % pointwise confidence bounds are shown while for the Bayesian analysis, 95 % pointwise credible bounds are shown. As shown in Fig. 5b, the Bayesian credible intervals were tighter than the frequentist confidence intervals. As described below, treatment effect was estimated using these exposure-response relationships, frequentist and Bayesian approaches, and three different methods based on the probability of a successful response at free-drug AUC:MIC ratios of 0.01 and 25.

For Method 1, treatment effect was calculated as the difference in point estimates of the probability of clinical success at AUC:MIC ratios of 0.01 and 25. For Method 2, treatment effect was calculated as the difference between the upper limit of a 95 % interval for the probability of clinical success at an AUC:MIC ratio of 0.01 and the lower limit of a 95 % interval for the probability of clincal success at an AUC:MIC ratio of 25. This approach is analogous to the current practice for estimating treatment effect for the design of non-inferiority clinical trials for antimicrobial agents [41]. Figure 6 shows a schematic for calculating treatment effect

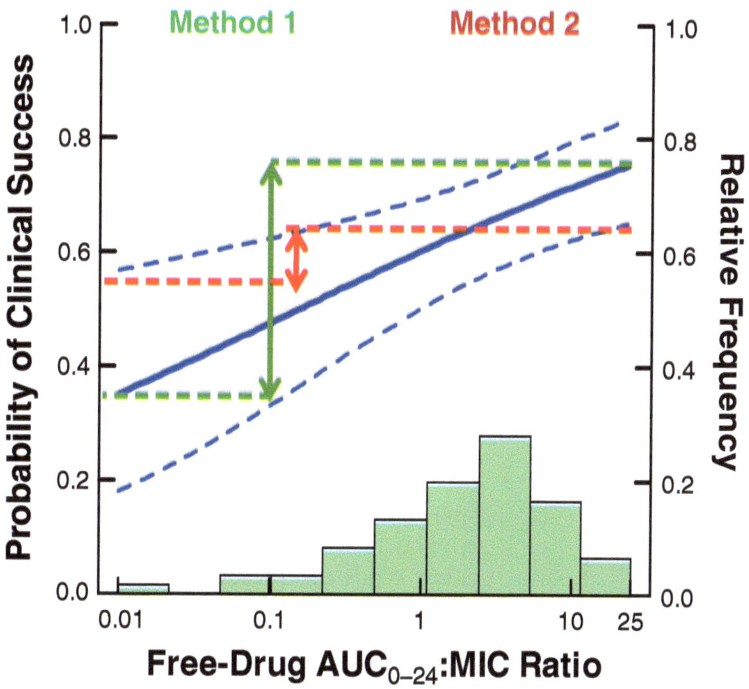

Fig. 6 Schematic showing the calculation of treatment effect based on an exposure-response relationship for efficacy using two methods

based on the relationship between the probability of clinical success and free-drug AUC:MIC ratio using Bayesian logistic regression and Methods 1 and 2. Finally, for Method 3, 95 % lower bounds for the treatment effect were obtained by using 1000 bootstrap samples and the bias-correcting acceleration method.

Estimates of the treatment effect for clinical response as determined using frequentist and Bayesian logistic regression and each of the above-described three methods are summarized in Table 1. Differences in point estimates of the treatment effect for clinical response (Method 1) were larger using the frequentist compared to the Bayesian approach. However, the comparatively tighter Bayesian credible intervals were indicative of increased certainty with the latter approach. For Methods 2 and 3, treatment effect was greater for the Bayesian analyses. These results demonstrate the utility of frequentist and Bayesian-based analyses to quantify treatment effect, an endpoint which is important for powering clinical trials. And while not illustrative of the benefits of a Bayesian approach, these results also demonstrated that irrespective of the type of approach, use of bootstrapping to obtain lower bounds for the treatment effect served to improve upon an overly imprecise and arbitrary practice of taking the difference between the lower bound of the interval for the maximal effect and the upper bound of the interval for the minimal effect.

Table 1
Estimates of treatment effect for clinical response as determined using frequentist and Bayesian logistic regression and three different methods[a]

	Treatment effect estimated by method		
Approach	1	2	3
Frequentist logistic regression	0.672	0.043	0.211
Bayesian logistic regression	0.405	0.085	0.314

[a]Based on the probability of clinical success at free-drug AUC:MIC ratios of 0.01 and 25.

While the above-described example was based on the evaluation of an exposure-response relationship using a dichotomous efficacy endpoint and logistic regression, a Bayesian approach can be applied to the evaluation of exposure-response relationships using other types of efficacy endpoints. Regardless of the type of endpoints or statistical analyses undertaken, consideration of prior data using a Bayesian approach could increase the certainty in the findings. However, whether certainty can be increased or the degree to which it can be increased by a Bayesian approach will depend on the quality and careful quantification of the prior information.

7 Applications of Exposure-Response Analyses for Efficacy

The current paradigm for identifying dosing regimens for further clinical study and establishing interpretive criteria for in vitro susceptibility testing for antimicrobial agents involves the use of population PK models based on Phase 1 PK data, PK-PD targets based on preclinical data, surveillance data, and Monte Carlo simulation [6, 10, 42, 43]. Using these inputs and statistical approach, the probability of simulated patients achieving PK-PD targets associated with efficacy over a MIC distribution for a relevant pathogen and by MIC value are determined. By evaluating PK-PD target attainment over a MIC distribution, the performance of a dosing regimen can be assessed from a population perspective, weighting the probability of isolates at different MIC values in accordance with the likelihood of their occurrence. By evaluating probabilities of PK-PD target attainment by MIC value, a susceptibility breakpoint, which is defined as the highest MIC value at which a high probability of PK-PD target attainment is achieved, can be identified.

In later stages of drug development, there is an opportunity to use Phase 2 and/or 3 data to refine the population PK and potentially the PK-PD target inputs. Such PK-PD targets, which represent thresholds that divide patients with higher PK-PD indices achieving greater efficacy compared to those with lower PK-PD indices achieving less efficacy, can be identified. Approaches to identify PK-PD targets include the use of recursive partitioning (e.g., classification and regression tree analysis), constructing receiver operating characteristic (ROC) curves, or using a PK-PD index associated with a given magnitude of the efficacy endpoint. However, as described below, the assessment of PK-PD target attainment based on clinically-derived PK-PD targets suffers from an important limitation [44, 45] and does not make full use of the available data.

The limitation of PK-PD target attainment analyses is that failure to achieve a PK-PD target, as evidenced by a low probability of PK-PD target attainment at a given MIC value, does not necessarily imply that the probability of a successful response will also be low at that same MIC value. Similarly, a high probability of PK-PD target attainment at a given MIC value does not necessarily imply a high probability of a successful response. The basis for this lack of correlation is that other patient factors besides drug exposure and pathogen susceptibility, such as underlying medical illnesses or severity of illness, also influence response. Thus, to overcome this limitation and make better use of the information provided by the exposure-response relationship for efficacy, model-predicted probabilities of response rather than probabilities of PK-PD target attainment can be assessed by MIC value. To demonstrate this point, the results of an exposure-response analysis conducted using data from clinical trials for 82 quinolone-treated patients with CABP can be examined [46]. Results of classification tree analysis demonstrated that a free-drug AUC:MIC ratio of 33.8 was predictive of a successful clinical response. The probability of a successful clinical response for patients with free-drug AUC:MIC ratios at and above versus below this breakpoint was 95 % and 67 %, respectively. Thus, despite 100 % of patients achieving the PK-PD target, the percentage of successful clinical responses was less than 100 %. Also, rather than clinical response approaching 0 % for those patients who did not achieve the PK-PD index, the percentage of successful clinical responses was 67 %, which was similar to the estimate of 69 % for the *y*-intercept (E_0 which is the drug effect in the presence of no drug) for the Hill-type function that was used to describe this exposure-response relationship. Instead of merely assessing PK-PD target attainment, an exposure-response relationship derived using clinical data can be used together with the population PK model and Monte Carlo simulation to generate probabilities of model-predicted response. By using an exposure-response relationship to determine the probability of achieving an efficacy endpoint at given MIC values, such predictions are likely to be more aligned with observed successful response than probabilities of PK-PD target attainment at that MIC.

Differences between the percent probabilities of PK-PD target attainment and model-predicted clinical response by MIC were demonstrated for tigecycline in an evaluation of the interpretive criteria for in vitro susceptibility testing for Enterobacteriaceae [44].

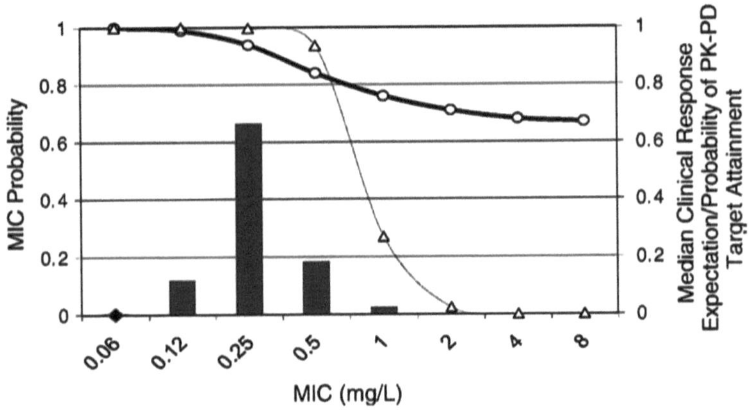

Fig. 7 Probabilities of PK-PD target attainment (*open triangles*) and the median model-predicted probabilities of clinical success (*open circles*) by MIC value overlaid on the MIC distribution (*gray bars*) of tigecycline against *E. coli* ($n = 440$). Reproduced from ref. 44 with permission from Elsevier

The PK-PD target and model for clinical response were based on the previously-described exposure-response relationship for efficacy based on tigecycline-treated patients with cIAI [26]. The results of this assessment showed that a total-drug AUC:MIC ratio of 6.96 was associated with a higher probability of achieving a positive clinical response; total-drug AUC:MIC ratios ≥6.96 were associated with 94 % of patients having a successful clinical response while total-drug AUC:MIC ratios <6.96 were associated with 60 % of patients having a successful clinical response ($p = 0.04$). Figure 7 shows probabilities of PK-PD target attainment (open triangles) and the median model-predicted probabilities of clinical success (open circles) by MIC value overlaid on the MIC distribution (gray bars) of tigecycline against *E. coli* ($n = 440$). At MIC values of 0.25 mg/L or less, both sets of probabilities were high. However, for a MIC value of 1 mg/L, the probability of PK-PD target attainment was 0.27 while the model-predicted probability of clinical success was 0.76. Regardless of which set of results one examines, results of these analyses do not support the current US FDA susceptibility breakpoint for tigecycline against Enterobacteriaceae of 2 mg/L [37].

In conclusion, PK-PD target attainment analyses supporting the selection of dose or susceptibility breakpoints that are conducted later in drug development should be conducted using exposure-response relationships when such data are available.

8 PK-PD Analyses for Safety

The favorable safety and tolerability profile for a number of classes of antimicrobial agents [19, 20], including beta-lactam agents, has allowed for the administration of higher doses of such agents to patients with serious infections arising from potentially resistant bacterial pathogens. Characterization of exposure-response relationships for safety endpoints has, therefore, been limited to select agents and/or subclasses of agents which have demonstrated a narrow therapeutic window. For such agents, safety signals based on dose-ranging clinical data can be used to define the upper bound for dosing. This method of investigation, as described below for tigecycline, is a common practice during early clinical drug development. For other agents, alternate dosing strategies may allow for administration of the antimicrobial agent in a manner that reduces the likelihood of the occurrence of the safety event. Such was the case for aminoglycosides, principles as described below that were better understood decades after these agents had been introduced into clinical practice.

In this section, three examples of exposure-response analyses for safety are reviewed [21, 47, 48]. In the first example, data demonstrating the relationships between tigecycline exposure and the probability of nausea and vomiting were examined [47]. The result of such analyses, which were based on Phase 1 data, helped identify the upper limit of tigecycline dosing. For the second example, exposure-response relationships for both safety and efficacy are examined for aminoglycosides. Such dual considerations allowed for the identification of an optimal exposure window [21]. In the third example, exposure-response relationships for three endpoints, safety, efficacy, and emergence of resistance, and the application of these relationships to inform dose selection for daptomycin [48], are reviewed.

The wide exposure range provided through the conduct of dose-ranging Phase 1 studies provides the opportunity to characterize dose- and/or exposure-response relationships for safety endpoints early in clinical development. Passarell and colleagues used data from 136 subjects enrolled in three Phase 1 studies to evaluate relationships between tigecycline exposure and the probability of nausea and vomiting [47]. Subjects received one of seven single IV tigecycline doses ranging from 12.5 to 300 mg. Significant relationships between AUC from 0 to infinity ($AUC_{0-\infty}$) and the probability of the first occurrence of nausea and vomiting ($p < 0.0001$ for each), which were based on logistic regression models, are shown in Fig. 8a, b, respectively. The 25th to 75th percentiles of the $AUC_{0-\infty}$ range at each dose level are shown by the vertical bars. At the median $AUC_{0-\infty}$ values of 2.6 mg•h/L for 50 mg and 4.7 mg•h/L for 100 mg (the approved maintenance and loading dose, respectively), model-predicted percent probabilities of nausea were 26 and 33 %, respectively. At these same exposures, model-predicted percent probabilities of vomiting were 7.5 and 11 %, respectively. The percent probability of nausea increased dramatically with higher doses. For tigecycline doses greater than or equal to 200 mg, the percent probability of nausea was greater

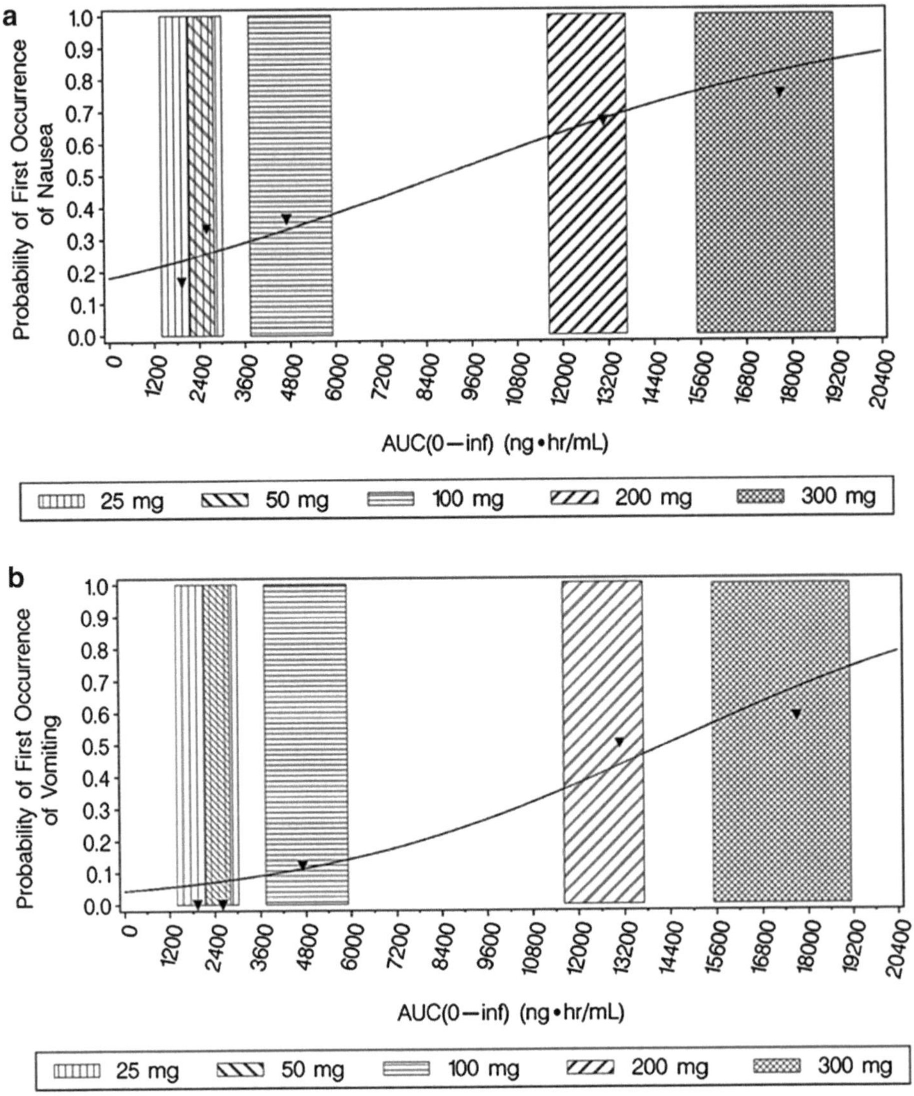

Fig. 8 Relationships between the probability of $AUC_{0-\infty}$ and the first occurrence of nausea (**a**) and vomiting (**b**) based on data from subjects who received single IV doses of tigecycline. The 25th to 75th percentiles of the $AUC_{0-\infty}$ range at each dose level are shown by the *vertical bars*. The *line* represents the model-based probability of the first occurrence of nausea and vomiting. The *triangles* represent the observed probability of nausea and vomiting in each dose group. Reproduced from ref. [47] with permission from Elsevier

than 60 %. For vomiting, the percent probability was greater than 30 %. Despite the single doses studied, the above-described model-predicted percent probabilities were consistent with rates of nausea and vomiting among tigecycline-treated patients with ABSSSI (nausea, 24.4 %; vomiting, 19.2 %) and cIAI (nausea, 34.5 %; vomiting, 19.6 %) enrolled in Phase 3 clinical trials [49, 50]. Perhaps as would be expected given that 28.1 % of patients had VABP, rates of these events were lower among patients with HABP or VABP (nausea, 15.4 %; vomiting, 12.6 %) [33]. Although nausea and vomiting were the most frequently reported adverse events among tigecycline-treated patients, such events rarely led to the discontinuation of the drug [33, 49, 50]. The results of the above-described exposure-response analyses for nausea and vomiting supported the decision to limit Phase 3 tigecycline dosing regimens to 100 mg administered as a loading dose following by 50 mg once daily. When available early in clinical development, data from exposure-response analyses for safety endpoints can be combined with preclinical PK-PD targets associated with efficacy to identify dosing regimens that will have a high likelihood of being well tolerated and efficacious.

The dual examination of exposure-response relationships for safety and efficacy endpoints allows for the evaluation of risk versus benefit for a given dosing regimen. For aminoglycosides, a class of agents for which exposure-response relationships for safety and efficacy have been the focus of investigation for several decades, results of such analyses [51, 52] have allowed for the identification of an optimal exposure window [21]. As described for this example, the integration of exposure-response analyses for safety and efficacy in this manner allows for the understanding of the impact of MIC and the chosen dosing regimen on the probabilities of achieving safety and efficacy endpoints. However, as a prelude to these data, it is useful to review earlier insights gathered from non-clinical and clinical data that led to the use of less fractionated aminoglycoside dosing regimens.

Preclinical observations of saturable aminoglycoside uptake by proximal renal tubular epithelial cells [53–55] led to the conduct of in vivo and clinical studies to compare drug uptake of different dosing schedules [56, 57]. Results of such studies demonstrated that more fractionated dosing regimens resulted in higher drug concentrations in the proximal renal tubular epithelial cells. Subsequent clinical studies were initiated to test the hypothesis that less frequent aminoglycoside administration, which would result in less aminoglycoside uptake, would lead to a lower rate of nephrotoxicity for patients treated with shorter courses of therapy [51, 58]. These data demonstrated a significant reduction in the occurrence of nephrotoxicity for once-daily versus more frequent administration of netilmicin [58]. Similarly, Rybak et al. [51], who evaluated exposure-response relationships for aminoglycosides, reported a significantly lower likelihood of nephrotoxicity for administration of therapy once daily versus every 12 h. Additional studies provided further data to support earlier observations of reduced rates of nephrotoxicity [59]. Since AUC:MIC ratio and Cmax:MIC ratio were the PK-PD indices that are most predictive of efficacy [25], administration of less fractionated aminoglycoside dosing regimens was not predicted to be associated with less efficacy than more fractionated dosing regimens. Ultimately, the above-described data changed the clinical practice for administering aminoglycosides [60, 61].

Using the results of the exposure-response analyses for the probability of nephrotoxicity of aminoglycosides reported by Ryak et al. based on data from 74 patients with Gram-negative bacterial infections, together with the results of the exposure-response relationship for the probability of temperature defervescence reported by Kashuba et al. based on data from 78 patients with nosocomial pneumonia [51, 52] who received aminoglycosides, Drusano et al. examined exposure windows based on scenarios with different MIC values [21]. Figure 9 shows the relationships between the AUC for gentamicin or tobramycin and the probability of nephrotoxicity (red-colored functions) and the probability of temperature defervescence (black-colored functions) shown as a function of three different MIC values, 0.25, 0.5, and 1.0 mg/L, in panels a, b, and c, respectively. The aminoglycoside dosing regimen was gentamicin or tobramycin 5 mg/kg per day administered as 2.5 mg/kg dose every 12 h. In this example, a weight of 80 kg was assumed and a dose of 200 mg was administered every 12 h. In each panel, the horizontal lines represent the values at which the probability of temperature defervescence is 0.9 and the probability of nephrotoxicity is 0.1. The vertical lines represent the optimal exposure window which was defined as the AUC values associated with probabilities of temperature defervescence ≥0.9 and probabilities of nephrotoxicity ≤0.1.

As can be seen in Fig. 9a, a broad exposure window exists for probabilities of 0.9 and 0.1 for temperature defervescence and nephrotoxicity, respectively, when the gentamicin or tobramycin MIC value is 0.25 mg/L. As shown in Fig. 9b, the exposure window narrows markedly when the MIC value increases to 0.5 mg/L. At an MIC of 1.0 mg/L (Fig. 9c), a probability of 0.9 for temperature defervescence cannot be achieved without a consequent probability of nephrotoxicity that approaches 60 %. In order to achieve a probability of 0.1 for nephrotoxicity, the probability of temperature defervescence would be approximately 0.75. Given that the use of aminoglycosides has become more common to treat infected patients for whom other antimicrobials are not an option, the goal for individualizing therapy is to achieve the highest probability of efficacy while keeping the probability of nephrotoxicity reasonably low.

In the last example, results of an analysis for daptomycin are discussed [48]. This analysis involved the integration of exposure-response relationships for the following three endpoints in order to evaluate the risk versus benefit of different dosing regimens: (1) the probability of CPK elevation, (2) the probability of clinical success, and (3) the time to decreased susceptibility. The clinical data used to derive these relationships were obtained from a Phase 3 clinical trial

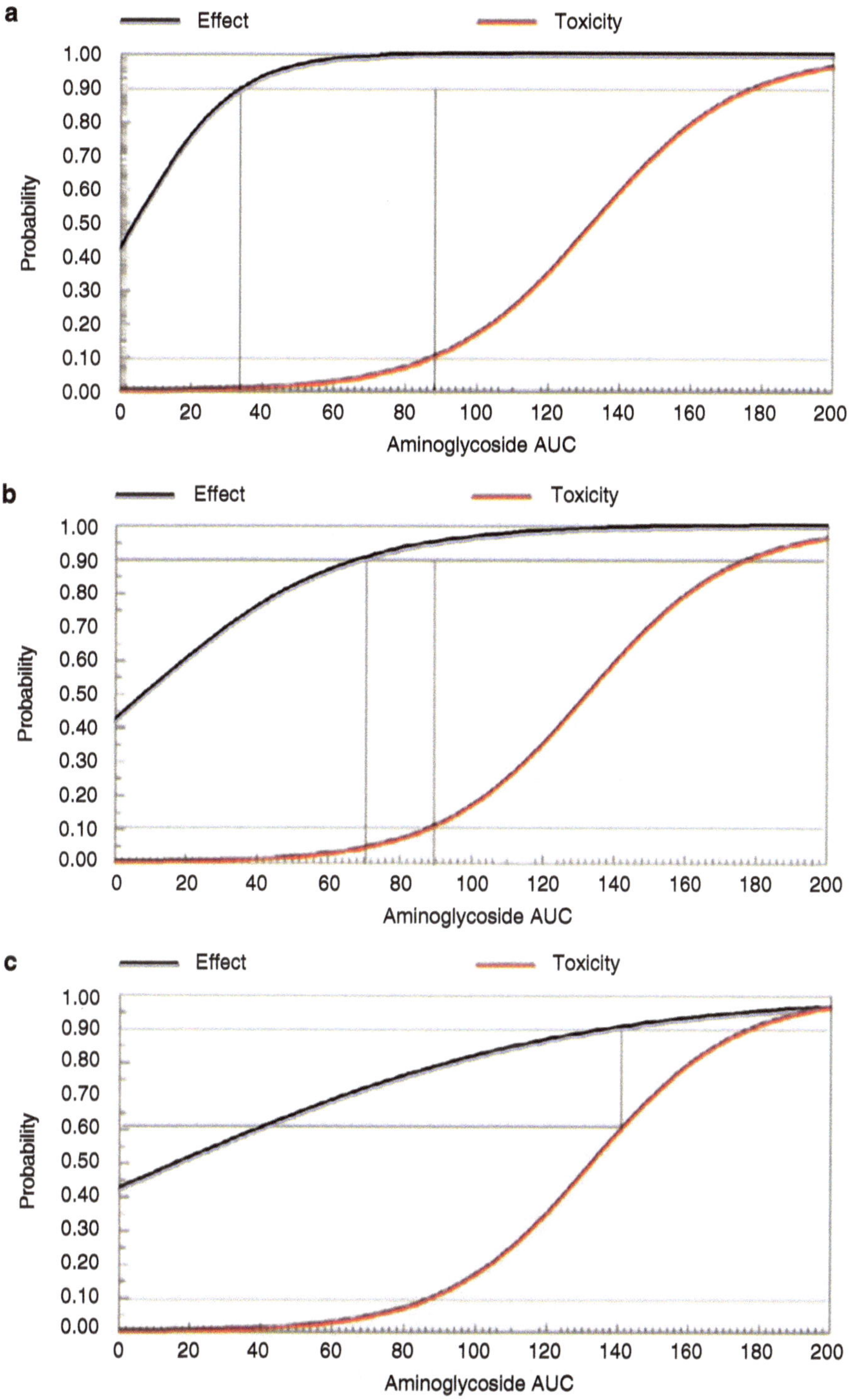

Fig. 9 The relationships between the AUC for gentamicin or tobramycin and the probability of nephrotoxicity (*red-colored functions*) and the probability of temperature defervescence (*black-colored functions*) shown as a function of three different MIC values, 0.25, 0.5, and 1.0 mg/L, in panels (**a**), (**b**), and (**c**), respectively. Reproduced from ref. [21] with permission from Oxford University Press

in which patients with *Staphylococcus aureus* bacteremia with or without infective endocarditis received daptomycin 6 mg/kg/day [62]. The analysis of the exposure-response relationships for CPK elevation demonstrated that daptomycin trough concentrations ≥24.3 mg/L were associated with a higher probability of CPK elevation [63]. Exposure-response relationships identified for the probability of clinical response and time to decreased daptomycin susceptibility during therapy were both non-monotonic in nature. The relationship between the probability of clinical success and AUC:MIC ratio resembled a U shape (i.e., the probability of a positive clinical success was low in the middle of the AUC:MIC ratio distribution and high at low and high ends of the distribution). An inverted U shape was evident for the relationship between time to decreased daptomycin susceptibility and AUC:MIC ratio. At 30 days after the start of therapy, the probability of patients with decreased susceptibility was 0, 0.278, and 0.081 in patients with low, intermediate, and high AUC:MIC ratios, respectively. Similar such exposure-response relationships for efficacy and the resistance amplification of quinolones have been described based on in vitro PK-PD system and clinical data [64, 65].

Using the above-described relationships and Monte Carlo simulation [48], probabilities of each endpoint by MIC for daptomycin 6 and 8 mg/kg/day were calculated. Impressive improvements for probabilities of clinical success and decreased susceptibility at 30 days were not evident for 6 versus 8 mg/kg/day. The probability of CPK elevation was modestly lower for the 6 versus 8 mg/kg/day dosing regimen (0.073 versus 0.114). However, the risk of CPK elevation, which is reversible, should be assessed in the context of the mortality and severe morbidity associated with these serious infections. The assessment of the joint probability of favorable outcomes (i.e., clinical success, no change in susceptibility, and no CPK elevation) was also consistent with the above-described findings and did not reveal impressive differences between dosing regimens. Although impressive differences between dosing regimens were not identified, the assessment of these probabilities by clinical scenarios defined by the combination of four independent variables included in the multivariable model (creatinine clearance, AUC:MIC ratio, albumin, and diagnosis category for bacteremia with or without infective endocarditis) served to identify populations of patients for which optimal daptomycin exposure had the greatest and least impact.

While the identification of exposure-response relationships based on data from patients who received one dose level represented an important limitation of the above-described analyses for daptomycin, the paradigm to assess risk versus benefit of different dosing regimens in this manner is instructive. Exposure-response relationships for antimicrobials have three potential axes. While efficacy and safety endpoints are typically considered, the probability of antimicrobial resistance which is measured on the third axis is a less commonly elucidated endpoint. However, by understanding the nature of exposure-response relationship for changes in MIC, outcomes for patient populations can be favorably impacted. Preserving the ability to use an antimicrobial agent is an important objective from a societal perspective. In conclusion, by applying exposure-response relationships to predict the probability of good outcomes, clinicians can make informed decisions regarding the risk versus benefit ratio for the administration of a given antimicrobial dosing regimen. Future evaluations of such relationships using multivariable analyses will allow clinicians to further understand the patient populations at greater risk and the impact of suboptimal antimicrobial exposure on each of the above-described endpoints.

9 Prospectus

The evaluation of the relationships between exposure and both efficacy and safety endpoints for antimicrobial agents using clinical data from patients provides valuable information that can be used to guide decisions during and after a drug is approved. As described herein, data from exposure-response relationships for efficacy and safety have been used to support decisions about dose selection early and late in clinical development and even after a drug has been approved. Results of clinical exposure-response analyses can also be used to inform decisions about in vitro susceptibility test interpretive criteria and to answer other questions related to the study design of clinical trials.

The next frontier is to use the concepts described herein at the patient bedside to support decisions when selecting antimicrobial therapy. By applying population PK models for which patient covariates explain a reasonable amount of variability in the PK of the antimicrobial agent, the distribution of expected drug exposures for groups of patients can be better predicted. Using these data together with expected or actual MIC values or appropriate MIC distributions for suspected or known infecting pathogens and exposure-response relationships for efficacy and/or safety endpoints, tools to be used at the patient's bedside can be developed to determine the probability that a given antimicrobial dosing regimen will achieve adequate drug exposure relative to PK-PD targets associated with positive outcomes. Such information can be used by clinicians, together with other patient-specific data, to better discriminate among choices of antimicrobial agents. In an era of increasing rates of resistance for bacterial pathogens and thus, fewer choices of antimicrobial agents, the use of PK-PD principles at the patient bedside to select optimal dosing regimens has never been needed more.

References

1. Dubois A, Lavielle M, Gsteiger S, Pigeolet E, Mentré F (2011) Model-based analyses of bioequivalence crossover trials using the stochastic approximation expectation maximization algorithm. Stat Med 30:2582–2600
2. Food and Drug Administration, U.S. Department of Health and Human Services (1999) Guidance for industry: population pharmacokinetics (Clinical Pharmacology)
3. Steimer JL, Mallet A, Golmard JL, Boisvieux JF (1984) Alternative approaches to estimation of population pharmacokinetic parameters: comparison with the nonlinear mixed-effect model. Drug Metab Rev 15: 265–292
4. Ette EI, Williams PJ (2004) Populations pharmacokinetics I: background, concepts, and models. Ann Pharmacother 38:1702–1706
5. Sheiner LB, Rosenberg B, Marathe VV (1977) Estimation of population characteristics of pharmacokinetic parameters from routine clinical data. J Pharmacokinet Biopharm 5: 445–479
6. Bhavnani SM, Hammel JP, Cirincione BB, Wikler MA, Ambrose PG (2005) Use of pharmacokinetic-pharmacodynamics target attainment analyses to support Phase 2 and 3 dosing strategies for doripenem. Antimicrob Agents Chemother 49:3944–3947
7. Van Wart SA, Andes DR, Ambrose PG, Bhavnani SM (2009) Pharmacokinetic-pharmacodynamic modeling to support doripenem dose regimen optimization for critically ill patients. Diagn Microbiol Infect Dis 63:409–414
8. Bhavnani SM, Lehoux D, Rubino CM, Moeck G, Okusanya OO, Forrest A, Parr TR Jr., Ambrose PG. Use of pharmacokinetics-pharmacodynamics to support oritavancin dose selection for patients with complicated skin and skin-structure infections. Clinical confirmation of proof of concept. In: Abstracts of the 49th interscience conference on antimicrobial agents and chemotherapy, San Francisco, CA, 12–15 September 2009, Abstract No. A1-1288
9. Bhavnani SM, Rubino CM, Hammel JP, Forrest A, Shlaes DM, Horn PT, Ambrose PG. Pharmacokinetics-pharmacodynamics and dose selection analyses for eravacycline using Phase 2 data from patients with community-acquired complicated intra-abdominal infections. In: Abstracts of the 53rd interscience conference on antimicrobial agents and chemotherapy, Denver, CO, 10–13 September 2013, Abstract No. A-293
10. Okusanya OO, Bhavnani SM, Forrest A, Bulik CC, Oldach D, Fernandes P, Ambrose PG. Population pharmacokinetics and pharmacokinetic-pharmacodynamic target attainment analyses for solithromycin to support intravenous dose selection in patients with community-acquired bacterial pneumonia. In: 52nd interscience conference on antimicrobial agents and chemotherapy, San Francisco, CA, 9–12 September 2012, Abstract No. A-1269
11. Wakefield J, Bennett J (1996) The Bayesian modeling of covariates for population pharmacokinetic models. J Am Stat Assoc 91:917–927
12. Preston SL, Drusano GL, Berman AL, Fowler CL, Chow AT, Dornseif B, Reichl V, Natarajan J, Wong FA, Corrado M (1998) Levofloxacin population pharmacokinetics and creation of a demographic model for prediction of individual drug clearance in patients with serious community-acquired infection. Antimicrob Agents Chemother 42:1098–1104
13. Li C, Kuti JL, Nightingale CH, Nicolau DP (2006) Population pharmacokinetic analysis and dosing regimen optimization of meropenem in adult patients. J Clin Pharmacol 46:1171–1178
14. Van Wart SA, Forrest A, Khariton T, Rubino CM, Bhavnani SM, Reynolds DK, Riccobene T, Ambrose PG (2013) Population pharmacokinetics of ceftaroline in patients with acute bacterial skin and skin structure infections or community-acquired bacterial pneumonia. J Clin Pharmacol 53:1155–1167
15. D'Argenio DZ (1981) Optimal sampling times for pharmacokinetic experiments. J Pharmacokinet Biopharm 9:739–756
16. Reed MD (1999) Optimal sampling theory: an overview of its application to pharmacokinetic studies in infants and children. Pediatrics 104:627–632
17. Drusano GL, Forrest A, Snyder MJ, Reed MD, Blumer JL (1988) An evaluation of optimal sampling strategy and adaptive study design. Clin Pharmacol Ther 44:232–238
18. Forrest A, Ballow CH, Nix DE, Birmingham MC, Schentag JJ (1993) Development of a population pharmacokinetic model and optimal sampling strategies for intravenous ciprofloxacin. Antimicrob Agents Chemother 37:1065–1072
19. Owens RC Jr (2008) An overview of harms associated with β-lactam antimicrobials: where do the carbapenems fit in? Crit Care 12(Suppl 4):S3–S13
20. Mohr JF III (2008) Update on the efficacy and tolerability of meropenem in the treat-

ment of serious bacterial infections. Clin Infect Dis 47:S41–S51

21. Drusano GL, Ambrose PG, Bhavnani SM, Bertino JS, Nafziger AN, Louie A (2007) Back to the future: using aminoglycosides again and how to dose them optimally. Clin Infect Dis 45:753–776
22. Guidance for Industry. Exposure-response analyses – Study design, data analysis, and regulatory applications. U.S. Department of Health and Human Services, Food and Drug Administration, Center for Drug Evaluation and Research (CDER), Center for Biologics Evaluation and Research (CBER), April 2003
23. Craig WA (1998) Pharmacokinetic/pharmacodynamic parameters: rationale for antibacterial dosing of mice and men. Clin Infect Dis 26:1–10
24. Ambrose PG, Bhavnani SM, Ellis-Grosse EJ, Drusano GL (2010) Pharmacokinetic-pharmacodynamic considerations in the design of hospital-acquired or ventilator-associated bacterial pneumonia studies: look before you leap! Clin Infect Dis 51:S103–S110
25. Craig WA (2007) Pharmacodynamics of antimicrobials: general concepts and application. In: Nightingale GH et al (eds) Antimicrobial pharmacodynamics in theory and clinical practice, 2nd edn. Informa Healthcare, New York
26. Passarell JA, Meagher AK, Liolios K, Cirincione BB, Van Wart SA, Babinchak T, Ellis-Grosse EJ, Ambrose PG (2008) Exposure-response analyses of tigecycline efficacy in patients with complicated intra-abdominal infections. Antimicrob Agents Chemother 52:204–210
27. Forrest A, Nix DE, Ballow CH, Goss TF, Birmingham MC, Schentag JJ (1993) Pharmacodynamics of intravenous ciprofloxacin in seriously ill patients. Antimicrob Agents Chemother 37:1073–1081
28. Drusano GL, Preston SL, Fowler C, Corrado M, Weisinger B, Kahn J (2004) Relationship between fluoroquinolone area under the curve: minimum inhibitory concentration ratio and the probability of eradication of the infecting pathogen, in patients with nosocomial pneumonia. J Infect Dis 189:1590–1597
29. U.S. Department of Health and Human Services, Food and Drug Administration. Guidance for Industry; Community-Acquired Bacterial Pneumonia: Developing drugs for treatment. Draft Guidance. January 2014
30. U.S. Department of Health and Human Services, Food and Drug Administration. Guidance for Industry; Acute bacterial skin and skin structure infections: Developing drugs for treatment. Draft guidance. August 2010
31. Ambrose PG (2008) Use of Pharmacokinetics and pharmacodynamics in a failure analysis of community-acquired pneumonia: implications for future clinical trial study design. Clin Infect Dis 47:S225–S231
32. Bhavnani SM, Rubino CM, Hammel JP, Forrest A, Dartois N, Cooper CA, Korth-Bradley J, Ambrose PG (2012) Pharmacological and patient-specific response determinants in patients with hospital-acquired pneumonia treated with tigecycline. Antimicrob Agents Chemother 56:1065–1072
33. Freire AT, Melnyk V, Kim MJ, Datsenko O, Dzyublik O, Glumcher F, Chuang YC, Maroko RT, Dukart G, Cooper CA, Korth-Bradley JM, Dartois N, Gandjini H, 311 Study Group (2010) Comparison of tigecycline with imipenem/cilistatin for the treatment of hospital-acquired pneumonia. Diagn Microbiol Infect Dis 68:140–151
34. van Ogtrop ML, Andes D, Stamstad TJ, Conklin B, Weiss WJ, Craig WA, Vesga O (2000) *In vivo* pharmacodynamic activities of two glycylcyclines (GAR-936 and WAY 152,288) against various Gram-positive and Gram-negative bacteria. Antimicrob Agents Chemother 44:943–949
35. Eliopoulos GM, Wennersten CB, Cole G, Moellering RC (1994) *In vitro* activities of two glycylcyclines against Gram-positive bacteria. Antimicrob Agents Chemother 38:534–541
36. Wise R, Andrews JM (1994) *In vitro* activities of two glycylcyclines. Antimicrob Agents Chemother 38:1096–1102
37. Tygacil tigecycline injection, powder, lyophilized, for solution. Product label. Wyeth Pharmaceuticals, Inc. A subsidiary of Pfizer Inc. Philadelphia, PA. December 2014
38. Meagher AK, Passarell JA, Cirincione BB, Van Wart SA, Liolios K, Babinchak T, Ellis-Grosse EJ, Ambrose PG (2007) Exposure-response analyses of tigecycline efficacy in patients with complicated skin and skin-structure infections. Antimicrob Agents Chemother 51:1939–1945
39. Bhavnani SM, Rubino CM, Ambrose PG, Babinchak TJ, Korth-Bradley JM, Drusano GL (2010) Impact of different factors on the probability of clinical response in tigecycline-treated patients with intra-abdominal infections. Antimicrob Agents Chemother 54:1207–1212
40. Ambrose PG, Hammel JP, Bhavnani SM, Rubino CM, Ellis-Grosse EJ, Drusano GL (2012) Frequentist and Bayesian pharmacometric-based approaches to facilitate critically needed new antibiotic development:

overcoming lies, damn lies, and statistics. Antimicrob Agents Chemother 56:1466–1470
41. U.S. Department of Health and Human Services, Food and Drug Administration. Guidance for Industry; Non-Inferiority Clinical Trials. Draft guidance. March 2010
42. Dudley MN, Ambrose PG, Bhavnani SM, Craig WA, Ferraro MJ, Jones RN (2013) Background and rationale for revised Clinical and Laboratory Standards Institute interpretive criteria (breakpoints) for Enterobacteriaceae and *Pseudomonas aeruginosa*: I. cephalosporins and aztreonam. Clin Infect Dis 56:1301–1309
43. Drusano GL, Preston SL, Hardalo C, Hare R, Banfield C, Andes D, Vesga O, Craig WA (2001) Use of preclinical data for selection of a Phase II/III dose for evernimicin and identification of a preclinical MIC breakpoint. Antimicrob Agents Chemother 45:13–22
44. Ambrose PG, Meagher AK, Passarell JA, Van Wart SA, Cirincione BB, Rubino CM, Korth-Bradley JM, Babinchak T, Ellis-Grosse E (2009) Use of a clinically derived exposure-response relationship to evaluate potential tigecycline-Enterobacteriaceae susceptibility breakpoints. Diagn Microbiol Infect Dis 63:38–42
45. Ambrose PG, Meagher AK, Passarell JA, Van Wart SA, Cirincione BB, Bhavnani SM, Ellis-Grosse E (2009) Application of patient population-derived pharmacokinetic-pharmacodynamic relationships to tigecycline breakpoint determination for staphylococci and streptococci. Diagn Microbiol Infect Dis 63:155–159
46. Bhavnani SM, Forrest A, Hammel JP, Drusano GL, Rubino CM, Ambrose PG (2008) Pharmacokinetics-pharmacodynamics of quinolones against *Streptococcus pneumoniae* in patients with community-acquired pneumonia. Diagn Microbiol Infect Dis 62:99–101
47. Passarell J, Ludwig E, Liolios K, Meagher AK, Grasela TH, Babinchak T, Ellis-Grosse EJ (2009) Exposure-response analyses of tigecycline tolerability in healthy subjects. Diagn Microbiol Infect Dis 65:123–129
48. Bhavnani SM, Ambrose PG, Hammel JP, Rubino CM, Drusano GL (2016) Evaluation of daptomycin exposure and efficacy and safety endpoints to support risk versus benefit considerations. Antimicrob Agents Chemother 60(3): 1600–1607. doi:10.1128/AAC.02967-15
49. Ellis-Grosse EJ, Babinchak T, Dartois N, Rose G, Loh E (2005) The efficacy and safety of tigecycline in the treatment of skin and skin structure infections: results of 2 double-blind Phase 3 comparison studies with vancomycin-aztreonam. Clin Infect Dis 41(Suppl 5):S341–S353
50. Babinchak T, Ellis-Grosse E, Dartois N, Rose GM, Loh E (2005) The efficacy and safety of tigecycline for the treatment of complicated intra-abdominal infections: analysis of pooled clinical trial data. Clin Infect Dis 41(Suppl 5):S354–S367
51. Rybak MJ, Abate BJ, Kang SL, Ruffing MJ, Lemer SA, Drusano GL (1999) Prospective evaluation of the effect of an aminoglycoside dosing regimen on rates of observed nephrotoxicity and ototoxicity. Antimicrob Agents Chemother 43:1549–1555
52. Kashuba AD, Nafziger AN, Drusano GL, Bertino JS Jr (1999) Optimizing aminoglycoside therapy for nosocomial pneumonia caused by Gram-negative bacteria. Antimicrob Agents Chemother 43:623–629
53. Mingeot-Leclercq MP, Tulkens PM (1999) Aminoglycosides: nephrotoxicity. Antimicrob Agents Chemother 43:1003–1012
54. Whelton A (1979) Aminoglycoside renal cortical kinetics: a clue to mechanisms of nephrotoxicity. Prog Clin Biol Res 35:33–41
55. Whelton A, Carter GG, Bryant HH, Fox L, Walker WG (1976) Therapeutic implications of gentamicin accumulation in severely diseased kidneys. Arch Intern Med 135:172–177
56. Guiliano RA, Verpooten GA, Verbist L, Weeden R, DeBroe ME (1986) *In vivo* uptake kinetics of aminoglycosides in the kidney cortex of rats. J Pharmacol Exp Ther 236:470–475
57. DeBroe ME, Verbist L, Verpooten GA (1991) Influence of dosage schedule on renal accumulation of amikacin and tobramycin in man. J Antimicrob Chemother 27(Suppl C):41–47
58. ter Braak EW, de Vries PJ, Bouter KP, van der Vegt SG, Dorrestein GC, Nortier JW, van Dijk A, Verkooyen RP, Verbrugh HA (1990) Once-daily dosing regimen for aminoglycoside plus β-lactam combination therapy of serious bacterial infections: comparative trial of netilmicin plus ceftriaxone. Am J Med 89:58–66
59. Nicolau DP, Freeman CD, Belliveau PP, Nightingale CH, Ross JW, Quintiliani R (1995) Experience with a once-daily aminoglycoside program administered to 2,184 adult patients. Antimicrob Agents Chemother 39:650–655
60. American Thoracic Society and The Infectious Diseases Society of America (2005) Guidelines for the management of adults with hospital-acquired, ventilator-associated, and healthcare-associated pneumonia. Am J Respir Crit Care Med 171:388–416
61. Mandell LA, Wunderink RG, Anzueto A, Bartlett JG, Campbell GD, Dean NC, Dowell

SF, File TM Jr, Musher DM, Niederman MS, Torres A, Whitney CG (2007) Infectious Diseases Society of America/American Thoracic Society consensus guidelines on the management of community-acquired pneumonia in adults. Clin Infect Dis 44:S27–S72

62. Fowler VG Jr, Boucher HW, Corey GR, Abrutyn E, Karchmer AW, Rupp ME, Levine DP, Chambers HF, Tally FP, Vibliani GA, Cabell CH, Link AS, DeMeyer I, Filler SG, Zervos M, Cook P, Parsonnet J, Bernstein JM, Price CS, Forrest GN, Fatkenheuer G, Gareca M, Rehm SJ, Brodt HR, Tice A, Cosgrove SE (2006) Daptomycin versus standard therapy for bacteremia and endocarditis caused by *Staphylococcus aureus*. N Engl J Med 355:653–665

63. Bhavnani SM, Rubino CM, Ambrose PG, Drusano GL (2010) Daptomycin exposure and the probability of elevations in the creatine phosphokinase level: data from a randomized trial of patients with bacteremia and endocarditis. Clin Infect Dis 50:1568–1574

64. Tam VH, Louie A, Deziel MR, Liu W, Drusano GL (2007) The relationship between quinolone exposures and resistance amplification is characterized by an inverted U: a new paradigm for optimizing pharmacodynamics to counterselect resistance. Antimicrob Agents Chemother 51:744–747

65. Thwaites GE, Bhavnani SM, Chau TT, Hammel JP, Torok ME, Van Wart SA, Mai PP, Reynolds DK, Caws M, Dung NT, Hien TT, Kulawy R, Farrar J, Ambrose PG (2011) Randomized pharmacokinetic and pharmacodynamic comparison of fluoroquinolones for tuberculous meningitis. Antimicrob Agents Chemother 55:3244–3253

Chapter 7

Toxicokinetics and Toxicodynamics of Anti-infective Agents

David E. Nix

Abstract

Toxicokinetics (TK) is an essential component of preclinical toxicology assessment. The primary objective is to characterize systemic exposure (blood, plasma, or serum) to add relevance to toxicological findings. Parameters such as Cmax and AUC allow comparison of exposures between species and different studies to clarify the relationship between toxic effects and dosimetry. Further information can be gained by considering toxicodynamics (TD) in conjunction with TK, and results can be summarized descriptively or with a model-based strategy. This chapter provides a description of TK/TD and provides examples of the application of TK/TD principles in the development of anti-infective agents.

Key words Toxicokinetics, Toxicodynamics, TK/TD, Anti-infectives, Preclinical toxicology, Drug development

1 Introduction

The term toxicokinetics (TK) was first used in the early 1970s referring to in vivo kinetics of toxic substances. TK applied pharmacokinetic techniques to the study of substances of known toxic properties. Originally, TK was concerned with all aspects of kinetics including absorption, disposition, metabolism, and excretion (ADME), and some toxicologists still use the term to indicate application of kinetic methods to study toxic substances. Around 1990, there was a gradual evolution of the term to include nonclinical study of drug substances [1]. A European Federation of Pharmaceutical Industry Associations Working Group defined TK as "the generation of pharmacokinetic data as an integral component in the conduct of nonclinical toxicity studies and the use of these data in the interpretation of toxicological findings and their relevance to clinical safety issues." This definition changed slightly for the ICH S3A document of 1994 where TK was defined as "the generation of pharmacokinetic data, either as an integral component in the conduct of non-clinical toxicology studies or in

John C. Rotschafer et al. (eds.), *Antibiotic Pharmacodynamics*, Methods in Pharmacology and Toxicology,
DOI 10.1007/978-1-4939-3323-5_7, © Springer Science+Business Media New York 2016

specially designed supportive studies in order to assess systemic exposure. These data may be used in the interpretation of toxicologic findings and their relevance to clinical safety issues" [2]. TK information is used to ensure that relevant exposure is attained in animal species with application to minimize potential toxicity in humans [3].

In the drug development arena, the primary objective of TK is to describe the systemic exposure achieved in animals and its relationship to the dose level and time course of toxicity. The most commonly used measures of systemic exposure are Cmax, Tmax, and AUC as determined from serum, plasma, or whole blood. Secondary objectives include "relating the exposure achieved in toxicity studies to toxicologic findings and contributing to assessing the relevance of these findings to clinical safety; and providing information which in conjunction with toxicity findings contributes to the design of subsequent non-clinical toxicity studies" (http://www.fda.gov/downloads/Drugs/GuidanceComplianceRegulatoryInformation/Guidances/UCM074937.pdf; accessed 3/18/2014). Most applications of TK have employed simple descriptive measures of exposure; however, sophisticated modeling methods may be used. Physiologically based models have been used to predict target organ concentrations in situations where systemic drug exposure is unable to serve as a link between dose and biological effects [4].

While pharmacodynamics refers to the time course of pharmacologic effect, toxicodynamics (TD) is an analogous term which relates to toxic effects. More generally, TD falls within the context of safety and tolerance. In the nonclinical setting, TD is an evolving science that provides one basis for risk assessment. Understanding intraspecies and interspecies toxicodynamic variability provides a framework for quantitative extrapolation to humans [5, 6]. A pharmacodynamic (PD) study may involve the integration of pharmacokinetics (PK) either formally or in a supportive role and be referred to as a PK/PD study. Likewise, TK and TD (TK/TD) may be incorporated into preclinical toxicology studies or performed in parallel. TK/TD is useful in the preclinical setting to explore the relevance of toxicity findings and to predict dose target range in humans [7]. The TK/TD assessment should include an across-species analysis of preclinical acute and chronic toxicity studies with the goal of predicting outcomes [3]. For situations, where toxicity is predictable across species and is exposure related, modeling can be quite valuable in planning early human studies. Much of the nonclinical experience is handled as proprietary information and used to support drug development leading to substantial publication bias. Some of the information becomes publically available at the time of drug approval; however, methodologic details are often omitted and the results are often redacted.

TK assessments may be used to support the use of biomarkers, provide data for interspecies scaling, and explore the value of non-plasma drug concentrations [8]. Other investigators have used TK principles as a marker of dosimetry involving environmental exposures in fetuses and children [9–11]. Throughout clinical development and even post-marketing, TK/TD studies may be conducted to explore ways to manage drug toxicity and refine dose recommendations. Sex differences in TK and TD may be explored in the nonclinical setting to differentiate causes of observed differences in toxicity [12].

This chapter is intended to address the principles and application of TK/TD in anti-infective drug development. The bulk of this manuscript will focus on examples of how TK/TD has been useful to support toxicology studies.

2 Glycopeptides and Lipopeptides

Vancomycin and teicoplanin were studied in rats for acute toxicity [13]. Both drugs were administered by intra-jugular injection at several doses, and the TK endpoints included plasma urea nitrogen, creatinine, alanine aminotransferase, and aspartate aminotransferase over an 8-h period. Results were presented as AUC from time 0 to 8 h. The vancomycin dose ranged from 40 to 250 mg/kg. The first finding was that exposure, vancomycin AUC (0–8 h), increased more than proportional to dose. Relative exposure was 1.4× and 4.5× the expected exposure for the 100 mg/kg and 250 mg/kg doses, respectively, using a 40 mg/kg reference dose. This magnified exposure was due to dose-related acute kidney injury and reduced vancomycin clearance. Cmax was more than an order of magnitude higher in this model than achieved with clinical use. The endpoint in this case was the integrated creatinine $AUC_{0-8\ h}$. Creatinine AUC was 4.6 mg h/dl for 40 mg/kg, 5.5 mg h/dl for 100 mg/kg, and 11.5 mg h/dl for 250 mg/kg dose [13]. Given that no control animals were included, it is impossible to determine a no-effect dose level; however, given the degree of increase in just 8 h, acute renal failure is evident. Vancomycin-induced nephrotoxicity is poorly characterized in terms of mechanism. Acute renal failure is observed with doses in the range of 200 mg/kg. Evidence suggests that vancomycin can accumulate in proximal renal tubular cells and localize in lysosomes similar to that seen with aminoglycosides. However, vancomycin is less nephrotoxic than aminoglycosides. The acute kidney injury would need to be rapid and severe which is not consistent with the proposed mechanism. Vancomycin can induce histamine release in rats by causing mast cell degranulation similar to the red man syndrome described in humans [14, 15]. This may be associated with hypotension and renal artery constriction. Considering that vancomycin was administered as a IV bolus and this would be expected to cause extensive release of histamine and potentially other mediators, hemodynamic changes might explain the acute renal injury. The vancomycin AUC (0–8) ranged from 68 to 1510 μg h/ml [13]. Typical clinical use involves target average steady-state concentrations of 15–35 μg/ml, an 8-h AUC of 120–280 μg h/ml, and use of a slow infusion over 1 to 2 h to minimize the risk of red man syndrome. Consequently, the TK data may not directly relate to vancomycin use in humans.

Teicoplanin was studied in the same model as above with intrajugular doses ranging from 10 to 60 mg/kg. There was again evidence of dose-dependent pharmacokinetics with relative exposure based on AUC (0–8 h) of 1.3× for 30–40 mg/kg, 1.6× for 50 mg/kg, and 2.2× for 60 mg/kg using the 10 mg/kg dose as a reference. Unlike the acute kidney injury seen with vancomycin, no changes in integrated plasma creatinine over 8 h were observed; however, there was a dose-dependent increase in ALT and AST with doses of at least 40 mg/kg. Teicoplanin appears to exhibit less nephrotoxicity than vancomycin in clinical use but has not specifically been associated with hepatotoxicity.

The primary concern with daptomycin is development of myopathy for which creatine phosphokinase (CPK) is the most validated biomarker. A major breakthrough in the nonclinical setting was the discovery that dosing interval has major effects on the risk of myopathy [16]. In the clinical setting, development of significant CPK elevation is associated with minimum serum concentrations >24.3 μg/ml [17].

2.1 Aminoglycosides

Aminoglycosides produce ototoxicity and nephrotoxicity in humans and animals alike [18]. Interpretation of the relationship between nephrotoxicity and aminoglycoside exposure is complicated by toxicity to the organ responsible for aminoglycoside elimination. Toxicity was not apparent based on serum creatinine for gentamicin doses of 16 mg/kg Q 8 h for 6 days in rats. TK was assessed after the first dose and the average predicted exposure (24 h AUC) was 81 μg h/ml [19]. Note that typical human doses provide a 24-h AUC target of 70–100 μg h/ml for gentamicin. Dose-dependent nephrotoxicity was seen for the higher doses studied including 25 and 40 mg/kg Q 8 h [19, 20]. As toxicity produces reduced gentamicin clearance, exposure would be expected to increase with these higher doses over the observation period. With 12 days of dosing, the maximum dose administered without increases in serum creatinine was 10 mg/kg Q 8 h [19]. There also appears to be a subgroup of rats that exhibit increased susceptibility to nephrotoxicity although the mechanism of enhanced sensitivity is not clear.

In dogs, administration of 3 mg/kg every 8 h for 14 days did not produce functional nephrotoxicity. This dose regimen based on drug clearance would provide a 24-h AUC of about 40 μg h/ml. The same dose administered to ¾ to 7/8 subtotal nephrectomized dogs was estimated to provide a 24-h AUC of 107–176 μg h/ml. Four of six of these dogs developed nephrotoxicity characterized by increased serum creatinine. When the dose was reduced to 1–1.5 mg/kg Q 8 h (estimating a 24-h AUC of 36–54 μg h/ml), nephrotoxicity was still seen in three of six nephrectomized dogs, but overall less severe than with the higher dose. Interestingly, no nephrotoxicity was observed when 3 mg/kg was administered with an extended interval of 16–24 h [21]. This study appears to be the origin of our current dosing strategy for aminoglycosides [20].

In the case of ototoxicity, animals are most susceptible to permanent high-frequency sensorineural hearing loss. This hearing loss is associated with damage to hair cells and neurons in the cochlea. In contrast, vestibular toxicity may be temporary [22]. Using a guinea pig model, amikacin was administered using continuous infusion with varying dose rates. Hearing loss correlated with the total dose administered and cumulative total exposure (AUC); however, the total cumulative AUC was the best predictor of magnitude of hearing loss. As an example, the total AUC associated with 10 % incidence of at least 15 dB loss at 8000 mHz frequency was 305 μg d/ml [23]. With current dose recommendations, the typical AUC of amikacin in humans is in the range of 7.3–10 μg d/ml. Based on extrapolation, more than 30 days of therapy in humans would be needed to reach a 10 % incidence of ototoxicity at the upper range of frequencies that are applicable for hearing function in daily life. The ratio between perilymph and plasma concentrations is quite variable, averaging about 0.5, without evidence of accumulation over time [24]. Direct measurement of amikacin concentration in the tissue compartment associated with ototoxicity is not possible; thus a theoretical tissue compartment termed "ototoxic pool" was created. Amikacin enters into the "ototoxic pool" at a rate that is proportional to the plasma concentration and dose rate. Loss of amikacin from the "ototoxic pool" is first order with a half-life in the order of 80 days and results in accumulation of amikacin over the period of treatment. Given the persistence of amikacin, delayed ototoxicity noted within 2 weeks after discontinuing treatment is commonly observed and is occasionally observed, up to 8 weeks after discontinuing treatment [25].

The TK/TD model developed using the guinea pig model provides a framework to design human studies. It is clear that total exposure including duration of therapy is relevant to development of ototoxicity. Given the persistence of amikacin in the "ototoxic pool," repeated treatment courses within a year will likely lower the threshold needed to cause hair cell damage and once the hair cells are lost, the loss is permanent [26]. Also, some patients are more sensitive than others to the ototoxic effects of aminoglycosides, and this may be explained by genetic differences or mutations [22].

2.2 Fluoroquinolone

Toxicity concerns with fluoroquinolones generally involve the central nervous system (seizures), joints (cartilage damage), heart (QT prolongation), or skin (phototoxicity). One of the few published examples of TK added to a standard chronic toxicology studies involves prulifloxacin. Prulifloxacin is a prodrug that is rapidly converted to ulifloxacin after oral administration. The authors suggest that toxicity involving lungs, liver, stomach, and joints may be related to higher tissue concentrations. Their use of the word accumulation in several contexts is confusing. However, the persistence of ulifloxacin in various tissues 14 days after the end of drug administration is unexplained based on pharmacokinetic properties [27].

Seizures have been investigated using a mouse model based on an intravenous continuous infusion of fluoroquinolone. The average serum and brain concentration at the point in which convulsions developed was approximately 247 μg/ml and 34 μg/g for enoxacin, and 362 μg/ml and 22 μg/g for ciprofloxacin, respectively, in different mouse breeds [28]. Imipenem induced clonic convulsions at an ip dose of 1–1.5 g/kg. Fluoroquinolone pretreatment (250 μmol/kg) resulted in increased sensitivity to imipenem-induced convulsions. The ip dose of imipenem required to induce clonic convulsions in 50 % of mice was lowered to 0.5–0.8 g/kg following treatment with pefloxacin, ciprofloxacin, enoxacin, or ofloxacin [29]. The lack of TK assessment makes interpretation difficult. From mice pharmacokinetic studies, mice require 10–20 times the human dose (mg/kg) to achieve similar exposure. The equivalent human dose would be in the range of 50–200 mg/kg for imipenem alone and 25–100 mg/kg following the fluoroquinolone pretreatment [30]. Even with correction for exposure (AUC), Cmax would be much higher in the mice. The adult human dose is usually in the range of 7–13 mg/kg. A similar investigation was conducted with cefazolin where the ED_{50} was 0.91 g/kg for cefazolin alone and 0.35–0.65 g/kg after pretreatment with these same fluoroquinolones [31]. The findings support clinical experience in that seizures are rarely reported with fluoroquinolones and usually occur in cases where there are confounding factors [32]. Sitafloxacin and levofloxacin have been studied using injection of drug into the lateral cerebral ventricle. The dose required to induce convulsions was 50.6 nmol for sitafloxacin and 76.7 nmol for levofloxacin, indicating that the two fluoroquinolones have weak convulsant activity. Furthermore the convulsant activity was not enhanced with concurrent administration of anti-inflammatory drugs including aspirin, acetaminophen, and various nonsteroidal anti-inflammatory drugs [33].

Fluoroquinolones inhibit I(Kr) slow potassium channels of heart muscle cells leading to prolongation of the QT interval. The extent of QT prolongation is directly related to plasma concentration. Moxifloxacin is the best studied FQ, having fairly predictable pharmacokinetics and consistent effect on QT interval [34–36]. As such, moxifloxacin is used as a positive control for thorough QT studies in humans. Moxifloxacin increases QT interval by an average of 3.1 ms (mean change of 1.6–4.8 ms across different studies) per μg/ml plasma concentration [34]. A variety of animal models have been used to assess risk of QT prolongation and ventricular arrhythmias [37–43]. Given the direct relationship between plasma drug concentrations and QT prolongation, one only needs to consider plasma concentrations achieved in relationship to concentrations observed in humans with usual doses. Efforts to produce a "humanized" pharmacokinetic profile are useful. Although QT interval is an accepted surrogate marker of risk for torsades de pointes, there are drugs that prolong QT interval without being associated with torsades de pointes. Drugs that have known risk for causing torsades de pointes generally produce a decrease in the delay between end of QT interval and end of mechanical systole (A.K.A. the E-M window) [40]. QT dispersion may also be more predictive of cardiac risk than QT interval prolongation [44].

Ciprofloxacin was shown to cause lesions in cartilage of weight-bearing joints in immature dogs. The chondrotoxicity is dose dependent with no toxicity at 10 mg/kg/day, minimal lesions at 30 mg/kg/day, and extensive lesions with joint symptoms at 90 mg/kg/day. Signs of joint symptoms resolved within a few weeks after the 14-day treatment period. Dogs given 10 mg/kg/day of ciprofloxacin also did not develop any delayed cartilage lesions or joint symptoms [45]. Although TK were not studied, an estimate of exposure was derived from a study of adult dogs using allometric scaling [46]. The total CL of ciprofloxacin for a 10 mg/kg dose in a 5.7 kg immature beagle dog was estimated to be 5.6 l/h. The 24-h AUC (~10 μg h/ml for 10 mg/kg) in this model is somewhat less than the 24-h AUC observed with the maximum recommended dose in humans which is ~50 μg h/ml. Using a rat model, the chondrotoxic dose of sparfloxacin was 300 times the human therapeutic dose (1800 mg/kg versus 6 mg/kg) and after correction for exposure was 15 times the typical human exposure. However, this model demonstrated cartilage lesions with a single 1800 mg/kg dose and no toxicity with 600 mg/kg/day for up to 8 days [47]. Fluoroquinolone-induced chondrotoxicity involves weight-bearing joints, appears to be species and dose dependent, and is detected in immature animals with an open growth plate. Although publication bias may be an issue, TK assessment may be useful to better characterize susceptibility differences by species. Fluoroquinolone use in children has been restricted for more than

30 years based on these animal findings without evidence of the same toxicity pattern in humans [48, 49]. However, arthralgia is more common with levofloxacin than with comparator (non-fluoroquinolone) antibiotics in children [49].

Phototoxicity has been reported with some fluoroquinolones in the clinical setting. In humans, fleroxacin, lomefloxacin, and sparfloxacin have been associated with severe skin lesions, and lomefloxacin and sparfloxacin were removed from the market after FDA approval. In one human comparison, enoxacin and sparfloxacin produced moderate to severe phototoxic lesions and in particular sparfloxacin caused severe lesions over a broad range of UV and visible light exposure. Sitafloxacin was associated with mild lesions, while no phototoxicity was seen with levofloxacin [50]. Animal models were developed to evaluate relative differences and to explore mechanisms. One model involved BALB/c mice that were administered drug followed by 4-h exposure to UV light or artificial sunlight. Phototoxicity was measured by observing the ears and measuring thickness over 7 days post-drug and -UV light exposure. Minimal or no phototoxicity was seen with sparfloxacin, sitafloxacin, or lomefloxacin at doses of 10 mg/kg. With sparfloxacin, erythema was seen at 30, 40, and 100 mg/kg, with the addition of swelling at 40–100 mg/kg [51, 52]. The overall exposure (24-h AUC) for the 40 mg/kg dose was only 1/3 of that in humans with usual doses. Lomefloxacin produced erythema and swelling at the 40, 100, and 300 mg/kg doses, and the exposure for the 100 mg/kg dose was similar to a typical human exposure. Interestingly, the auricular tissue concentrations for both drugs were 6.0–8.9 times the corresponding plasma concentrations [51, 52]. A similar study was done with trovafloxacin using lomefloxacin as a positive control. Lomefloxacin, 71 mg/kg, caused pronounced erythema and swelling of the auricle. Erythema was noted for trovafloxacin with 90 and 250 mg/kg doses; however, swelling was absent even at the highest dose. The ratio of trovafloxacin concentration in skin (dorsal area) to serum was <0.4 [53]. Retinal degeneration was documented in a BALB/c mouse model which showed retinal degeneration following sitafloxacin + UV light exposure. The magnitude of retinal damage was associated with sitafloxacin peak concentration which is in contrast to the relationship between AUC and toxicity for the auricular phototoxicity [54].

2.3 Beta-lactams

The most common problems with beta-lactam antibiotics are allergic disorders which are idiosyncratic and non-concentration dependent. However, there are issues with neurotoxicity that can be considered from a TK/TD perspective. One model that assesses neurotoxicity involves microinjection into the lateral cerebral ventricles of rats to determine the dose required to induce clonus in 50 % of animals. Table 1 provides the relative potencies of selected

Table 1

Relative potency of selected beta-lactam antibacterial required to induce clonic seizures in a rat intraventricular injection model

Drug	Relative potency (penicillin G = 100)
Cefazolin	294
Penicillin G	100
Imipenem	71
Aztreonam	42
Ampicillin	21
Ceftazidime	17
Meropenem	16
Ceftriaxone	12
Piperacillin	11
Cefotaxime	8.8
Cefoxitin	1.8

For comparison, penicillin G was assigned an arbitrary potency of 100 [55]

beta-lactam agents using penicillin G as a reference with an arbitrary value of 100 assigned. The actual ED_{50} required was 0.05 µmol per injection for penicillin G [55]. Considering that a normal volume of the lateral ventricle is in the order of 10 µl [56], the concentration required to induce seizures would be approximately 1672 µg/ml. However, direct injection into the ventricle is an over-simplification of the pathogenic sequence. Cefazolin was the most potent seizure-inducing beta-lactam following intraventricular injection; however, this cephalosporin is known to have poor penetration into cerebrospinal fluid. In one study, cefazolin was administered to rats at a rate of 3.2 g/h and continued until seizures developed. At that point, drug concentration was determined in serum, brain tissue, and CSF. Seizures occurred at a serum concentration of 16,800 µg/ml, brain concentration of 178 µg/ml, and CSF concentration of 81 µg/ml. The brain and CSF penetration was only 1 % and 0.5 %, respectively. Cases of beta-lactam-induced seizures typically occur in patients with excessively high doses in the face of impaired elimination leading to accumulation of drug in the CNS. Brain tissue concentrations correlate with toxicity more directly than CSF concentrations [57], and patients often have other factors that contribute to development of seizures. In rats, seizures occurred following administration of 2.5 to 5 million units of penicillin per kg by IP injection, although there was no TK assessment [58]. In another model, ip injection of pentylenetetrazole, 50 mg/kg, was administered with and without beta-lactam pretreatment. Pentylenetetrazole alone caused seizures in 30 % of rats, but in 100 % of rats following pretreatment with imipenem/cilastatin (400/400 mg/kg). Cefazolin had less effect of lower seizure threshold and required a dose of 800 mg/kg to increase seizure frequency to 80 % [59]. Again, no TK data was captured to help sort out relevance of these findings.

2.4 Azole Antifungal Drugs

All of the azole antifungal drugs have been associated with hepatotoxicity. Rabbits given single 40–160 mg/kg doses of ketoconazole develop dose-dependent increases in alanine aminotransferase and aspartate aminotransferase, and liver tissue necrosis. The liver toxicity correlates with AUC which was 85 μg h/ml for 40 mg/kg, 158 μg h/ml for 80 mg/kg, and 623 μg h/ml for 160 mg/kg. Note that saturable clearance occurs with a dose greater than 80 mg/kg [60]. For comparison, the AUC in humans following a 200 mg dose (tablet) is 14.7 μg h/ml [61]; thus 15 mg/kg (1125 mg/day) in humans would be approximately equal in exposure to 40 mg/kg in rabbits. The FDA-approved label includes a box warning about hepatoxicity including fatal hepatotoxicity (Nizoral prescribing information, Janssen Pharmaceuticals Inc., 7/2013). In a study involving combined voriconazole and anidulafungin, voriconazole, 10 mg/kg/day, caused increased serum gamma glutamyltransferase in female juvenile rats only. The 24-h AUC for voriconazole was about 20 μg h/ml [62]. In clinical practice, doses of 200–2000 mg have been described; however, toxicity limits doses greater than 400 mg/day. In this limited experience, increases in serum transaminases were seen in about 5 % of patients and was not explained by dose and/or exposure [63].

Prolonged QT interval is another concern for antifungal azoles. Ketoconazole, 200 mg/kg, administered orally failed to increase QT interval in a guinea pig model; however, the combination of terbinafine and ketoconazole substantially reduced heart rate and prolonged QTc by almost 30 % [64]. This study shows the implications of omitting TK data. Readers are left with the question of whether exposure was relevant in terms of plasma concentration achieved. With ketoconazole there is always the concern of poor bioavailability and validation of the dose formulation is critical. Fluconazole is classified as a weak inhibitor of hERG current with an IC_{50} of 48.2 μM. Doses of 400 mg daily at steady state result in average peak plasma concentrations near this IC_{50} [65].

Itraconazole adverse events in relation to serum concentration have been examined in humans. Adverse event frequency was positively associated with exposure and a concentration of 17.1 μg/ml was associated with a 50 % frequency of adverse events. The most common adverse effects included fluid retention, nausea, vomiting, abdominal pain, flatulence, or diarrhea. There was a 2 % frequency of liver toxicity with bilirubin concentrations at least three times normal with or without an increase in alkaline phosphatase. Serum transaminase increases were not mentioned [66].

2.5 Amphotericin B

Dose-limiting nephrotoxicity is the most common toxicity seen with amphotericin B. Early studies in patients revealed a mild-moderate reduction in renal function in the majority of patients receiving treatment; however, the renal failure generally stabilized and was reversible in the months following treatment [67].

In acute toxicity studies, the LD_{50} of amphotericin B deoxycholate is approximately 2.3 mg/kg and 1.6 mg/kg in mice and rats, respectively. Much higher doses of liposomal amphotericin B were tolerated and the LD_{50}s were 175 mg/kg and 50 mg/kg, respectively. Mice were able to tolerate 25–50 mg/kg/day of liposomal amphotericin B for 14 days, although there was initial weight loss. By the end of the treatment period, weight had stabilized and was increasing. The same pattern was seen in rats given liposomal amphotericin B for 30 days. The lowest weight was recorded on day 8, and weight increased towards baseline by 30 days. Renal failure was not seen in the rats, but there was a very large increase in serum transaminases on day 2 of dosing. The transaminases fell to near the upper limit of normal on subsequent days. In comparing tissue concentrations of liposomal formulation (5 mg/kg) to conventional amphotericin B (1 mg/kg), the ratio of amphotericin B was 1.1 for kidney, 2.3 for lung, 4.3 for brain, 10.7 for spleen, and 10.9 for liver [68].

Liposomal amphotericin B was evaluated in dogs with doses ranging from 0.25 to 16 mg/kg/day administered for 30 days. Toxicological findings were similar to those seen with conventional amphotericin B; however, much higher plasma concentrations were required to produce the same effects. Minimal effects were seen on the kidney at 1 mg/kg/day with a 0.3 mg/dl increase in serum creatinine. Moderate renal toxicity was seen with doses of 4 and 8 mg/kg/day where a 3.3- to 3.8-fold increase in serum creatinine was observed. Renal tubular necrosis and severe toxicity were seen with the 16 mg/kg/day dose. A strong relationship between renal effects and the renal tissue concentration of amphotericin B was observed. Dogs given the two highest doses (8 or 16 mg/kg/day) developed vomiting, anorexia, and weight loss exceeding 25 % of the initial body weight. Increases in spleen, kidney, and liver weights were observed with doses of at least 4 mg/kg/day. There was saturable clearance noted throughout the concentration range studied and time-dependent accumulation of drug in plasma. If the 4 mg/kg/day dose is taken as the highest tolerated dose, plasma 24-h AUC was 143 μg h/ml on day 1, 728 μg h/ml on day 14, and 1452 μg h/ml on day 30. Nearly all of the plasma amphotericin B was associated with liposomes or bound to plasma proteins since amphotericin B was not detectable in plasma ultrafiltrate [69]. A 3-month chronic toxicity study was conducted in rats with doses ranging from 1 to 12 mg/kg/day. Amphotericin B plasma clearance averaged 12 ml/h/kg, 5.4 ml/h/kg, and 3.5 ml/h/kg in the rats with doses of 1 mg/kg, 4 mg/kg, and 12 mg/kg, respectively [70]. In dogs, the clearance averaged 8.7 ml/h/kg, 1.8 ml/h/kg, 1.7 ml/h/kg, and 1.4 ml/h/kg with doses of 1 mg/kg, 4 mg/kg, 8 mg/kg, and 16 mg/kg, respectively [69]. Toxicities in mice were similar qualitatively to those observed in dogs, but somewhat less severe for the same exposure level. Despite accumulation of drug and increasing plasma concentration over time, toxicologic manifestations were noted early and became stable during the dosing period [70].

3 Conclusion

TK/TD modeling has proven to be an extremely valuable tool for increasing the relevance of toxicology findings and adding predictive potential. Further evolution of this tool is likely as pharmacometrics and predictive modeling and simulation techniques become more integrated into drug development.

References

1. Case D (1994) Toxicokinetics: some definitions. Drug Inf J 28:145–148
2. Anon (1995) Toxicokinetics: the assessment of systemic exposure in toxicity studies. ICH Guidence of Industry, vol S3A
3. Dahlem AM, Allerheiligen SR, Vodicnik MJ (1995) Concomitant toxicokinetics – techniques for and interpretation of exposure data obtained during the conduct of toxicology studies. Toxicol Pathol 23(2):170–178
4. Dixit R, Riviere J, Krishnan K, Andersen ME (2003) Toxicokinetics and physiologically based toxicokinetics in toxicology and risk assessment. J Toxicol Environ Health B Crit Rev 6(1):1–40
5. Heinrich-Hirsch B, Madle S, Oberemm A, Gundert-Remy U (2001) The use of toxicodynamics in risk assessment. Toxicol Lett 120(1–3):131–141
6. Hoshino-Yoshino A, Kato M, Nakano K, Ishigai M, Kudo T, Ito K (2011) Bridging from preclinical to clinical studies for tyrosine kinase inhibitors based on pharmacokinetics/pharmacodynamics and toxicokinetics/toxicodynamics. Drug Metab Pharmacokinet 26(6):612–620. doi:10.2133/dmpk.DMPK-11-RG-043
7. Welling PG (1995) Differences between pharmacokinetics and toxicokinetics. Toxicol Pathol 23(2):143–147
8. Baldrick P (2003) Toxicokinetics in preclinical evaluation. Drug Discov Today 8(3):127–133
9. Daston G, Faustman E, Ginsberg G, Fenner-Crisp P, Olin S, Sonawane B, Bruckner J, Breslin W, McLaughlin TJ (2004) A framework for assessing risks to children from exposure to environmental agents. Environ Health Perspect 112(2):238–256
10. Ginsberg G, Slikker W Jr, Bruckner J, Sonawane B (2004) Incorporating children's toxicokinetics into a risk framework. Environ Health Perspect 112(2):272–283
11. Mason H, Wilson K (1999) Biological monitoring: the role of toxicokinetics and physiologically based pharmacokinetic modeling. Am Ind Hyg Assoc J 60(2):237–242
12. Gochfeld M (2007) Framework for gender differences in human and animal toxicology. Environ Res 104(1):4–21. doi:10.1016/j.envres.2005.12.005
13. Yoshida M, Matzno S, Namba H, Nishikata M, Matsuyama K (2006) Statistical analysis of the adverse effects of glycopeptide antibiotics, based on pharmacokinetics and toxicokinetics

(PK/TK). J Infect Chemother 12(3):114–118. doi:10.1007/s10156-006-0437-z
14. Horinouchi Y, Abe K, Kubo K, Oka M (1993) Mechanisms of vancomycin-induced histamine-release from rat peritoneal mast-cells. Agents Actions 40(1–2):28–36. doi:10.1007/bf01976748
15. Shuto H, Sueyasu M, Otsuki S, Hara T, Tsuruta Y, Kataoka Y, Oishi R (1999) Potentiation of vancomycin-induced histamine release by muscle relaxants and morphine in rats. Antimicrob Agents Chemother 43(12):2881–2884
16. Oleson FB, Berman CL, Kirkpatrick JB, Regan KS, Lai JJ, Tally FP (2000) Once-daily dosing in dogs optimizes daptomycin safety. Antimicrob Agents Chemother 44(11):2948–2953. doi:10.1128/aac.44.11.2948-2953.2000
17. Bhavnani SM, Rubino CM, Ambrose PG, Drusano GL (2010) Daptomycin exposure and the probability of elevations in the creatine phosphokinase level: data from a randomized trial of patients with bacteremia and endocarditis. Clin Infect Dis 50(12):1568–1574. doi:10.1086/652767
18. Welles JS, Emmerson JL, Gibson WR, Nickander R, Owen NV, Anderson RC (1973) Preclinical toxicology studies with tobramycin. Toxicol Appl Pharmacol 25(3):398–409
19. Carver MP, Shy-Modjeska JS, Brown TT, Rogers RA, Riviere JE (1985) Dose-response studies of gentamicin nephrotoxicity in rats with experimental renal dysfunction. I. Subtotal surgical nephrectomy. Toxicol Appl Pharmacol 80(2):251–263
20. Riviere JE, Dix LP, Carver MP, Frazier DL (1986) Identification of a subgroup of Sprague-Dawley rats highly sensitive to drug-induced renal toxicity. Fundam Appl Toxicol 7(1):126–131
21. Riviere JE, Carver MP, Coppoc GL, Carlton WW, Lantz GC, Shy-Modjeska J (1984) Pharmacokinetics and comparative nephrotoxicity of fixed-dose versus fixed-interval reduction of gentamicin dosage in subtotal nephrectomized dogs. Toxicol Appl Pharmacol 75(3):496–509
22. Guthrie OW (2008) Aminoglycoside induced ototoxicity. Toxicology 249(2–3):91–96. doi:10.1016/j.tox.2008.04.015
23. Beaubien AR, Desjardins S, Ormsby E, Bayne A, Carrier K, Cauchy MJ, Henri R, Hodgen M, Salley J, St Pierre A (1989) Incidence of amikacin ototoxicity: a sigmoid function of total drug exposure independent of plasma levels. Am J Otolaryngol 10(4):234–243
24. Desjardins-Giasson S, Beaubien AR (1984) Correlation of amikacin concentrations in perilymph and plasma of continuously infused guinea pigs. Antimicrob Agents Chemother 26(1):87–90
25. Beaubien AR, Karpinski K, Ormsby E (1995) Toxicodynamics and toxicokinetics of amikacin in the guinea pig cochlea. Hear Res 83(1–2):62–79
26. Steyger PS, Karasawa T (2008) Intra-cochlear trafficking of aminoglycosides. Commun Integr Biol 1(2):140–142
27. Nandi U, Roy B, Das AK, Pal TK (2012) Correlation among the toxicity profiling (28-days repeated oral dose toxicity), toxicokinetics and tissue distribution data of ulifloxacin, the active metabolite of prulifloxacin in Wistar albino rats. Environ Toxicol Pharmacol 34(2):588–607. doi:10.1016/j.etap.2012.07.001
28. Matsuo H, Ryu M, Nagata A, Uchida T, Kawakami JI, Yamamoto K, Iga T, Sawada Y (1998) Neurotoxicodynamics of the interaction between ciprofloxacin and foscarnet in mice. Antimicrob Agents Chemother 42(3):691–694
29. De Sarro A, Ammendola D, De Sarro G (1994) Effects of some quinolones on imipenem-induced seizures in DBA/2 mice. Gen Pharmacol 25(2):369–379
30. Fluckiger U, Segessenmann C, Gerber AU (1991) Integration of pharmacokinetics and pharmacodynamics of imipenem in a human-adapted mouse model. Antimicrob Agents Chemother 35(9):1905–1910
31. De Sarro A, Zappala M, Chimirri A, Grasso S, De Sarro GB (1993) Quinolones potentiate cefazolin-induced seizures in DBA/2 mice. Antimicrob Agents Chemother 37(7):1497–1503
32. Tome AM, Filipe A (2011) Quinolones: review of psychiatric and neurological adverse reactions. Drug Saf 34(6):465–488. doi:10.2165/11587280-000000000-00000
33. Hori S (2009) Convulsant activity of sitafloxacin and its interactions with anti-inflammatory drugs in mice. J Infect Chemother 15(4):266–268. doi:10.1007/s10156-009-0693-9
34. Florian JA, Tornoe CW, Brundage R, Parekh A, Garnett CE (2011) Population pharmacokinetic and concentration – QTc models for moxifloxacin: pooled analysis of 20 thorough QT studies. J Clin Pharmacol 51(8):1152–1162. doi:10.1177/0091270010381498
35. Mason JW, Florian JA Jr, Garnett CE, Moon TE, Selness DS, Spaulding RR (2010) Pharmacokinetics and pharmacodynamics of

three moxifloxacin dosage forms: implications for blinding in active-controlled cardiac repolarization studies. J Clin Pharmacol 50(11):1249–1259. doi:10.1177/0091270009356298
36. Watson KJ, Gorczyca WP, Umland J, Zhang Y, Chen X, Sun SZ, Fermini B, Holbrook M, Van Der Graaf PH (2011) Pharmacokinetic-pharmacodynamic modelling of the effect of moxifloxacin on QTc prolongation in telemetered cynomolgus monkeys. J Pharmacol Toxicol Methods 63(3):304–313. doi:10.1016/j.vascn.2011.03.002
37. Akita M, Shibazaki Y, Izumi M, Hiratsuka K, Sakai T, Kurosawa T, Shindo Y (2004) Comparative assessment of prurifloxacin, sparfloxacin, gatifloxacin and levofloxacin in the rabbit model of proarrhythmia. J Toxicol Sci 29(1):63–71
38. Anderson ME, Mazur A, Yang T, Roden DM (2001) Potassium current antagonist properties and proarrhythmic consequences of quinolone antibiotics. J Pharmacol Exp Ther 296(3):806–810
39. Chiba K, Sugiyama A, Hagiwara T, Takahashi S, Takasuna K, Hashimoto K (2004) In vivo experimental approach for the risk assessment of fluoroquinolone antibacterial agents-induced long QT syndrome. Eur J Pharmacol 486(2):189–200. doi:10.1016/j.ejphar.2003.12.014
40. Guns PJ, Johnson DM, Van Op den Bosch J, Weltens E, Lissens J (2012) The electromechanical window in anaesthetized guinea pigs: a new marker in screening for Torsade de Pointes risk. Br J Pharmacol 166(2):689–701. doi:10.1111/j.1476-5381.2011.01795.x
41. Lacroix P, Crumb WJ, Durando L, Ciottoli GB (2003) Prulifloxacin: in vitro (HERG current) and in vivo (conscious dog) assessment of cardiac risk. Eur J Pharmacol 477(1):69–72
42. Satoh Y, Sugiyama A, Chiba K, Tamura K, Hashimoto K (2000) QT-prolonging effects of sparfloxacin, a fluoroquinolone antibiotic, assessed in the in vivo canine model with monophasic action potential monitoring. J Cardiovasc Pharmacol 36(4):510–515
43. Takahara A, Sugiyama A, Satoh Y, Hashimoto K (2003) Effects of mexiletine on the canine model of sparfloxacin-induced long QT syndrome. Eur J Pharmacol 476(1–2):115–122
44. Chiba K, Sugiyama A, Takasuna K, Hashimoto K (2004) Comparison of sensitivity of surrogate markers of drug-induced torsades de pointes in canine hearts. Eur J Pharmacol 502(1–2):117–122. doi:10.1016/j.ejphar.2004.08.035
45. von Keutz E, Ruhl-Fehlert C, Drommer W, Rosenbruch M (2004) Effects of ciprofloxacin on joint cartilage in immature dogs immediately after dosing and after a 5-month treatment-free period. Arch Toxicol 78(7):418–424. doi:10.1007/s00204-004-0551-6
46. Cester CC, Toutain PL (1997) A comprehensive model for enrofloxacin to ciprofloxacin transformation and disposition in dog. J Pharm Sci 86(10):1148–1155. doi:10.1021/js9603461
47. Stahlmann R, Zippel U, Forster C, Schwabe R, Shakibaei M, Merker HJ, Borner K (1998) Chondrotoxicity and toxicokinetics of sparfloxacin in juvenile rats. Antimicrob Agents Chemother 42(6):1470–1475
48. Grady R (2003) Safety profile of quinolone antibiotics in the pediatric population. Pediatr Infect Dis J 22(12):1128–1132. doi:10.1097/01.inf.0000101994.25947.12
49. Noel GJ, Bradley JS, Kauffman RE, Duffy CM, Gerbino PG, Arguedas A, Bagchi P, Balis DA, Blumer JL (2007) Comparative safety profile of levofloxacin in 2523 children with a focus on four specific musculoskeletal disorders. Pediatr Infect Dis J 26(10):879–891. doi:10.1097/INF.0b013e3180cbd382
50. Dawe RS, Ibbotson SH, Sanderson JB, Thomson EM, Ferguson J (2003) A randomized controlled trial (volunteer study) of sitafloxacin, enoxacin, levofloxacin and sparfloxacin phototoxicity. Br J Dermatol 149(6):1232–1241
51. Matsumoto N, Akimoto A, Kawashima H, Kim S (2010) Comparative study of skin phototoxicity with three drugs by an in vivo mouse model. J Toxicol Sci 35(1):97–100
52. Shimoda K, Ikeda T, Okawara S, Kato M (2000) Possible relationship between phototoxicity and photodegradation of sitafloxacin, a quinolone antibacterial agent, in the auricular skin of albino mice. Toxicol Sci 56(2):290–296
53. Mayne JT, Johnson NJ, Kluwe WM, Lencoski DL, Polzer RJ (1997) A study of the phototoxic potential of trovafloxacin in BALB/c mice. J Antimicrob Chemother 39(Suppl B):67–73
54. Shimoda K, Okawara S, Kato M (2001) Phototoxic retinal degeneration and toxicokinetics of sitafloxacin, a quinolone antibacterial agent, in mice. Arch Toxicol 75(7):395–399
55. De Sarro A, Ammendola D, Zappala M, Grasso S, De Sarro GB (1995) Relationship between structure and convulsant properties of some beta-lactam antibiotics following intracerebroventric-

ular microinjection in rats. Antimicrob Agents Chemother 39(1):232–237. doi:10.1128/aac.39.1.232

56. Basati S, Desai B, Alaraj A, Charbel F, Linninger A (2012) Cerebrospinal fluid volume measurements in hydrocephalic rats. J Neurosurg Pediatr 10(4):347–354. doi:10.3171/2012.6.PEDS11457
57. Chow KM, Hui AC, Szeto CC (2005) Neurotoxicity induced by beta-lactam antibiotics: from bench to bedside. Eur J Clin Microbiol Infect Dis 24(10):649–653. doi:10.1007/s10096-005-0021-y
58. Chen RC, Huang YH, How SW (1986) Systemic penicillin as an experimental model of epilepsy. Exp Neurol 92(3):533–540
59. Williams PD, Bennett DB, Comereski CR (1988) Animal model for evaluating the convulsive liability of beta-lactam antibiotics. Antimicrob Agents Chemother 32(5):758–760. doi:10.1128/aac.32.5.758
60. Ma YM, Ma ZQ, Gui CQ, Yao JS, Sun RY (2003) Hepatotoxicity and toxicokinetics of ketoconazole in rabbits. Acta Pharmacol Sin 24(8):778–782
61. Huang YC, Colaizzi JL, Bierman RH, Woestenborghs R, Heykants J (1986) Pharmacokinetics and dose proportionality of ketoconazole in normal volunteers. Antimicrob Agents Chemother 30(2):206–210
62. Cross DM, Chmielewski G, Lewis EM, Liu L, Modesitt MS, Ripp SL, Sawaryn CM, Bowman CJ (2012) Non-clinical safety assessment and toxicokinetics of voriconazole and anidulafungin in the juvenile rat: a combination study design in support of a Paediatric Investigation Plan. Regul Toxicol Pharmacol 63(1):29–39. doi:10.1016/j.yrtph.2012.02.004
63. Sugar AM, Alsip SG, Galgiani JN, Graybill JR, Dismukes WE, Cloud GA, Craven PC, Stevens DA (1987) Pharmacology and toxicity of high-dose ketoconazole. Antimicrob Agents Chemother 31(12):1874–1878
64. Rajput SK, Singh JN, Sharma SS (2010) Evaluation of terfenadine and ketoconazole-induced QT prolongation in conscious telemetered guinea pigs. Pharmacol Rep 62(4):683–688
65. Han S, Zhang Y, Chen Q, Duan Y, Zheng T, Hu X, Zhang Z, Zhang L (2011) Fluconazole inhibits hERG K(+) channel by direct block and disruption of protein trafficking. Eur J Pharmacol 650(1):138–144. doi:10.1016/j.ejphar.2010.10.010
66. Lestner JM, Roberts SA, Moore CB, Howard SJ, Denning DW, Hope WW (2009) Toxicodynamics of itraconazole: implications for therapeutic drug monitoring. Clin Infect Dis 49(6):928–930. doi:10.1086/605499
67. Bennett JE (1964) Amphotericin B toxicity; review of selected aspects of pharmacology. Ann Intern Med 61:335–340
68. Proffitt RT, Satorius A, Chiang SM, Sullivan L, Adler-Moore JP (1991) Pharmacology and toxicology of a liposomal formulation of amphotericin B (AmBisome) in rodents. J Antimicrob Chemother 28(Suppl B):49–61, Erratum appears in J Antimicrob Chemother 1992 Mar;29(3):355
69. Bekersky I, Boswell GW, Hiles R, Fielding RM, Buell D, Walsh TJ (1999) Safety and toxicokinetics of intravenous liposomal amphotericin B (AmBisome) in beagle dogs. Pharm Res 16(11):1694–1701
70. Bekersky I, Boswell GW, Hiles R, Fielding RM, Buell D, Walsh TJ (2000) Safety, toxicokinetics and tissue distribution of long-term intravenous liposomal amphotericin B (AmBisome): a 91-day study in rats. Pharm Res 17(12):1494–1502

Part II

Pharmacodynamics of Antibacterial Agents

Chapter 8

Pharmacodynamics of Fluoroquinolones

Ramy H. Elshaboury, Thomas J. Dilworth, and John C. Rotschafer

Abstract

Fluoroquinolones are a ubiquitous class of broad-spectrum antibacterials used to treat a multitude of bacterial infections in both the inpatient and outpatient settings. Pharmacodynamic research has played an integral role in the drug development and approval process for fluoroquinolones. There exists a wealth of fluoroquinolone pharmacodynamic literature and, despite considerable heterogeneity among studies, the results are almost universally the same: f-AUC_{24}/MIC ratio is most predictive of microbiologic and clinical efficacy; >30 for gram-positive and >125 for gram-negative organisms. However, rising rates of fluoroquinolone resistance, particularly among gram-negative pathogens, may challenge these established pharmacodynamic indices. This chapter discusses the pharmacodynamics of fluoroquinolones with particular focus on the commonly used agents in current clinical practice: ciprofloxacin, levofloxacin, and moxifloxacin.

Key words Fluoroquinolones, Pharmacokinetics, Pharmacodynamics, Fluoroquinolones pharmacodynamics, Levofloxacin, Ciprofloxacin, Moxifloxacin

1 Introduction and History of Development

The first quinolones were developed nearly 50 years ago, including nalidixic acid, and had good activity against aerobic and facultative gram-negative organisms. At that time, their utility was limited to urinary tract infections due to low serum and tissue drug concentrations [1]. Newer compounds with structural-related modifications exhibited enhanced activity against a broad range of gram-negative organisms, *Mycobacteria* and *Chlamydia* spp. Ultimately, second and third generation fluoroquinolones were developed and exhibit additional activity against gram-positive organisms such as streptococci, including penicillin-resistant strains of *Streptococcus pneumoniae*, and methicillin-susceptible *Staphylococcus aureus* (MSSA), as well as compounds with activity against anaerobic organisms.

Fluoroquinolones represent the first class of antibiotics where the science of pharmacodynamics was prospectively applied in vitro, in vivo, and clinically in the antibiotic development and licensing process [2–4]. Pharmacodynamic research incorporating

John C. Rotschafer et al. (eds.), *Antibiotic Pharmacodynamics*, Methods in Pharmacology and Toxicology,
DOI 10.1007/978-1-4939-3323-5_8, © Springer Science+Business Media New York 2016

this new class of antimicrobials challenged the traditional scientific and regulatory status quo as the science offered insight where clinical data were sparse or could not be obtained in a timely, practical, or economic fashion. Moreover, there was a remarkable agreement between in vitro, in vivo, and clinical data [2–4]. Pharmacodynamics research was a key tool in identifying quantitated outcome parameters that predicted microbiologic and clinical success for fluoroquinolones and specific bacterial pathogens.

As pharmacodynamics became more engrained and accepted in the scientific and medical communities, the concepts articulated became fodder for pharmaceutical company marketing and detailing strategies as the industry attempted to use pharmacodynamic concepts to distinguish specific drug products against a growing marketplace of fluoroquinolone compounds. Managed care and hospital formulary committees would also use pharmacodynamic concepts to identify which fluoroquinolone products would become part of a contract bidding strategy that would ultimately determine which specific fluoroquinolone(s) would or would not be available to prescribers and patients in specific hospitals or health plans.

Depending upon the specific fluoroquinolone compound, this class of drugs offered clinical coverage of gram-positive, gram-negative, anaerobic, *S. aureus*, *Pseudomonas aeruginosa*, and other difficult-to-treat gram-negative infections with oral dosing. Interestingly while the free area under the concentration–time curve (*f*-AUC) to the pathogen minimum inhibitory concentration (MIC) (*f*-AUC/MIC) ratios seem to be the best overall pharmacodynamic outcome parameter for fluoroquinolones against a spectrum of pathogens, the quantitative value of this parameter is not the same for all pathogens [2–4]. Also of note is that the pharmacodynamic action of fluoroquinolones may be concentration-dependent (time-independent) against gram-negative pathogens, while for gram-positive and anaerobic pathogens their action is reported as concentration-independent (time-dependent) [3, 4].

Adverse events associated with fluoroquinolones were unique to specific products while others were class related. Thus far, there does not appear to be a toxicodynamic predictor of phototoxicity, QTc prolongation, spontaneous tendon rupture, glucose hemostasis, liver toxicity, tendonitis, arthropathy, or other fluoroquinolone side effects. There have been a number of US Food and Drug Administration (FDA) black box adverse event warnings that have been issued over the years, with many being directed at the entire marketed class of fluoroquinolone products, but none include toxicodynamic markers.

Fluoroquinolones are generally highly regarded by prescribers due to their versatility of use in a wide range of infections, the ease of administration as a once or twice a day product, and their overall safety record. While many of the fluoroquinolones entered the market as oral agents, parenteral forms generally emerged a few years later. Clinicians quickly learned that they could essentially generate the same fluoroquinolone serum concentration–time curve orally or parentally [3–8]. As such, parenteral to oral switch programs became commonplace and fluoroquinolones challenged the widely held belief that acutely ill patients require antibiotic management solely with parenteral drugs [3]. While fluoroquinolone resistance is certainly part of our current landscape, the magnitude of resistance for the most part falls short of expectations considering the widespread use and antibiotic pressure generated by fluoroquinolones both in the hospital and the community.

While a substantial number of fluoroquinolone compounds were screened and entered clinical testing, only a small fraction of these compounds were actually marketed and of those drugs only a handful survived the rigors of the marketplace. As such, we primarily limit the discussion of the fluoroquinolones to ciprofloxacin, ofloxacin/levofloxacin, and moxifloxacin.

2 Mechanism of Action and Pharmacokinetics

2.1 Mechanism of Action and Spectrum of Activity

Quinolones are synthetic compounds that act by inhibiting the activity of type II topoisomerases (DNA gyrase and topoisomerase IV), resulting in rapid bactericidal activity. These enzymes help maintain the negative configuration of the supercoiled DNA helix and the ability of the DNA to appropriately uncoil for translation [3, 9]. The interaction of quinolones with DNA and topoisomerase enzymes subsequently leads to the formation of a stable ternary compound ahead of the replication fork, halting the normal replication processes [5, 10].

2.2 Absorption and Oral Bioavailability

Following oral administration, ciprofloxacin, levofloxacin, and moxifloxacin exhibit rapid oral absorption and excellent bioavailability with little to no significant first pass metabolism (Table 1) [4–8]. Furthermore, ciprofloxacin peak plasma concentrations (C_{max}) and 24-h area under the curve (AUC_{24}) show linear relationships with escalating oral doses [11]. Time to peak serum concentration (T_{max}) in healthy volunteers typically ranges from 60–90 min following the oral administration of moxifloxacin, while ciprofloxacin and levofloxacin exhibit values of approximately 60 min [6, 12, 13]. Comparable doses of levofloxacin and moxifloxacin yield significantly higher C_{max} than those of ciprofloxacin [6]. Fluoroquinolones are administered without regard to food; however, their oral absorption is negatively affected by the presence of divalent cations and iron due to chelation effects [14–16]. A non-blinded, randomized, crossover study in 24 healthy male volunteers showed moxifloxacin oral absorption was significantly affected by the co-administration of magnesium- and aluminum-containing antacid, but not ranitidine [17]. In two similar studies,

Table 1
Pharmacokinetic parameters of commonly prescribed fluoroquinolones [4–8]

Agent	Ciprofloxacin	Levofloxacin	Moxifloxacin
Daily dose (mg)	500	500	400
C_{max} (mcg/mL)	2.4	6	3.25–4.5
T_{max} (hours)	1.2	1–1.2	1–1.5
Half-life (hours)[a]	3–5	6	12
Protein binding (%)	30–35	30	50–55
Renal elimination (%)	40–50	90–95	20
Oral bioavailability (%)	70–85	99	90
AUC_{0-24} (mg h/L)	21–42	47–48	31–48

[a]Assumes adults with baseline normal renal function

the rate of oral moxifloxacin absorption was reduced when co-administered with calcium-containing dairy products; yet the extent of oral absorption was not clinically affected [18, 19].

The reliable oral absorption of fluoroquinolones makes these agents ideal for numerous systemic infections including pulmonary, genitourinary, intra-abdominal, and skin and soft tissue infections. Additionally, fluoroquinolones that exhibit in vivo activity against *P. aeruginosa* are the only available oral treatments for pseudomonal infections in current clinical practice.

2.3 Distribution and Tissue Penetration

Currently available fluoroquinolones exhibit a large volume of distribution (V_d) consistent with significant penetration into extravascular and tissue compartments. The observed V_d values typically range from 1 to >5 L/kg [5, 6]. Additionally, these compounds exhibit moderate plasma protein binding, possibly contributing to larger volume of distribution. Ciprofloxacin and levofloxacin show mild protein binding (20–40 %), while moxifloxacin shows moderately higher affinity to plasma proteins (40–50 %) [4, 20]. Owing to the extensive tissue penetration, tissue concentrations are often higher than corresponding serum concentrations. For example, ciprofloxacin exhibits tissue-to-serum concentration ratios of 1.6, 2.1, 1.2, 13.3, and 30 in bronchial, lung, blister fluid, kidneys, and bile; respectively [20, 21]. Levofloxacin and moxifloxacin exhibit similar tissue penetration and tissue-to-serum concentration ratios to ciprofloxacin, with the exception of low urinary concentrations with moxifloxacin [22–25].

A multiple-dose study compared epithelial lining fluid and alveolar macrophage concentrations of levofloxacin and ciprofloxacin following the administration of comparable oral doses. Levofloxacin achieved higher intra-pulmonary distribution and a higher steady-state concentration in epithelial lining fluid than ciprofloxacin [26]. In a single-dose pharmacokinetic study following the intravenous (IV) administration of 400 mg of moxifloxacin, serial plasma and pleural fluid samples were collected during a 24-h interval. The maximum concentration of moxifloxacin in pleural fluid of patients with empyema or parapneumonic effusion was 2.23 mcg/mL, detected 7.5 h after the initiation of the infusion. A similar moxifloxacin peak concentration was measured in patients with malignant pleural effusion (2.96 mcg/mL), but detected only 3.58 h after the initiation of the infusion. Ratios of moxifloxacin pleural fluid to simultaneous serum concentrations were 1.11 and 1.17 for patients with empyema or parapneumonic effusion and those with malignant effusions, respectively [27]. Fluoroquinolones have been also studied as alternative agents for central nervous system (CNS) infections due to penicillin-resistant *S. pneumoniae* and gram-negative organisms such as *P. aeruginosa*. Mean CSF-to-serum AUC_{0-24} ratios in un-inflamed or mildly inflamed meninges for ciprofloxacin, levofloxacin, and moxifloxacin were approximately 0.25, 0.75, and 0.45; respectively. Higher CSF distribution values were demonstrated in strongly inflamed meninges [28]. Owing to their extensive distribution, tissue concentrations of these agents are expected to exceed MIC values for most pathogens following therapeutic doses in adult patients (Table 2) [29].

2.4 Elimination

Renal clearance is considered the major route of elimination for ciprofloxacin and levofloxacin, while the hepatic route constitutes the main elimination pathway for moxifloxacin. In a comparative crossover study of healthy volunteers, levofloxacin demonstrated the highest renal recovery (approximately 76 %), while 41 % and 20 % of ciprofloxacin and moxifloxacin doses, respectively, were recovered in the urine [6]. Moxifloxacin is metabolized through phase-II sulfate and glucuronide-conjugation to inactive metabolites. In a study of nine patients with severe liver insufficiency (Child–Pugh Class C), pharmacokinetic parameters of moxifloxacin were not significantly different than in healthy patients [30]. Consequently, no moxifloxacin dosage adjustments are recommended for patients with severe liver impairment. Due to significant renal elimination of ciprofloxacin and levofloxacin, dosage adjustments are recommended for patients with renal impairment or those undergoing renal replacement therapy.

3 Pharmacodynamics of Fluoroquinolones

The following section will discuss in detail the available pharmacodynamic data of fluoroquinolones against several groups of organisms, and primarily limit the discussion of the fluoroquinolones to ciprofloxacin, ofloxacin/levofloxacin, and moxifloxacin.

Table 2
CLSI susceptibility breakpoints (mcg/mL) for ciprofloxacin, levofloxacin, and moxifloxacin[a] [29]

	Ciprofloxacin	Levofloxacin	Moxifloxacin
Gram-negative organisms			
N. meningitidis	≤0.03	≤0.03	–
N. gonorrhoeae	≤0.06	–	–
M. cattarhalis	≤1	≤2	
H. influenzae	≤1	≤2	≤1
P. aeruginosa	≤1	≤2	–
Enterobacteriaceae (except for *Salmonella* spp.)	≤1	≤2	–
Salmonella spp.	≤0.06	≤0.12	–
Gram-positive organisms			
Staphylococcus spp.	≤1	≤1	≤0.5
S. pneumoniae	–	≤2	≤1
Other			
Anaerobes	–	–	≤2

CLSI Clinical and Laboratory Standards Institute
[a]Blank cells indicate no susceptibility breakpoint available

3.1 Basics of In Vitro Models and Monte Carlo Simulations

The in vitro models that have been used to examine fluoroquinolones pharmacodynamics have utilized one compartment, two compartment and planktonic systems. However, heterogeneity exists among these studies with respect to the following experimental parameters: starting inoculum, method of susceptibility testing, duration of experiments, growth media and oxygen use. There are differences between outcome measures as well. Methods used for animal models also exhibit similar heterogeneity. These differences in both study design and outcome measures are well summarized by Wright *et al.* [4]. Despite the various in vitro and in vivo experiments used, the studies have all yielded similar pharmacodynamic indices to be predictive of fluoroquinolone efficacy.

The *f*-AUC/MIC ratio has been shown to be the pharmacodynamic index most predictive of fluoroquinolone efficacy. A 24-h free area under the curve to MIC ratio (f-AUC_{24}/MIC) of 30 or more has been shown to be predictive of efficacy against gram-positive bacteria [31]. For gram-negative bacteria, the f-AUC_{24}/MIC predictive of efficacy is higher, and usually cited as 125 (Table 3) [32]. These two accepted AUC_{24}/MIC ratios have proved highly useful as in vitro and animal models can be used to help predict fluoroquinolone activity in less common, or difficult to study, clinical scenarios.

Table 3
Pharmacodynamics of fluoroquinolones

Organisms	Action	Parameter
Gram negative	Concentration-dependent	f-AUC_{24}/MIC ≥125
Gram positive	Concentration-independent	f-AUC_{24}/MIC ≥30
Anaerobes	Concentration-independent	f-AUC_{24}/MIC ~50

Monte Carlo simulations have also been used to examine fluoroquinolone pharmacodynamics. These simulations attempt to estimate the probability of obtaining pharmacodynamic parameters by using MIC data in combination with human pharmacokinetic data. With respect to fluoroquinolones, thousands of AUC_{24}/MIC estimates are generated using available pharmacokinetic and MIC data, which yield the probability of obtaining a desired f-AUC_{24}/MIC value(s). The majority of these studies have examined the pharmacodynamics of fluoroquinolones against either *S. pneumoniae* or various gram-negative pathogens, including but not limited to: *Escherichia coli*, *Klebsiella pneumoniae*, *P. aeruginosa*, and *Acinetobacter baumannii*. Some studies have focused on the probability of obtaining currently accepted AUC_{24}/MIC breakpoints. Other studies have examined both accepted AUC_{24}/MIC breakpoints as well as higher breakpoints in order to determine the probability of preventing the selection of fluoroquinolone-resistant mutants. The results of *S. pneumoniae* Monte Carlo simulations are more encouraging for clinicians than similar studies involving gram-negative pathogens. The latter body of literature has shown that fluoroquinolones have a lower probability of target AUC_{24}/MIC attainment against gram-negative pathogens, especially those with higher MIC.

3.2 Gram-Negative Organisms

Pharmacodynamic properties of fluoroquinolones against gram-negative organisms have been extensively studied, and were incorporated in the early drug development process. A review of available in vitro and animal infection models by Schentag *et al.* suggested three main breakpoints to describe the antimicrobial effects of fluoroquinolones: AUC_{24}/MIC values of 30–50 represent bacteriostatic effects, values above 100 but less than 250 represent bactericidal effects, while values above 250 represent rapid and maximal bactericidal action. Additionally, the emergence of resistance most closely correlated with an AUC_{24}/MIC ratio of less than 100 [33]. This section outlines available in vitro, animal and human data to mainly characterize the antimicrobial effect of ciprofloxacin, levofloxacin, and moxifloxacin against gram-negative pathogens.

3.2.1 In Vitro Simulations

Early in vitro models by Blaser and colleagues using netilmicin and enoxacin against gram-positive and gram-negative organisms demonstrated bacterial regrowth within 24 h unless the C_{max}/MIC ratio was above 8. Moreover, regrowing bacteria exhibited four- to eightfold higher MIC values with little bactericidal activity of study agents with subsequent dosing [34]. A C_{max}/MIC ratio of <8 was also shown to increase the selection of ciprofloxacin-resistant colonies of *P. aeruginosa* in a separate in vitro, two-compartment model of infection [35]. Further research aimed to determine whether C_{max}/MIC or AUC_{24}/MIC ratio most accurately predict microbiologic outcomes. In a study of ciprofloxacin and oflaxacin activity against *P. aeruginosa*, investigators showed microbiologic outcomes better correlated with AUC_{24}/MIC ratios of $\geq$100, when compared to other pharmacodynamic parameters such as AUC_{24} and C_{max}/MIC ratios [36].

More recently, an in vitro model simulated the human free non-protein bound concentrations of 400 mg IV moxifloxacin daily, 500 mg IV levofloxacin daily and 750 mg IV levofloxacin daily against strains of *S. pneumoniae*, *S. aureus*, *K. pneumoniae*, and *E. coli* with variable susceptibilities. An AUC_{24}/MIC of 100 and a C_{max}/MIC of 10 were shown to produce maximal bactericidal effect for levofloxacin and moxifloxacin [37]. Finally, an in vitro model explored the pharmacodynamics of escalating doses moxifloxacin against a high inoculum (10^8 colony forming units/mL) of three wild-type strains of *E. coli* (MIC of 0.0625 mcg/mL). Bacterial regrowth and resistance amplification were observed between AUC_{24}/MIC ratios of 47 and 117, while sustained bacterial suppression was achieved at AUC_{24}/MIC ratio of 180; illustrating the potential impact of inoculum size on fluoroquinolone antibacterial activity [38].

As in vitro models continued to show varying AUC_{24}/MIC thresholds, further research compared different endpoints to describe the antibacterial effects of fluoroquinolones. Ultimately, the intensity of antimicrobial effect (I_E) was shown to be an accurate descriptor endpoint of fluoroquinolones antibacterial activity [39–42]. Defined as the area between the control growth in the absence of antibiotics and the antibiotic-induced time-kill/regrowth curves [43], I_E describes the area between the control and time-kill curves from time zero to the time when bacterial counts with antibiotic exposure reach the same maximal numbers as in the absence of antibiotic; which typically exceeds the dosing interval of a given agent [44]. This approach overcomes the limitations of traditional endpoints such as area between the control growth and time-kill curves and area under the time-kill curve, which describe the antimicrobial effects over a prespecified dosing interval without regard to the actual duration of effect. It also allows investigators to account for the differences seen amongst various agents based on their individual duration of antimicrobial effects. Subsequently, this approach was studied and validated in both single- and multiple dose simulations [40, 42].

In a simulation of single doses of moxifloxacin and levofloxacin against two isolates of *S. aureus* and one each of *E. coli* and *K. pneumoniae*, the predicted equivalent AUC_{24}/MIC ratios for moxifloxacin and levofloxacin were estimated at 80 and 130, respectively, indicating important differences in the antimicrobial effects between the two agents [40]. These breakpoints were predicted to be equivalent to previously reported breakpoints of ciprofloxacin AUC_{24}/MIC values of 125 against gram-negative organisms [33, 45]. Similarly, an in vitro dynamic model simulated human plasma levels after single oral doses of 1000 mg of ciprofloxacin, 320 mg gemifloxacin, 500 mg levofloxacin or 400 mg moxifloxacin against one isolate of *Moraxella catarrhalis*. Using traditional dosing interval-dependent endpoint, the time-kill/regrowth curves demonstrated similar patterns with all study agents, while effect of moxifloxacin as expressed by the I_E was 30, 55, and 120 % greater than gemifloxacin, levofloxacin, and ciprofloxacin, respectively [44].

When considering resistant subpopulations and the concept of mutant prevention concentration (MPC), defined as the concentration required to prevent the emergence of resistant mutants, an in vitro kinetic model by Olofsson and colleagues studied six simulated clinical doses of norfloxacin, ciprofloxacin, and moxifloxacin against *E. coli* mixed cultures containing fluoroquinolone-resistant subpopulations. All six simulated regimens eradicated the-wild type population at AUC_{24}/MIC values above 100, while AUC_{24}/MPC values of 35 were effective at preventing the growth of the resistant single mutant strain [46].

Despite varying methodologies of in vitro models used, these experiments offer important predictions of the antibacterial effects of various fluoroquinolones against a wide range of gram-negative organisms.

3.2.2 Animal Infection Models

Similar to in vitro models, the pharmacodynamic properties of various fluoroquinolones have been evaluated in animal infection models. Leggett and colleagues studied the impact of dosing interval on the relative efficacy of various antibiotics, including ciprofloxacin, in neutropenic murine thigh and pulmonary infection models using *P. aeruginosa* and *K. pneumoniae*, respectively. Dosing interval in this study was shown to have minimal effect on the antibacterial effect of ciprofloxacin [47]. Similarly, in a neutropenic rat infection model of *P. aeruginosa* sepsis, lomefloxacin C_{max}/MIC ratios of 10–20 were significantly associated with survival when compared with AUC_{24}/MIC ratios and fraction of the time drug levels were maintained above the MIC. Furthermore, when C_{max}/MIC ratios were <10, AUC_{24}/MIC ratio most closely predicted the outcome [48]. Unfortunately, C_{max}/MIC ratios of above 10–20 may be difficult to replicate in human subjects as the

MIC of the offending pathogen approaches or exceeds 1 mcg/mL, as in the case of *P. aeruginosa* (Tables 1 and 2) [4–8, 29].

Craig and colleagues presented composite data of studies using strains of gram-positive and gram-negative organisms in pneumonia, peritonitis and sepsis infection models performed in mice, rats, and guinea pigs treated for at least 2 days. AUC_{24}/MIC ratios of <30 were associated with >50 % mortality, while values above 100 were associated with minimal mortality [49]. More recently, investigators studied a murine model of pneumonia using levofloxacin against one strain of *P. aeruginosa*. Levofloxacin levels in the epithelial lining fluid (ELF) and corresponding AUC_{ELF}/MIC ratios were measured between 0 and 6 h after an intraperitoneal dose. AUC_{ELF}/MIC ratios of 12.4, 31.2, 62.8, and 127.6 were required to drive bacteriostatic, 1-, 2-, and 3-$\log_{10}$ (colony forming units/g) kills [50]. In the same study, resistance suppression occurred when the AUC_{24}/MIC ratio was greater than 64 [50].

Similar to in vitro research, animal infection models are not without heterogeneity, that stems from varying study designs and methodologies, organisms used, and the duration each model observed the antimicrobial effects of study fluoroquinolones.

3.2.3 Human Data

In 1989, Peloquin and colleagues studied 50 acutely ill patients with gram-negative lower respiratory tract infections treated with IV ciprofloxacin 200 mg twice daily. C_{max}/MIC ratios below 10 were associated with development of resistance while on treatment in 10 of 13 (76.9 %) patients with *P. aeruginosa* pneumonia, lung abscess or bronchiectasis [51]. Antibacterial effects of ciprofloxacin for serious infections due to gram-negative pathogens were further demonstrated in a study of 70 patients treated with various IV doses. Both clinical and microbiologic cures were significantly associated with AUC_{24}/MIC values of 125 or more. The probability of clinical and microbiologic cures when achieving AUC_{24}/MIC values above 125 were 80 % and 82 %, compared with 42 % and 26 % when AUC_{24}/MIC values were below 125. Additionally, the median times to microbiologic eradication also differed significantly between treatment groups. At AUC_{24}/MIC values above 250, time to microbiologic eradication was approximately 1.9 days, as compared with 32 days when corresponding values were below 125 and 6.6 days when values were between 125 and 250 [32]. In an open-label multicenter trial of 134 patients who had a pathogen isolated from the primary site of infection and an available MIC to levofloxacin, C_{max}/MIC ratios of 12.2 or more correlated with both clinical and microbiologic endpoints [2]. To further characterize the impact of pharmacodynamic indices on the risk of developing resistance during treatment, investigators combined the results of four trials of patients with nosocomial lower respiratory tract infections. Thirty-two of the 128 (25 %) initially fluoroquinolone-susceptible strains, the majority of which were gram-negative organisms, ultimately developed resistance during treatment. The probability of developing resistance among study patients significantly correlated with AUC_{24}/MIC ratios less than 100 (80 % probability). In cases when AUC_{24}/MIC values exceeded 100, the probability of developing resistance was <10 % [52]. Results of above studies are in line with various in vitro and animal models suggesting an AUC_{24}/MIC ratio of at least 125 is required to optimize antibacterial activity of fluoroquinolones and decrease the risk of selecting resistant strains while on treatment. Conversely, Zelenitsky and Ariano recently called into question the validity of AUC_{24}/MIC breakpoints of 125 for treating Enterobacteriaceae bloodstream infections. Clinical and microbiological data were collected from 42 patients with bloodstream infections due to *E. coli*, *Klebsiella* spp., *Enterobacter* spp., or *Serratia* spp. treated with ciprofloxacin. Patients with ciprofloxacin AUC_{24}/MIC of <250 were 27.8 times (95 % CI 2.1–333, $p = 0.011$) more likely to experience treatment failure, and the probability of attaining an AUC_{24}/MIC of at least 250 was 88 % using intravenous doses of 400 mg every 12 h [53].

As the aforementioned AUC_{24}/MIC breakpoints became widely acceptable, focus shifted to studying the likelihood of achieving adequate serum and tissue concentrations using various intravenous and oral doses. To demonstrate the probability of target attainment, a study of three ciprofloxacin dosing regimens against *P. aeruginosa* using clinical outcome-based Monte Carlo simulations showed higher ciprofloxacin doses of 400 mg IV every 8 h should be used to ensure target attainment. However, as the authors conclude, even higher doses may be ineffective in ensuring target attainment as the MIC of offending pathogens approaches 1 mcg/mL [54]. Similarly, in a study of critically ill patients with severe community-acquired pneumonia undergoing mechanical ventilation, a levofloxacin intravenous dose of 500 mg once daily achieved a C_{max}/MIC of 10 or more and AUC_{24}/MIC of at least 125 in both serum and epithelial lining fluid when the MIC of the isolated pathogen was 1 mcg/mL or less. However, doses of 500 mg twice daily were needed to achieve the same pharmacodynamic indices when the corresponding MIC exceeded 1 mcg/mL [22]. These observations were validated in other studies demonstrating the impact of higher fluoroquinolone MICs (≥1 mcg/mL) on the probability of target attainment. Conil and colleagues showed ciprofloxacin AUC_{24}/MIC thresholds were rarely reached in intensive-care patients when the MIC was 1 mcg/mL, particularly in those with increased renal elimination of ciprofloxacin [55]. A prospective, randomized, two-way crossover trial of ten patients with gram-negative bacilli bacteremia evaluated consecutive intravenous ciprofloxacin doses of 400 mg every 8 h for four doses followed by 400 mg every 12 h for four doses. Both dosing regimens achieved adequate AUC_{24}/MIC breakpoints (at least

100) for pathogens with MIC of 0.5 mcg/mL. However, for pathogens with MIC of 1 mcg/mL, only higher daily doses provided AUC_{24}/MIC greater than 100 with no observed increase in adverse effects [56]. Finally, in a study of hospitalized patients treated with ciprofloxacin, 21 % and 75 % of study patients did not achieve AUC_{24}/MIC breakpoint of at least 125 when the MICs were 0.25 and 0.5 mcg/mL, respectively. Furthermore, a computer simulation showed a decrease in those percentages to 1 % and 37 %, respectively, when higher doses (400 mg every 8 h) were utilized [57].

3.3 *Streptococcus pneumoniae*

Fluoroquinolones are often used to treat upper and lower respiratory tract infections of which *S. pneumoniae* is often the causative pathogen. Fluoroquinolone pharmacodynamics against *S. pneumoniae* has been extensively studied, including in vitro, animal and human studies, as well as Monte Carlo simulations. The data from numerous studies indicate that AUC_{24}/MIC ratio of at least 30 is necessary for bactericidal activity [58, 59]. It should be noted that this AUC_{24}/MIC value has often been described with respect to wild-type *S. pneumoniae*. Also, this was not always the accepted AUC_{24}/MIC value for fluoroquinolones against *S. pneumoniae*. After an AUC_{24}/MIC of 125 was shown to be necessary for the eradication of gram-negative pathogens, this pharmacodynamic breakpoint was extrapolated to *S. pneumoniae* [32]. Bedos *et al.* examined ciprofloxacin and sparfloxacin in a murine model of *S. pneumoniae* pneumonia and found AUC_{24}/MIC of greater than 160 was required to achieve 100 % survival [60]. Lister and colleagues then examined levofloxacin against five *S. pneumoniae* isolates using an in vitro, two-compartment, dynamic model and found that a levofloxacin AUC_{24}/MIC of 32–64 corresponded to bacterial eradication. In the same study, a ciprofloxacin AUC_{24}/MIC of at least 44 correlated with bactericidal activity against *S. pneumoniae* [61].

These lower AUC_{24}/MIC values were substantiated by Ambrose and colleagues who evaluated the pharmacodynamics of ciprofloxacin among 58 patients treated for documented *S. pneumoniae* respiratory tract infections; either community-acquired pneumonia or an exacerbation of chronic bronchitis. The authors dichotomized the probability of microbiologic eradication around an AUC_{24}/MIC of 33.7 and found that ratios greater than 33.7 led to a 100 % probability of microbiologic eradication. While patients with a ciprofloxacin AUC_{24}/MIC less than 33.7 had only a 64 % probability of microbiologic eradication. Additionally, the clinical cure rate was 92 % when the AUC_{24}/MIC was above 40 [31]. In a prospective trial of levofloxacin for the treatment of urinary tract, respiratory, and skin and soft tissue infections, Preston et al. found the C_{max}/MIC to be most predictive of microbiologic and clinical outcomes [2]. In this study, a C_{max}/MIC of 12.2

correlated with clinical success and microbiologic eradication. The authors also found a high degree of correlation between C_{max}/MIC and AUC_{24}/MIC. This finding is not surprising because C_{max} and AUC are directly related; as C_{max} increases so does the AUC and vice versa. While these human data are compelling, most pharmacodynamic examinations of fluoroquinolones against *S. pneumoniae* have utilized in vitro models.

Using in vitro kinetic models, Odenholt and Cars studied levofloxacin and moxifloxacin against *S. pneumoniae, S. aureus,* and *E. coli* isolates with varying degrees of susceptibility to each antibiotic. The authors found that an AUC_{24}/MIC ratio of at least 100 and a C_{max}/MIC ratio of 10 or more led to a maximum antibacterial activity for both levofloxacin and moxifloxacin [37]. Both pharmacodynamic indices were higher for moxifloxacin than levofloxacin against the *S. pneumoniae* isolates studied. This is counterintuitive as moxifloxacin 400 mg daily has lower C_{max} than levofloxacin 500 mg and 750 mg daily. However, the levofloxacin MICs for *S. pneumoniae* in this study were at least fourfold higher than the moxifloxacin MICs. Nevertheless, moxifloxacin 400 mg daily, levofloxacin 500 mg daily and levofloxacin 750 mg daily attained at least a four-log kill against a *S. pneumoniae* strain harboring a single fluoroquinolone resistance mutation (*parC*) [37]. The associated AUC_{24}/MIC values against this isolate were 102, 40, and 52 for moxifloxacin 400 mg, levofloxacin 500 mg and levofloxacin 750 mg, respectively. None of these three regimens attained bactericidal activity against a *S. pneumoniae* strain harboring both *parC* and *gyrA* mutations. The AUC_{0-24}/MIC values for all antibiotic regimens tested against this resistant strain were 5–13 [37]. MacGowan and colleagues examined the impact of moxifloxacin pharmacodynamics against *S. pneumoniae* on the emergence of fluoroquinolone-resistant mutants. The mean moxifloxacin AUC_{24}/MIC was 45 with a standard deviation of 22, and there was no development of moxifloxacin-resistant *S. pneumoniae* mutants [62]. The results of these studies may explain the minimal increase in *S. pneumoniae* resistance worldwide despite an increase in fluoroquinolone resistance among gram-negative pathogens [63]. Moxifloxacin, levofloxacin, and ciprofloxacin should obtain an AUC_{24}/MIC of at least 40 if the *S. pneumoniae* MIC is ≤ 1 mcg/mL, the MIC range for the majority of *S. pneumoniae* isolates [63]. However, up to 30 % of *S. pneumoniae* isolates possess a single *parC*, a "first-step mutation," which is not detected by conventional laboratory susceptibility testing [63, 64]. These single mutations in the quinolone resistance-determining region allow the bacteria to develop additional resistance mutations rapidly in the mutant selection window [63].

The emergence of fluoroquinolone-resistant mutants depends on the bacterial species, the duration of exposure and drug exposure [62]. For many *S. pneumoniae* isolates, the mutant prevention concentration (MPC) lies between four and eight times the MIC [65]. Even after the antibiotic concentration drops below the MPC, it takes time for bacteria to enter logarithmic growth phase. This delay in bacterial recovery and growth is called the post-antibiotic effect. Fluoroquinolones have a post-antibiotic effect of approximately 3 h or less against *S. pneumoniae* [66, 67].

Allen and colleagues found that first and second step mutations were selected after *S. pneumoniae* isolates were exposed to levofloxacin in an in vitro dynamic model [68]. In the same study, moxifloxacin also selected for a second-step mutant when a first-step *gyrA* mutant was present. Florea et al. studied moxifloxacin and levofloxacin against *S. pneumoniae* isolates harboring a *parC* mutation using an in vitro model simulating epithelial lining fluid pharmacokinetics of each antibiotic [69]. There was no selection of resistant mutants in the moxifloxacin experiments. However, levofloxacin 500 mg daily failed to achieve bacterial eradication or prevent the emergence of resistant mutants despite AUC_{24}/MIC values above 100. Building on that study, a similar study was performed in which levofloxacin and moxifloxacin were tested against *parC*-containing mutants using an in vitro dynamic model simulating epithelial lining fluid concentrations of both antibiotics [70]. Regimens simulating levofloxacin 500 and 750 mg daily experienced regrowth and acquisition of a second-step *gyrA* mutation in 100 and 50 % of isolates tested, respectively. Moxifloxacin 400 mg daily demonstrated sustained bactericidal activity without acquisition of second-step mutants. The authors concluded that an AUC_{24}/MIC of 200 for levofloxacin and 400 for moxifloxacin were needed to prevent the acquisition of second-step fluoroquinolone resistance mutations [70]. The results of these studies are important but, because clinical microbiology laboratories do not routinely test for first-step fluoroquinolone resistance mutations, their clinical applicability remains in question.

In Monte Carlo simulations, both levofloxacin and moxifloxacin have shown high probabilities of attaining the accepted AUC_{24}/MIC of 30 or more against *S. pneumoniae.* Jones and colleagues performed a 10,000 patient Monte Carlo simulation using the *S. pneumoniae* isolates from the SENTRY Antimicrobial Surveillance Program. The authors found that levofloxacin 500 mg daily would achieve an AUC_{24}/MIC of 30 in 79 % of patients [71]. However, levofloxacin 500 mg daily had only a 15 % probability of attaining an AUC_{24}/MIC of 120. Frei and Burgess examined the pharmacodynamics of levofloxacin 500 and 750 mg daily against 7,866 *S. pneumoniae* isolates with varying susceptibility to penicillin including 1,287 penicillin-resistant strains [72]. The authors evaluated time above MIC and AUC_{24}/MIC using accepted and elevated AUC_{24}/MIC values. Levofloxacin 500 and 750 mg daily had a high probability of attaining an AUC_{24}/MIC of 30 (90 and 99 %, respectively); however, as the AUC_{24}/MIC value increased the probability of attainment decreased. For example, the probability of levofloxacin 750 mg daily attaining an AUC_{24}/MIC of 70 or more was less than 40 % [72]. Noreddin et al. examined the probability of moxifloxacin 400 mg daily achieving an AUC_{24}/MIC of 30, 40, 100, and 120 against *S. pneumoniae* MIC data from patients hospitalized with community-acquired pneumonia. The authors performed their analyses using pharmacokinetic data from human serum and human epithelial lining fluid and the MIC_{90} value for the *S. pneumoniae* isolates. Moxifloxacin 400 mg daily had a 97 % probability or greater of attaining an AUC_{24}/MIC of 30, 40, 100, and 120 in the serum and greater than 97 % probability of attaining AUC_{24}/MIC of 30 and 40 in the epithelial lining fluid. The probabilities of moxifloxacin 400 mg daily attaining an AUC_{24}/MIC of 100 and 120 in the epithelial lining fluid were slightly lower (87.3 and 86.2 %, respectively) [73]. This decrease in AUC_{24}/MIC target attainment in the epithelial lining fluid may be noteworthy as the epithelial lining fluid could be a better determinant of fluoroquinolone efficacy in respiratory infections than corresponding serum values.

These Monte Carlo simulation data suggest that both levofloxacin and moxifloxacin have a high probability of attaining an AUC_{24}/MIC of 30. The probability of these agents attaining higher AUC_{24}/MIC ratios remains in question, as does the clinical significance of attaining these higher ratios. The fact that levofloxacin and, to a lesser extent, moxifloxacin have a lower probability of attaining higher AUC_{24}/MIC values is concerning for the selection of fluoroquinolone-resistant *S. pneumoniae*.

3.4 Staphylococcus aureus

Fluoroquinolones possess activity against *S. aureus*, but are not routinely used to treat invasive *S. aureus* infections. Pharmacodynamic studies have shown that fluoroquinolones are bactericidal against *S. aureus* when the AUC_{24}/MIC is greater than 30 [37, 74, 75]. Fluoroquinolones have also been found to behave differently against *S. aureus* depending on whether the conditions are anaerobic or aerobic. Lewin and colleagues found fluoroquinolones to be bacteriostatic against *S. aureus* under anaerobic conditions. The authors stated this finding may have resulted from decreased fluoroquinolone uptake into *S. aureus* cells in the absence of oxygen [76]. However, other investigators found that numerous fluoroquinolones were bactericidal against *S. aureus* under anaerobic conditions [77, 78]. The rate of kill was slower under anaerobic conditions in the study by Zabinski et al. [78]. Wright and colleagues found that moxifloxacin and levofloxacin achieved bactericidal activity within 12 h against methicillin-sensitive and methicillin-resistant strains of *S. aureus* and *S. epidermidis* under anaerobic conditions [77]. Regrowth was not observed in any of the aforementioned experiments. Notably, in experiments with moxifloxacin, the mean survival times were much longer for methicillin-resistant *S. aureus* and *S. epidermidis* under anaerobic conditions compared with aerobic conditions [77].

Using a two-compartment in vitro model of levofloxacin against *S. aureus*, Zhang et al. found AUC_{24}/MIC above 25 was predictive of antibacterial activity, and AUC_{24}/MPC of ≥2.2 predicted resistance outcomes [74]. Lister compared levofloxacin 500 mg daily and moxifloxacin 400 mg daily against three *S. aureus* and three *S. epidermidis* strains using an in vitro hollow fiber model [75]. Two of the three strains for each *Staphylococcus* spp. studied were resistant to ciprofloxacin (MIC of 4 and 16 mcg/mL) and methicillin (MIC of 1 mcg/mL for both). Both levofloxacin and moxifloxacin achieved bactericidal activity within 8 h, but this was sustained only with moxifloxacin. Levofloxacin experienced regrowth after 8 h when tested against the four *Staphylococcus* strains that were resistant to ciprofloxacin, irrespective of the ciprofloxacin MIC. Resistant subpopulations with elevated levofloxacin MIC emerged in all four of these experiments for which the AUC_{24}/MIC values ranged from 8 to 32. Moxifloxacin sustained bactericidal activity for the duration of the experiment against all strains except the *S. epidermidis* strain with a ciprofloxacin MIC of 16 mcg/mL. Against that strain, moxifloxacin achieved bactericidal activity at 4 h after which there was regrowth [75]. Nevertheless, the final inoculum was more than 2 log_{10} colony forming units/mL below the starting inoculum and no resistant mutants were detected. Moxifloxacin AUC_{24}/MIC values ranged from 54 to 108. Notably, the AUC_{24}/MIC ratio for moxifloxacin was 54 against both ciprofloxacin-resistant strains of *S. epidermidis*. These results, similar to those for *S. pneumoniae*, may suggest that moxifloxacin has better antibacterial activity than levofloxacin against *S. aureus*. However, this may have little clinical importance, as fluoroquinolone mono-therapy is not often utilized to treat infections due to *S. aureus*.

3.5 Anaerobic Infections

The first FDA-approved fluoroquinolone antibiotics (norfloxacin, ciprofloxacin, ofloxacin, and later levofloxacin) contained no indication for the management of anaerobic infections [79]. However, with the introduction of trovafloxacin and moxifloxacin, as well as several other fluoroquinolones that did not receive FDA approval, there was clear evidence of bactericidal action against a number of clinically relevant anaerobes. Both trovafloxacin and moxifloxacin had/have FDA-approved indications for the management of intra-abdominal and complicated skin infections [80, 81]. Moxifloxacin, the only remaining marketed fluoroquinolone with anaerobic activity, is used clinically off label in a variety of situations where mixed flora including anaerobes is likely. There is also data linking some of the newer fluoroquinolones as a risk factor for *Clostridium difficile* infections [79].

Fluoroquinolones appear to kill anaerobes in a concentration independent (time dependent) fashion [82]. Most investigators identify AUC_{24}/MIC ratio as the best predictor of antibiotic performance and the quantitative value of this parameter may vary for different anaerobic species. Peterson and colleagues reported that an AUC_{24}/MIC ratio ≥40 is required to maximize the fluoroquinolone antibacterial effect against *Bacteroides fragilis* [82, 83]. There are reports that suboptimal exposures (AUC_{24}/MIC ratio <44) against anaerobic bacteria can foster fluoroquinolone resistance depending upon species, fluoroquinolone, and the magnitude of the AUC_{24}/MIC ratio [82, 83].

Peterson et al., when conducting preliminary in vitro dynamic experiments attempting to quantitate the impact of five different fluoroquinolones against *B. fragilis*, noticed curious phenomena with sparfloxacin. Initially the anaerobic pathogens were susceptible to sparfloxacin and caused a significant reduction in the anaerobic population at clinically relevant concentrations of the drug. While the inoculum was initially susceptible, a sampling at the end of the 24-h experiment demonstrated a significant rise in the sparfloxacin MIC [82, 83]. Other fluoroquinolones were also studied to determine if this phenomenon was limited to sparfloxacin only or was a class effect. Results of these additional in vitro experiments demonstrated these findings to be a class effect and irreversible after 10 days of serial passage. Later studies proved the mechanism of resistance was due to alterations in *gyrA* and *gyrB* [84, 85].

Hospitals and health plans, as a result of pharmaceutical contracting, became either ciprofloxacin /moxifloxacin or levofloxacin institutions heavily promoting specific fluoroquinolone usage according to their respective contracts. This may have created a scenario of unrecognized collateral damage for patient anaerobic flora. Often in complicated skin and intra-abdominal infections, cultures are not performed due to the likely multitude of bacteria present. Even if anaerobes are recovered most hospitals do not perform routine anaerobic antimicrobial susceptibility studies for fluoroquinolones so the significance of this antibiotic pressure is unknown. Edlund et al. have reported that fluoroquinolones have a selective effect on intestinal flora, primarily affecting the Enterobacteriaceae, but also having a minor impact on anaerobes [86]. However, Golan et al. reported a dramatic increase in fluoroquinolone-resistant *Bacteroides* spp. from 1994 to 2001 and Betriu et al. made a similar observation with moxifloxacin and trovafloxacin over a 6-year period from 1997 to 2002 [87, 88].

4 Summary

Fluoroquinolones continue to be a cornerstone of antibacterial treatments for a wide range of infectious diseases in the inpatient and outpatient settings. The breadth of fluoroquinolone pharmacodynamics knowledge has greatly improved our understanding of appropriate dosing to optimize clinical outcomes and limit the likelihood of selecting for resistant isolates. To date, available research has identified distinct pharmacodynamic indices to predict the antimicrobial effects of fluoroquinolones against gram-positive, gram-negative, and anaerobic pathogens. In the era of increased bacterial resistance to a multitude of antibacterial agents, including fluoroquinolones, dose optimization based on pharmacodynamic principles will undoubtedly direct daily clinical practice in the near future.

References

1. Oliphant CM, Green GM (2002) Quinolones: a comprehensive review. Am Fam Physician 65(3):455–464
2. Preston SL, Drusano GL, Berman AL, Fowler CL, Chow AT, Dornseif B et al (1998) Pharmacodynamics of levofloxacin: a new paradigm for early clinical trials. JAMA 279(2):125–129
3. Rotschafer JC, Ullman MA, Sullivan CJ (2011) Optimal use of fluoroquinolones in the intensive care unit setting. Crit Care Clin 27(1):95–106
4. Wright DH, Brown GH, Peterson ML, Rotschafer JC (2000) Application of fluoroquinolone pharmacodynamics. J Antimicrob Chemother 46(5):669–683
5. Brighty K, Gootz T (2000) Chemistry and mechanism of action of the quinolone antibacterials. In: Andriole VT (ed) The quinolones, 3rd edn. Academic, San Diego, pp 33–97
6. Lubasch A, Keller I, Borner K, Koeppe P, Lode H (2000) Comparative pharmacokinetics of ciprofloxacin, gatifloxacin, grepafloxacin, levofloxacin, trovafloxacin, and moxifloxacin after single oral administration in healthy volunteers. Antimicrob Agents Chemother 44(10):2600–2603
7. Turnidge J (1999) Pharmacokinetics and pharmacodynamics of fluoroquinolones. Drugs 58(Suppl 2):29–36
8. Walker RC (1999) The fluoroquinolones. Mayo Clin Proc 74(10):1030–1037
9. Drlica K, Zhao X (1997) DNA *gyrase*, topoisomerase IV, and the 4-quinolones. Microbiol Mol Biol Rev 61(3):377–392
10. Hawkey PM (2003) Mechanisms of quinolone action and microbial response. J Antimicrob Chemother 51(Suppl 1):29–35
11. Bergan T, Thorsteinsson SB, Solberg R, Bjornskau L, Kolstad IM, Johnsen S (1987) Pharmacokinetics of ciprofloxacin: intravenous and increasing oral doses. Am J Med 82(4A):97–102
12. Sullivan JT, Woodruff M, Lettieri J, Agarwal V, Krol GJ, Leese PT et al (1999) Pharmacokinetics of a once-daily oral dose of moxifloxacin (bay 12-8039), a new enantiomerically pure 8-methoxy quinolone. Antimicrob Agents Chemother 43(11):2793–2797
13. Stass H, Kubitza D, Schuhly U (2001) Pharmacokinetics, safety and tolerability of moxifloxacin, a novel 8-methoxyfluoroquinolone, after repeated oral administration. Clin Pharmacokinet 40(Suppl 1):1–9
14. Stass H, Kubitza D (2001) Effects of iron supplements on the oral bioavailability of moxifloxacin, a novel 8-methoxyfluoroquinolone, in humans. Clin Pharmacokinet 40(Suppl 1):57–62
15. Lettieri J, Vargas R, Agarwal V, Liu P (2001) Effect of food on the pharmacokinetics of a single oral dose of moxifloxacin 400 mg in healthy male volunteers. Clin Pharmacokinet 40(Suppl 1):19–25
16. Teng R, Dogolo LC, Willavize SA, Friedman HL, Vincent J (1997) Oral bioavailability of trovafloxacin with and without food in healthy volunteers. J Antimicrob Chemother 39(Suppl B):87–92
17. Stass H, Bottcher MF, Ochmann K (2001) Evaluation of the influence of antacids and h2 antagonists on the absorption of moxifloxacin after oral administration of a 400 mg dose to healthy volunteers. Clin Pharmacokinet 40(Suppl 1):39–48
18. Stass H, Wandel C, Delesen H, Moller JG (2001) Effect of calcium supplements on the oral bioavailability of moxifloxacin in healthy male volunteers. Clin Pharmacokinet 40(Suppl 1):27–32

19. Stass H, Kubitza D (2001) Effects of dairy products on the oral bioavailability of moxifloxacin, a novel 8-methoxyfluoroquinolone, in healthy volunteers. Clin Pharmacokinet 40(Suppl 1):33–38
20. Aminimanizani A, Beringer P, Jelliffe R (2001) Comparative pharmacokinetics and pharmacodynamics of the newer fluoroquinolone antibacterials. Clin Pharmacokinet 40(3):169–187
21. Vance-Bryan K, Guay DR, Rotschafer JC (1990) Clinical pharmacokinetics of ciprofloxacin. Clin Pharmacokinet 19(6):434–461
22. Boselli E, Breilh D, Rimmele T, Djabarouti S, Saux MC, Chassard D et al (2005) Pharmacokinetics and intrapulmonary diffusion of levofloxacin in critically ill patients with severe community-acquired pneumonia. Crit Care Med 33(1):104–109
23. Rink AD, Stass H, Delesen H, Kubitza D, Vestweber KH (2008) Pharmacokinetics and tissue penetration of moxifloxacin in intervention therapy for intra-abdominal abscess. Clin Drug Investig 28(2):71–79
24. Ober MC, Hoppe-Tichy T, Koninger J, Schunter O, Sonntag HG, Weigand MA et al (2009) Tissue penetration of moxifloxacin into human gallbladder wall in patients with biliary tract infections. J Antimicrob Chemother 64(5):1091–1095
25. Krasemann C, Meyer J, Tillotson G (2001) Evaluation of the clinical microbiology profile of moxifloxacin. Clin Infect Dis 32(Suppl 1):S51–S63
26. Gotfried MH, Danziger LH, Rodvold KA (2001) Steady-state plasma and intrapulmonary concentrations of levofloxacin and ciprofloxacin in healthy adult subjects. Chest 119(4):1114–1122
27. Chatzika K, Manika K, Kontou P, Pitsiou G, Papakosta D, Zarogoulidis K et al (2014) Moxifloxacin pharmacokinetics and pleural fluid penetration in patients with pleural effusion. Antimicrob Agents Chemother 58(3): 1315–1319
28. Nau R, Sorgel F, Eiffert H (2010) Penetration of drugs through the blood-cerebrospinal fluid/blood-brain barrier for treatment of central nervous system infections. Clin Microbiol Rev 23(4):858–883
29. Clinical and Laboratory Standards Institute (2013) M100-S23. Performance standards for antimicrobial susceptibility testing: 23rd informational supplement. Clinical and Laboratory Standards Institute, Wayne, PA
30. Barth J, Jager D, Mundkowski R, Drewelow B, Welte T, Burkhardt O (2008) Single- and multiple-dose pharmacokinetics of intravenous moxifloxacin in patients with severe hepatic impairment. J Antimicrob Chemother 62(3):575–578
31. Ambrose PG, Bhavnani SM, Owens RC Jr (2003) Clinical pharmacodynamics of quinolones. Infect Dis Clin North Am 17(3):529–543
32. Forrest A, Nix DE, Ballow CH, Goss TF, Birmingham MC, Schentag JJ (1993) Pharmacodynamics of intravenous ciprofloxacin in seriously ill patients. Antimicrob Agents Chemother 37(5):1073–1081
33. Schentag JJ, Meagher AK, Forrest A (2003) Fluoroquinolone AUIC break points and the link to bacterial killing rates. Part 2: human trials. Ann Pharmacother 37(10):1478–1488
34. Blaser J, Stone BB, Groner MC, Zinner SH (1987) Comparative study with enoxacin and netilmicin in a pharmacodynamic model to determine importance of ratio of antibiotic peak concentration to MIC for bactericidal activity and emergence of resistance. Antimicrob Agents Chemother 31(7):1054–1060
35. Dudley MN, Blaser J, Gilbert D, Mayer KH, Zinner SH (1991) Combination therapy with ciprofloxacin plus azlocillin against *Pseudomonas aeruginosa*: effect of simultaneous versus staggered administration in an in vitro model of infection. J Infect Dis 164(3):499–506
36. Madaras-Kelly KJ, Ostergaard BE, Hovde LB, Rotschafer JC (1996) Twenty-four-hour area under the concentration-time curve/MIC ratio as a generic predictor of fluoroquinolone antimicrobial effect by using three strains of *Pseudomonas aeruginosa* and an in vitro pharmacodynamic model. Antimicrob Agents Chemother 40(3):627–632
37. Odenholt I, Cars O (2006) Pharmacodynamics of moxifloxacin and levofloxacin against *Streptococcus pneumoniae*, *Staphylococcus aureus*, *Klebsiella pneumoniae* and *Escherichia coli*: simulation of human plasma concentrations after intravenous dosage in an in vitro kinetic model. J Antimicrob Chemother 58(5):960–965
38. Singh R, Ledesma KR, Chang KT, Hou JG, Prince RA, Tam VH (2009) Pharmacodynamics of moxifloxacin against a high inoculum of *Escherichia coli* in an in vitro infection model. J Antimicrob Chemother 64(3):556–562
39. Firsov AA, Vostrov SN, Shevchenko AA, Cornaglia G (1997) Parameters of bacterial killing and regrowth kinetics and antimicrobial effect examined in terms of area under the concentration-time curve relationships: action of ciprofloxacin against *Escherichia coli* in an

in vitro dynamic model. Antimicrob Agents Chemother 41(6):1281–1287

40. Firsov AA, Lubenko IY, Vostrov SN, Kononenko OV, Zinner SH, Portnoy YA (2000) Comparative pharmacodynamics of moxifloxacin and levofloxacin in an in vitro dynamic model: prediction of the equivalent AUC/MIC breakpoints and equiefficient doses. J Antimicrob Chemother 46(5):725–732
41. Firsov AA, Zinner SH (2001) Use of modeling techniques to aid in antibiotic selection. Curr Infect Dis Rep 3(1):35–43
42. Firsov AA, Zinner SH, Vostrov SN, Portnoy YA, Lubenko IY (2002) AUC/MIC relationships to different endpoints of the antimicrobial effect: multiple-dose in vitro simulations with moxifloxacin and levofloxacin. J Antimicrob Chemother 50(4):533–539
43. Firsov AA, Vasilov RG, Vostrov SN, Kononenko OV, Lubenko IY, Zinner SH (1999) Prediction of the antimicrobial effects of trovafloxacin and ciprofloxacin on staphylococci using an in-vitro dynamic model. J Antimicrob Chemother 43(4):483–490
44. Firsov AA, Zinner SH, Lubenko IY, Portnoy YA, Vostrov SN (2002) Simulated in vitro quinolone pharmacodynamics at clinically achievable AUC/MIC ratios: advantage of I E over other integral parameters. Chemotherapy 48(6):275–279
45. Schentag JJ, Meagher AK, Forrest A (2003) Fluoroquinolone AUIC break points and the link to bacterial killing rates. Part 1: in vitro and animal models. Ann Pharmacother 37(9):1287–1298
46. Olofsson SK, Marcusson LL, Stromback A, Hughes D, Cars O (2007) Dose-related selection of fluoroquinolone-resistant *Escherichia coli*. J Antimicrob Chemother 60(4):795–801
47. Leggett JE, Ebert S, Fantin B, Craig WA (1990) Comparative dose-effect relations at several dosing intervals for beta-lactam, aminoglycoside and quinolone antibiotics against gram-negative bacilli in murine thigh-infection and pneumonitis models. Scand J Infect Dis Suppl 74:179–184
48. Drusano GL, Johnson DE, Rosen M, Standiford HC (1993) Pharmacodynamics of a fluoroquinolone antimicrobial agent in a neutropenic rat model of pseudomonas sepsis. Antimicrob Agents Chemother 37(3):483–490
49. Craig WA (1998) Pharmacokinetic/pharmacodynamic parameters: rationale for antibacterial dosing of mice and men. Clin Infect Dis 26(1):1–10, quiz 11–12
50. Louie A, Fregeau C, Liu W, Kulawy R, Drusano GL (2009) Pharmacodynamics of levofloxacin in a murine pneumonia model of *Pseudomonas aeruginosa* infection: determination of epithelial lining fluid targets. Antimicrob Agents Chemother 53(8):3325–3330
51. Peloquin CA, Cumbo TJ, Nix DE, Sands MF, Schentag JJ (1989) Evaluation of intravenous ciprofloxacin in patients with nosocomial lower respiratory tract infections. Impact of plasma concentrations, organism, minimum inhibitory concentration, and clinical condition on bacterial eradication. Arch Intern Med 149(10):2269–2273
52. Thomas JK, Forrest A, Bhavnani SM, Hyatt JM, Cheng A, Ballow CH et al (1998) Pharmacodynamic evaluation of factors associated with the development of bacterial resistance in acutely ill patients during therapy. Antimicrob Agents Chemother 42(3):521–527
53. Zelenitsky SA, Ariano RE (2010) Support for higher ciprofloxacin AUC_{24}/MIC targets in treating enterobacteriaceae bloodstream infection. J Antimicrob Chemother 65(8):1725–1732
54. Zelenitsky S, Ariano R, Harding G, Forrest A (2005) Evaluating ciprofloxacin dosing for *Pseudomonas aeruginosa* infection by using clinical outcome-based Monte Carlo simulations. Antimicrob Agents Chemother 49(10):4009–4014
55. Conil JM, Georges B, de Lussy A, Khachman D, Seguin T, Ruiz S et al (2008) Ciprofloxacin use in critically ill patients: pharmacokinetic and pharmacodynamic approaches. Int J Antimicrob Agents 32(6):505–510
56. Saengsuwan P, Jaruratanasirikul S, Jullangkoon M, Aeinlang N (2010) Comparative study of pharmacokinetics/ pharmacodynamics of ciprofloxacin between 400 mg intravenously every 8 h and 400 mg intravenously every 12 h in patients with gram negative bacilli bacteremia. J Med Assoc Thai 93(7):784–788
57. Haeseker M, Stolk L, Nieman F, Hoebe C, Neef C, Bruggeman C et al (2013) The ciprofloxacin target AUC: MIC ratio is not reached in hospitalized patients with the recommended dosing regimens. Br J Clin Pharmacol 75(1):180–185
58. Ambrose PG, Grasela DM, Grasela TH, Passarell J, Mayer HB, Pierce PF (2001) Pharmacodynamics of fluoroquinolones against *Streptococcus pneumoniae* in patients with community-acquired respiratory tract infections. Antimicrob Agents Chemother 45(10): 2793–2797

59. Lacy MK, Lu W, Xu X, Tessier PR, Nicolau DP, Quintiliani R et al (1999) Pharmacodynamic comparisons of levofloxacin, ciprofloxacin, and ampicillin against *Streptococcus pneumoniae* in an in vitro model of infection. Antimicrob Agents Chemother 43(3):672–677
60. Bedos JP, Azoulay-Dupuis E, Moine P, Muffat-Joly M, Veber B, Pocidalo JJ et al (1998) Pharmacodynamic activities of ciprofloxacin and sparfloxacin in a murine pneumococcal pneumonia model: relevance for drug efficacy. J Pharmacol Exp Ther 286(1):29–35
61. Lister PD, Sanders CC (1999) Pharmacodynamics of levofloxacin and ciprofloxacin against *Streptococcus pneumoniae*. J Antimicrob Chemother 43(1):79–86
62. MacGowan AP, Rogers CA, Holt HA, Bowker KE (2003) Activities of moxifloxacin against, and emergence of resistance in, *Streptococcus pneumoniae* and *Pseudomonas aeruginosa* in an in vitro pharmacokinetic model. Antimicrob Agents Chemother 47(3):1088–1095
63. Dalhoff A (2012) Global fluoroquinolone resistance epidemiology and implications for clinical use. Interdiscip Perspect Infect Dis 2012:976273
64. Lim S, Bast D, McGeer A, de Azavedo J, Low DE (2003) Antimicrobial susceptibility breakpoints and first-step parc mutations in *Streptococcus pneumoniae*: redefining fluoroquinolone resistance. Emerg Infect Dis 9(7):833–837
65. Blondeau JM, Zhao X, Hansen G, Drlica K (2001) Mutant prevention concentrations of fluoroquinolones for clinical isolates of *Streptococcus pneumoniae*. Antimicrob Agents Chemother 45(2):433–438
66. Licata L, Smith CE, Goldschmidt RM, Barrett JF, Frosco M (1997) Comparison of the post-antibiotic and postantibiotic sub-MIC effects of levofloxacin and ciprofloxacin on *Staphylococcus aureus* and *Streptococcus pneumoniae*. Antimicrob Agents Chemother 41(5):950–955
67. Odenholt-Tornqvist I, Lowdin E, Cars O (1992) Postantibiotic sub-MIC effects of vancomycin, roxithromycin, sparfloxacin, and amikacin. Antimicrob Agents Chemother 36(9):1852–1858
68. Allen GP, Kaatz GW, Rybak MJ (2003) Activities of mutant prevention concentration-targeted moxifloxacin and levofloxacin against *Streptococcus pneumoniae* in an in vitro pharmacodynamic model. Antimicrob Agents Chemother 47(8):2606–2614
69. Florea NR, Tessier PR, Zhang C, Nightingale CH, Nicolau DP (2004) Pharmacodynamics of moxifloxacin and levofloxacin at simulated epithelial lining fluid drug concentrations against *Streptococcus pneumoniae*. Antimicrob Agents Chemother 48(4):1215–1221
70. Deryke CA, Du X, Nicolau DP (2006) Evaluation of bacterial kill when modelling the bronchopulmonary pharmacokinetic profile of moxifloxacin and levofloxacin against parc-containing isolates of *Streptococcus pneumoniae*. J Antimicrob Chemother 58(3):601–609
71. Jones RN, Rubino CM, Bhavnani SM, Ambrose PG (2003) Worldwide antimicrobial susceptibility patterns and pharmacodynamic comparisons of gatifloxacin and levofloxacin against *Streptococcus pneumoniae*: report from the antimicrobial resistance rate epidemiology study team. Antimicrob Agents Chemother 47(1):292–296
72. Frei CR, Burgess DS (2005) Pharmacodynamic analysis of ceftriaxone, gatifloxacin, and levofloxacin against *Streptococcus pneumoniae* with the use of Monte Carlo simulation. Pharmacotherapy 25(9):1161–1167
73. Noreddin AM, Reese AA, Ostroski M, Hoban DJ, Zhanel GG (2007) Comparative pharmacodynamics of garenoxacin, gemifloxacin, and moxifloxacin in community-acquired pneumonia caused by *Streptococcus pneumoniae*: a Monte Carlo simulation analysis. Clin Ther 29(12):2685–2689
74. Liang B, Bai N, Cai Y, Wang R, Drlica K, Zhao X (2011) Mutant prevention concentration-based pharmacokinetic/pharmacodynamic indices as dosing targets for suppressing the enrichment of levofloxacin-resistant subpopulations of *Staphylococcus aureus*. Antimicrob Agents Chemother 55(5):2409–2412
75. Lister PD (2001) Pharmacodynamics of moxifloxacin and levofloxacin against *Staphylococcus aureus* and *Staphylococcus epidermidis* in an in vitro pharmacodynamic model. Clin Infect Dis 32(Suppl 1):S33–S38
76. Lewin CS, Morrissey I, Smith JT (1991) The mode of action of quinolones: the paradox in activity of low and high concentrations and activity in the anaerobic environment. Eur J Clin Microbiol Infect Dis 10(4):240–248
77. Wright DH, Gunderson BW, Hovde LB, Ross GH, Ibrahim KH, Rotschafer JC (2002) Comparative pharmacodynamics of three newer fluoroquinolones versus six strains of staphylococci in an in vitro model under aerobic and anaerobic conditions. Antimicrob Agents Chemother 46(5):1561–1563
78. Zabinski RA, Walker KJ, Larsson AJ, Moody JA, Kaatz GW, Rotschafer JC (1995) Effect of aerobic and anaerobic environments on antistaphylococcal activities of five fluoroqui-

nolones. Antimicrob Agents Chemother 39(2):507–512

79. Stein GE, Goldstein EJ (2006) Fluoroquinolones and anaerobes. Clin Infect Dis 42(11):1598–1607
80. Bayer HealthCare Pharmaceuticals (2008) Avelox prescribing information. Bayer HealthCare Pharmaceuticals, Wayne. NJ
81. Pfizer Corporation (2000) Trovan prescribing information. Pfizer Corporation, New York, NY
82. Peterson ML, Hovde LB, Wright DH, Brown GH, Hoang AD, Rotschafer JC (2002) Pharmacodynamics of trovafloxacin and levofloxacin against *Bacteroides fragilis* in an in vitro pharmacodynamic model. Antimicrob Agents Chemother 46(1):203–210
83. Peterson ML, Hovde LB, Wright DH, Hoang AD, Raddatz JK, Boysen PJ et al (1999) Fluoroquinolone resistance in *Bacteroides fragilis* following sparfloxacin exposure. Antimicrob Agents Chemother 43(9):2251–2255
84. Peterson ML, Rotschafer JC, Piddock LJ (2003) Plasmid-mediated complementation of *gyr*A and *gyr*B in fluoroquinolone-resistant *Bacteroides fragilis*. J Antimicrob Chemother 52(3):481–484
85. Ricci V, Peterson ML, Rotschafer JC, Wexler H, Piddock LJ (2004) Role of topoisomerase mutations and efflux in fluoroquinolone resistance of *Bacteroides fragilis* clinical isolates and laboratory mutants. Antimicrob Agents Chemother 48(4):1344–1346
86. Edlund C, Nord CE (1988) A review on the impact of 4-quinolones on the normal oropharyngeal and intestinal human microflora. Infection 16(1):8–12
87. Golan Y, McDermott LA, Jacobus NV, Goldstein EJ, Finegold S, Harrell LJ et al (2003) Emergence of fluoroquinolone resistance among *Bacteroides* species. J Antimicrob Chemother 52(2):208–213
88. Betriu C, Rodriguez-Avial I, Gomez M, Culebras E, Picazo JJ (2005) Changing patterns of fluoroquinolone resistance among *Bacteroides fragilis* group organisms over a 6-year period (1997-2002). Diagn Microbiol Infect Dis 53(3):221–223

Chapter 9

Aminoglycoside Pharmacodynamics

Dana R. Bowers, Amy N. Schilling, and Vincent H. Tam

Abstract

Aminoglycosides are antimicrobial agents traditionally derived from natural sources. They exhibit potent in vitro bactericidal activity against a broad spectrum of pathogens. Over the years, the clinical use of the aminoglycosides has changed considerably. With a narrow therapeutic index, there is a need for individualized therapy based on patient specific pharmacokinetics and pathogen susceptibility, especially if prolonged therapy is indicated. With an improved understanding of resistance mechanisms, synthetic structural analogs are under clinical development. These agents could have a unique role in the management of infections due to multidrug-resistant bacteria.

Key words Aminoglycosides, Antimicrobial resistance, Concentration-dependent activity, Tobramycin, Gentamicin, Amikacin

1 A Brief History

Aminoglycosides have been available for clinical use since the 1960s. Early agents in the family are natural products derived from various soil microorganisms. Subsequently, synthetic derivatives with improved susceptibility profiles were obtained by chemical modification of natural agents. The development of resistance was expected to decrease as structural alteration mediated by bacterial enzymes was reduced.

Aminoglycosides are highly polar compounds with excellent water solubility; the pharmacokinetics could be reasonably predicted by their physicochemical properties. They exhibit concentration-dependent bactericidal activity against gram-negative bacteria and a significant post-antibiotic effect has been reported. Despite impressive in vitro activity, toxicity remains a concern for many clinicians and is a major hindrance to widespread use of these agents.

In the 1990s, we entered a new paradigm of anti-infective chemotherapy. Dosing regimen design based on concepts integrating pharmacokinetics and pharmacodynamics of antimicrobial agents appeared in the literature, which led to a more individualized approach to bedside dosing. The optimization of benefit-to-risk

John C. Rotschafer et al. (eds.), *Antibiotic Pharmacodynamics*, Methods in Pharmacology and Toxicology,
DOI 10.1007/978-1-4939-3323-5_9,

ratio of antimicrobial therapy was eventually widely accepted and applied clinically.

Over the years, the use of aminoglycosides as monotherapy has become less popular; they are increasingly used in combination with other agents (e.g., beta-lactams or fluoroquinolones) to broaden the spectrum of empiric coverage and only for a short duration of time. New agent(s) in clinical development may have a better safety profile and could have a unique role in the management of infections due to multidrug-resistant bacteria. This chapter provides an overview of the aminoglycosides in terms of chemical structures, pharmacokinetics, mechanism of action, resistance mechanisms, optimal dosing, and clinical use for different infections.

2 Chemical Structure

The aminoglycosides are a class of antibiotics whose main components include two or more aminosugar molecules linked via glycosidic bonds to an aminocyclitol ring (streptidine or deoxystretamine) [1] (Fig. 1). The aminoglycosides can be derived naturally (from

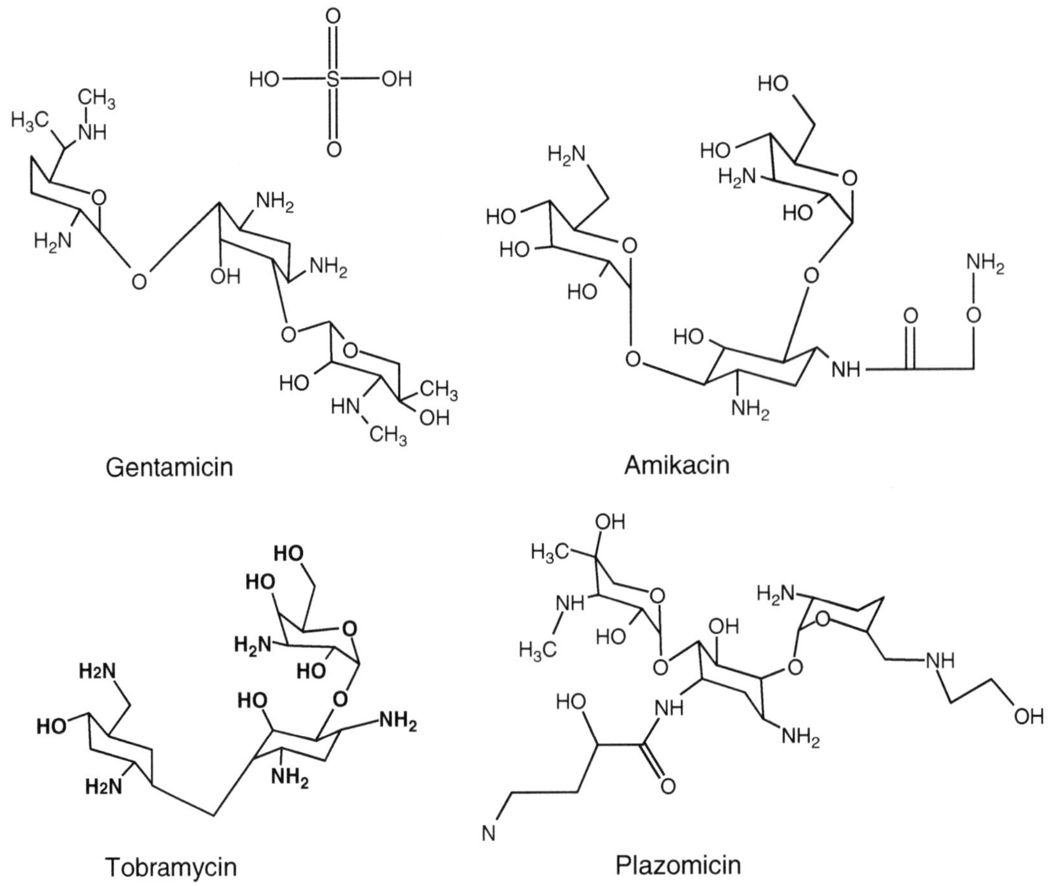

Fig. 1 Chemical structure of selected aminoglycosides

Table 1
Aminoglycoside characteristics

Aminoglycoside	Chemical formula/ structure	MW	Isolated from	Notes
Amikacin	C22H43N5O13	585.6	Derivative of kanamycin	Presence of AHB side chain helps amikacin retain activity against gentamicin-and tobramycin-resistant GNB
Gentamicin	C1 C21H43N5O7 C1a C19H39N5O7 C2C20H41N5O7	C1 477 C1a 449 C2 463	*Micromonospora purpurea*	
Isepamicin	C22H43N5O12	667.7	Semisynthetic derivative of gentamicin	
Kanamycin	C18H36N4O11	484.5	*Streptomyces kanamyceticus*	Reserved for MDR TB
Neomycin B	C23H46N6O13	614	*Streptomyces fradiae*	Very toxic, not used systemically
Netilmicin	C21H37N5O7	475.6	Semisynthetic derivative of sisomicin	Retains some activity against gentamicin-resistant strains
Plazomicin	C25H48N6O10	592	Dervivative of sisomicin	Currently under clinical investigation
Paromomycin	C23H47N5o18S	713.7		Used for parasitic infection
Sisomicin	C19H37N5O7	447.5	*Micromonospora inyoesis*	More active than gentamicin b but not as active as tobramycin for PA. Available in Europe
Streptomycin	C42H84N14O36S3	1457.4	*Streptomycin griseus*	Reserved for resistant tuberculosis or MAC
Tobramycin	C18H37N5O9	467.5	*Streptomyces tenebrarius*	Best intrinsic activity against PA

AHB s-4 amino 2 hydroxybutyryl, *GNB* gram-negative bacilli, *MDR-TB* multidrug-resistant tuberculosis, *MAC* mycobacteria avium complex, *PA Pseudomonas aeruginosa*

Streptomyces spp. or *Micromonospora* spp.) or synthetically. Almost all the aminoglycosides are used clinically as their sulfate salts. In clinical practice, the most frequently used aminoglycosides are gentamicin, tobramycin, amikacin, and occasionally streptomycin. The other aminoglycosides are mentioned for completeness (Table 1); however, the remainder of the chapter focuses on aminoglycosides that are used most commonly within the USA.

3 Pharmacokinetics

The pharmacokinetics of the aminoglycosides are generally predictable based on their physicochemical properties. As highly polar compounds, minimal oral bioavailability is expected of the aminoglycosides. Consequently, the oral route of administration is not preferred for the treatment of systemic infections. However, there may be a unique role for oral administration of "non-absorbable antibiotics" in certain clinical situations such as in selective digestive tract decontamination preoperatively, in critically ill patients, and for patients with hepatic encephalopathy or intestinal parasites [2–5].

Binding of aminoglycosides to serum proteins are low [6]. Despite low protein binding, the drugs primarily remain in extracellular space in view of their polar nature (poor diffusion across cell membrane). Volume of distribution resembles that of the extracellular fluid compartment (approximately 25–35 % of body weight). Generally speaking, the volume of distribution is proportional to body weight up to a certain threshold, where further increase in body weight is more likely contributed by adipose tissues. It can also be expected to be larger in patients who are fluid overloaded, ascitic or pregnant. Consequently, one can expect the aminoglycosides to have low volume of distribution, poor penetration into epithelial lining fluid in the lungs [7, 8] and oxygen-poor environments (e.g., abscesses). Inhaled (aerosolized) therapy may be necessary to achieve therapeutic concentrations, and to reduce/eradicate bacterial colonization in cystic fibrosis patients. The aminoglycosides are also known to be preferentially accumulated in the renal cortex and inner ear (perilymph and endolymph). The accumulation of aminoglycosides into the renal cortex is mediated by transporters [9]. Drug accumulation and nephrotoxicity could be minimized by using an extended dosing interval [10, 11]. The uptake of drug by the inner ear tissues of rats was also found to be dose dependent, saturable and associated with an extended residence, which could have implications to ototoxicity especially after prolonged exposure [12, 13].

Aminoglycosides are not metabolized; they are primarily excreted unchanged in the urine. Total body clearance is correlated to glomerular filtration rate. Relatively short elimination half-lives (2–3 h) are expected to be in patients with normal renal function, which could be significantly prolonged in renal insufficiency. Although these are typically considered standard pharmacokinetic parameters for the aminoglycosides, these parameters have been shown to exhibit wide intra- and inter-patient variability [14, 15]. Adjustment in dosing regimen is recommended in patients with renal impairment and premature infants to prevent excessive drug accumulation. As the major route of elimination, aminoglycosides are highly concentrated in the urine, which could be used to treat localized cystitis due to pathogens with low to intermediate level resistance.

In view of their physicochemical properties, aminoglycosides are effectively removed by conventional/high flux hemodialysis and various forms of continuous renal replacement therapy [16, 17]. Consequently, supplemental doses are commonly given post-dialysis to patients with acute kidney injury or end-stage renal diseases to maintain an adequate systemic drug exposure. However, based on our understanding of the pharmacokinetics and pharmacodynamics of the aminoglycosides, novel pre-dialysis dosing strategies have been proposed [18]. The rationale is to expose the patient to a high drug concentration for a brief period of time and take advantage of the concentration-dependent bactericidal activity, then quickly remove a significant proportion of the dose with dialysis. While the theoretical benefits appear to be sound and supported by computer simulations [19], more favorable outcomes have not been conclusively demonstrated in a clinical study.

4 Mechanism of Action

The use of these agents has changed significantly since their initial introduction due to increased knowledge from basic and clinical research. The primary mechanism of action of aminoglycosides occurs via the irreversible binding of ribosomes resulting in inhibition of protein synthesis [20, 21]. Aminoglycosides are taken up into cells across the outer membrane of gram-negative bacteria by disruption of magnesium bridges between adjacent lipopolysaccharide molecules. The energy-dependent phase I (EDP-I), which is dependent on electron transport, allows the transport of aminoglycosides across the cytoplasmic membrane. This rate-limiting step is inhibited by divalent cations, hyperosmolarity, low pH, and anaerobic metabolism. The binding of the 30S subunit of ribosomes takes place in the cytosol through the energy-dependent phase II (EDP-II), which is thought to be related to the bactericidal activity of aminoglycosides [20, 22, 23]. The bactericidal aminoglycosides are thought to cause amino acid substitutions during protein synthesis resulting in inaccurate reading of the genetic code. The actual lethal event is unknown but many theories exist [23].

4.1 Concentration-Dependent Killing

Aminoglycosides are rapidly bactericidal and exhibit concentration-dependent killing against gram-negative organisms, in which more rapid killing is observed as drug concentrations increase [24, 25]. There is a small window between therapeutic and toxic levels for the aminoglycosides. Studies show serum levels above ten times the MIC for the isolated gram-negative organisms is more effective than lower peak to MIC ratios [26, 27]. Most drug concentrations achieved in the infected tissues are lower than those attained in the serum with the exception of bacteremia and in infections of the urinary tract [26]. It is important to take this into consideration when monitoring aminoglycoside levels for the treatment of infections.

While aminoglycosides are known to exhibit concentration-dependent killing and post antibiotic effect against gram-negative pathogens, the limited data available suggests that this is not the case in gram-positive infections and that higher doses of aminoglycosides may not improve bacterial kill rates [28, 29]. Aminoglycoside activity against gram-positive organisms, particularly *Enterococcus* sp., is related to its synergistic activity in the presence of cell-wall active agents. The cell-wall active agent, such as beta-lactams, is thought to increase the uptake of the aminoglycoside in the treatment of severe, complicated infections such as endocarditis [30].

4.2 Post Antibiotic Effect

The post antibiotic effect (PAE) is a period of time in which no bacterial growth is observed following the complete removal of an antimicrobial agent. The ribosomal binding of aminoglycosides is thought to contribute to the PAE of these agents as it may be attributed to the time required for synthesis of new ribosomes [21]. This suppression can occur even after a limited exposure to an antimicrobial agent [31]. The presence of PAE can be affected by the antimicrobial agent, organism, and environmental conditions. The aminoglycosides exhibit a long PAE against gram-negative organisms. Longer PAE can be observed in vivo than in vitro due to environmental conditions including the presence of neutrophils, drug concentration, area under the concentration-time curve, and duration of exposure [31, 32]. The PAE of aminoglycosides allows for longer dosing intervals because bacterial growth is inhibited even when serum and tissue drug concentrations fall below the minimum inhibitory concentration (MIC) [31]. The PAE is reduced in gram-negative bacilli in the setting of a larger inoculum [21]. Studies had shown that efficacy of aminoglycosides was associated with the total amount of drug given rather than how frequently it was administered [31].

4.3 Aminoglycoside in Combination with Cell Wall Active Agents

Aminoglycosides are synergistic in combination with cell wall active agents against gram-negative and gram-positive bacteria. Using agents with different mechanisms of action results in enhanced bacterial killing. The synergistic combination of beta-lactams and aminoglycosides is thought to be related to the cell-wall disturbance caused by beta-lactams, which facilitates the entry of aminoglycosides into the periplasmic space [23, 33]. Improved clinical outcomes were demonstrated when aminoglycosides were used with antipseudomonal penicillins, especially in the management of immunocompromised hosts [34–36]. In cases of enterococcal endocarditis, concurrent use of cell wall active agents allow for increased uptake of aminoglycosides.

5 Resistance Mechanisms

As with many other antimicrobials, resistance to aminoglycosides has emerged since their introduction. Common mechanisms of resistance for aminoglycosides include: (1) aminoglycoside modifying enzymes, (2) decreased uptake or accumulation of the drug in bacteria, and (3) aminoglycoside ribosomal target modification [20, 37, 38]. A majority of these resistance mechanisms are encoded on bacterial plasmids and transposons, resulting in the opportunity for rapid spread of resistance between bacteria [37]. Some resistance mechanisms can also be chromosomally encoded and constitutively expressed, as those found in *Providencia* and *Serratia* species [33].

The most common mechanism of aminoglycoside resistance is associated with aminoglycoside modifying enzymes [39]. A larger number of aminoglycoside modifying enzymes are found in aminoglycoside producing bacteria such as *Streptomyces* spp. and *Micromonospora* spp.; there is also evidence that the genetic elements can be transferred between gram-positive and gram-negative bacteria allowing for the rapid spread of these enzymes [37]. A variety of phenotypes have been determined, with several distinct proteins resulting in similar aminoglycoside modifying activity [20]. These enzymes modify aminoglycosides by N-acetylation, O-adenylation, or O-phosphorylation which, when they are present concurrently, can result in a broad spectrum of aminoglycoside resistance [39, 40].

In the presence of aminoglycoside modifying enzymes, the energy dependent interactions between an aminoglycoside and ribosomes will not occur, resulting in an inability to inhibit protein synthesis [37]. This covalent modification of amino or hydroxyl functions results in high-level aminoglycoside resistance. Subsequent to initial studies where aminoglycoside resistance was associated with a single modifying enzyme, complex phenotypes and many genotypes have emerged, some related to local patterns of aminoglycoside use [20, 41]. These factors have led to more complicated decisions regarding the choice of empiric aminoglycoside therapy, including the use of local epidemiological data and institution-specific antibiograms.

While the mechanism for the decreased uptake of aminoglycosides by gram-negative bacilli is not fully understood, it is likely due to membrane impermeability [20]. Anaerobic bacteria are intrinsically resistant to aminoglycosides. The uptake of aminoglycosides by bacteria is mediated by an oxygen-dependent electron transport system. The transport system required for the aminoglycosides uptake is absent in anaerobic bacteria, and therefore the aminoglycosides do not reach their ribosomal target [42]. Bacteria exposed to aminoglycosides can potentially have an alteration in gene regulation of the anaerobic respiratory pathway and membrane protein changes. Active efflux of certain aminoglycosides has also been described [43].

Finally, the modification of the aminoglycoside target, the bacterial ribosomal RNA and proteins including the 16S ribosomal subunit, by mutation or nucleotide methylation has been described [23, 39]. Target modification is a less common mechanism of aminoglycoside resistance, primarily reported in *Mycobacterium* [43].

While aminoglycosides are commonly affected by aminoglycoside modifying enzymes and alterations in membrane permeability, *Pseudomonas aeruginosa* displays intrinsic aminoglycoside resistance associated with proteolysis [44–46]. *P. aeruginosa* also displays adaptive resistance in which a decreased susceptibility is exhibited following frequent exposure to an antimicrobial agent. Combinations of these resistance mechanisms can result in an increase in the spectrum of aminoglycoside resistance. As aminoglycoside usage has increased over time, these resistance mechanism combinations do not seem to correlate with the specific aminoglycoside usage but rather a more general increased overall use of these agents [47].

With the increasing resistance to broad-spectrum antibiotics, including beta-lactams and fluoroquinolones, new sisomycin analogs have been developed. These drug candidates could potentially be used to treat infections due to organisms that harbor aminoglycoside resistance mechanisms, including the three most common aminoglycoside-modifying enzymes. Plazomicin (ACHN-490) is one of these agents being developed clinically due to its promising in vitro susceptibility results [40]. Plazomicin exhibits in vitro activity against resistant gram-negative and gram-positive bacteria [48, 49]. The ability to evade common resistance mechanisms is related to its structure. The basic sisomicin structure lacks hydroxyl groups, thus these analogs are poor substrate for certain aminoglycoside modifying enzymes. Specific to the plazomicin structure, the addition at the $N-1$ position of a hydroxyl-aminobutyric acid substituent and a hydroxyethyl substituent addition block many aminoglycoside modifying enzymes without compromising the activity of the drug. These structure modifications allow for activity against amikacin- and gentamicin-resistant isolates. Plazomicin has been shown to retain activity against resistant clinical isolates, including *K. pneumoniae*, *E. coli* and *Enterobacter* spp. [50]. However, plazomicin remains susceptible to resistance mediated by 16S rRNA methylases [49].

6 Optimizing the Use of Aminoglycosides

6.1 Dosing Regimens

6.1.1 Traditional Dosing

Aminoglycoside dosing conventionally is given 3–6 mg/kg/day divided every 8 h for gentamicin and tobramycin. Amikacin is usually administered 15 mg/kg daily divided every 8 or 12 h. Patients with renal dysfunction require further adjustments based on the degree of renal impairment in addition to their severity of infection. Individual dosing regimens are often used utilized to account for patient variability. Since alternative dosing strategies have not been studied extensively in all populations and certain populations such as patients with extensive burns or gram-positive infections were excluded from extended interval daily aminoglycoside nomograms [51–53], traditional dosing is still recommended for these patients.

6.1.2 Peak Concentration to Minimum Inhibitory Concentration Ratio (Cmax/MIC)

The aminoglycosides demonstrate concentration-dependent killing; their killing effect is a function of their peak concentration (Cmax). Optimal bacterial killing for the aminoglycosides occurs when the Cmax is approximately ten times greater than the minimum inhibitory concentration (MIC) of the pathogen [54–57]. In a study by Moore et al., efficacy in patients with gram-negative bacterial infections was correlated to the Cmax/MIC ratio. For example, when the gentamicin Cmax/MIC was 2, the clinical efficacy reported was approximately 50 %. However, when the Cmax/MIC was 10, the observed efficacy increased to around 90 % [27]. It is important to note that the majority of the efficacy results were from patients with urinary tract infections, where favorable outcomes could generally be expected. However, the killing profile of the aminoglycosides could be different depending on the type of bacteria. It has been observed when the concentration of gentamicin is twice the MIC or greater, the extent of bacterial killing of *S. aureus* is not increased [29]. In this situation, gentamicin does not appear to have concentration-dependent but rather time-dependent bacterial killing. Therefore, some experts recommend administering aminoglycosides as a single daily dose for gram-negative infections and as multiple daily doses for gram-positive infections [58].

6.1.3 Extended Interval Aminoglycoside Dosing (EIAD)

The rationale behind using EIAD of aminoglycoside (administering one large dose daily) is to maximize concentration-dependent bacterial killing and prolonging its post-antibiotic effect, while theoretically minimizing dose-dependent toxicity. Gentamicin and tobramycin are typically administered as 5–7 mg/kg and amikacin is dosed at 15–20 mg/kg once daily. Various nomograms have been developed and used clinically [51, 53, 54, 59]. Caution is recommended with any nomogram as they almost always assume that the patients' volume of distribution is constant throughout treatment and may not be appropriate for all patients. Most patients studied were treated for intra-abdominal, genitourinary, pulmonary, and skin or soft tissue infections and the patients had a non-significant change in volume of distribution [51–53]. Experience in patients with changing volume of distribution (e.g., pregnant, pediatric, or burn patients), spinal cord injury or gram-positive infections remains limited.

6.1.4 Comparison of EIAD vs. Traditional Dosing Strategies

There have been many studies comparing different dosing strategies of aminoglycosides, including several meta-analyses [60–64]. One meta-analysis showed no difference in bacteriologic cure, mortality, ototoxicity, or nephrotoxicity between EIAD and traditional dosing [61]. An explanation for the results is that many of the traditionally dosed patients could have achieved an optimal peak/MIC ratio, i.e., if the peak was 6 mg/mL and the MIC was 0.5 mg/mL, this would result in a ratio of 12. Most of the meta-analyses have shown comparable ototoxicity or a decreased trend of ototoxicity with EIAD. Another meta-analysis by Barza et al. demonstrated lower nephrotoxicity with EIAD. Another study examining nephrotoxicity suggested that nephrotoxicity developed later in a course of therapy with the EIAD compared with traditional dosing, but with similar incidence for prolonged treatment courses [65].

6.2 Toxicity

6.2.1 Nephrotoxicity

Aminoglycosides concentrate preferentially within renal cortical cells. The uptake of aminoglycosides is nonlinear and saturable [66]. Phosphatidylinositol phospholipase A1 and A2 are inhibited by aminoglycosides causing lamellar body formation [67]. This causes both functional and structural damage within the proximal tubules. High concentration of aminoglycosides results in acute tubular necrosis [68], which has been reported in 5–15 % of patients after aminoglycoside therapy [69].

Nephrotoxicity has been well described with aminoglycosides and usually manifests as an increase in serum creatinine, mild proteinuria, hypophosphatemia, hypokalemia and hypocalcemia [70]. Rougier et al. sought to characterize the predictors for nephrotoxicity as a single toxicity effect model [71]. The model demonstrated with more frequently administered doses, the onset of nephrotoxicity was rapid, the extent pronounced, and the duration was prolonged. Interestingly, the authors also found a temporal association with nephrotoxicity where administration during periods of activity was associated with decreased nephrotoxicity.

Patient characteristics that have been associated with increased risk for nephrotoxicity are prolonged high trough levels >2 mg/L, duration of treatment greater than 2 weeks, underlying renal dysfunction, elderly, concomitant use of other nephrotoxic agents such as loop diuretics and vancomycin [72]. Aminoglycoside-associated nephrotoxicity is typically reversible after adequate hydration and discontinuation of therapy.

6.2.2 Ototoxicity

Treatment with aminoglycosides can lead to permanent hearing loss that is often bilateral. Hair cells and cochlear neurons are susceptible to aminoglycoside-induced oxidative damage due to the formation of reactive oxygen species [73]. High frequency hearing loss usually manifests before lower frequency hearing loss and can occur as soon as 4 h post treatment [74]. Vestibular dysfunction such as disequilibrium, nausea, vertigo and nystagmus can occur along with hearing loss. However, unlike hearing loss, vestibular dysfunction is often reversible [75].

The likelihood of aminoglycoside ototoxicity is dependent on various factors such as route of administration, genetic susceptibility, and comorbid conditions. Administration through the tympanic membrane for the treatment of Meniere's disease is less ototoxic compared with systemic administration [76, 77]. There have been a few studies suggesting a genetic predisposition to aminoglycoside ototoxicity. The most common genetic component is a mitrochondrial mutation, A1555G, found on the 12S ribosomal RNA gene. In China, it was estimated that this mutation accounts for 33–59 % of all aminoglycoside ototoxicity [78]. Another report from South Africa described a family who received streptomycin and was subsequently deafened. Molecular investigations revealed the same mitochondrial mutation [79]. While genetic testing before treatment with aminoglycosides may identify patients at risk for ototoxicity, it is currently not well established for routine clinical use.

6.2.3 Neuromuscular

Although rare, the aminoglycosides can cause neuromuscular toxicity or blockade. Presentation can include respiratory failure or muscle weakness. The mechanism of kanamycin induced neuromuscular toxicity is believed to involve the interference of calcium and acetylcholine release presynaptically [80]. Additionally, there have been reports of gentamicin exacerbating or unmasking myasthenia gravis [81], as well as prolonging the effect of *Clostridium botulism* toxin [82, 83]. Patients should be screened for coadministration of other neuromuscular blockers prior to aminoglycoside administration; special attention is also warranted for patients who receive aminoglycosides perioperatively.

6.2.4 Others

Hypersensitivity reactions are uncommon, but they can occur with both systemically and topically administered aminoglycosides [84]. Hematological side effects such as leukopenia and agranulocytosis are rare but have been reported [85].

6.3 Therapeutic Drug Monitoring

Therapeutic drug monitoring (TDM) is often used to maximize the benefit to risk ratio of antimicrobial therapy. Utilizing TDM for an individual patient is a way to personalize therapy, aiming to increase the probability of achieving therapeutic success and minimizing the risk for toxicity [54, 86].

6.3.1 Drug Serum Concentrations

The aminoglycosides have a narrow therapeutic range and TDM of aminoglycosides is often performed clinically. When traditional dosing is used, typically both pre-infusion and post-infusion concentrations are measured. Post-infusion levels are usually drawn 15–30 min after the end of the infusion and pre-infusion levels are drawn 15–30 min prior to the next scheduled administration time under steady-state conditions. Several studies have suggested that patient mortality is reduced if post-infusion concentrations are above 5–7 mg/L within the first few days of treatment [27, 87, 88]. For efficacy, studies recommend serum post-infusion concentrations of 6–10 mg/L for gentamicin and tobramycin, and 20–40 mg/L for amikacin. For example, in patients with pneumonia caused by gram-negative pathogens, Moore et al. found post-infusion levels >7 mg/L (gentamicin or tobramycin) or >28 mg/L (amikacin) increased the likelihood for therapeutic success compared with post-infusion that were below these thresholds [88]. To reduce the likelihood of toxicity, the recommended pre-infusion concentrations were <2 mg/L for gentamicin and tobramycin, or <7 mg/L for amikacin [89, 90].

EIAD of aminoglycosides does not require measurement of a peak but rather a serum concentration somewhere between 6 h post dose and the end of the dosing interval. Peaks are not usually required but some experts recommend checking a peak in patients with less predictable volume of distribution such as critically ill, obese, or burn patients [91]. It is important to keep in mind which type of dosing when ordering laboratory tests and interpreting the results. The time of the blood sampling also needs to be accurately reported in order to appropriately assess the level.

6.3.2 Toxicity Monitoring

Monitoring for nephrotoxicity includes measuring baseline serum creatinine and at least 2–3 times weekly thereafter. Changes greater than 0.5 mg/dL may indicate potential nephrotoxicity. Monitoring of renal tubular markers (urinary casts and enzymes) has been proposed to detect early renal damage and prevent further damage [92, 93]. However, due to the lack of specificity of these markers, they are not widely used. Patients who experience an increase in serum creatinine should be reevaluated whether aminoglycoside therapy should be continued or an alternate antibiotic is indicated.

According to the Academy of Audiology, patients who receive aminoglycosides should have pure-tone audiograms to monitor thresholds for conventional (8 kHz and below) and high-frequency regions (8–20 kHz) at baseline, once or twice weekly, then after drug discontinuation for several months [94]. Monitoring for vestibular toxicity usually includes tests of vestibular-ocular reflex, vestibular autorotation or full-frequency rotary chair testing [95].

6.4 Special Populations

6.4.1 Pediatrics/Neonates

New born infants, especially premature neonates, have underdeveloped end organ functions and dynamic change in physiologic function that can predispose them to toxicity. A meta-analysis concluded that EIAD might be superior to traditional dosing in treating sepsis in neonates greater than 32 weeks gestation [96]. Another review reported that EIAD in neonates was safe and efficacious, with a reduced risk of having peak and trough levels outside the therapeutic range [97].

For pediatric patients, a meta-analysis showed no difference in efficacy, nephrotoxicity, or ototoxicity between EIAD and multiple daily dosing [98].

6.4.2 Cystic Fibrosis (CF)

Patients with CF often require higher daily doses of aminoglycoside compared to patients without CF due to their increased drug clearance [99]. Several meta-analyses have been completed by the Cochrane Collaborate [100–102]. The conclusions from these studies are that aminoglycosides administered once daily or multiple times daily are equally efficacious in treating pulmonary exacerbations in CF. Also, there is evidence to support less nephrotoxicity in children given aminoglycosides once daily compared to three times daily [101].

6.4.3 Pregnancy

During the later stages of pregnancy, increases in extracellular fluid, cardiac output, total body water, renal blood flow, and glomerular filtration up to 50 % can occur [103]. Aminoglycoside distribution and elimination are both affected by pregnancy, making aminoglycoside pharmacokinetics widely variable [104, 105]. Pregnancy is often an exclusion criterion to many dosing nomograms [53, 106, 107]. EIAD of aminoglycosides has been studied in postpartum women for endometritis with gentamicin doses ranging from 4 to 5 mg/kg [108–111]. Although there is a risk for fetal toxicity, some experts recommend aminoglycoside use in patients with chorioamnionitis, postpartum endometritis, pyelonephritis, pelvic inflammatory disease, and other life threatening infections where the benefits outweigh the risks [103].

6.4.4 Renal Impairment

Dosing aminoglycosides in patients with chronic kidney disease on dialysis presents its own challenges. These patients lack intrinsic renal function and are not candidates for extended interval dosing of aminoglycosides due to reduced aminoglycoside clearance. One strategy that has been studied recently is to administer aminoglycoside shortly before hemodialysis. Patients who received this dosing still achieved high peak concentrations followed by aminoglycoside removal during dialysis, thus mimicking EIAD [18]. Using simulated patient data, studies suggest that predialysis dosing is able to achieve a Cmax of 8 mg/L and AUC between 10 and 70 mg h/L over 24 h [16, 112].

6.4.5 Burn Patients

Burn patients are often in a hypermetabolic state with altered protein binding, drug distribution and clearance [113]. Burn patients have an extremely high rate of aminoglycoside elimination [114–116]. These patients may require more frequent dosing intervals to achieve adequate drug concentrations [117, 118].

7 Clinical Uses: Specific Infections

In the era of multidrug resistance, aminoglycosides are commonly used empirically along with another agent (beta-lactams or fluoroquinolones) for sepsis, nosocomial pneumonia, and complicated intra-abdominal infections suspected to be caused by gram-negative bacilli. Once susceptibilities are available, aminoglycosides are often discontinued if the organism(s) are susceptible to other agents. Data have shown that combination therapy may not always be necessary in *Pseudomonas aeruginosa* bacteremia as long as the pathogen is susceptible to one of the antibiotics [119, 120].

7.1 Broadening Empiric Spectrum

Aminoglycosides are used frequently in combination for empiric therapy of serious gram-negative infections. The addition of a second agent, such as an aminoglycoside, has been shown to increase the probability of achieving appropriate empiric antibiotic therapy [121]. Local susceptibility patterns should be considered when using combination therapy. Some experts recommend the addition of an aminoglycoside to broad-spectrum antibiotics when local resistance patterns demonstrate significantly less than 90 % susceptibility for broad spectrum beta-lactams alone [122].

7.2 Gram-Positive Synergism

Aminoglycosides are used in the treatment of gram-positive endocarditis. This is based on in vitro data demonstrating synergy between penicillin and either gentamicin or streptomycin [123, 124]. There have been randomized controlled trials for *Staphylococcus aureus* and *Streptococcus viridians* [125–129], but no randomized controlled trials for enterococcal endocarditis. A cell-wall active agent (ampicillin, penicillin, or vancomycin) plus gentamicin 1 mg/kg three times daily given for 4–6 weeks are recommended for susceptible enterococcal endocarditis [130]. A recent, pilot study reported using once daily gentamicin (3 mg/kg) for a shorter course (2 weeks) [131]. Although additional studies are still needed, the authors found this regimen to be efficacious and less toxic than the previously recommended regimen of gentamicin for 4–6 weeks.

According to the Infectious Diseases Society of America and American Thoracic Society treatment guidelines on endocarditis, EIDA is not recommended due to the conflicting data in animal models of endocarditis [130]. Therefore, the use of the Hartford nomogram is not recommended in the setting of endocarditis.

The role of gentamicin in *S. aureus* endocarditis is less certain. Current recommendations are for gentamicin of 2 weeks in the presence of prosthetic material and 3–5 days in the absence of prosthetic material [130]. However, recent data have challenged the use of initial low dose aminoglycosides in *S. aureus* endocarditis due to increased nephrotoxicity [132, 133].

7.3 Pneumonia

Aminoglycosides are often used in pneumonia despite their poor penetration and variable concentration at the site of infection [134]. Currently, aminoglycosides are recommended in combination therapy with an antipseudomonal beta-lactam as an alternative to fluoroquinolones in patients with health-care-associated pneumonia, health-care-acquired pneumonia, or ventilator-associated pneumonia [135]. Due to their poor penetration into the lungs, local instillation or aerosolization of aminoglycosides have been used in addition to systemic therapy and should be considered for patients with suspected pseudomonal infection or who are not responding to systemic therapy [135].

7.4 Intra-abdominal Infections

Although aminoglycosides lack activity against anaerobic pathogens, they are commonly used in combination with anaerobic agent for intra-abdominal infections. Aminoglycosides are currently recommended for health-care-acquired intra-abdominal infections in adults but not community acquired infections in favor of less toxic agents [136]. A meta-analysis was conducted to compare the efficacies of aminoglycoside based regimens with newer agents for intra-abdominal infections [137]. However, due to their toxicity, the authors did not recommend aminoglycosides as first-line therapy [137]. A Cochrane Collaborative review of different antibiotic regimens for secondary peritonitis of gastrointestinal origin in adults found that aminoglycosides in addition to an anaerobic agent had a significantly lower response rate compared to all other regimens (OR 0.65, 95 % CI 0.46–0.92; $p=0.02$) [138]. These data suggest that aminoglycoside combination therapies should not be used first-line when alternative therapies are available.

7.5 Urinary Tract Infections

Approximately 85–95 % of an aminoglycoside dose is excreted unchanged renally and a high concentration is achieved in the urine [139]. However, in lieu of safer agents, currently aminoglycosides are only recommended as alternative therapy in acute uncomplicated cystitis [140]. There is an ongoing debate whether or not aminoglycoside monotherapy is appropriate. According to a meta-analysis, urinary tract infections are the only place where aminoglycosides can be used as monotherapy [141].

8 Conclusion

With a better understanding of the pharmacokinetics, pharmacodynamics, and toxicity, the clinical use of aminoglycosides has changed over the years. It represents one of the first bedside applications of pharmacokinetics to individualized therapy. Landmark studies by legendary investigators have paved for how antibiotics would be used and save lives in the modern era. In most critically ill patients, they are commonly used to broaden the spectrum of empiric coverage. Various nomograms have been proposed to facilitate empiric dosing. When the aminoglycosides are used for definitive therapy, a more personalized approach to dosing (based on pathogen susceptibility and prospective monitoring of drug concentrations) is widely adopted. Optimal dosing is expected to maximize the likelihood of efficacy and minimize (delaying the onset of) toxicity. With a better understanding of the resistance mechanisms, better synthetic analogs are under (clinical) development. These next-generation aminoglycosides are expected to have better antimicrobial activity against contemporary drug-resistant pathogens.

References

1. Rinehart KL Jr (1969) Comparative chemistry of the aminoglycoside and aminocyclitol antibiotics. J Infect Dis 119:345–350
2. Melsen WG, de Smet AM, Kluytmans JA, Bonten MJ (2012) Selective decontamination of the oral and digestive tract in surgical versus non-surgical patients in intensive care in a cluster-randomized trial. Br J Surg 99:232–237
3. Roos D, Dijksman LM, Oudemans-van Straaten HM, de Wit LT, Gouma DJ, Gerhards MF (2011) Randomized clinical trial of perioperative selective decontamination of the digestive tract versus placebo in elective gastrointestinal surgery. Br J Surg 98:1365–1372
4. Pedretti G, Calzetti C, Missale G, Fiaccadori F (1991) Rifaximin versus neomycin on hyperammoniemia in chronic portal systemic encephalopathy of cirrhotics. A double-blind, randomized trial. Ital J Gastroenterol 23:175–178
5. Davidson RN, den Boer M, Ritmeijer K (2009) Paromomycin. Trans R Soc Trop Med Hyg 103:653–660
6. Bailey DN, Briggs JR (2004) Gentamicin and tobramycin binding to human serum in vitro. J Anal Toxicol 28:187–189
7. Panidis D, Markantonis SL, Boutzouka E, Karatzas S, Baltopoulos G (2005) Penetration of gentamicin into the alveolar lining fluid of critically ill patients with ventilator-associated pneumonia. Chest 128:545–552
8. Carcas AJ, Garcia-Satue JL, Zapater P, Frias-Iniesta J (1999) Tobramycin penetration into epithelial lining fluid of patients with pneumonia. Clin Pharmacol Ther 65:245–250
9. Nagai J, Tanaka H, Nakanishi N, Murakami T, Takano M (2001) Role of megalin in renal handling of aminoglycosides. Am J Physiol Renal Physiol 281:F337–F344
10. De Broe ME, Verbist L, Verpooten GA (1991) Influence of dosage schedule on renal cortical accumulation of amikacin and tobramycin in man. J Antimicrob Chemother 27(Suppl C):41–47
11. Rybak MJ, Abate BJ, Kang SL, Ruffing MJ, Lerner SA, Drusano GL (1999) Prospective evaluation of the effect of an aminoglycoside dosing regimen on rates of observed nephrotoxicity and ototoxicity. Antimicrob Agents Chemother 43:1549–1555
12. Tran Ba Huy P, Bernard P, Schacht J (1986) Kinetics of gentamicin uptake and release in the rat. Comparison of inner ear tissues and fluids with other organs. J Clin Invest 77:1492–1500
13. Singer C, Smith C, Krieff D (1996) Once-daily aminoglycoside therapy: potential ototoxicity. Antimicrob Agents Chemother 40:2209–2211
14. Zaske DE, Cipolle RJ, Rotschafer JC, Solem LD, Mosier NR, Strate RG (1982) Gentamicin pharmacokinetics in 1,640 patients: method for control of serum concentrations. Antimicrob Agents Chemother 21:407–411

15. Fuhs DW, Mann HJ, Kubajak CA, Cerra FB (1988) Intrapatient variation of aminoglycoside pharmacokinetics in critically ill surgery patients. Clin Pharm 7:207–213
16. Sowinski KM, Magner SJ, Lucksiri A, Scott MK, Hamburger RJ, Mueller BA (2008) Influence of hemodialysis on gentamicin pharmacokinetics, removal during hemodialysis, and recommended dosing. Clin J Am Soc Nephrol 3:355–361
17. Trotman RL, Williamson JC, Shoemaker DM, Salzer WL (2005) Antibiotic dosing in critically ill adult patients receiving continuous renal replacement therapy. Clin Infect Dis 41:1159–1166
18. Kamel Mohamed OH, Wahba IM, Watnick S, Earle SB, Bennett WM, Ayres JW, Munar MY (2007) Administration of tobramycin in the beginning of the hemodialysis session: a novel intradialytic dosing regimen. Clin J Am Soc Nephrol 2:694–699
19. Veinstein A, Venisse N, Badin J, Pinsard M, Robert R, Dupuis A (2013) Gentamicin in hemodialyzed critical care patients: early dialysis after administration of a high dose should be considered. Antimicrob Agents Chemother 57:977–982
20. Mingeot-Leclercq MP, Tulkens PM (1999) Aminoglycosides: nephrotoxicity. Antimicrob Agents Chemother 43:1003–1012
21. Zhanel GG, Craig WA (1994) Pharmacokinetic contributions to postantibiotic effects. Focus on aminoglycosides. Clin Pharmacokinet 27:377–392
22. Benveniste R, Davies J (1973) Structure-activity relationships among the aminoglycoside antibiotics: role of hydroxyl and amino groups. Antimicrob Agents Chemother 4:402–409
23. Hancock RE (1981) Aminoglycoside uptake and mode of action--with special reference to streptomycin and gentamicin. I. Antagonists and mutants. J Antimicrob Chemother 8:249–276
24. Turnidge J (2003) Pharmacodynamics and dosing of aminoglycosides. Infect Dis Clin North Am 17:503–528, v
25. Lacy MK, Nicolau DP, Nightingale CH, Quintiliani R (1998) The pharmacodynamics of aminoglycosides. Clin Infect Dis 27:23–27
26. Holm SE, Hill B, Lowestad A, Maller R, Vikerfors T (1983) A prospective, randomized study of amikacin and gentamicin in serious infections with focus on efficacy, toxicity and duration of serum levels above the MIC. J Antimicrob Chemother 12:393–402
27. Moore RD, Lietman PS, Smith CR (1987) Clinical response to aminoglycoside therapy: importance of the ratio of peak concentration to minimal inhibitory concentration. J Infect Dis 155:93–99
28. Schafer JA, Hovde LB, Rotschafer JC (2006) Consistent rates of kill of Staphylococcus aureus by gentamicin over a 6-fold clinical concentration range in an in vitro pharmacodynamic model (IVPDM). J Antimicrob Chemother 58:108–111
29. Tam VH, Kabbara S, Vo G, Schilling AN, Coyle EA (2006) Comparative pharmacodynamics of gentamicin against Staphylococcus aureus and Pseudomonas aeruginosa. Antimicrob Agents Chemother 50:2626–2631
30. Ramos MC, Grayson ML, Eliopoulos GM, Bayer AS (1992) Comparison of daptomycin, vancomycin, and ampicillin-gentamicin for treatment of experimental endocarditis caused by penicillin-resistant enterococci. Antimicrob Agents Chemother 36:1864–1869
31. Craig WA (1993) Post-antibiotic effects in experimental infection models: relationship to in-vitro phenomena and to treatment of infections in man. J Antimicrob Chemother 31(Suppl D):149–158
32. Fantin B, Carbon C (1990) Importance of the aminoglycoside dosing regimen in the penicillin-netilmicin combination for treatment of Enterococcus faecalis-induced experimental endocarditis. Antimicrob Agents Chemother 34:2387–2391
33. Miller MH, Feinstein SA, Chow RT (1987) Early effects of beta-lactams on aminoglycoside uptake, bactericidal rates, and turbidimetrically measured growth inhibition in Pseudomonas aeruginosa. Antimicrob Agents Chemother 31:108–110
34. Fass RJ (1982) Comparative in vitro activities of beta-lactam-tobramycin combinations against Pseudomonas aeruginosa and multidrug-resistant gram-negative enteric bacilli. Antimicrob Agents Chemother 21:1003–1006
35. Giamarellou H (1986) Aminoglycosides plus beta-lactams against gram-negative organisms. Evaluation of in vitro synergy and chemical interactions. Am J Med 80:126–137
36. Hooton TM, Blair AD, Turck M, Counts GW (1984) Synergism at clinically attainable concentrations of aminoglycoside and beta-lactam antibiotics. Antimicrob Agents Chemother 26:535–538
37. Davies J, Wright GD (1997) Bacterial resistance to aminoglycoside antibiotics. Trends Microbiol 5:234–240
38. Doi Y, Wachino J, Yamane K, Shibata N, Yagi T, Shibayama K, Kato H, Arakawa Y (2004) Spread of novel aminoglycoside resistance

gene aac(6′)-Iad among Acinetobacter clinical isolates in Japan. Antimicrob Agents Chemother 48:2075–2080
39. Wright GD (1999) Aminoglycoside-modifying enzymes. Curr Opin Microbiol 2:499–503
40. Aggen JB, Armstrong ES, Goldblum AA, Dozzo P, Linsell MS, Gliedt MJ, Hildebrandt DJ, Feeney LA, Kubo A, Matias RD, Lopez S, Gomez M, Wlasichuk KB, Diokno R, Miller GH, Moser HE (2010) Synthesis and spectrum of the neoglycoside ACHN-490. Antimicrob Agents Chemother 54:4636–4642
41. Davies J, Brzezinska M, Benveniste R (1971) The problems of drug-resistant pathogenic bacteria. R factors: biochemical mechanisms of resistance to aminoglycoside antibiotics. Ann N Y Acad Sci 182:226–233
42. Rasmussen BA, Bush K, Tally FP (1997) Antimicrobial resistance in anaerobes. Clin Infect Dis 24(Suppl 1):S110–S120
43. Hermann T (2007) Aminoglycoside antibiotics: old drugs and new therapeutic approaches. Cell Mol Life Sci 64:1841–1852
44. Hinz A, Lee S, Jacoby K, Manoil C (2011) Membrane proteases and aminoglycoside antibiotic resistance. J Bacteriol 193:4790–4797
45. Shawar RM, MacLeod DL, Garber RL, Burns JL, Stapp JR, Clausen CR, Tanaka SK (1999) Activities of tobramycin and six other antibiotics against Pseudomonas aeruginosa isolates from patients with cystic fibrosis. Antimicrob Agents Chemother 43:2877–2880
46. Westbrock-Wadman S, Sherman DR, Hickey MJ, Coulter SN, Zhu YQ, Warrener P, Nguyen LY, Shawar RM, Folger KR, Stover CK (1999) Characterization of a Pseudomonas aeruginosa efflux pump contributing to aminoglycoside impermeability. Antimicrob Agents Chemother 43:2975–2983
47. Miller GH, Sabatelli FJ, Hare RS, Glupczynski Y, Mackey P, Shlaes D, Shimizu K, Shaw KJ (1997) The most frequent aminoglycoside resistance mechanisms--changes with time and geographic area: a reflection of aminoglycoside usage patterns? Aminoglycoside Resistance Study Groups. Clin Infect Dis 24(Suppl 1):S46–S62
48. Lin G, Ednie LM, Appelbaum PC (2010) Antistaphylococcal activity of ACHN-490 tested alone and in combination with other agents by time-kill assay. Antimicrob Agents Chemother 54:2258–2261
49. Livermore DM, Mushtaq S, Warner M, Zhang JC, Maharjan S, Doumith M, Woodford N (2011) Activity of aminoglycosides, including ACHN-490, against carbapenem-resistant Enterobacteriaceae isolates. J Antimicrob Chemother 66:48–53
50. Galani I, Souli M, Daikos GL, Chrysouli Z, Poulakou G, Psichogiou M, Panagea T, Argyropoulou A, Stefanou I, Plakias G, Giamarellou H, Petrikkos G (2012) Activity of plazomicin (ACHN-490) against MDR clinical isolates of Klebsiella pneumoniae, Escherichia coli, and Enterobacter spp. from Athens, Greece. J Chemother 24:191–194
51. Sawchuk RJ, Zaske DE, Cipolle RJ, Wargin WA, Strate RG (1977) Kinetic model for gentamicin dosing with the use of individual patient parameters. Clin Pharmacol Ther 21:362–369
52. Duffull SB, Kirkpatrick CM, Begg EJ (1997) Comparison of two Bayesian approaches to dose-individualization for once-daily aminoglycoside regimens. Br J Clin Pharmacol 43:125–135
53. Nicolau DP, Freeman CD, Belliveau PP, Nightingale CH, Ross JW, Quintiliani R (1995) Experience with a once-daily aminoglycoside program administered to 2,184 adult patients. Antimicrob Agents Chemother 39:650–655
54. Begg EJ, Barclay ML, Kirkpatrick CJ (1999) The therapeutic monitoring of antimicrobial agents. Br J Clin Pharmacol 47:23–30
55. Davis BD (1987) Mechanism of bactericidal action of aminoglycosides. Microbiol Rev 51:341–350
56. Ebert SC, Craig WA (1990) Pharmacodynamic properties of antibiotics: application to drug monitoring and dosage regimen design. Infect Control Hosp Epidemiol 11:319–326
57. Keating MJ, Bodey GP, Valdivieso M, Rodriguez V (1979) A randomized comparative trial of three aminoglycosides--comparison of continuous infusions of gentamicin, amikacin and sisomicin combined with carbenicillin in the treatment of infections in neutropenic patients with malignancies. Medicine (Baltimore) 58:159–170
58. Durante-Mangoni E, Grammatikos A, Utili R, Falagas ME (2009) Do we still need the aminoglycosides? Int J Antimicrob Agents 33:201–205
59. MacGowan A, Reeves D (1994) Serum aminoglycoside concentrations: the case for routine monitoring. J Antimicrob Chemother 34:829–837
60. Munckhof WJ, Grayson ML, Turnidge JD (1996) A meta-analysis of studies on the safety and efficacy of aminoglycosides given either once daily or as divided doses. J Antimicrob Chemother 37:645–663
61. Hatala R, Dinh T, Cook DJ (1996) Once-daily aminoglycoside dosing in immunocompetent adults: a meta-analysis. Ann Intern Med 124:717–725
62. Barza M, Ioannidis JP, Cappelleri JC, Lau J (1996) Single or multiple daily doses of ami-

noglycosides: a meta-analysis. BMJ 312:338–345
63. Bailey TC, Little JR, Littenberg B, Reichley RM, Dunagan WC (1997) A meta-analysis of extended-interval dosing versus multiple daily dosing of aminoglycosides. Clin Infect Dis 24:786–795
64. Ali MZ, Goetz MB (1997) A meta-analysis of the relative efficacy and toxicity of single daily dosing versus multiple daily dosing of aminoglycosides. Clin Infect Dis 24:796–809
65. Rougier F, Ducher M, Maurin M, Corvaisier S, Claude D, Jelliffe R, Maire P (2003) Aminoglycoside dosages and nephrotoxicity: quantitative relationships. Clin Pharmacokinet 42:493–500
66. Giuliano RA, Verpooten GA, De Broe ME (1986) Kinetics of the renal cortical uptake and release of aminoglycosides: a rational approach to the understanding and prevention of their nephrotoxicity. Dev Toxicol Environ Sci 14:105–114
67. Laurent G, Kishore BK, Tulkens PM (1990) Aminoglycoside-induced renal phospholipidosis and nephrotoxicity. Biochem Pharmacol 40:2383–2392
68. Appel GB, Neu HC (1977) The nephrotoxicity of antimicrobial agents (first of three parts). N Engl J Med 296:663–670
69. Streetman DS, Nafziger AN, Destache CJ, Bertino AS Jr (2001) Individualized pharmacokinetic monitoring results in less aminoglycoside-associated nephrotoxicity and fewer associated costs. Pharmacotherapy 21:443–451
70. de Jager P, van Altena R (2002) Hearing loss and nephrotoxicity in long-term aminoglycoside treatment in patients with tuberculosis. Int J Tuberc Lung Dis 6:622–627
71. Rougier F, Claude D, Maurin M, Sedoglavic A, Ducher M, Corvaisier S, Jelliffe R, Maire P (2003) Aminoglycoside nephrotoxicity: modeling, simulation, and control. Antimicrob Agents Chemother 47:1010–1016
72. Maglio D, Nightingale CH, Nicolau DP (2002) Extended interval aminoglycoside dosing: from concept to clinic. Int J Antimicrob Agents 19:341–348
73. Hinojosa R, Lerner SA (1987) Cochlear neural degeneration without hair cell loss in two patients with aminoglycoside ototoxicity. J Infect Dis 156:449–455
74. Boettcher FA, Henderson D, Gratton MA, Danielson RW, Byrne CD (1987) Synergistic interactions of noise and other ototraumatic agents. Ear Hear 8:192–212
75. Minor LB (1998) Gentamicin-induced bilateral vestibular hypofunction. JAMA 279:541–544
76. Bottrill I, Wills AD, Mitchell AL (2003) Intratympanic gentamicin for unilateral Meniere's disease: results of therapy. Clin Otolaryngol Allied Sci 28:133–141
77. Wu IC, Minor LB (2003) Long-term hearing outcome in patients receiving intratympanic gentamicin for Meniere's disease. Laryngoscope 113:815–820
78. Usami S, Abe S, Akita J, Namba A, Shinkawa H, Ishii M, Iwasaki S, Hoshino T, Ito J, Doi K, Kubo T, Nakagawa T, Komiyama S, Tono T, Komune S (2000) Prevalence of mitochondrial gene mutations among hearing impaired patients. J Med Genet 37:38–40
79. Gardner JC, Goliath R, Viljoen D, Sellars S, Cortopassi G, Hutchin T, Greenberg J, Beighton P (1997) Familial streptomycin ototoxicity in a South African family: a mitochondrial disorder. J Med Genet 34:904–906
80. Finegold SM (1966) Toxicity of kanamycin in adults. Ann N Y Acad Sci 132:942–956
81. Argov Z, Mastaglia FL (1979) Drug therapy: disorders of neuromuscular transmission caused by drugs. N Engl J Med 301:409–413
82. Santos JI, Swensen P, Glasgow LA (1981) Potentiation of Clostridium botulinum toxin aminoglycoside antibiotics: clinical and laboratory observations. Pediatrics 68:50–54
83. Schwartz RH, Eng G (1982) Infant botulism: exacerbation by aminoglycosides. Am J Dis Child 136:952
84. Ristuccia AM, Cunha BA (1982) The aminoglycosides. Med Clin North Am 66:303–312
85. Chang JC, Reyes B (1975) Agranulocytosis associated with gentamicin. JAMA 232:1154–1155
86. Roberts JA, Field J, Visser A, Whitbread R, Tallot M, Lipman J, Kirkpatrick CM (2010) Using population pharmacokinetics to determine gentamicin dosing during extended daily diafiltration in critically ill patients with acute kidney injury. Antimicrob Agents Chemother 54:3635–3640
87. Noone P, Parsons TM, Pattison JR, Slack RC, Garfield-Davies D, Hughes K (1974) Experience in monitoring gentamicin therapy during treatment of serious gram-negative sepsis. Br Med J 1:477–481
88. Moore RD, Smith CR, Lietman PS (1984) Association of aminoglycoside plasma levels with therapeutic outcome in gram-negative pneumonia. Am J Med 77:657–662
89. Neu HC (1987) New antibiotics: areas of appropriate use. J Infect Dis 155:403–417
90. Burton ME, Vasko MR, Brater DC (1985) Comparison of drug dosing methods. Clin Pharmacokinet 10:1–37

91. Roberts JA, Norris R, Paterson DL, Martin JH (2012) Therapeutic drug monitoring of antimicrobials. Br J Clin Pharmacol 73:27–36
92. Davey PG, Geddes AM, Cowley DM (1983) Study of alanine aminopeptidase excretion as a test of gentamicin nephrotoxicity. J Antimicrob Chemother 11:455–465
93. Schentag JJ, Plaut ME (1980) Patterns of urinary beta 2-microglobulin excretion by patients treated with aminoglycosides. Kidney Int 17:654–661
94. American Academy of Audiology (2009) American Academy of Audiology Position state and clinical practice guidelines ototoxicity monitoring. American Academy of Audiology, Reston, VA
95. Xie J, Talaska AE, Schacht J (2011) New developments in aminoglycoside therapy and ototoxicity. Hear Res 281:28–37
96. Rao SC, Srinivasjois R, Hagan R, Ahmed M (2011) One dose per day compared to multiple doses per day of gentamicin for treatment of suspected or proven sepsis in neonates. Cochrane Database Syst Rev (11): CD005091
97. Nestaas E, Bangstad HJ, Sandvik L, Wathne KO (2005) Aminoglycoside extended interval dosing in neonates is safe and effective: a meta-analysis. Arch Dis Child Fetal Neonatal Ed 90:F294–F300
98. Contopoulos-Ioannidis DG, Giotis ND, Baliatsa DV, Ioannidis JP (2004) Extended-interval aminoglycoside administration for children: a meta-analysis. Pediatrics 114: e111–e118
99. de Groot R, Smith AL (1987) Antibiotic pharmacokinetics in cystic fibrosis. Differences and clinical significance. Clin Pharmacokinet 13:228–253
100. Smyth AR, Bhatt J (2010) Once-daily versus multiple-daily dosing with intravenous aminoglycosides for cystic fibrosis. Cochrane Database Syst Rev (1): CD002009
101. Smyth AR, Bhatt J (2012) Once-daily versus multiple-daily dosing with intravenous aminoglycosides for cystic fibrosis. Cochrane Database Syst Rev 2: CD002009
102. Smyth AR, Tan KH (2006) Once-daily versus multiple-daily dosing with intravenous aminoglycosides for cystic fibrosis. Cochrane Database Syst Rev (6): CD002009
103. Ward K, Theiler RN (2008) Once-daily dosing of gentamicin in obstetrics and gynecology. Clin Obstet Gynecol 51:498–506
104. Zaske DE, Cipolle RJ, Strate RG, Malo JW, Koszalka MF Jr (1980) Rapid gentamicin elimination in obstetric patients. Obstet Gynecol 56:559–564
105. Wiesenfeld HC, Heine RP (1998) The use of once-daily dosing of gentamicin in obstetrics and gynecology. Infect Dis Obstet Gynecol 6:155–159
106. Prins JM, Weverling GJ, de Blok K, van Ketel RJ, Speelman P (1996) Validation and nephrotoxicity of a simplified once-daily aminoglycoside dosing schedule and guidelines for monitoring therapy. Antimicrob Agents Chemother 40:2494–2499
107. Wallace AW, Jones M, Bertino JS Jr (2002) Evaluation of four once-daily aminoglycoside dosing nomograms. Pharmacotherapy 22: 1077–1083
108. Del Priore G, Jackson-Stone M, Shim EK, Garfinkel J, Eichmann MA, Frederiksen MC (1996) A comparison of once-daily and 8-hour gentamicin dosing in the treatment of postpartum endometritis. Obstet Gynecol 87:994–1000
109. Livingston JC, Llata E, Rinehart E, Leidwanger C, Mabie B, Haddad B, Sibai B (2003) Gentamicin and clindamycin therapy in postpartum endometritis: the efficacy of daily dosing versus dosing every 8 hours. Am J Obstet Gynecol 188:149–152
110. Mitra AG, Whitten MK, Laurent SL, Anderson WE (1997) A randomized, prospective study comparing once-daily gentamicin versus thrice-daily gentamicin in the treatment of puerperal infection. Am J Obstet Gynecol 177:786–792
111. Sunyecz JA, Wiesenfeld HC, Heine RP (1998) The pharmacokinetics of once-daily dosing with gentamicin in women with postpartum endometritis. Infect Dis Obstet Gynecol 6:160–162
112. Teigen MM, Duffull S, Dang L, Johnson DW (2006) Dosing of gentamicin in patients with end-stage renal disease receiving hemodialysis. J Clin Pharmacol 46:1259–1267
113. Blanchet B, Jullien V, Vinsonneau C, Tod M (2008) Influence of burns on pharmacokinetics and pharmacodynamics of drugs used in the care of burn patients. Clin Pharmacokinet 47:635–654
114. Zaske DE, Sawchuk RJ, Strate RG (1978) The necessity of increased doses of amikacin in burn patients. Surgery 84:603–608
115. Zaske DE, Sawchuk RJ, Gerding DN, Strate RG (1976) Increased dosage requirements of gentamicin in burn patients. J Trauma 16:824–828
116. Loirat P, Rohan J, Baillet A, Beaufils F, David R, Chapman A (1978) Increased glomerular filtration rate in patients with major burns and its effect on the pharmacokinetics of tobramycin. N Engl J Med 299:915–919
117. Roberts JA, Lipman J (2006) Antibacterial dosing in intensive care: pharmacokinetics, degree of disease and pharmacodynamics of sepsis. Clin Pharmacokinet 45:755–773

118. Udy AA, Roberts JA, Boots RJ, Paterson DL, Lipman J (2010) Augmented renal clearance: implications for antibacterial dosing in the critically ill. Clin Pharmacokinet 49:1–16
119. Bowers DR, Liew YX, Lye DC, Kwa AL, Hsu LY, Tam VH (2013) Outcomes of appropriate empiric combination versus monotherapy for Pseudomonas aeruginosa bacteremia. Antimicrob Agents Chemother 57:1270–1274
120. Pena C, Suarez C, Ocampo-Sosa A, Murillas J, Almirante B, Pomar V, Aguilar M, Granados A, Calbo E, Rodriguez-Bano J, Rodriguez F, Tubau F, Oliver A, Martinez-Martinez L (2013) Effect of adequate single-drug vs combination antimicrobial therapy on mortality in Pseudomonas aeruginosa bloodstream infections: a post Hoc analysis of a prospective cohort. Clin Infect Dis 57:208–216
121. Micek ST, Lloyd AE, Ritchie DJ, Reichley RM, Fraser VJ, Kollef MH (2005) Pseudomonas aeruginosa bloodstream infection: importance of appropriate initial antimicrobial treatment. Antimicrob Agents Chemother 49:1306–1311
122. Leibovici L, Vidal L, Paul M (2009) Aminoglycoside drugs in clinical practice: an evidence-based approach. J Antimicrob Chemother 63:246–251
123. Robbins WC, Tompsett R (1951) Treatment of enterococcal endocarditis and bacteremia; results of combined therapy with penicillin and streptomycin. Am J Med 10:278–299
124. Jawetz E, Gunnison JB, Coleman VR (1950) The combined action of penicillin with streptomycin or chloromycetin on enterococci in vitro. Science 111:254–256
125. Abrams B, Sklaver A, Hoffman T, Greenman R (1979) Single or combination therapy of staphylococcal endocarditis in intravenous drug abusers. Ann Intern Med 90:789–791
126. Rajashekaraiah KR, Rice T, Rao VS, Marsh D, Ramakrishna B, Kallick CA (1980) Clinical significance of tolerant strains of Staphylococcus aureus in patients with endocarditis. Ann Intern Med 93:796–801
127. Korzeniowski O, Sande MA (1982) Combination antimicrobial therapy for Staphylococcus aureus endocarditis in patients addicted to parenteral drugs and in nonaddicts: a prospective study. Ann Intern Med 97:496–503
128. Ribera E, Gomez-Jimenez J, Cortes E, del Valle O, Planes A, Gonzalez-Alujas T, Almirante B, Ocana I, Pahissa A (1996) Effectiveness of cloxacillin with and without gentamicin in short-term therapy for right-sided Staphylococcus aureus endocarditis. A randomized, controlled trial. Ann Intern Med 125:969–974
129. Sexton DJ, Tenenbaum MJ, Wilson WR, Steckelberg JM, Tice AD, Gilbert D, Dismukes W, Drew RH, Durack DT (1998) Ceftriaxone once daily for four weeks compared with ceftriaxone plus gentamicin once daily for two weeks for treatment of endocarditis due to penicillin-susceptible streptococci. Endocarditis Treatment Consortium Group. Clin Infect Dis 27:1470–1474
130. Baddour LM, Wilson WR, Bayer AS, Fowler VG Jr, Bolger AF, Levison ME, Ferrieri P, Gerber MA, Tani LY, Gewitz MH, Tong DC, Steckelberg JM, Baltimore RS, Shulman ST, Burns JC, Falace DA, Newburger JW, Pallasch TJ, Takahashi M, Taubert KA (2005) Infective endocarditis: diagnosis, antimicrobial therapy, and management of complications: a statement for healthcare professionals from the Committee on Rheumatic Fever, Endocarditis, and Kawasaki Disease, Council on Cardiovascular Disease in the Young, and the Councils on Clinical Cardiology, Stroke, and Cardiovascular Surgery and Anesthesia, American Heart Association: endorsed by the Infectious Diseases Society of America. Circulation 111:e394–e434
131. Dahl A, Rasmussen RV, Bundgaard H, Hassager C, Bruun LE, Lauridsen TK, Moser C, Sogaard P, Arpi M, Bruun NE (2013) Enterococcus faecalis infective endocarditis: a pilot study of the relationship between duration of gentamicin treatment and outcome. Circulation 127:1810–1817
132. Cosgrove SE, Vigliani GA, Fowler VG Jr, Abrutyn E, Corey GR, Levine DP, Rupp ME, Chambers HF, Karchmer AW, Boucher HW (2009) Initial low-dose gentamicin for Staphylococcus aureus bacteremia and endocarditis is nephrotoxic. Clin Infect Dis 48:713–721
133. Bayer AS, Murray BE (2009) Initial low-dose aminoglycosides in Staphylococcus aureus bacteremia: good science, urban legend, or just plain toxic? Clin Infect Dis 48:722–724
134. Rodvold KA, George JM, Yoo L (2011) Penetration of anti-infective agents into pulmonary epithelial lining fluid: focus on antibacterial agents. Clin Pharmacokinet 50:637–664
135. American Thoracic Society; Infectious Diseases Society of America (2005) Guidelines for the management of adults with hospital-acquired, ventilator-associated, and healthcare-associated pneumonia. Am J Respir Crit Care Med 171:388–416
136. Solomkin JS, Mazuski JE, Bradley JS, Rodvold KA, Goldstein EJ, Baron EJ, O'Neill PJ, Chow AW, Dellinger EP, Eachempati SR,

Gorbach S, Hilfiker M, May AK, Nathens AB, Sawyer RG, Bartlett JG (2010) Diagnosis and management of complicated intra-abdominal infection in adults and children: guidelines by the Surgical Infection Society and the Infectious Diseases Society of America. Clin Infect Dis 50:133–164
137. Bailey JA, Virgo KS, DiPiro JT, Nathens AB, Sawyer RG, Mazuski JE (2002) Aminoglycosides for intra-abdominal infection: equal to the challenge? Surg Infect (Larchmt) 3:315–335
138. Wong PF, Gilliam AD, Kumar S, Shenfine J, O'Dair GN, Leaper DJ (2005) Antibiotic regimens for secondary peritonitis of gastrointestinal origin in adults. Cochrane Database Syst Rev (2): CD004539
139. Evans WE, Schentag JJ, Jusko WJ (1992) Applied pharmacokinetics. Lippincott Williams and Wilkins, Vancouver, BC
140. Gupta K, Hooton TM, Miller L (2011) Managing uncomplicated urinary tract infection--making sense out of resistance data. Clin Infect Dis 53:1041–1042
141. Vidal L, Gafter-Gvili A, Borok S, Fraser A, Leibovici L, Paul M (2007) Efficacy and safety of aminoglycoside monotherapy: systematic review and meta-analysis of randomized controlled trials. J Antimicrob Chemother 60:247–257

Chapter 10

Polymyxin Pharmacokinetics and Pharmacodynamics

Soon-Ee Cheah, Jian Li, Phillip J. Bergen, and Roger L. Nation

Abstract

Polymyxin B and E (the latter more commonly known as colistin) were originally introduced into clinical medicine in the late 1950s for the treatment of infections caused by gram-negative pathogens. They fell into relative disuse during the next decade as concern about their potential to cause nephrotoxicity grew and other new antibiotics regarded at the time as less toxic became available. In more recent times, the polymyxins have been resurrected as an important component of the therapeutic armamentarium because of rising rates of resistance to other available antibiotics and the limited number of new antibacterial agents with activity against gram-negative pathogens emerging from the drug development pipeline. At the time of their original regulatory approval for clinical use the rigor of drug development and approval processes was substantially less than it is today and there was little information to guide clinicians in the optimal use of these agents. Over the last decade, the polymyxins have been subject to a "redevelopment" process, led by academic researchers and clinicians, and funded largely by public grant bodies around the world. The result has been a considerable increase in knowledge of the preclinical and clinical pharmacology of the polymyxins. This chapter reviews key aspects of the chemistry, microbiology, and especially the pharmacokinetics and pharmacodynamics of both of the clinically available polymyxins. The similarities and differences between colistin and polymyxin B are highlighted as are the clinical implications for use of these important last-line antibiotics.

Key words Colistin, Colistin methanesulfonate, Polymyxin B, Pharmacodynamics, Pharmacokinetics, Dose optimization, *P. aeruginosa*, *A. baumannii*, *K. pneumoniae*, Multidrug resistance

1 Introduction

The polymyxins are a family of antimicrobial peptides (polymyxins A, B, C, D, E, F, M, P, S, and T) first discovered in the 1940s from the soil bacterium *Paenibacillus polymyxa* [1–3]. Colistin, first described in 1950 and obtained from *Pa. polymyxa* ssp. *colistinus* [4], was subsequently determined to be identical with polymyxin E [5–7]. Preclinical investigations demonstrated severe renal toxicity from polymyxins A, C, and D, and consequently only polymyxin B and colistin (polymyxin E) were further developed [8–12]. These two polymyxins were used clinically beginning in the late 1950s whereupon reports of nephrotoxicity and neurotoxicity following

John C. Rotschafer et al. (eds.), *Antibiotic Pharmacodynamics*, Methods in Pharmacology and Toxicology, DOI 10.1007/978-1-4939-3323-5_10, © Springer Science+Business Media New York 2016

parenteral administration began to emerge [13–21]. These safety concerns led to declining use of the polymyxins in the 1970s as newer, supposedly safer antibiotics such as the aminoglycosides began to replace them in the clinic. Colistin first began making a comeback in the 1980s when reintroduced to manage respiratory infection or colonization by *Pseudomonas aeruginosa* in patients with cystic fibrosis (CF) [22]. More recently the increasing incidence of infections caused by multidrug-resistant (MDR) gram-negative organisms generally [23, 24], coupled with a lack of novel antimicrobial agents in development [25, 26], has led to a resurgence in interest in polymyxins as a last-line treatment. However, owing to their discovery prior to the modern era of drug development there was a major paucity of pharmacological and other scientific information with which to guide their reintroduction into the clinic. This situation has started to change over the last decade or so as modern drug development procedures have begun to be applied to the polymyxins. While significant gaps still remain in our understanding of polymyxins and their optimal use, much progress has been made over this time.

This chapter reviews the current state of microbiological and pharmacological knowledge of the clinically used polymyxins, especially in relation to their pharmacokinetics (PK) and pharmacodynamics (PD). The chemistry of the polymyxins, especially in the case of colistin, has a profound impact on both the PK and PD behavior of these antibiotics and is also reviewed briefly. Clinical efficacy is not reviewed in this chapter; readers interested in this area may consult other sources of information [27–31].

2 Chemistry

2.1 Colistin and Polymyxin B

Knowledge of the chemical structures of the polymyxins is essential for an understanding of their mechanism(s) of antibacterial activity and resistance. Both polymyxin B and colistin consist of a mixture of D- and L-amino acids arranged as a cyclic heptapeptide with a tripeptide side chain covalently linked to a fatty acyl tail; each differs from the other by a single amino acid residue within their heptapeptide ring (Fig. 1). At physiological pH, 5 of the L-α,γ-diaminobutyric acid (Dab) residues contained within the polymyxin structure are protonated, which in combination with the fatty acyl tail and other hydrophobic domains give polymyxins an amphipathic nature. As the polymyxins are of biological origin each consists of a mixture of products with differing amino acids and fatty acyl tails [32–35]. Variations in fatty acyl tail composition give rise to polymyxin B1 and B2 and colistin A and B which combined account for approximately 85 % of total polymyxin B and colistin, respectively, in commercially available products [32, 33, 36]. The ratios of polymyxin components within commercial products exhibit inter-batch and -supplier variability [36, 37].

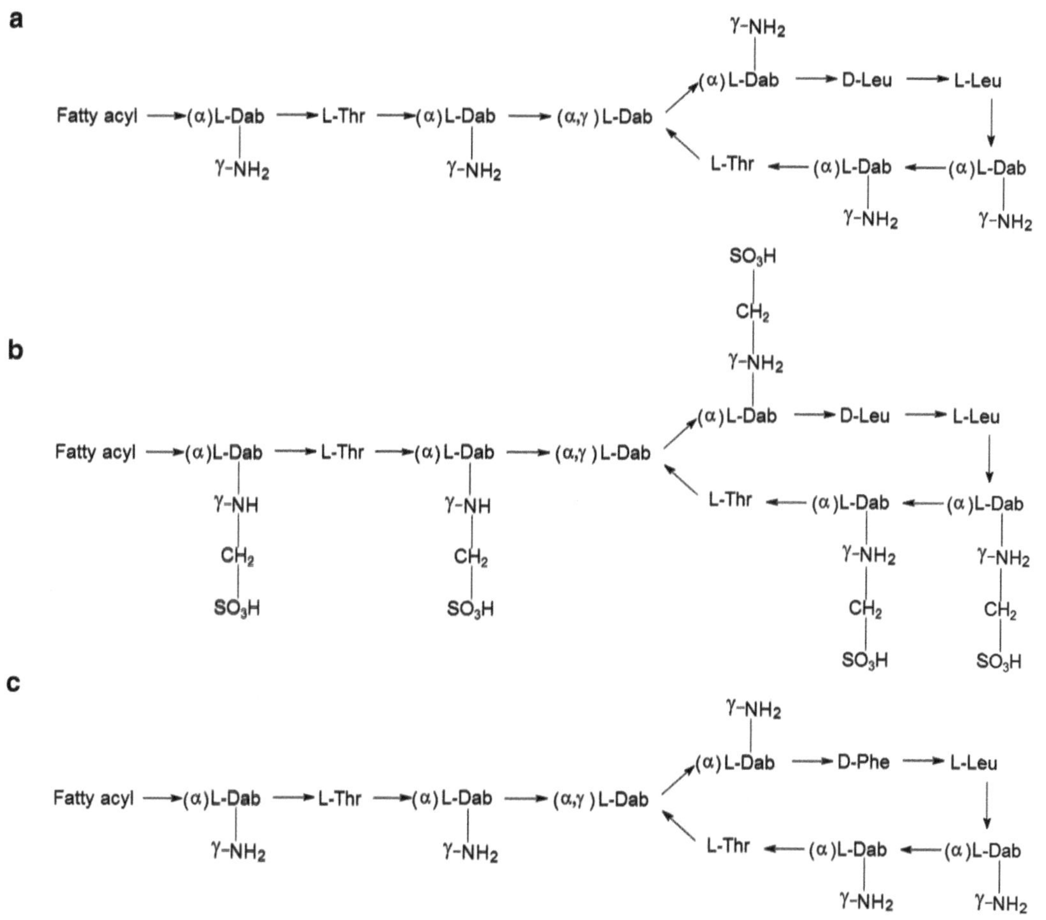

Fig. 1 The chemical structure of colistin (**a**), colistin methanesulfonate (**b**) and polymyxin B (**c**). Colistin A/ polymyxin B1: fatty acyl—6-methyloctanoic acid, colistin B/polymyxin B2: fatty acyl—6-methylheptanoic acid. Dab—L-α,γ-diaminobutyric acid

Harmonized limits on the minimum amount of colistin A and B together with three minor components in colistin products (≥77 % of the total content) have been established in the European (Ph. Eur) and British Pharmacopoeias (BP) [38, 39]. Similar limits have been established for polymyxin B, with both the Ph. Eur and BP establishing that no less than 80 % of total content is to consist of polymyxin B1, B2, and two minor components [38, 39]. Notably, similar composition limits for colistin or polymyxin B are absent from the United States Pharmacopeia (USP) [40].

2.2 Colistin Methanesulfonate: An Inactive Prodrug of Colistin

An important distinction between the two clinically used polymyxins is their administered form. Polymyxin B is administered parenterally as its sulfate salt while colistin is administered as the sodium salt of colistin methanesulfonate (CMS; also called colistimethate sodium, pentasodium colistimethanesulfate, and colistin sulfonyl methate) (Fig. 1) [41]. CMS is not a colistin salt but rather a derivative of colistin where free γ-amino groups of L-

Dab residues within colistin are reacted with formaldehyde followed by sodium bisulfite [42, 43]. Variations in the number and position of γ-amino groups substituted by methanesulfonate (32 possible variations arising from five available substitution sites), coupled with the variability in the ratios of colistin components (Sect. 2.1) contribute to the complexity of CMS as a prodrug. Currently, none of the Ph. Eur, BP, and USP has established limits on the minimum or maximum amount of each potential sulfomethylated derivative within a CMS product. Differences in the composition of CMS products may be responsible for the observed variability in PK of formed colistin following intravenous administration of different CMS products [44]. In aqueous media including plasma, the methanesulfonate groups on CMS are cleaved to yield a mixture of partially sulfomethylated colistin derivatives and colistin itself [44–55]. Importantly, CMS does not exhibit any antimicrobial activity with observed antibacterial effects attributable to the gradual conversion of CMS to colistin via cleavage of methanesulfonate groups [46]; CMS is thus an inactive prodrug of colistin. Stability studies conducted with CMS have shown that it undergoes conversion to colistin at physiological temperatures (20 % conversion to colistin within 12 h at 37 °C) and even at temperatures as low as −20 °C (a sample initially containing 2.0 μg/mL CMS and no detectable colistin when stored for 2 months at −20 °C was found to contain ~0.4 μg/mL colistin and ~1.4 μg/mL CMS) [56]. Thus, CMS can undergo conversion to colistin not only in vivo but also in vitro. This complicates the quantification of CMS and colistin in biological fluids. Specifically, unless care is taken ongoing conversion of the inactive prodrug CMS to the active drug colistin elevates colistin concentrations and lowers CMS concentrations within samples, which has the potential to lead to spurious conclusions about the PK and PD of CMS/colistin [56]. Inaccurate PK and PD data relating to CMS/colistin from studies which have not prevented in vitro CMS conversion, in particular those studies employing microbiological assays for measurement of "colistin" concentrations, remain in the published literature [57–59] and the Product Information for parenteral products of CMS. The PK and PD implications arising from the chemistry of CMS and the conversion of this inactive prodrug to colistin are discussed in detail in Sect. 4.

3 Spectrum of Activity, and Mechanisms of Antibacterial Activity, Resistance, and Toxicology

3.1 Spectrum of Activity and Susceptibility Testing

It is important to recognize that although colistin is administered parenterally as CMS, activity results from the formation of colistin, not CMS or its partially sulfomethylated derivatives [46]. As both colistin and polymyxin B are structurally very similar (Sect. 2.1), they share similar in vitro potencies (as measured by minimum inhibitory concentrations [MIC]) [60]. They are active against a range of common gram-negative organisms but have limited activity against gram-positive organisms. The binding selectivity of polymyxins to lipopolysaccharide (LPS), which is present in the outer membrane (OM) of gram-negative organisms but absent in gram-positive organisms, is the likely cause of poor activity against gram-positive bacteria [61].

In recently conducted large-scale surveillance studies of antimicrobial susceptibility (Table 1), polymyxins demonstrated excellent antimicrobial activity ($MIC_{90} \leq 2$ mg/L) against problematic multidrug-resistant organisms such as *P. aeruginosa*, *Acinetobacter* spp., and *Klebsiella* spp. [60, 62–64]. Polymyxins are also active ($MIC_{90} \leq 2$ mg/L) against a number of other bacterial species including *Escherichia coli*, *Enterobacter* spp. and *Citrobacter freundii* [60, 62, 64, 65]. It should be noted that although resistance rates to colistin and polymyxin B remained stable against most clinical isolates between 2006 and 2009, a minor increase in resistance rates for *K. pneumoniae* was reported in Latin America and Asia [60]; it is possible that a lack of PK/PD knowledge resulting in suboptimal use of polymyxins contributed to this increase. The incorporation of novel PK/PD insights into therapy with polymyxins will be critical to the ongoing maintenance of their activity against problematic nosocomial pathogens [66].

3.2 Mode of Action

As colistin and polymyxin B are structurally very similar (Sect. 2.1) and display a high degree of cross-resistance [12, 60, 67–69], they are believed to share the same mechanism of antibacterial action. References to the "polymyxins" in this section thus apply to both colistin and polymyxin B. Although the mechanism of action of polymyxin antibiotics has not been fully elucidated, several interactions critical to polymyxin activity have been identified. The initial target of the polymyxins against gram-negative bacteria is LPS, the principal component of the outer leaflet of the OM. Interaction is initiated by electrostatic attraction between the cationic amine functionalities on polymyxin Dab amino acid residues and the anionic phosphate and carboxylate functionalities on the lipid A and core-oligosaccharide LPS domains [70–72]. The electrostatic attraction of polymyxins for LPS is at least three orders of magnitude higher than the native divalent cations (Ca^{2+} and Mg^{2+}) which stabilize the OM [73, 74], competitively displacing them from lipid A and enabling the hydrophobic fatty acyl tail and D-Phe-L-Leu (polymyxin B) or D-Leu-L-Leu (colistin) hydrophobic domains of the polymyxin molecule to be inserted into the OM. Although subsequent events are not completely understood this process is believed to weaken the packing of adjacent lipid A fatty acyl chains causing considerable disruption and further permeabilization of the membrane, including to the peptide itself, a process termed

Table 1
Summary of large-scale antimicrobial surveillance studies published from 2010 to 2014

Reference	Year	Polymyxin form	Method	Species	No. of isolates	MIC breakpoint used (mg/L) S	MIC breakpoint used (mg/L) R	No. of resistant isolates (%)		MIC_{50} (mg/L)	MIC_{90} (mg/L)	Range (mg/L)
Hawser et al. [63]	2010	Colistin	Broth microdilution	*Klebsiella pneumoniae*	303	≤2	>2	8	(2.6)	0.25	0.5	≤0.12–>4.0
Gales et al. [60]	2011	Colistin	Broth microdilution	*Acinetobacter* spp.	4686	≤2	≥4	42	(0.9)	≤0.5	1.0	–
				E. coli	17,035	≤2	>2	34	(0.2)	≤0.5	≤0.5	–
				Klebsiella spp.	9774	≤2	>2	147	(1.5)	≤0.5	≤0.5	–
				P. aeruginosa	9130	≤2	>4	37	(0.4)	1	1	–
		Polymyxin B	Broth microdilution	*Acinetobacter* spp.	4686	≤2	≥4	37	(0.8)	≤0.5	≤0.5	–
				E. coli	17,035	≤2	>2	17	(0.1)	≤0.5	≤0.5	–
				Klebsiella spp.	9774	≤2	>2	137	(1.4)	≤0.5	≤0.5	–
				P. aeruginosa	9130	≤2	>4	9	(0.1)	1	1	–
Lee et al. [205]	2011	Colistin	Broth microdilution	*P. aeruginosa*	215	≤2	≥8	16	(7.4)	2	2	–
		Polymyxin B	Broth microdilution	*P. aeruginosa*	215	≤2	≥8	0	(0.0)	1	2	–
Gales et al. [62]	2012	Colistin	Not specified	*Acinetobacter* spp.	845	≤2	≥4	10	(1.2)	≤0.5	1	≤0.5–>4
				Enterobacter spp.	451	≤2	>2	78	(17.3)	≤0.5	>4	≤0.5–>4
				E. coli	1517	≤2	>2	3	(0.2)	≤0.5	≤0.5	≤0.5–>4
				Klebsiella spp.	1052	≤2	≥8	32	(3.0)	≤0.5	≤0.5	≤0.5–>4
				P. aeruginosa	1099	≤2	≥8	1	(0.1)	1	2	≤0.5–>4

Queenan et al. [206]	2012	Colistin	Broth microdilution	*Acinetobacter* spp.	514	≤2	≥4	27	(5.3)	1	2	0.12–>32
Jones et al. [207]	2013	Colistin	Broth microdilution	*P. aeruginosa*	586	≤2	≥8	0	(0.0)	1	2	≤0.25–4
Zhanel et al. [65]	2013	Colistin	Broth microdilution	*E. coli*	5451	–	–	–	–	0.25	0.5	≤0.06–>16
				ESBL *E. coli*	231	–	–	–	–	0.5	1	≤0.06–4
				P. aeruginosa	2183	≤2	≥8	24	(1.1)	2	2	≤0.06–>16
				K. pneumoniae	1659	–	–	–	–	0.5	1	≤0.06–>16
				E. cloacae	637	–	–	–	–	0.5	>16	≤0.06–>16
				P. mirabilis	415	–	–	–	–	>16	>16	0.5–>16
				K. oxytoca	411	–	–	–	–	0.5	1	0.12–>16
				S. marcescens	412	–	–	–	–	>16	>16	0.5–>16
				S. maltophilia	378	–	–	–	–	8	>16	0.25–>16
				E. aerogenes	163	–	–	–	–	0.5	1	0.12–16
				C. freundii	123	–	–	–	–	0.5	0.5	0.12–1
				A. baumannii	104	≤2	≥4	3	(3.2)	1	2	0.25–>16
Nakamura et al. [64]	2014	Colistin	Broth microdilution	*E. coli*	174	≤2	>2	7	(4.0)	0.5	2	–
				K. pneumoniae	37	≤2	>2	5	(13.5)	0.5	2	–

"self-promoted uptake" [75]. That polymyxin B nonapeptide (which does not contain a fatty acyl tail) and CMS (which has methanesulfonate moieties masking the primary amines) are devoid of antimicrobial activity highlights the importance of both the hydrophobic and electrostatic interactions between polymyxins and the bacterial OM. Once the OM has been breached, polymyxins interact with anionic phospholipids of the cytoplasmic membrane in a process driven by electrostatic and hydrophobic interactions [71, 76, 77]. This once again is believed to lead to membrane disruption and increased permeability, causing membrane depolarization and leakage of cell contents [61].

While it was originally proposed that the permeabilization of bacterial cell membranes and subsequent leakage of cell contents was the sole mode of action of the polymyxins, alternative mechanisms of action have been suggested [71, 76, 78–86]. In an effort to better understand the mechanism(s) of action, several studies have examined the potential downstream effects of polymyxins following uptake into bacterial cells. Notably, inhibition by polymyxin B of enzymes critical for cellular respiration such as NADH-quinone oxidoreductase and NADH dehydrogenase [78], as well as inhibition of translation [85] have been demonstrated and proposed as additional mechanisms of action. The formation of reactive oxygen species (ROS) has also been implicated as a potential mechanism of action for polymyxins [79], although doubts about the importance of ROS to antimicrobial activity have been raised [87]. The loss of the compositional specificity of each membrane resulting in an osmotic imbalance in the absence of cell lysis or cytoplasmic leakage [80–83] and the arrest of cell proliferation [84] have also been suggested as possible mechanisms of action. However, the precise mechanism(s) by which polymyxins ultimately kill bacterial cells is still unknown and awaits further investigations.

3.3 Mechanisms of Resistance

Mechanisms of polymyxin resistance were initially investigated in the 1970s and revisited recently following the increase in clinical use of polymyxins. To date the resistance mechanisms identified in gram-negative bacteria have focused on attenuation of the initial binding between polymyxins and LPS (see Sect. 3.1); although resistance via the synthesis of colistinase has been reported in *Pa polymyxa* ssp. *colistinus*, this resistance mechanism has not been identified in any other bacterial strain [88]. The similarities in the mechanism of action between polymyxin B and colistin give rise to cross-resistance between the two antibiotics [12, 60, 67–69].

In *K. pneumoniae*, upregulation in capsule polysaccharide gene expression led to increased polymyxin resistance [89]. It has been proposed that capsule polysaccharide functions as a barrier preventing binding of polymyxins to LPS situated on the OM of gram-negative bacteria [90]. Modifications to the composition of the OM have also been shown to confer resistance to polymyxins. The first involves the substitution of phosphate groups on the lipid A component of LPS with 4-amino-4-deoxy-L-arabinose or phosphoethanolamine, reducing the overall negative charge on lipid A and attenuating the initial electrostatic interaction between the bacterium and polymyxin [91–93]. As a consequence, binding to the outer membrane and subsequent self-promoted uptake is reduced or inhibited. This substitution has been shown to be regulated by two-component regulatory systems such as PhoP-PhoQ and PmrA-PmrB [94–96], that are upregulated in response to polymyxins and elevated cation concentrations, and have been observed in *Acinetobacter baumannii*, *P. aeruginosa*, *K. pneumoniae*, *Salmonella enterica*, and *E. coli*. A second mechanism which to date has only been observed in *A. baumannii* involves the total loss of LPS from the OM caused by a point mutation in the *lpx* gene [97]. Polymyxin heteroresistance (the presence of preexisting resistant subpopulations within an isolate that is susceptible based upon its minimum inhibitory concentration [MIC]) has been identified in *A. baumannii*, *P. aeruginosa*, *Enterobacter cloacae*, and *K. pneumoniae* [98–105]. As discussed in Sect. 5.2, the resistant subset of the bacterial population is amplified during polymyxin treatment resulting in significant bacterial regrowth [99, 105, 106].

3.4 Toxicity

Nephrotoxicity, though almost always reversible, represents the key dose-limiting toxicity associated with polymyxin therapy [107–109]. Concerns regarding nephrotoxicity were primarily responsible for the decline in polymyxin use in the 1970s as newer classes of antibiotics such as the aminoglycosides were introduced into the clinical setting. Studies in critically ill patients have reported a wide range of nephrotoxicity rates. However recent studies report rates of acute kidney injury of ~30–55 % with standard CMS dosages [108, 110–112] and a rate of ~14–42 % for polymyxin B [31, 113–115]. In a study of 173 critically ill patients that compared the incidence of nephrotoxicity following administration of either CMS ($n = 106$) or polymyxin B ($n = 67$), Akajagbor et al. [114] demonstrated lower rates of nephrotoxicity for polymyxin B compared with that of CMS (41.8 % vs. 60.4 %, $p = 0.02$). Another comparative study of CMS and polymyxin B by Phe et al. [115] involving 225 patients with normal renal function (CMS, $n = 121$; polymyxin B, $n = 104$) showed a similar trend, with nephrotoxicity occurring in 23.1 % of polymyxin B treated patients compared with 33.9 % in patients receiving CMS ($p = 0.08$).

While the exact mechanism by which polymyxins cause nephrotoxicity is unknown, studies with polymyxin B have indicated that it induces apoptosis in kidney proximal tubular cells in a concentration-dependent manner [116, 117]. It has been postulated that extensive tubular reabsorption of polymyxin increases intracellular exposure in kidney cells, leading to the nephrotoxicity observed in clinical settings [118]. In animal models various agents including *N*-acetylcysteine, melatonin, ascorbic acid, and heme oxygenase-1 have been reported to have nephroprotective properties when co-administered with polymyxins [119–122]. However, clinical investigations into the co-administration of nephroprotective agents with polymyxins have not been reported and as such the implications of these findings are unclear.

A second but less frequently reported toxicity associated with polymyxins is neurotoxicity including dizziness, weakness, polyneuropathy, facial and peripheral paresthesia, partial deafness, vertigo, visual disturbance, confusion, ataxia, and neuromuscular blockade which can lead to respiratory failure and apnea [123]. Several reports of polymyxin-induced respiratory apnea following intramuscular administration were published in the late 1960s [16, 124, 125], but only three case reports (two for polymyxin B and one for colistin) of neurotoxicity (paraesthesia and apnea) have been published in the last 10 years [126, 127]. However, neurotoxicity may be underreported as many patients requiring polymyxins are sedated and under mechanical ventilation which makes assessment difficult [27]. It has been proposed that polymyxins act presynaptically by interfering with the release of acetylcholine, giving rise to neurotoxicity in a dose-dependent manner [128].

There remains a need to gain a greater understanding of the factors which contribute to both nephrotoxicity and neurotoxicity arising from the polymyxins and to investigate potential strategies for minimizing or removing the risk of toxicity. This would increase the therapeutic index of these agents and allow administration of higher daily doses to more effectively kill bacteria and suppress emergence of resistance.

4 Pharmacokinetics

The majority of investigations into the PK of polymyxins have examined CMS and colistin and can be broadly classified by polymyxin quantification methods. Prior to the relatively recent introduction of high-performance liquid chromatography (HPLC) and liquid chromatography tandem mass spectrometry (LC-MS and LC-MS/MS) assays for the quantification of polymyxin concentrations [129–137], measurements were performed using microbiological assays [57, 58]. However, quantification by microbiological assay of either "CMS" or "colistin" following administration of CMS is unable to differentiate between colistin present in the sample at the time of collection from that formed subsequently from CMS during the incubation period of the assay [46]. Such a situation results in an underestimation of the concentration of CMS in the sample and, most importantly, an overestimation of the colistin concentration. A second key shortcoming in microbiological assays is their poor specificity, particularly in samples containing one or more co-administered antibiotics which are commonplace in critically ill patients. As the information provided by microbiological assays may not be a true reflection of the time-course of polymyxin plasma concentrations, only research articles that have utilized chromatographic polymyxin quantification methods have been included in this review.

4.1 Polymyxin Pharmacokinetics in Animals

The PK of polymyxins in animals has been primarily characterized in rodents, which are routinely used to investigate polymyxin microbiological activity and nephrotoxicity. As is the case in humans (discussed below), both colistin and polymyxin B are cleared primarily via non-renal routes of elimination (Figs. 2 and 3) [47, 48, 50, 118, 138, 139]. In rats, intravenously administered colistin (sulfate; 1 mg/kg) was shown to undergo extensive reabsorption in the renal tubules by a carrier-mediated process,

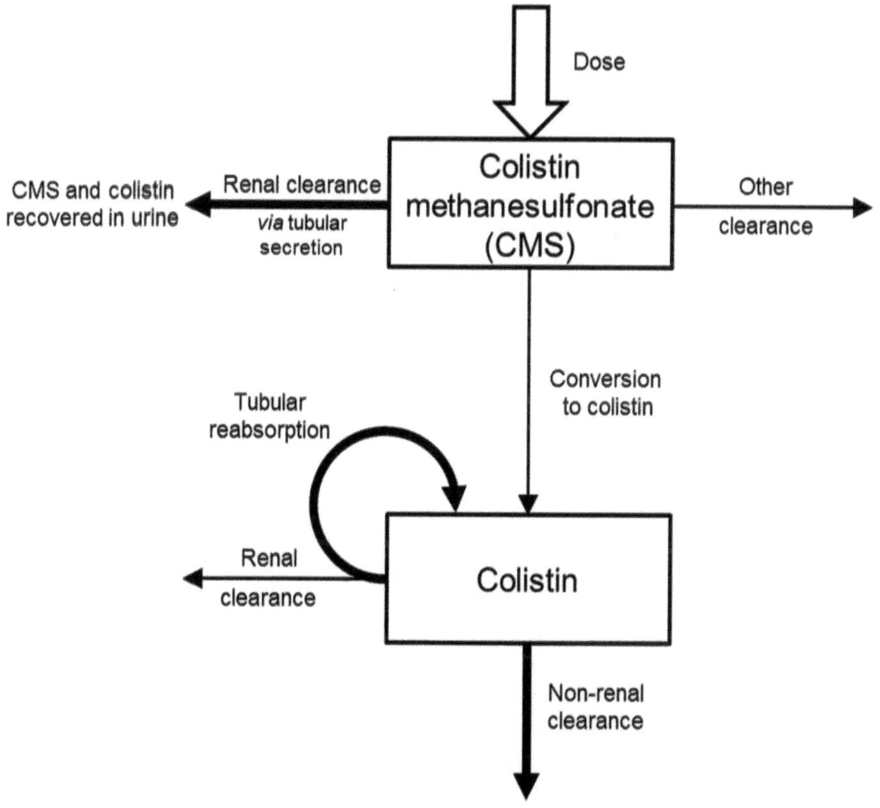

Fig. 2 Schematic of the processes that influence the disposition of formed colistin following administration of CMS. The relative magnitudes of pathways when kidney function is normal are indicated by the thickness of the *arrows*

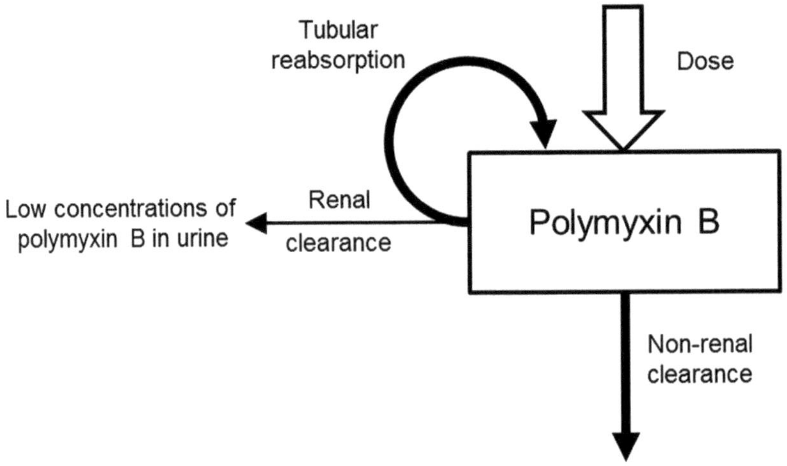

Fig. 3 Schematic of the processes that influence the disposition of polymyxin B. The relative magnitudes of pathways when kidney function is normal are indicated by the thickness of the *arrows*

resulting in less than 1 % of the intravenously administered dose of colistin being recovered in urine [138]. The mean peak colistin concentration (C_{max}) achieved was ~2.5 mg/L at 10 min, which declined to ~0.2 mg/L at 240 min; the mean half-life ($t_{½}$) was ~75 min. A similarly minor contribution of renal clearance to total clearance for polymyxin B has been observed in rats, with less than 1 % of administered polymyxin B (4 mg/kg intravenously; polymyxin B1 free base quantified in urine collected over 48 h) recovered unchanged in urine; the $t_{½}$ was very similar to that of colistin (~87 min) [140]. In mice, Dudhani et al. [141] reported the $t_{½}$ and C_{max} of unbound colistin following subcutaneous administration of colistin (sulfate; dose range 5–40 mg/kg/day) ranged between ~18 min and 85 min and ~0.3 mg/L and 9 mg/L, respectively, increasing in a dose-dependent manner.

Unlike colistin and polymyxin B, it is apparent that CMS undergoes tubular secretion and is predominantly renally cleared (Fig. 2). Subsequent to the initial study by Li et al. [138], where colistin was directly administered to rats, the same authors conducted further studies in which rats were administered CMS intravenously (single intravenous bolus of 15 mg/kg) [47]. The C_{max} of formed colistin was achieved within 10 min indicating rapid conversion of CMS to colistin. The terminal $t_{½}$ of formed colistin was approximately twice that of the administered CMS (55.7 ± 19.3 min versus 23.6 ± 3.9 min) indicating the elimination of colistin is not rate limited by its formation from CMS, and was similar to the $t_{½}$ of colistin administered directly [47, 138]. Comparison of the dose-normalized area under the concentration–time curve (AUC) of colistin which formed following administration of CMS with that of colistin administered directly enabled the fraction of the dose of CMS converted systemically to colistin to be estimated. This comparison revealed that only a very small proportion (~7 %) of administered CMS was converted systemically to colistin. Subsequently, the disposition of formed colistin following CMS administration in rats has shown high inter-manufacturer variability [44, 47, 49]. In a study examining the disposition of formed colistin following administration of CMS from four different manufacturers from three different continents, He et al. [44] observed statistically significant ($p = 0.0121$) differences in colistin $AUC_{0-180\,min}$ between the various CMS manufacturers. The ratio of $AUC_{0-\infty}$ of formed colistin to CMS displayed up to twofold variation between manufacturers (1.68 ± 0.35–3.29 ± 0.43 %). This variation may arise from differences in sulfomethylated colistin derivative content within commercial CMS products, with each derivative potentially having a different elimination or conversion rate. This was an important observation as it demonstrated the different brands of CMS gave rise to different exposures to the microbiologically active formed colistin despite each having similar elemental compositions. Notably, the conversion of CMS to colistin appeared to occur at a faster rate compared to in vitro conversion, suggesting the potential contribution of mechanisms other than spontaneous chemical hydrolysis toward the in vivo conversion of CMS to colistin [44, 47].

4.2 Clinical Pharmacokinetics of Polymyxins

Both CMS and polymyxin B are most commonly administered to patients intravenously, especially in the case of critically ill patients. The largest published clinical PK study ($n = 105$) examining the disposition of colistin following intravenous CMS administration in critically ill patients (median daily dose of colistin base activity [CBA], 200 mg; range, 75–410 mg) identified an inverse relationship between average steady-state concentrations ($C_{ss,avg}$) of formed colistin and creatinine clearance (CrCL) [50]. This relationship stems from a reduction in the renal clearance of CMS increasing its availability for conversion to colistin; thus the apparent clearance of formed colistin correlates with creatinine clearance. However, renal impairment did not have any direct influence on colistin elimination, with a terminal $t_{½}$ of ~10–13 h across a wide range of CrCL values. The terminal $t_{½}$ of colistin was longer than that of CMS resulting in smaller peak to trough fluctuations when compared to CMS (Fig. 4), with the $C_{ss,avg}$ for formed colistin in patients ranging from 0.48 to 9.38 mg/L (median, 2.36 mg/L). Smaller-scale studies investigating the PK of colistin following intravenous administration of CMS in critically ill patients found no association with renal function, probably due to the smaller sample sizes and exclusion of patients with low creatinine clearance values [52, 53]. In these studies the reported $t_{½}$ of CMS was ~2.2 h and for colistin between 14.4 and 18.0 h. A notable exception is the study by Imberti et al. [55] in critically ill patients ($n = 13$)

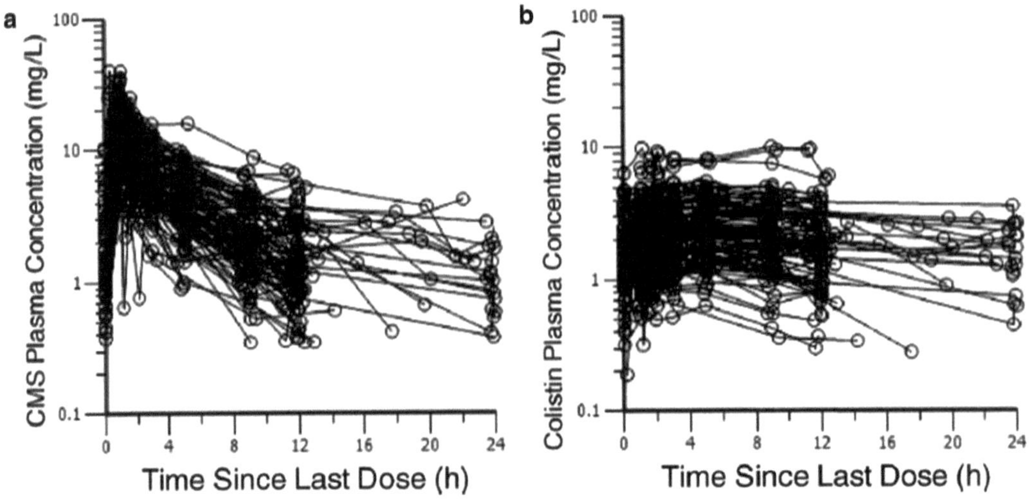

Fig. 4 Steady-state plasma concentration–time profiles of CMS (**a**) and formed colistin (**b**) in 105 critically ill patients (89 not on renal replacement, 12 on intermittent hemodialysis and four on continuous renal replacement therapy), illustrating the relatively level PK profiles for formed colistin concentrations in contrast to the pronounced peak and trough seen in CMS concentrations [50]. Copyright © 2011, American Society for Microbiology. All Rights Reserved

where a comparatively short $t_{½}$ of 5.9 ± 2.6 h for formed colistin was reported.

Differences in the disposition of colistin have been observed in various patient groups other than the critically ill. In burns patients administered CMS, the population $t_{½}$ of formed colistin was 6.6 h, shorter than observed in critically ill patients [54]. Li et al. [48] investigated 12 patients with CF receiving intravenous CMS (1–2 million IU [equivalent to 30–60 mg CBA] 8-hourly). Colistin was rapidly formed in vivo, while steady-state C_{max} ($C_{max,SS}$) ranges for CMS and colistin in plasma were 3.6–13.2 mg/L and 1.2–3.1 mg/L, respectively. The $t_{½}$ of formed colistin at steady state was approximately twice that of the administered CMS (4.2 ± 1.3 h versus 2.1 ± 0.87 h) and considerably shorter than reported in critically ill patients. In healthy young adult volunteers administered CMS (1 million IU [equivalent to 30 mg CBA] infused over 1 h), the mean $t_{½}$ of CMS and colistin was 2 h and 3 h respectively, with corresponding C_{max} values of 4.8 and 0.83 mg/L [142]. Importantly, in this study ~70 % of the administered dose of CMS was excreted in the urine as both CMS and colistin, the latter very likely having formed in the urinary tract. This is a very similar finding to that of Li et al. [47] in rats and arises because the renal clearance of CMS is substantially higher than the conversion clearance of CMS to colistin. In light of these findings, conclusions arising from PK studies conducted using CMS/colistin are not applicable to polymyxin B, as the latter is not administered as a prodrug. Across all reviewed articles, reported plasma colistin concentrations following intravenous administration of CMS in patients tended to range between 1.0 and 10.0 mg/L, with the majority of measured concentrations below 5.0 mg/L [48, 50, 52–54].

Polymyxins may also be administered by inhalation, a route of administration common in patients with CF but also increasingly used for patients suffering pneumonia [143, 144]. Following administration by inhalation, both CMS and colistin are well localized in the lungs, although a small amount of systemic absorption may occur [145–147]. Consequently, high colistin concentrations are achieved within bronchoalveolar lavage (BAL) fluid or sputum with significantly lower concentrations observed systemically. A pharmacokinetic study examining CMS (2 million IU; equivalent to ~60 mg CBA) inhalation in CF patients reported peak concentrations of formed colistin (polymyxin E1 quantified) (C_{max}) in sputum and plasma of ~40 mg/L and 0.17 mg/L, respectively [148], while a separate study investigating the disposition of colistin after inhalation of CMS (1 million IU; equivalent to ~30 mg CBA) in critically ill patients observed a colistin C_{max} in epithelial lining fluid of 6.7 and 1.6 mg/L in plasma [149]. In a crossover study that compared the disposition of formed colistin following intravenous (dose equivalent to 150 mg CBA) and inhaled CMS (two dose levels equivalent to 60 and 120 mg CBA) in 6 CF patients, Yapa et al. [147] evaluated the ratio of dose normalized $AUC_{0-12\,h}$ in sputum and plasma following nebulized CMS administration divided by the same ratio following intravenous administration to obtain a drug targeting index (DTI). Nebulization of CMS resulted in relatively high sputum concentrations of CMS and formed colistin compared to those resulting from IV administration, with a DTI of 15952 and 31 for CMS and formed colistin, respectively. This result demonstrated the effective targeting of CMS and formed colistin delivery to the lungs in CF patients via inhalation, with very low exposure to these compounds in the systemic circulation thereby potentially sparing the kidneys.

Compared to CMS/colistin, far fewer clinical studies have examined the PK of intravenous polymyxin B in critically ill patients. The largest published clinical PK study ($n = 24$) reported a population mean $t_{½}$ for polymyxin B of 11.9 h, with a population $C_{ss,avg}$ of 2.79 ± 0.9 mg/L (range 0.68–4.88 mg/L) [118]; the dose range of intravenous polymyxin B in this study was 0.45–3.38 mg/kg/day. Similar results have been reported in several smaller clinical studies [139, 150, 151]. Sandri et al. [139] examined the disposition of polymyxin B in 2 patients on renal replacement therapy and found that the PK of polymyxin B in this patient group and non-renally impaired patients [118] were similar. Clearly, there is an urgent need for larger studies on the clinical PK of polymyxin B. Additionally, there is also a significant gap in information available pertaining to the disposition of polymyxin B following inhalation and further research is required to ensure its judicious use in the treatment of pneumonia [152].

The difference in the administered form of the two polymyxins has a profound impact on their overall disposition in patients. Specifically, colistin formation and thus exposure (as measured by AUC_{0-t}) is dependent upon the interplay between the in vivo conversion of colistin from CMS and the relatively more efficient renal clearance of the prodrug (Fig. 2). This situation leads to a slow rise in colistin plasma concentrations after initiation of CMS therapy, even when loading doses are employed [52]. In contrast the disposition of polymyxin B is relatively simple (Fig. 3) compared to that of CMS/colistin owing to its administration in the form of the active species. This enables steady-state concentrations of polymyxin B to be rapidly achieved with loading doses [118]. Given the importance of AUC to the activity of polymyxins (Sect. 5.3), it has been proposed that compared to CMS/colistin, the clinical PK properties of polymyxin B are better suited to achieving optimal polymyxin activity for those infections where it is important to rapidly and reliably attain antibacterial concentrations in the systemic circulation [41]. CMS may be expected to be a better option than polymyxin B for treatment of urinary tract infections due to the relatively high concentrations of CMS (and subsequently formed colistin) within the urinary tract (Fig. 2) [41]. Further clinical studies are required to examine and identify potential differences in the relative clinical efficacy between the two polymyxins for different types of infections.

5 Pharmacodynamics of Polymyxins

5.1 Susceptibility Testing

At present, globally harmonized susceptibility breakpoints for polymyxins have not been established and there remains variation in the breakpoints set between laboratory standards organizations for various bacterial species (Table 2). This situation is further complicated by a lack of standardization of in vitro testing methods. MIC determinations are routinely performed for polymyxins by disk diffusion, agar dilution, broth microdilution, and E-test methods, with the latter three methods showing high concordance [98, 153–155]. CMS should not be used for MIC determination as it is an inactive prodrug which undergoes gradual conversion to colistin (Sect. 2.2); all currently available breakpoints for colistin susceptibility are for colistin sulfate.

5.2 In Vitro Pharmacodynamics of Polymyxins

The majority of in vitro studies examining the PD of polymyxins (both static and dynamic [PK/PD] time-kill models) have used colistin. The rate and extent of polymyxin-induced bacterial killing

Table 2
Summary of susceptibility breakpoints for colistin and polymyxin B

Laboratory Organization	Version (Year)	Drug	*Entero bacteriaceae* S	I	R	*Pseudomonas* spp.[a] S	I	R	*Acinetobacter* spp. S	I	R	Other Non-*Entero bacteriaceae* S	I	R
			Susceptibility breakpoints (mg/L)[b]											
EUCAST	Ver. 4.0 (2014)	Colistin	≤2	–	>2	≤4	–	>4	≤2	–	>2	–	–	–
CLSI	M100-S23 (2013)	Colistin and Polymyxin B	–	–	–	≤2	4	≥8	≤2	–	≥4	≤2	4	≥8
BSAC	Ver. 12 (2013)	Colistin	≤2	–	>2	≤4	–	>4	≤2	–	>2	–	–	–

[a]CLSI M100-S23 contains separate sections for *P. aeruginosa* and *Pseudomonas* spp. with identical breakpoints; either breakpoint may be altered in future versions of CLSI M100
[b]*S* susceptible, *I* intermediate, *R* resistant, – no breakpoint determined

increases in a concentration-dependent manner [67, 99, 105, 106, 156–159]. At concentrations near or above the MIC of an isolate rapid bacterial killing of several Log_{10} colony forming units per mL (CFU/mL) is observed within as little as 5 min; this is shown in Fig. 5 for *K. pneumoniae* and is similar in other relevant gram-negative pathogens such as *P. aeruginosa* and *A. baumannii* [99, 105, 106]. Polymyxins are subject to an inoculum effect such that both the rate and extent of killing are markedly attenuated at high bacterial inocula [67, 103, 160–163]. Through the use of mathematical modeling Bulitta et al. [160] found that the rate of bacterial killing by colistin against *P. aeruginosa* decreased with increasing inocula, with killing of susceptible bacterial populations sixfold slower at an inoculum of 10^8 CFU/mL and 23-fold slower at an inoculum of 10^9 CFU/mL compared to an inoculum of 10^6 CFU/mL. Additionally, the concentration of colistin required to achieve a ≥3-Log_{10} CFU/mL reduction in the bacterial population was up to 32-fold higher at the 10^9 CFU/mL inoculum compared to the 10^6 CFU/mL inoculum. The inoculum effect remains in need of further investigation as neither the biological mechanisms which underpin this effect nor its clinical implications are fully understood. However, the existing data suggest a potential need for higher colistin exposure or combination regimens when treating infections with high inocula.

Despite initial rapid and extensive bacterial killing a consistent finding with polymyxin monotherapy is bacterial regrowth following a delay of between 6 and 24 h, even at exposures well beyond

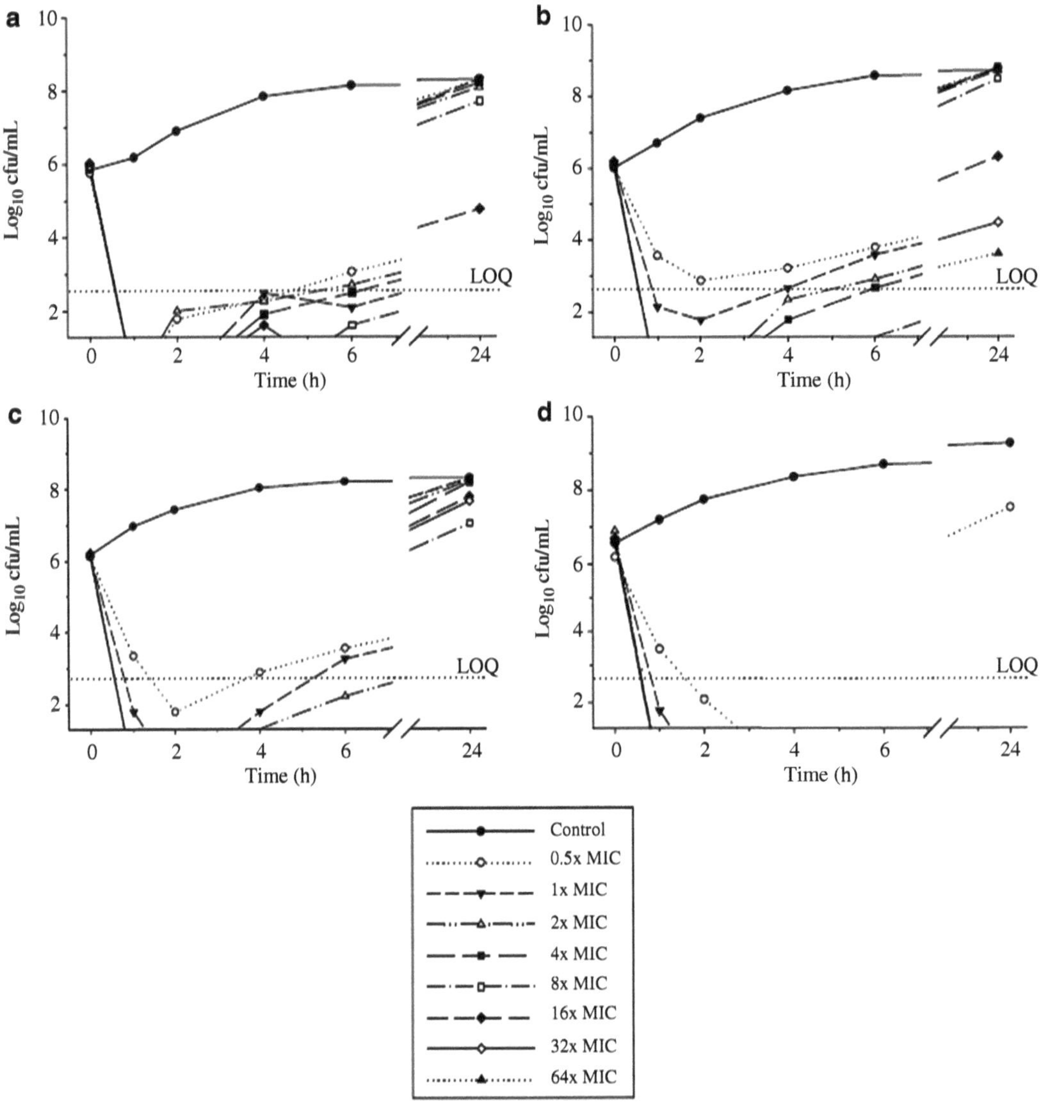

Fig. 5 Killing curves of colistin against four colistin-susceptible or -heteroresistant isolates of *K. pneumoniae*: (**a**) colistin-heteroresistant reference strain (ATCC 13883, MIC of 1 mg/L), (**b**) colistin-heteroresistant clinical isolate (MIC of 0.125 mg/L), (**c**) colistin-heteroresistant clinical isolate (MIC of 1 mg/L), and (**d**) colistin-susceptible clinical isolate (MIC of 1 mg/L). The *y*-axis begins from the limit of detection and the limit of quantification (LOQ) is indicated by the *dotted horizontal line*. Reproduced from Poudyal et al. [99] with permission from Oxford University Press

clinically achievable concentrations (e.g., up to 200 mg/L) [156]. Such regrowth has been reported for *P. aeruginosa* [67, 103, 160, 163, 164], *K. pneumoniae* [99, 101, 162] and *A. baumannii* [100, 106, 158, 161, 165]. In these and other bacterial species, population analysis profiles have revealed a small proportion of preexistent colistin-resistant cells in many clinical isolates deemed susceptible based upon MIC testing (i.e., colistin heteroresistance). The combined contribution of constitutive (amplification of preexisting resistant subpopulations—see Sect. 3.3) and adaptive resistance mechanisms have been proposed by the authors of these studies as an explanation for the observed regrowth [67, 99, 105, 106, 156, 157]. Such observations suggest that emergence of colistin resistance may occur with colistin monotherapy. As discussed below, polymyxin combination therapy has been suggested as a means to enhance bacterial killing and minimize the emergence of resistance [50, 166–168].

The magnitude of the post-antibiotic effect (PAE) following polymyxin exposure varies between bacterial species. A modest PAE has been reported with high concentrations of colistin against *P. aeruginosa* and *K. pneumoniae* [99, 106, 157], while uncertainty surrounds the presence of a PAE for colistin against *A. baumannii* [106, 169]. Against *P. aeruginosa*, a PAE of 2–3 h was noted in three isolates at colistin concentrations of 16× MIC after a 15 min exposure [157]. In *K. pneumoniae*, a smaller PAE of 1.6 h was reported against reference strain ATCC 13883 at 64× MIC while no PAE was observed in any of 21 clinical isolates tested [99, 169]. Conflicting PAE values have been published in the literature for *A. baumannii* [106]. Owen et al. [106] reported a modest PAE (1.0 h at 16× MIC, 2.3 h at 32× MIC, and 3.5 h at 64× MIC) for colistin against *A. baumannii* ATCC 19606 following a 20-min exposure, but negative PAE values (−0.8 to −8.15 h) in 5 clinical isolates examined. In contrast, Plachouras et al. [169] observed a significant PAE (3.9 h at 1× MIC and 4.48 h at 4× MIC across 19 isolates) against *A. baumannii* following a 5-h exposure to colistin. It should be noted that the length of colistin exposure differed significantly between the two studies, which may have contributed to the variation in magnitude of the PAE. Clinically, the implications of polymyxin PAE are unclear particularly as both colistin and polymyxin B have a long $t_{½}$ that reduces the magnitude of fluctuations in polymyxin plasma concentration.

In addition to static time-kill experiments, a small number of studies have utilized dynamic in vitro PK/PD models to simulate the PK of polymyxins in critically ill patients and patients with CF [67, 158, 164]. These experimental models provide critical insights into the influence of dosing regimens on polymyxin PD during therapy, simulating the peaks and troughs in drug concentrations seen during intermittent dosing [170]. In a hollow-fiber infection model Tam et al. [67] investigated the effect of three different polymyxin B dosage regimens involving 8, 12, and 24 h dosage intervals (C_{max} of 5.3 mg/L, 8.0 mg/L, and 16.0 mg/L, respectively) on activity against *P. aeruginosa*. Following extensive initial bacterial killing, substantial regrowth was observed with all regimens even with exposures eight times the recommended daily dose; additionally, the emergence of polymyxin B-resistant colonies was observed following 72 h of polymyxin exposure. Similar observations were made by Bergen et al. [164] and Tan et al. [158] using colistin in a one-compartment PK/PD model against *P. aeruginosa* and *A. baumannii*, respectively. In both these studies overall bacterial killing with three intermittent dosage regimens involving 8, 12, and 24 h dosage intervals (C_{max} of 3.0 mg/L, 4.5 mg/L, or 9.0 mg/L respectively) was similar for each species, although regrowth was much more rapid for *A. baumannii*. Against *P. aeruginosa*, colistin resistance emerged gradually over the 72 h duration of the experiment and was greater with dosing regimens incorporating higher doses of colistin administered less frequently [164]. In contrast, there was rapid and extensive emergence of resistant subpopulations of *A. baumannii* irrespective of the colistin dosage regimen [158].

5.3 Correlation of Pharmacokinetic/Pharmacodynamic Indices with Antibacterial Activity

The dynamic in vitro model studies discussed above highlighted the potential shortfalls of polymyxin monotherapy and provided strong initial evidence that area under the unbound concentration curve to MIC ratio (*f*AUC/MIC) is the PK/PD index most closely correlated with polymyxin activity [67, 158, 164]. That *f*AUC/MIC and not the fC_{max}/MIC or $fT_{>MIC}$ (time for which the unbound concentrations exceed the MIC) was indeed most closely correlated with polymyxin activity (as measured by Log_{10} CFU/mL reductions in the bacterial population) was subsequently confirmed in in vitro [159] and in vivo [141, 165, 171] experiments discussed below. Of these experiments, investigations by Bergen et al. [159] and Dudhani et al. [141, 165] took account of protein binding and employed a dose-fractionation design to better characterize the relationship between the PK and PD of colistin. That bacterial killing for the polymyxins is most closely associated with the *f*AUC/MIC indicates that the time-averaged exposure to polymyxins is more important than attainment of high peak concentrations achieved through the use of larger doses administered less frequently.

Bergen et al. [159] examined 37 different dosage regimens with various colistin C_{max} and dosage intervals (including intermittent dosing and continuous infusion regimens) in an in vitro PK/PD model against three strains of *P. aeruginosa* including a colistin-susceptible MDR strain. Bacterial killing was best correlated with the *f*AUC/MIC ($R^2=0.931$), with weaker correlations observed for $fT_{>MIC}$ ($R^2=0.785$) and fC_{max}/MIC ($R^2=0.868$). For the reference strain *P. aeruginosa* ATCC 27853, the magnitudes of *f*AUC/MIC required to achieve 1- and 2-log_{10} reductions in the area under the CFU/mL curve relative to growth control were determined to be 22.6 and 30.4, respectively. In two in vivo dose-fractionation studies, Dudhani et al. [141, 165] examined colistin against three strains each of *P. aeruginosa* and *A. baumannii* (including MDR but colistin-susceptible strains and, for *A. bau-*

mannii, colistin-heteroresistant strains) in neutropenic murine thigh and lung infection models. Against *P. aeruginosa* colistin exposure induced significant bacterial killing (>3 Log_{10} CFU/mL) over 24 h, with the *f*AUC/MIC (Thigh, $R^2 = 87$ %; Lung, $R^2 = 89$ %) more closely correlated with bacterial killing than the fC_{max}/MIC (Thigh, $R^2 = 66$ %; Lung, $R^2 = 71$ %) and $fT_{>MIC}$ (Thigh, $R^2 = 84$ %; Lung, $R^2 = 88$ %) in both infection models (Fig. 6) [141]. Against *A. baumannii*, initial killing was similarly extensive with the *f*AUC/MIC (Thigh, $R^2 = 90$ %) once again most predictive of antibacterial effect in both the thigh and lung [165]. In this study the emergence of colistin-resistant subpopulations, which was not examined in the study involving *P. aeruginosa* [141], occurred in all three isolates following 24 h of colistin exposure. Against both bacterial species, the target *f*AUC/MIC values to obtain 2 Log_{10} CFU/mL killing were similar to those determined in vitro against *P. aeruginosa* by Bergen et al. [159], although somewhat higher values were required to achieve maximal killing in the lung.

Wang et al. [171] investigated the activity of colistin against both planktonic and biofilm-embedded *P. aeruginosa* in a murine lung biofilm infection model. Unlike the studies of Bergen et al. [159] and Dudhani et al. [141, 165] discussed above, where analysis was based upon unbound or free indices, protein binding was not measured in this study and results were reported based on the time-course of total colistin concentrations. In line with previously published results, the AUC/MIC was most closely correlated with killing of planktonic bacteria; for biofilm-embedded cells, the AUC/minimum biofilm inhibitory concentration [MIBC] best predicted bacterial killing. Notably, the target AUC/MIBC values required to achieve substantial bactericidal activity were significantly higher (~4- to 5-fold) for biofilm-embedded cells compared to the AUC/MIC values for planktonic cells. The differences in bacterial killing observed between planktonic and biofilm-embedded cells in this study, and between thigh and lung infection sites in the investigations by Dudhani et al. [141, 165] indicate that different dosage regimens may be required depending upon the nature and/or site of the infection.

5.4 Polymyxin Combination Therapy

The use of polymyxins in combination with one or more additional antibiotics is increasingly being reported [172–177], although systematic investigations have occurred only recently. As outlined above, regrowth and the emergence of resistance is commonly reported with polymyxin monotherapy even with concentrations far in excess of those which are clinically achievable [48, 50, 52–54, 118, 139, 150, 151]. The amplification of polymyxin-resistant subpopulations in heteroresistant isolates, i.e., isolates which are susceptible to polymyxins based upon their MICs but which contain preexisting resistant subpopulations, is a known contributor

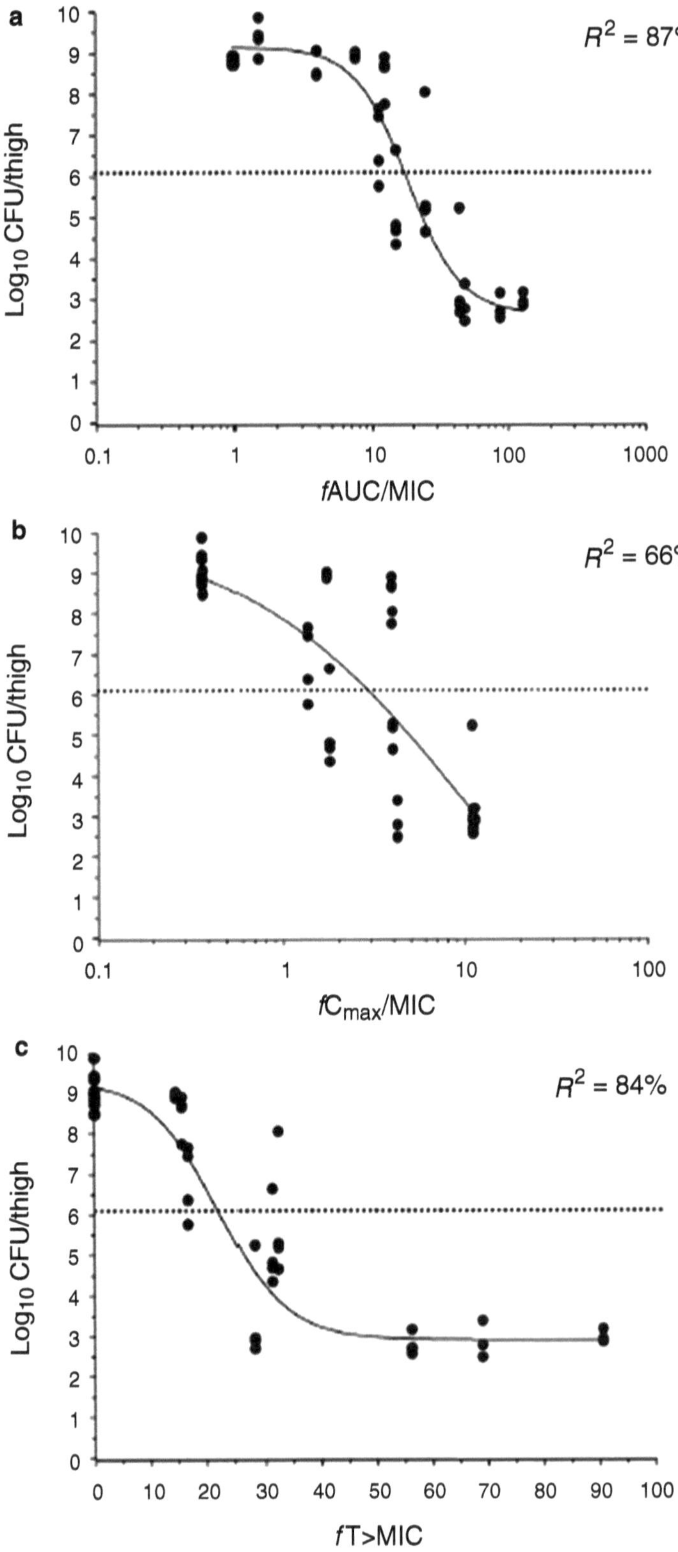

Fig. 6 Relationships for *P. aeruginosa* ATCC 27853 between Log_{10} CFU per thigh at 24 h and the PK/PD indices *f*AUC/MIC (**a**), fC_{max}/MIC (**b**), and $fT_{>MIC}$ (**c**), highlighting the superior predictive performance of *f*AUC/MIC [141].

to the observed regrowth following monotherapy and has been reported for *P. aeruginosa* [67, 103, 160, 163, 164], *K. pneumoniae* [99, 101, 162], and *A. baumannii* [100, 106, 158, 161, 165]; in many of these studies, polymyxin concentrations were well above those of the MIC. These observations suggest selective eradication of the susceptible bacterial population with unopposed regrowth of resistant subpopulations (for example, LPS-deficient *A. baumannii* [97]). Given this situation it is not surprising that polymyxin combination therapy has been suggested as a possible means by which to increase antimicrobial activity and reduce the development of resistance [50, 166–168]. Such a view has been bolstered by the unexpected finding that colistin-resistant strains of MDR *A. baumannii* have increased susceptibility to most tested antibiotics, including those that are normally active only against gram-positive bacteria [178]. It has been suggested that the increased susceptibility of these polymyxin-resistant organisms to antibiotics usually considered effective against only gram-positive bacteria may be due to changes in the outer membrane associated with polymyxin resistance, increasing access of the second antibiotic to its target site [178]. Given these observations two mechanisms have been proposed whereby polymyxins combinations may provide an enhanced PD effect, namely "subpopulation synergy" (where one drug kills the resistant subpopulation(s) of the other drug, and vice versa) and "mechanistic synergy" (two drugs acting on different cellular pathways to increase the rate and/or extent of killing) [179]. Given the "last resort" status of colistin and increasing resistance, systematic investigations of the effect of combination therapy on the emergence of colistin resistance, including on heteroresistant strains, will be crucial for optimal dosage regimen design.

5.4.1 Preclinical Investigations

Only a small number of preclinical studies have examined polymyxin combination therapy in vivo and many of these suffer from a number of significant shortcomings [59, 180–187]. These include ambiguity in the form of colistin administered (colistin sulfate or CMS) and a failure to account for animal scaling in the design of polymyxin dosage regimens. On this latter point the majority of doses administered appear to have been chosen to reflect human doses on a mg/kg basis, failing to take into account the dissimilarities in PK across species from such an approach (specifically, substantially lower plasma concentrations in the preclinical models). Additionally, PK data are almost never provided for the polymyxin or combination drug(s), preventing comparisons with PK profiles achieved in patients. As a result of these major deficiencies animal studies are not considered here.

Numerous in vitro investigations have utilized the fractional inhibitory concentration (FIC) index and Etest methods to examine the PD of polymyxin combination therapy. However, these methods are less discriminatory than other more sophisticated in vitro methods (e.g., static or dynamic [PK/PD] time-kill models; discussed below) for assessing the interactions of antimicrobial agents and are not discussed here [188, 189]. Of the various studies that have utilized static or dynamic time-kill methods to examine polymyxins in combination, the majority have employed colistin against *P. aeruginosa*, *A. baumannii*, or *K. pneumoniae*. The most common antibiotics combined with the polymyxins are the carbapenems [103, 162, 163, 182, 190–195] and rifampicin [59, 161, 192, 193, 195, 196]; others include (but are not limited to) ampicillin/sulbactam [195], ceftazidime [156], ciprofloxacin [59, 156], aminoglycosides [59, 186, 197], glycopeptides [104, 193, 198] and fosfomycin [186, 192, 199]. As summarized above for animal models, there are a number of limitations with many of the in vitro studies. These include use of a single, generally low inoculum (~10^6 CFU/mL or lower), an emphasis on "synergy" as a marker of the success of a particular combination without consideration of the overall antimicrobial activity of the combination, and use of antibiotic concentrations as multiples of the MIC with little reference to, or discussion of, the clinical relevance of the actual concentrations used. Importantly, relatively few studies take into consideration polymyxin heteroresistance or the effect of combinations on the development of polymyxin resistance [103, 161–163, 200]; as these investigations represent the major systematic investigations into polymyxin (specifically colistin) combination therapy and additionally address the other shortcomings noted above, they are the focus of the remainder of this section.

Bergen et al. systematically examined colistin in combination with imipenem (static time-kill model) [103] or doripenem (PK/PD model) [163] at multiple inocula (~10^6 and ~10^8 CFU/mL) against *P. aeruginosa*. Colistin heteroresistant and non-heteroresistant strains and MDR and non-MDR strains were investigated, and a range of clinically achievable concentrations was employed (e.g., constant colistin concentrations of 0.5 or 2 mg/L plus doripenem C_{max} of 2.5 or 25 mg/L every 8 h; half-life, 1.5 h were employed in the PK/PD model). The addition of either imipenem or doripenem to colistin at both inocula generally resulted in substantial improvements in bacterial killing over equivalent monotherapy against MDR *P. aeruginosa* isolates resistant to either antibiotic. An interesting finding across these two studies was the difference in the emergence of colistin resistance with the varying study designs. Using static time-kill methodology, the emergence of colistin-resistant subpopulations with the colistin/imipenem combination generally resulted in a similar increase in colistin-resistant subpopulations across the duration of the experiment (48 h) as observed with equivalent colistin monotherapy [103]. However, when colistin was combined with doripenem in a PK/PD model simulating the unbound (free) plasma concentration–time profiles of each drug in critically ill patients (constant colistin concentrations of 0.5 or 2 mg/L; doripenem C_{max} of 2.5 or 25 mg/L every 8 h; half-life, 1.5 h), the emergence of colistin resistance was greatly reduced across 96 h [163]. While the antibiotics and their concentrations between these two studies are not directly comparable, the activity of colistin combined with either imipenem or doripenem was similar across 48 h (the duration of the colistin/imipenem study) at both inocula against a hetero-resistant reference strain. Together with the differences observed in the emergence of colistin-resistant colonies these observations highlight the importance of simulating PK profiles when assessing the activity and emergence of resistance to antimicrobial therapy.

Subsequent investigations utilizing the same PK/PD model design as Bergen et al. [163] against MDR isolates of *K. pneumoniae* (constant colistin concentrations of 0.5 or 2 mg/L plus doripenem C_{max} of 2.5 or 25 mg/L every 8 h; half-life, 1.5 h) [162] and *A. baumannii* (constant colistin concentrations of 0.5, 2 or 5 mg/L plus rifampicin C_{max} of 5 mg/L every 24 h; half-life, 3 h) [161] likewise resulted in similar substantial (and in many cases dramatic) improvements in bacterial killing at both inocula with synergy ($\geq$2-$\log_{10}$ decrease in the number of CFU/mL between the combination and its most active component) or additivity (a 1.0- to <2-$\log_{10}$ decrease in the number of CFU/mL between the combination and its most active component) observed at the majority of time points at both inocula across the 72 h duration. As was observed against *P. aeruginosa* [163] the colistin–doripenem combination all but eliminated the emergence of colistin-resistant subpopulations against *K. pneumoniae*, with resistant colonies only detected at the lowest concentration combination tested (colistin 0.5 mg/L plus doripenem 2.5 mg/L) at the high (~10^8 CFU/mL) inoculum. Remarkably, all three colistin/rifampicin regimens (colistin 0.5, 2 or 5 mg/L plus rifampicin 5 mg/L) completely suppressed the emergence of colistin-resistant subpopulations in a MDR-colistin-susceptible clinical isolate of *A. baumannii* [161]. Similar findings have recently been reported with a colistin–doripenem combination against both planktonically growing and biofilm-embedded *P. aeruginosa* using a PK/PD biofilm model [200].

One further combination study deserves particular mention. Clancy et al. [201] examined colistin (2 mg/L) in combination with doripenem (8 mg/L) against 23 KPC-2-producing strains of *K. pneumoniae*, each of which contained a variant mutant *opmK35* porin gene. The colistin–doripenem combination was significantly more active against the four strains with doripenem MICs of ≤8 mg/L, whereas there was little difference in killing for strains with doripenem MICs >8 mg/L; improvements in antimicrobial activity were unaffected by colistin MICs (≤2 mg/L or >2 mg/L).

Importantly, while certain variants (e.g., those with insertions encoding glycine and aspartic acid at amino acid (aa) positions 134 and 135 (ins aa134-135 GD; $n = 8$)) were associated with significantly higher doripenem MICs and reduced efficacy of the combination, other mutant/wild-type ompK36 strains demonstrated increased killing with the combination even with elevated doripenem MICs. These results suggest that despite the potentially increased access of doripenem to target sites afforded by disruption of the outer membrane by the polymyxin, allowing hydrolysis by KPC to be overcome, OmpK36 porins may also be necessary for synergy.

In general, the results of the above and other in vitro studies with many drug combinations suggest a potential clinical benefit with polymyxin combination therapy. Two important findings across these studies are that substantial improvements in bacterial killing can be achieved with low (even sub-MIC), clinically achievable polymyxin concentrations even when resistance to one or more of the drugs in combination is present, and that this additionally holds true for many antibiotics that ordinarily have no effect on gram-negative organisms. It may therefore be possible to enhance bacterial killing with polymyxin combination therapy even in patients who achieve low plasma concentrations with standard dosage regimens or, alternatively, to utilize lower-than-normal polymyxin doses to allay toxicity concerns. Additionally, while enhanced bacterial killing in these in vitro models (which lack immune components) was sometimes absent with combination therapy at later time points (e.g., 24 or 48 h), this was often not the case with initial killing (e.g., up to 6 h). This initial response may thus be important in an immunocompetent host whereby the immune system can further facilitate bacterial clearance. On this point there is at least a theoretical difference between the use of colistin (administered as CMS in patients) and polymyxin B (administered as polymyxin B sulfate), with steady-state concentrations of the former attained far more slowly than the latter even with the use of a loading dose (Sect. 4.2). Finally, the study of Clancy et al. [201] cautions against a "one-size-fits-all" approach, highlighting that the specific resistance mechanisms present in different isolates of a bacterial species may dictate the efficacy of particular combination regimens.

5.4.2 Clinical Investigations

Although preclinical investigations suggest potential clinical benefits with polymyxin combination therapy the true value of such combinations must be determined in vivo with well-designed clinical studies. Unfortunately, practical and ethical considerations involved in the study of polymyxin combinations in patients have resulted in major limitations with published clinical studies in this area. These include the retrospective nature of many investigations, low patient numbers, lack of appropriate controls, heterogeneity in the definitions of outcomes (e.g., mortality, bacteriological eradication or clinical cure), variability in dosing regimens and failure to stratify outcomes based on the site and/or severity of illness. Importantly, all but the most recent studies lack PK information on polymyxin B, CMS and formed colistin, and concomitant antibiotics. Such a situation precludes the drawing of strong conclusions from currently available clinical evidence and as a consequence clinical studies are considered here only briefly.

Using a retrospective cohort design, Falagas et al. [202] found no statistically significant difference in clinical response (cure and improvement) and occurrence of nephrotoxicity between patients with MDR gram-negative infections receiving CMS monotherapy ($n = 14$; mean dose of colistin of 4.6 ± 2.3 million international units (IU)/day, equivalent to ~138 ± 69 mg of CBA/day) or CMS–meropenem combination therapy ($n = 57$; mean dose of colistin of 5.5 ± 2.2 million IU/day, equivalent to ~165 ± 66 mg of CBA/day), although there was a favorable association between survival and treatment with CMS monotherapy compared to the CMS–meropenem combination. In a later retrospective cohort study by the same group involving 258 patients infected with MDR gram-negative organisms infection was cured in an equal proportion of patients (83.3 %) who received CMS monotherapy or CMS combined with meropenem, whereas patients treated with CMS combined with piperacillin/tazobactam, ampicillin/sulbactam or other agents had significantly lower rates of infection cure (64.7 %, 75.0 %, and 61.3 %, respectively) [203]. However, univariate analysis revealed that mortality among patients who received an average colistin daily dose of 3 million IU (38.6 %) was higher than among patients who received 6 million IU (27.8 %) or 9 million IU (21.7 %). In contrast, a much smaller review of studies involving a total of 18 patients with infection caused by KPC β-lactamase-producing *K. pneumoniae* treated with polymyxins (CMS or polymyxin B) alone or in combination reported infections were successfully treated in one (14.3 %) of seven patients receiving polymyxin monotherapy and eight (72.7 %) of 11 patients receiving combination therapy (mainly with tigecycline or gentamicin) [204].

More recently Batirel et al. [177] retrospectively investigated various colistin-based therapies against bloodstream infections caused by extremely drug-resistant (XDR) *Acinetobacter* spp.; XDR was defined as non-susceptibility to at least one agent in all but two or more antimicrobial categories. Thirty-six patients received colistin monotherapy (administered as CMS) whereas 214 patients received colistin in combination with another agent (colistin/carbapenem [imipenem, meropenem, or doripenem], $n = 102$; colistin/sulbactam, $n = 69$; colistin/other agent, $n = 43$). Patients with normal renal function received 5 mg CBA/kg/day divided into 2–3 doses; no loading doses were administered. The rates of cure (defined as recovery of all symptoms, signs, and laboratory finding of infection) and 14-day survival were relatively higher in the combination group compared to the monotherapy group (46.3 % vs. 30.6 % and 68.2 % vs. 55.5 %, respectively), and microbiological eradication was significantly higher in the combination group (79.9 % vs. 55.6 %). In-hospital mortality was also significantly lower in the combination group compared to the monotherapy group (52.3 % vs. 72.2 %). There was no significant difference in clinical and microbiological outcomes between the three combination groups. In a multicenter randomized study of 209 patients with infections caused by XDR *A. baumannii*, Durante-Mangoni et al. [174] found a significant increase in the rate of microbiological eradication in those patients receiving a combination of colistin plus rifampicin ($n=104$) compared to colistin "monotherapy" ($n=105$) (60.6 % vs. 44.8 %), although there was no difference in 30-day mortality, infection-related death and length of hospitalization between groups; however, the clinical failure rate was not reported. It should also be noted that the dose of colistin in this study (administered as CMS) was 2 million units every 8 h (equivalent to ~180 mg of CBA/day) without a loading dose, and that approximately 70 % of patients in either arm received other antibiotics concomitantly. Importantly, the dose used in this and many other polymyxin clinical studies is considerably lower than that of Batirel et al. [177] and low based upon the findings of Garonzik et al. [50].

Unfortunately, given the practical and ethical considerations involved when undertaking clinical investigations comparing polymyxin monotherapy and combination therapy, as mentioned previously, the existing clinical data on polymyxin combination therapy is inconclusive. Considering the potential for rapid development of resistance to polymyxins [100] and the unknown clinical implications of heteroresistance, further multicenter, randomized trials are urgently required to provide a more definitive answer regarding the role of polymyxin combination therapy as compared to monotherapy.

6 Conclusions

Polymyxins are one of the few classes of antibiotics that retain activity against problematic MDR gram-negative organisms. The last decade has seen significant gains in our understanding of polymyxin pharmacokinetics and pharmacodynamics. It is now evident that colistin (administered as its inactive prodrug CMS) and polymyxin B (administered in its active form) differ substantially in their respective pharmacokinetic profiles, suggesting potentially significant differences in the relative efficacy of the two polymyxins, which were previously thought to be interchangeable. The development of polymyxin resistance during monotherapy remains a key concern, and attention has begun to shift toward identifying antibiotic combinations that increase bacterial killing and suppress the emergence of resistance. As the threat presented by MDR gram-negative organisms continues to grow, ongoing research into the pharmacology of the polymyxins will be critical to maintaining their efficacy as a last-line therapy in patients.

References

1. Ainsworth GC, Brown AM, Brownlee G (1947) Aerosporin, an antibiotic produced by Bacillus aerosporus Greer. Nature 159(4060):263
2. Stansly PG, Shepherd RG, White HJ (1947) Polymyxin: a new chemotherapeutic agent. Bull Johns Hopkins Hosp 81(1):43–54
3. Benedict RG, Langlykke AF (1947) Antibiotic activity of Bacillus polymyxa. J Bacteriol 54(1):24
4. Koyama Y, Kurosawa A, Tsuchiya A, Takakuta K (1950) A new antibiotic "colistin" produced by spore-forming soil bacteria. J Antibiot (Tokyo) 3:457–458
5. Wilkinson S (1963) Identity of colistin and polymyxin E. Lancet 281(7287):922–923. doi:10.1016/s0140-6736(63)91694-5
6. Suzuki T, Hayashi K, Fujikawa K, Tsukamoto K (1965) The chemical structure of polymyxin E: the identities of polymyxin E1 with colistin a and of polymyxin E2 with colistin B. J Biochem 57(2):226–227
7. Dautrevaux M, Biserte G (1961) Structure of colimycin. Bull Soc Chim Biol (Paris) 43: 495–504
8. Brownlee G (1949) Antibiotics derived from bacillus polymyxa. Ann N Y Acad Sci 51(Art. 5):875–878
9. Brownlee G, Bushby SR, Short EI (1949) Comparative biological studies of polymyxin A and polymyxin D. Ann N Y Acad Sci 51(Art. 5):891–896.doi:10.1111/j.1749-6632.1949. tb27315.x
10. Brownlee G, Bushby SRM, Short EI (1952) The chemotherapy and pharmacology of the polymyxins. Br J Pharmacol Chemother 7(1):170–188. doi:10.1111/j.1476-5381.1952. tb00702.x
11. Nord NM, Hoeprich PD (1964) Polymyxin B and colistin. A critical comparison. N Engl J Med 270:1030–1035. doi:10.1056/NEJM196405142702002
12. Storm DR, Rosenthal KS, Swanson PE (1977) Polymyxin and related peptide antibiotics. Annu Rev Biochem 46:723–763. doi:10.1146/annurev.bi.46.070177.003451
13. Wolinsky E, Hines JD (1962) Neurotoxic and nephrotoxic effects of colistin in patients with renal disease. N Engl J Med 266(15):759–762. doi:10.1056/nejm196204122661505
14. Brown J, Dorman D, Roy L (1970) Acute renal failure due to overdosage of colistin. Med J Aust 14(2):923–924
15. Yow EM, Moyer JH (1953) Toxicity of polymyxin B. II. Human studies with particular reference to evaluation of renal function. AMA Arch Intern Med 92(2):248–257. doi:10.1001/archinte.1953.00240200098012
16. Lindesmith LA, Baines RD, Bigelow DB, Petty TL (1968) Reversible respiratory paralysis associated with polymyxin therapy. Ann Intern Med 68(2):318. doi:10.7326/0003-4819-68-2-318
17. Elwood CM, Lucas GD, Muehrcke RC (1966) Acute renal failure associated with sodium colistimethate treatment. Arch Intern Med 118(4):326. doi:10.1001/archinte.1966.00290160026006
18. Ryan KJ, Schainuck LI, Hickman RO, Striker GE (1969) Colistimethate toxicity. JAMA 207(11):2099. doi:10.1001/jama.1969.03150240119022
19. Koch-Weser J, Sidel VW, Federman EB, Kanarek P, Finer DC, Eaton AE (1970) Adverse effects of sodium colistimethate. Manifestations and specific reaction rates during 317 courses of therapy. Ann Intern Med 72(6):857–868
20. Price D, Graham D (1970) Effects of large doses of colistin sulphomethate sodium on renal function. Br Med J 4(5734):525
21. Duncan DA (1973) Colistin toxicity. Neuromuscular and renal manifestations. Two cases treated by hemodialysis. Minn Med 56(1):31–35
22. Nation RL, Li J (2009) Colistin in the 21st century. Curr Opin Infect Dis 22(6):535–543. doi:10.1097/QCO.0b013e328332e672

23. Boucher HW, Talbot GH, Bradley JS, Edwards JE, Gilbert D, Rice LB, Scheld M, Spellberg B, Bartlett J (2009) Bad bugs, no drugs: no ESKAPE! An update from the Infectious Diseases Society of America. Clin Infect Dis 48(1):1–12. doi:10.1086/595011
24. World Health Organization (2014) Anti microbial resistance: global report on surveillance 2014. World Health Organization, Geneva
25. Walker B, Barrett S, Polasky S, Galaz V, Folke C, Engstrom G, Ackerman F, Arrow K, Carpenter S, Chopra K, Daily G, Ehrlich P, Hughes T, Kautsky N, Levin S, Maler KG, Shogren J, Vincent J, Xepapadeas T, de Zeeuw A (2009) Environment. Looming global-scale failures and missing institutions. Science 325(5946):1345–1346. doi:10.1126/science.1175325
26. Boucher HW, Talbot GH, Benjamin DK Jr, Bradley J, Guidos RJ, Jones RN, Murray BE, Bonomo RA, Gilbert D, Infectious Diseases Society of America (2013) 10 x '20 Progress--development of new drugs active against gram-negative bacilli: an update from the Infectious Diseases Society of America. Clin Infect Dis 56(12):1685–1694. doi:10.1093/cid/cit152
27. Landman D, Georgescu C, Martin DA, Quale J (2008) Polymyxins revisited. Clin Microbiol Rev 21(3):449–465. doi:10.1128/CMR.00006-08
28. Li J, Nation RL, Turnidge JD, Milne RW, Coulthard K, Rayner CR, Paterson DL (2006) Colistin: the re-emerging antibiotic for multidrug-resistant Gram-negative bacterial infections. Lancet Infect Dis 6(9):589–601. doi:10.1016/S1473-3099(06)70580-1
29. Molina J, Pachón ECJ, Cordero E, Pachón J (2009) New information about the polymyxin/colistin class of antibiotics. Expert Opin Pharmacother 10(17):2811–2828
30. Florescu DF, Qiu F, McCartan MA, Mindru C, Fey PD, Kalil AC (2012) What is the efficacy and safety of colistin for the treatment of ventilator-associated pneumonia? A systematic review and meta-regression. Clin Infect Dis 54(5):670–680. doi:10.1093/cid/cir934
31. Ouderkirk JP, Nord JA, Turett GS, Kislak JW (2003) Polymyxin B nephrotoxicity and efficacy against nosocomial infections caused by multiresistant gram-negative bacteria. Antimicrob Agents Chemother 47(8):2659–2662. doi:10.1128/aac.47.8.2659-2662.2003
32. Orwa JA, Govaerts C, Busson R, Roets E, Van Schepdael A, Hoogmartens J (2001) Isolation and structural characterization of colistin components. J Antibiot (Tokyo) 54(7):595–599
33. Orwa JA, Govaerts C, Busson R, Roets E, Van Schepdael A, Hoogmartens J (2001) Isolation and structural characterization of polymyxin B components. J Chromatogr A 912(2):369–373
34. Govaerts C, Orwa J, Van Schepdael A, Roets E, Hoogmartens J (2002) Liquid chromatography–ion trap tandem mass spectrometry for the characterization of polypeptide antibiotics of the colistin series in commercial samples. J Chromatogr A 976(1-2):65–78. doi:10.1016/s0021-9673(02)00375-8
35. Govaerts C, Orwa J, Van Schepdael A, Roets E, Hoogmartens J (2002) Characterization of polypeptide antibiotics of the polymyxin series by liquid chromatography electrospray ionization ion trap tandem mass spectrometry. J Pept Sci 8(2):45–55. doi:10.1002/psc.367
36. He J, Ledesma KR, Lam WY, Figueroa DA, Lim TP, Chow DS, Tam VH (2010) Variability of polymyxin B major components in commercial formulations. Int J Antimicrob Agents 35(3):308–310. doi:10.1016/j.ijantimicag.2009.11.005
37. Decolin D, Leroy P, Nicolas A, Archimbault P (1997) Hyphenated liquid chromatographic method for the determination of colistin residues in bovine tissues. J Chromatogr Sci 35(12):557–564
38. European Pharmacopoeia Commission (2014) European pharmacopoeia, 8th edn. Council of Europe, Strasbourg
39. British Pharmacopoeia Commission (2014) British pharmacopoeia. Stationery Office, London
40. United States Pharmacopeial Convention (2013) United States Pharmacopoeia 36: National Formulary 31. United States Pharmacopeial Convention, Rockville, MD
41. Nation RL, Velkov T, Li J (2014) Colistin and polymyxin B: are they like peas in a pod or chalk and cheese? Clin Infect Dis 59:88. doi:10.1093/cid/ciu213
42. Barnett M, Bushby SR, Wilkinson S (1964) Sodium sulphomethyl derivatives of polymyxins. Br J Pharmacol Chemother 23:552–574
43. Beveridge EG, Martin AJ (1967) Sodium sulphomethyl derivatives of polymyxins. Br J Pharmacol Chemother 29(2):125–135
44. He H, Li JC, Nation RL, Jacob J, Chen G, Lee HJ, Tsuji BT, Thompson PE, Roberts K, Velkov T, Li J (2013) Pharmacokinetics of four different brands of colistimethate and formed colistin in rats. J Antimicrob Chemother 68(10):2311–2317. doi:10.1093/jac/dkt207
45. Li J, Milne RW, Nation RL, Turnidge JD, Coulthard K (2003) Stability of colistin and

colistin methanesulfonate in aqueous media and plasma as determined by high-performance liquid chromatography. Antimicrob Agents Chemother 47(4):1364–1370. doi:10.1128/aac.47.4.1364-1370.2003

46. Bergen PJ, Li J, Rayner CR, Nation RL (2006) Colistin methanesulfonate is an inactive prodrug of colistin against Pseudomonas aeruginosa. Antimicrob Agents Chemother 50(6):1953–1958. doi:10.1128/AAC.00035-06
47. Li J, Milne RW, Nation RL, Turnidge JD, Smeaton TC, Coulthard K (2004) Pharmacokinetics of colistin methanesulphonate and colistin in rats following an intravenous dose of colistin methanesulphonate. J Antimicrob Chemother 53(5):837–840. doi:10.1093/jac/dkh167
48. Li J, Coulthard K, Milne R, Nation RL, Conway S, Peckham D, Etherington C, Turnidge J (2003) Steady-state pharmacokinetics of intravenous colistin methanesulphonate in patients with cystic fibrosis. J Antimicrob Chemother 52(6):987–992. doi:10.1093/jac/dkg468
49. Marchand S, Lamarche I, Gobin P, Couet W (2010) Dose-ranging pharmacokinetics of colistin methanesulphonate (CMS) and colistin in rats following single intravenous CMS doses. J Antimicrob Chemother 65(8):1753–1758. doi:10.1093/jac/dkq183
50. Garonzik SM, Li J, Thamlikitkul V, Paterson DL, Shoham S, Jacob J, Silveira FP, Forrest A, Nation RL (2011) Population pharmacokinetics of colistin methanesulfonate and formed colistin in critically ill patients from a multicenter study provide dosing suggestions for various categories of patients. Antimicrob Agents Chemother 55(7):3284–3294
51. Markou N, Markantonis SL, Dimitrakis E, Panidis D, Boutzouka E, Karatzas S, Rafailidis P, Apostolakos H, Baltopoulos G (2008) Colistin serum concentrations after intravenous administration in critically ill patients with serious multidrug-resistant, gram-negative bacilli infections: a prospective, open-label, uncontrolled study. Clin Ther 30(1):143–151. doi:10.1016/j.clinthera.2008.01.015
52. Mohamed AF, Karaiskos I, Plachouras D, Karvanen M, Pontikis K, Jansson B, Papadomichelakis E, Antoniadou A, Giamarellou H, Armaganidis A, Cars O, Friberg LE (2012) Application of a loading dose of colistin methanesulfonate in critically ill patients: population pharmacokinetics, protein binding, and prediction of bacterial kill. Antimicrob Agents Chemother 56(8):4241–4249. doi:10.1128/aac.06426-11
53. Plachouras D, Karvanen M, Friberg LE, Papadomichelakis E, Antoniadou A, Tsangaris I, Karaiskos I, Poulakou G, Kontopidou F, Armaganidis A, Cars O, Giamarellou H (2009) Population pharmacokinetic analysis of colistin methanesulfonate and colistin after intravenous administration in critically ill patients with infections caused by gram-negative bacteria. Antimicrob Agents Chemother 53(8):3430–3436. doi:10.1128/AAC.01361-08
54. Lee J, Han S, Jeon S, Hong T, Song W, Woo H, Yim DS (2013) Population pharmacokinetic analysis of colistin in burn patients. Antimicrob Agents Chemother 57(5):2141–2146. doi:10.1128/aac.00271-13
55. Imberti R, Cusato M, Villani P, Carnevale L, Iotti GA, Langer M, Regazzi M (2010) Steady-state pharmacokinetics and BAL concentration of colistin in critically Ill patients after IV colistin methanesulfonate administration. Chest 138(6):1333–1339. doi:10.1378/chest.10-0463
56. Dudhani RV, Nation RL, Li J (2010) Evaluating the stability of colistin and colistin methanesulphonate in human plasma under different conditions of storage. J Antimicrob Chemother 65(7):1412–1415. doi:10.1093/jac/dkq134
57. Mackay DN, Kaye D (1964) Serum concentrations of colistin in patients with normal and impaired renal function. N Engl J Med 270:394–397. doi:10.1056/NEJM196402202700804
58. al-Khayyat AA, Aronson AL (1973) Pharmacologic and toxicologic studies with the polymyxins. II. Comparative pharmacologic studies of the sulfate and methanesulfonate salts of polymyxin B and colistin in dogs. Chemotherapy 19(2):82–97
59. Aoki N, Tateda K, Kikuchi Y, Kimura S, Miyazaki C, Ishii Y, Tanabe Y, Gejyo F, Yamaguchi K (2009) Efficacy of colistin combination therapy in a mouse model of pneumonia caused by multidrug-resistant Pseudomonas aeruginosa. J Antimicrob Chemother 63(3):534–542. doi:10.1093/jac/dkn530
60. Gales AC, Jones RN, Sader HS (2011) Contemporary activity of colistin and polymyxin B against a worldwide collection of Gram-negative pathogens: results from the SENTRY Antimicrobial Surveillance Program (2006-09). J Antimicrob Chemother 66(9):2070–2074. doi:10.1093/jac/dkr239

61. Velkov T, Thompson PE, Nation RL, Li J (2010) Structure-activity relationships of polymyxin antibiotics. J Med Chem 53(5):1898–1916. doi:10.1021/jm900999h
62. Gales AC, Castanheira M, Jones RN, Sader HS (2012) Antimicrobial resistance among Gram-negative bacilli isolated from Latin America: results from SENTRY Antimicrobial Surveillance Program (Latin America, 2008-2010). Diagn Microbiol Infect Dis 73(4):354–360. doi:10.1016/j.diagmicrobio.2012.04.007
63. Hawser SP (2010) Susceptibility of Klebsiella pneumoniae clinical isolates from 2007 to 2009 to colistin and comparator antibiotics. Int J Antimicrob Agents 36(4):383–384. doi:10.1016/j.ijantimicag.2010.06.004
64. Nakamura T, Komatsu M, Yamasaki K, Fukuda S, Higuchi T, Ono T, Nishio H, Sueyoshi N, Kida K, Satoh K, Toda H, Toyokawa M, Nishi I, Sakamoto M, Akagi M, Mizutani T, Nakai I, Kofuku T, Orita T, Zikimoto T, Natsume S, Wada Y (2014) Susceptibility of various oral antibacterial agents against extended spectrum beta-lactamase producing Escherichia coli and Klebsiella pneumoniae. J Infect Chemother 20(1):48–51. doi:10.1016/j.jiac.2013.08.004
65. Zhanel GG, Adam HJ, Baxter MR, Fuller J, Nichol KA, Denisuik AJ, Lagace-Wiens PR, Walkty A, Karlowsky JA, Schweizer F, Hoban DJ (2013) Antimicrobial susceptibility of 22746 pathogens from Canadian hospitals: results of the CANWARD 2007-11 study. J Antimicrob Chemother 68(Suppl 1):i7–i22. doi:10.1093/jac/dkt022
66. Bergen PJ, Landersdorfer CB, Zhang J, Zhao M, Lee HJ, Nation RL, Li J (2012) Pharmacokinetics and pharmacodynamics of 'old' polymyxins: what is new? Diagn Microbiol Infect Dis 74(3):213–223. doi:10.1016/j.diagmicrobio.2012.07.010
67. Tam VH, Schilling AN, Vo G, Kabbara S, Kwa AL, Wiederhold NP, Lewis RE (2005) Pharmacodynamics of polymyxin B against Pseudomonas aeruginosa. Antimicrob Agents Chemother 49(9):3624–3630. doi:10.1128/AAC.49.9.3624-3630.2005
68. Li J, Nation RL, Milne RW, Turnidge JD, Coulthard K (2005) Evaluation of colistin as an agent against multi-resistant Gram-negative bacteria. Int J Antimicrob Agents 25(1):11–25
69. Hirsch HA, McCarthy CG, Finland M (1960) Polymyxin B and colistin: activity, resistance and cross resistance in vitro. Exp Biol Med (Maywood) 103(2):338–342. doi:10.3181/00379727-103-25511
70. Hancock RE, Chapple DS (1999) Peptide antibiotics. Antimicrob Agents Chemother 43(6):1317–1323
71. Brogden KA (2005) Antimicrobial peptides: pore formers or metabolic inhibitors in bacteria? Nat Rev Microbiol 3(3):238–250. doi:10.1038/nrmicro1098
72. Pristovsek P, Kidric J (1999) Solution structure of polymyxins B and E and effect of binding to lipopolysaccharide: an NMR and molecular modeling study. J Med Chem 42(22):4604–4613
73. Katz M, Tsubery H, Kolusheva S, Shames A, Fridkin M, Jelinek R (2003) Lipid binding and membrane penetration of polymyxin B derivatives studied in a biomimetic vesicle system. Biochem J 375(Pt 2):405–413. doi:10.1042/BJ20030784
74. Wiese A, Münstermann M, Gutsmann T, Lindner B, Kawahara K, Zähringer U, Seydel U (1998) Molecular mechanisms of polymyxin B-membrane interactions: direct correlation between surface charge density and self-promoted transport. J Memb Biol 162(2):127–138. doi:10.1007/s002329900350
75. Hancock RE (1984) Alterations in outer membrane permeability. Annu Rev Microbiol 38:237–264. doi:10.1146/annurev.mi.38.100184.001321
76. Hale JD, Hancock RE (2007) Alternative mechanisms of action of cationic antimicrobial peptides on bacteria. Expert Rev Anti Infect Ther 5(6):951–959. doi:10.1586/14787210.5.6.951
77. Hancock REW, Falla T, Brown M (1995) Cationic bactericidal peptides. Adv Microb Physiol 37:135–175. doi:10.1016/s0065-2911(08)60145-9
78. Mogi T, Murase Y, Mori M, Shiomi K, Omura S, Paranagama MP, Kita K (2009) Polymyxin B identified as an inhibitor of alternative NADH dehydrogenase and malate: quinone oxidoreductase from the Gram-positive bacterium Mycobacterium smegmatis. J Biochem 146(4):491–499
79. Sampson TR, Liu X, Schroeder MR, Kraft CS, Burd EM, Weiss DS (2012) Rapid killing of Acinetobacter baumannii by polymyxins is mediated by a hydroxyl radical death pathway. Antimicrob Agents Chemother 56(11):5642–5649. doi:10.1128/AAC.00756-12
80. Zhang L, Dhillon P, Yan H, Farmer S, Hancock RE (2000) Interactions of bacterial cationic peptide antibiotics with outer and cytoplasmic membranes of Pseudomonas aeruginosa. Antimicrob Agents Chemother

44(12):3317–3321. doi:10.1128/aac.44.12.3317-3321.2000

81. Cajal Y, Rogers J, Berg OG, Jain MK (1996) Intermembrane molecular contacts by polymyxin B mediate exchange of phospholipids. Biochemistry 35(1):299–308. doi:10.1021/bi9512408
82. Cajal Y, Ghanta J, Easwaran K, Surolia A, Jain MK (1996) Specificity for the exchange of phospholipids through polymyxin B mediated intermembrane molecular contacts. Biochemistry 35(18):5684–5695. doi:10.1021/bi952703c
83. Cajal Y, Berg OG, Jain MK (1995) Direct vesicle-vesicle exchange of phospholipids mediated by polymyxin B. Biochem Biophys Res Commun 210(3):746–752. doi:10.1006/bbrc.1995.1722
84. Mortensen NP, Fowlkes JD, Sullivan CJ, Allison DP, Larsen NB, Molin S, Doktycz MJ (2009) Effects of colistin on surface ultrastructure and nanomechanics of Pseudomonas aeruginosa cells. Langmuir 25(6):3728–3733. doi:10.1021/la803898g
85. McCoy LS, Roberts KD, Nation RL, Thompson PE, Velkov T, Li J, Tor Y (2013) Polymyxins and analogues bind to ribosomal RNA and interfere with eukaryotic translation in vitro. Chembiochem 14(16):2083–2086. doi:10.1002/cbic.201300496
86. Otvos L Jr (2005) Antibacterial peptides and proteins with multiple cellular targets. J Pept Sci 11(11):697–706. doi:10.1002/psc.698
87. Keren I, Wu Y, Inocencio J, Mulcahy LR, Lewis K (2013) Killing by bactericidal antibiotics does not depend on reactive oxygen species. Science 339(6124):1213–1216. doi:10.1126/science.1232688
88. Ito-Kagawa M, Koyama Y (1980) Selective cleavage of a peptide antibiotic, colistin by colistinase. J Antibiot (Tokyo) 33(12):1551–1555
89. Campos MA, Vargas MA, Regueiro V, Llompart CM, Alberti S, Bengoechea JA (2004) Capsule polysaccharide mediates bacterial resistance to antimicrobial peptides. Infect Immun 72(12):7107–7114. doi:10.1128/IAI.72.12.7107-7114.2004
90. Llobet E, Tomas JM, Bengoechea JA (2008) Capsule polysaccharide is a bacterial decoy for antimicrobial peptides. Microbiology 154(Pt 12):3877–3886. doi:10.1099/mic.0.2008/022301-0
91. Gunn JS, Lim KB, Krueger J, Kim K, Guo L, Hackett M, Miller SI (1998) PmrA-PmrB-regulated genes necessary for 4-aminoarabinose lipid A modification and polymyxin resistance. Mol Microbiol 27(6):1171–1182. doi:10.1046/j.1365-2958.1998.00757.x
92. McPhee JB, Lewenza S, Hancock REW (2003) Cationic antimicrobial peptides activate a two-component regulatory system, PmrA-PmrB, that regulates resistance to polymyxin B and cationic antimicrobial peptides in Pseudomonas aeruginosa. Mol Microbiol 50(1):205–217. doi:10.1046/j.1365-2958.2003.03673.x
93. Zhou Z, Ribeiro AA, Lin S, Cotter RJ, Miller SI, Raetz CR (2001) Lipid A modifications in polymyxin-resistant Salmonella typhimurium: PMRA-dependent 4-amino-4-deoxy-L-arabinose, and phosphoethanolamine incorporation. J Biol Chem 276(46):43111–43121. doi:10.1074/jbc.M106960200
94. Muller C, Plesiat P, Jeannot K (2011) A two-component regulatory system interconnects resistance to polymyxins, aminoglycosides, fluoroquinolones, and beta-lactams in Pseudomonas aeruginosa. Antimicrob Agents Chemother 55(3):1211–1221. doi:10.1128/AAC.01252-10
95. Fernandez L, Gooderham WJ, Bains M, McPhee JB, Wiegand I, Hancock RE (2010) Adaptive resistance to the "Last Hope" antibiotics polymyxin B and colistin in pseudomonas aeruginosa is mediated by the novel two-component regulatory system ParR-ParS. Antimicrob Agents Chemother 54(8):3372–3382
96. Adams MD, Nickel GC, Bajaksouzian S, Lavender H, Murthy AR, Jacobs MR, Bonomo RA (2009) Resistance to colistin in Acinetobacter baumannii associated with mutations in the PmrAB two-component system. Antimicrob Agents Chemother 53(9):3628–3634. doi:10.1128/AAC.00284-09
97. Moffatt JH, Harper M, Harrison P, Hale JD, Vinogradov E, Seemann T, Henry R, Crane B, Michael F, Cox AD, Adler B, Nation RL, Li J, Boyce JD (2010) Colistin resistance in acinetobacter baumannii is mediated by complete loss of lipopolysaccharide production. Antimicrob Agents Chemother 54(12):4971–4977
98. Lo-Ten-Foe JR, de Smet AM, Diederen BM, Kluytmans JA, van Keulen PH (2007) Comparative evaluation of the VITEK 2, disk diffusion, etest, broth microdilution, and agar dilution susceptibility testing methods for colistin in clinical isolates, including heteroresistant Enterobacter cloacae and Acinetobacter baumannii strains. Antimicrob Agents Chemother 51(10):3726–3730. doi:10.1128/AAC.01406-06

99. Poudyal A, Howden BP, Bell JM, Gao W, Owen RJ, Turnidge JD, Nation RL, Li J (2008) In vitro pharmacodynamics of colistin against multidrug-resistant Klebsiella pneumoniae. J Antimicrob Chemother 62(6):1311–1318. doi:10.1093/jac/dkn425
100. Hawley JS, Murray CK, Jorgensen JH (2008) Colistin heteroresistance in acinetobacter and its association with previous colistin therapy. Antimicrob Agents Chemother 52(1):351–352. doi:10.1128/AAC.00766-07
101. Meletis G, Tzampaz E, Sianou E, Tzavaras I, Sofianou D (2011) Colistin heteroresistance in carbapenemase-producing Klebsiella pneumoniae. J Antimicrob Chemother 66(4):946–947. doi:10.1093/jac/dkr007
102. Hermes DM, Pormann Pitt C, Lutz L, Teixeira AB, Ribeiro VB, Netto B, Martins AF, Zavascki AP, Barth AL (2013) Evaluation of heteroresistance to polymyxin B among carbapenem-susceptible and -resistant Pseudomonas aeruginosa. J Med Microbiol 62(Pt 8):1184–1189. doi:10.1099/jmm.0.059220-0
103. Bergen PJ, Forrest A, Bulitta JB, Tsuji BT, Sidjabat HE, Paterson DL, Li J, Nation RL (2011) Clinically relevant plasma concentrations of colistin in combination with imipenem enhance pharmacodynamic activity against multidrug-resistant Pseudomonas aeruginosa at multiple inocula. Antimicrob Agents Chemother 55(11):5134–5142. doi:10.1128/AAC.05028-11
104. Vidaillac C, Benichou L, Duval RE (2012) In vitro synergy of colistin combinations against colistin-resistant Acinetobacter baumannii, Pseudomonas aeruginosa, and Klebsiella pneumoniae isolates. Antimicrob Agents Chemother 56(9):4856–4861. doi:10.1128/AAC.05996-11
105. Li J, Rayner CR, Nation RL, Owen RJ, Spelman D, Tan KE, Liolios L (2006) Heteroresistance to colistin in multidrug-resistant Acinetobacter baumannii. Antimicrob Agents Chemother 50(9):2946–2950. doi:10.1128/AAC.00103-06
106. Owen RJ, Li J, Nation RL, Spelman D (2007) In vitro pharmacodynamics of colistin against Acinetobacter baumannii clinical isolates. J Antimicrob Chemother 59(3):473–477. doi:10.1093/jac/dkl512
107. Falagas ME, Kasiakou SK (2006) Toxicity of polymyxins: a systematic review of the evidence from old and recent studies. Crit Care 10(1):R27. doi:10.1186/cc3995
108. Hartzell JD, Neff R, Ake J, Howard R, Olson S, Paolino K, Vishnepolsky M, Weintrob A, Wortmann G (2009) Nephrotoxicity associated with intravenous colistin (colistimethate sodium) treatment at a tertiary care medical center. Clin Infect Dis 48(12):1724–1728. doi:10.1086/599225
109. Betrosian AP, Frantzeskaki F, Xanthaki A, Douzinas EE (2008) Efficacy and safety of high-dose ampicillin/sulbactam vs. colistin as monotherapy for the treatment of multidrug resistant Acinetobacter baumannii ventilator-associated pneumonia. J Infect 56(6):432–436. doi:10.1016/j.jinf.2008.04.002
110. Kwon JA, Lee JE, Huh W, Peck KR, Kim YG, Kim DJ, Oh HY (2010) Predictors of acute kidney injury associated with intravenous colistin treatment. Int J Antimicrob Agents 35(5):473–477. doi:10.1016/j.ijantimicag.2009.12.002
111. Deryke CA, Crawford AJ, Uddin N, Wallace MR (2010) Colistin dosing and nephrotoxicity in a large community teaching hospital. Antimicrob Agents Chemother 54(10):4503–4505. doi:10.1128/AAC.01707-09
112. Ko H, Jeon M, Choo E, Lee E, Kim T, Jun JB, Gil HW (2011) Early acute kidney injury is a risk factor that predicts mortality in patients treated with colistin. Nephron Clin Pract 117(3):c284–c288. doi:10.1159/000320746
113. Mendes CA, Cordeiro JA, Burdmann EA (2009) Prevalence and risk factors for acute kidney injury associated with parenteral polymyxin B use. Ann Pharmacother 43(12):1948–1955. doi:10.1345/aph.1M277
114. Akajagbor DS, Wilson SL, Shere-Wolfe KD, Dakum P, Charurat ME, Gilliam BL (2013) Higher incidence of acute kidney injury with intravenous colistimethate sodium compared with polymyxin B in critically ill patients at a tertiary care medical center. Clin Infect Dis 57(9):1300–1303. doi:10.1093/cid/cit453
115. Phe K, Lee Y, McDaneld PM, Prasad N, Yin T, Figueroa DA, Musick WL, Cottreau JM, Hu M, Tam VH (2014) In vitro assessment and multicenter cohort study of comparative nephrotoxicity rates associated with colistimethate versus polymyxin B therapy. Antimicrob Agents Chemother 58(5):2740–2746. doi:10.1128/AAC.02476-13
116. Azad MA, Finnin BA, Poudyal A, Davis K, Li J, Hill PA, Nation RL, Velkov T, Li J (2013) Polymyxin B induces apoptosis in kidney proximal tubular cells. Antimicrob Agents Chemother 57(9):4329–4335. doi: 10.1128/AAC.02587-12
117. Abdelraouf K, Braggs KH, Yin T, Truong LD, Hu M, Tam VH (2012) Characterization of polymyxin B-induced nephrotoxicity: implications for dosing regimen design. Antimicrob Agents Chemother 56(9):4625–4629. doi:10.1128/AAC.00280-12

118. Sandri AM, Landersdorfer CB, Jacob J, Boniatti MM, Dalarosa MG, Falci DR, Behle TF, Bordinhao RC, Wang J, Forrest A, Nation RL, Li J, Zavascki AP (2013) Population pharmacokinetics of intravenous polymyxin B in critically ill patients: implications for selection of dosage regimens. Clin Infect Dis 57(4):524–531. doi:10.1093/cid/cit334
119. Ozyilmaz E, Ebinc FA, Derici U, Gulbahar O, Goktas G, Elmas C, Oguzulgen IK, Sindel S (2011) Could nephrotoxicity due to colistin be ameliorated with the use of N-acetylcysteine? Intensive Care Med 37(1):141–146. doi:10.1007/s00134-010-2038-7
120. Yousef JM, Chen G, Hill PA, Nation RL, Li J (2011) Melatonin attenuates colistin-induced nephrotoxicity in rats. Antimicrob Agents Chemother 55(9):4044–4049. doi:10.1128/AAC.00328-11
121. Dezoti Fonseca C, Watanabe M, Vattimo Mde F (2012) Role of heme oxygenase-1 in polymyxin B-induced nephrotoxicity in rats. Antimicrob Agents Chemother 56(10):5082–5087. doi:10.1128/AAC.00925-12
122. Yousef JM, Chen G, Hill PA, Nation RL, Li J (2012) Ascorbic acid protects against the nephrotoxicity and apoptosis caused by colistin and affects its pharmacokinetics. J Antimicrob Chemother 67(2):452–459. doi:10.1093/jac/dkr483
123. Falagas ME, Kasiakou SK (2005) Colistin: the revival of polymyxins for the management of multidrug-resistant gram-negative bacterial infections. Clin Infect Dis 40(9):1333–1341. doi:10.1086/429323
124. Perkins RL (1964) Apnea with intramuscular colistin therapy. JAMA 190:421–424
125. Parisi AF (1965) Apnea during treatment with sodium colistimethate. JAMA 194(3):298. doi:10.1001/jama.1965.03090160076026
126. Weinstein L, Doan TL, Smith MA (2009) Neurotoxicity in patients treated with intravenous polymyxin B: two case reports. Am J Health Syst Pharm 66(4):345–347. doi:10.2146/ajhp080065
127. Wahby K, Chopra T, Chandrasekar P (2010) Intravenous and inhalational colistin-induced respiratory failure. Clin Infect Dis 50(6):e38–e40. doi:10.1086/650582
128. Zauder HL, Barton N, Bennett EJ, Lore J (1966) Colistimethate as a cause of postoperative apnoea. Can Anaesth Soc J 13(6):607–610. doi:10.1007/bf03002230
129. Li J, Milne RW, Nation RL, Turnidge JD, Coulthard K, Valentine J (2002) Simple method for assaying colistin methanesulfonate in plasma and urine using high-performance liquid chromatography. Antimicrob Agents Chemother 46(10):3304–3307. doi:10.1128/aac.46.10.3304-3307.2002
130. Li J, Milne RW, Nation RL, Turnidge JD, Coulthard K, Johnson DW (2001) A simple method for the assay of colistin in human plasma, using pre-column derivatization with 9-fluorenylmethyl chloroformate in solid-phase extraction cartridges and reversed-phase high-performance liquid chromatography. J Chromatogr B 761(2):167–175. doi:10.1016/S0378-4347(01)00326-7
131. Jansson B, Karvanen M, Cars O, Plachouras D, Friberg LE (2009) Quantitative analysis of colistin A and colistin B in plasma and culture medium using a simple precipitation step followed by LC/MS/MS. J Pharm Biomed Anal 49(3):760–767. doi:10.1016/j.jpba.2008.12.016
132. Gikas E, Bazoti FN, Katsimardou M, Anagnostopoulos D, Papanikolaou K, Inglezos I, Skoutelis A, Daikos GL, Tsarbopoulos A (2013) Determination of colistin A and colistin B in human plasma by UPLC-ESI high resolution tandem MS: application to a pharmacokinetic study. J Pharm Biomed Anal 83:228–236. doi:10.1016/j.jpba.2013.05.008
133. Cheng C, Liu S, Xiao D, Hollembaek J, Yao L, Lin J, Hansel S (2010) LC-MS/MS method development and validation for the determination of polymyxins and vancomycin in rat plasma. J Chromatogr B 878(28):2831–2838. doi:10.1016/j.jchromb.2010.08.037
134. Li J, Nation RL, Cao G, Ali FEA, Chiu F, Zavascki AP (2009) Development and validation of a reversed-phase high-performance liquid chromatography assay for polymyxin B in human plasma--authors' response. J Antimicrob Chemother 63(3):628–629. doi:10.1093/jac/dkn524
135. Dotsikas Y, Markopoulou CK, Koundourellis JE, Loukas YL (2011) Validation of a novel LC-MS/MS method for the quantitation of colistin A and B in human plasma. J Sep Sci 34(1):37–45. doi:10.1002/jssc.201000680
136. Cheah SE, Bulitta JB, Li J, Nation RL (2014) Development and validation of a liquid chromatography-mass spectrometry assay for polymyxin B in bacterial growth media. J Pharm Biomed Anal 92:177–182. doi:10.1016/j.jpba.2014.01.015
137. Cao G, Ali FE, Chiu F, Zavascki AP, Nation RL, Li J (2008) Development and validation of a reversed-phase high-performance liquid chromatography assay for polymyxin B in human plasma. J Antimicrob Chemother 62(5):1009–1014. doi:10.1093/jac/dkn343

138. Li J, Milne RW, Nation RL, Turnidge JD, Smeaton TC, Coulthard K (2003) Use of high-performance liquid chromatography to study the pharmacokinetics of colistin sulfate in rats following intravenous administration. Antimicrob Agents Chemother 47(5):1766–1770. doi:10.1128/aac.47.5.1766-1770.2003
139. Sandri AM, Landersdorfer CB, Jacob J, Boniatti MM, Dalarosa MG, Falci DR, Behle TF, Saitovitch D, Wang J, Forrest A, Nation RL, Zavascki AP, Li J (2013) Pharmacokinetics of polymyxin B in patients on continuous venovenous haemodialysis. J Antimicrob Chemother 68(3):674–677. doi:10.1093/jac/dks437
140. Abdelraouf K, He J, Ledesma KR, Hu M, Tam VH (2012) Pharmacokinetics and renal disposition of polymyxin B in an animal model. Antimicrob Agents Chemother 56(11):5724–5727. doi:10.1128/AAC.01333-12
141. Dudhani RV, Turnidge JD, Coulthard K, Milne RW, Rayner CR, Li J, Nation RL (2010) Elucidation of the pharmacokinetic/pharmacodynamic determinant of colistin activity against Pseudomonas aeruginosa in murine thigh and lung infection models. Antimicrob Agents Chemother 54(3):1117–1124. doi:10.1128/AAC.01114-09
142. Couet W, Gregoire N, Gobin P, Saulnier PJ, Frasca D, Marchand S, Mimoz O (2011) Pharmacokinetics of colistin and colistimethate sodium after a single 80-mg intravenous dose of CMS in young healthy volunteers. Clin Pharmacol Ther 89(6):875–879. doi:10.1038/clpt.2011.48
143. Jensen T, Pedersen SS, Garne S, Heilmann C, Høiby N, Koch C (1987) Colistin inhalation therapy in cystic fibrosis patients with chronic Pseudomonas aeruginosa lung infection. J Antimicrob Chemother 19(6):831–838. doi:10.1093/jac/19.6.831
144. Pereira GH, Muller PR, Levin AS (2007) Salvage treatment of pneumonia and initial treatment of tracheobronchitis caused by multidrug-resistant Gram-negative bacilli with inhaled polymyxin B. Diagn Microbiol Infect Dis 58(2):235–240. doi:10.1016/j.diagmicrobio.2007.01.008
145. Westerman EM, De Boer AH, Le Brun PP, Touw DJ, Roldaan AC, Frijlink HW, Heijerman HG (2007) Dry powder inhalation of colistin in cystic fibrosis patients: a single dose pilot study. J Cyst Fibros 6(4):284–292. doi:10.1016/j.jcf.2006.10.010
146. Westerman EM, de Boer AH, Le Brun PP, Touw DJ, Frijlink HW, Heijerman HG (2007) Dry powder inhalation of colistin sulphomethate in healthy volunteers: a pilot study. Int J Pharm 335(1-2):41–45. doi:10.1016/j.ijpharm.2006.11.021
147. W S Yapa S, Li J, Patel K, Wilson JW, Dooley MJ, George J, Clark D, Poole S, Williams E, Porter CJ, Nation RL, McIntosh MP (2014) Pulmonary and systemic pharmacokinetics of inhaled and intravenous colistin methanesulfonate in cystic fibrosis patients: targeting advantage of inhalational administration. Antimicrob Agents Chemother 58(5):2570–2579. doi:10.1128/AAC.01705-13
148. Ratjen F, Rietschel E, Kasel D, Schwiertz R, Starke K, Beier H, van Koningsbruggen S, Grasemann H (2006) Pharmacokinetics of inhaled colistin in patients with cystic fibrosis. J Antimicrob Chemother 57(2):306–311. doi:10.1093/jac/dki461
149. Athanassa ZE, Markantonis SL, Fousteri MZ, Myrianthefs PM, Boutzouka EG, Tsakris A, Baltopoulos GJ (2012) Pharmacokinetics of inhaled colistimethate sodium (CMS) in mechanically ventilated critically ill patients. Intensive Care Med 38(11):1779–1786. doi:10.1007/s00134-012-2628-7
150. Zavascki AP, Goldani LZ, Cao G, Superti SV, Lutz L, Barth AL, Ramos F, Boniatti MM, Nation RL, Li J (2008) Pharmacokinetics of intravenous polymyxin B in critically ill patients. Clin Infect Dis 47(10):1298–1304. doi:10.1086/592577
151. Kwa AL, Lim TP, Low JG, Hou J, Kurup A, Prince RA, Tam VH (2008) Pharmacokinetics of polymyxin B1 in patients with multidrug-resistant Gram-negative bacterial infections. Diagn Microbiol Infect Dis 60(2):163–167. doi:10.1016/j.diagmicrobio.2007.08.008
152. Zavascki AP, Goldani LZ, Li J, Nation RL (2007) Polymyxin B for the treatment of multidrug-resistant pathogens: a critical review. J Antimicrob Chemother 60(6):1206–1215. doi:10.1093/jac/dkm357
153. Behera B, Mathur P, Das A, Kapil A, Gupta B, Bhoi S, Farooque K, Sharma V, Misra MC (2010) Evaluation of susceptibility testing methods for polymyxin. Int J Infect Dis 14(7):e596–e601. doi:10.1016/j.ijid.2009.09.001
154. van der Heijden IM, Levin AS, De Pedri EH, Fung L, Rossi F, Duboc G, Barone AA, Costa SF (2007) Comparison of disc diffusion, Etest and broth microdilution for testing susceptibility of carbapenem-resistant P. aeruginosa to polymyxins. Ann Clin Microbiol Antimicrob 6:8. doi:10.1186/1476-0711-6-8
155. Maalej SM, Meziou MR, Rhimi FM, Hammami A (2011) Comparison of disc

diffusion, Etest and agar dilution for susceptibility testing of colistin against Enterobacteriaceae. Lett Appl Microbiol 53(5):546–551. doi:10.1111/j.1472-765X.2011.03145.x
156. Gunderson BW, Ibrahim KH, Hovde LB, Fromm TL, Reed MD, Rotschafer JC (2003) Synergistic activity of colistin and ceftazidime against multiantibiotic-resistant Pseudomonas aeruginosa in an in vitro pharmacodynamic model. Antimicrob Agents Chemother 47(3):905–909. doi:10.1128/aac.47.3.905-909.2003
157. Li J, Turnidge J, Milne R, Nation RL, Coulthard K (2001) In vitro pharmacodynamic properties of colistin and colistin methanesulfonate against Pseudomonas aeruginosa isolates from patients with cystic fibrosis. Antimicrob Agents Chemother 45(3):781–785. doi:10.1128/AAC.45.3.781-785.2001
158. Tan CH, Li J, Nation RL (2007) Activity of colistin against heteroresistant Acinetobacter baumannii and emergence of resistance in an in vitro pharmacokinetic/pharmacodynamic model. Antimicrob Agents Chemother 51(9):3413–3415. doi:10.1128/AAC.01571-06
159. Bergen PJ, Bulitta JB, Forrest A, Tsuji BT, Li J, Nation RL (2010) Pharmacokinetic/pharmacodynamic investigation of colistin against Pseudomonas aeruginosa using an in vitro model. Antimicrob Agents Chemother 54(9):3783–3789. doi:10.1128/AAC.00903-09
160. Bulitta JB, Yang JC, Yohonn L, Ly NS, Brown SV, D'Hondt RE, Jusko WJ, Forrest A, Tsuji BT (2010) Attenuation of colistin bactericidal activity by high inoculum of Pseudomonas aeruginosa characterized by a new mechanism-based population pharmacodynamic model. Antimicrob Agents Chemother 54(5):2051–2062. doi:10.1128/AAC.00881-09
161. Lee HJ, Bergen PJ, Bulitta JB, Tsuji B, Forrest A, Nation RL, Li J (2013) Synergistic activity of colistin and rifampin combination against multidrug-resistant Acinetobacter baumannii in an in vitro pharmacokinetic/pharmacodynamic model. Antimicrob Agents Chemother 57(8):3738–3745. doi:10.1128/AAC.00703-13
162. Deris ZZ, Yu HH, Davis K, Soon RL, Jacob J, Ku CK, Poudyal A, Bergen PJ, Tsuji BT, Bulitta JB, Forrest A, Paterson DL, Velkov T, Li J, Nation RL (2012) The combination of colistin and doripenem is synergistic against Klebsiella pneumoniae at multiple inocula and suppresses colistin resistance in an in vitro pharmacokinetic/pharmacodynamic model. Antimicrob Agents Chemother 56(10):5103–5112. doi:10.1128/AAC.01064-12
163. Bergen PJ, Tsuji BT, Bulitta JB, Forrest A, Jacob J, Sidjabat HE, Paterson DL, Nation RL, Li J (2011) Synergistic killing of multidrug-resistant Pseudomonas aeruginosa at multiple inocula by colistin combined with doripenem in an in vitro pharmacokinetic/pharmacodynamic model. Antimicrob Agents Chemother 55(12):5685–5695. doi:10.1128/AAC.05298-11
164. Bergen PJ, Li J, Nation RL, Turnidge JD, Coulthard K, Milne RW (2008) Comparison of once-, twice- and thrice-daily dosing of colistin on antibacterial effect and emergence of resistance: studies with Pseudomonas aeruginosa in an in vitro pharmacodynamic model. J Antimicrob Chemother 61(3):636–642. doi:10.1093/jac/dkm511
165. Dudhani RV, Turnidge JD, Nation RL, Li J (2010) fAUC/MIC is the most predictive pharmacokinetic/pharmacodynamic index of colistin against Acinetobacter baumannii in murine thigh and lung infection models. J Antimicrob Chemother 65(9): 1984–1990
166. Lister PD, Wolter DJ, Hanson ND (2009) Antibacterial-resistant Pseudomonas aeruginosa: clinical impact and complex regulation of chromosomally encoded resistance mechanisms. Clin Microbiol Rev 22(4):582–610. doi:10.1128/CMR.00040-09
167. Rahal JJ (2006) Novel antibiotic combinations against infections with almost completely resistant Pseudomonas aeruginosa and Acinetobacter species. Clin Infect Dis 43(Suppl 2):S95–S99. doi:10.1086/504486
168. Herrmann G, Yang L, Wu H, Song Z, Wang H, Hoiby N, Ulrich M, Molin S, Riethmuller J, Doring G (2010) Colistin-tobramycin combinations are superior to monotherapy concerning the killing of biofilm Pseudomonas aeruginosa. J Infect Dis 202(10):1585–1592. doi:10.1086/656788
169. Plachouras D, Giamarellos-Bourboulis EJ, Kentepozidis N, Baziaka F, Karagianni V, Giamarellou H (2007) In vitro postantibiotic effect of colistin on multidrug-resistant Acinetobacter baumannii. Diagn Microbiol Infect Dis 57(4):419–422. doi:10.1016/j.diagmicrobio.2006.10.006
170. Singh R, Tam VH (2011) Optimizing dosage to prevent emergence of resistance - lessons from in vitro models. Curr Opin Pharmacol 11(5):453–456. doi:10.1016/j.coph.2011.07.009

171. Hengzhuang W, Wu H, Ciofu O, Song Z, Hoiby N (2012) In vivo pharmacokinetics/pharmacodynamics of colistin and imipenem in Pseudomonas aeruginosa biofilm infection. Antimicrob Agents Chemother 56(5):2683–2690. doi:10.1128/AAC.06486-11
172. Petrosillo N, Giannella M, Antonelli M, Antonini M, Barsic B, Belancic L, Inkaya AC, De Pascale G, Grilli E, Tumbarello M, Akova M (2014) Clinical experience of colistin-glycopeptide combination in critically ill patients infected with Gram-negative bacteria. Antimicrob Agents Chemother 58(2):851–858. doi:10.1128/AAC.00871-13
173. Morelli P, Ferrario A, Tordato F, Piazza A, Casari E (2014) Successful treatment of post-neurosurgical multidrug-resistant Pseudomonas aeruginosa meningo-encephalitis with combination therapy of colistin, rifampicin and doripenem. J Antimicrob Chemother 69(3):857–859. doi:10.1093/jac/dkt437
174. Durante-Mangoni E, Signoriello G, Andini R, Mattei A, De Cristoforo M, Murino P, Bassetti M, Malacarne P, Petrosillo N, Galdieri N, Mocavero P, Corcione A, Viscoli C, Zarrilli R, Gallo C, Utili R (2013) Colistin and rifampicin compared with colistin alone for the treatment of serious infections due to extensively drug-resistant Acinetobacter baumannii: a multicenter, randomized clinical trial. Clin Infect Dis 57(3):349–358. doi:10.1093/cid/cit253
175. Ceccarelli G, Falcone M, Giordano A, Mezzatesta ML, Caio C, Stefani S, Venditti M (2013) Successful ertapenem-doripenem combination treatment of bacteremic ventilator-associated pneumonia due to colistin-resistant KPC-producing Klebsiella pneumoniae. Antimicrob Agents Chemother 57(6):2900–2901. doi:10.1128/AAC.00188-13
176. Aydemir H, Akduman D, Piskin N, Comert F, Horuz E, Terzi A, Kokturk F, Ornek T, Celebi G (2013) Colistin vs. the combination of colistin and rifampicin for the treatment of carbapenem-resistant Acinetobacter baumannii ventilator-associated pneumonia. Epidemiol Infect 141(6):1214–1222. doi:10.1017/S095026881200194X
177. Batirel A, Balkan II, Karabay O, Agalar C, Akalin S, Alici O, Alp E, Altay FA, Altin N, Arslan F, Aslan T, Bekiroglu N, Cesur S, Celik AD, Dogan M, Durdu B, Duygu F, Engin A, Engin DO, Gonen I, Guclu E, Guven T, Hatipoglu CA, Hosoglu S, Karahocagil MK, Kilic AU, Ormen B, Ozdemir D, Ozer S, Oztoprak N, Sezak N, Turhan V, Turker N, Yilmaz H (2014) Comparison of colistin-carbapenem, colistin-sulbactam, and colistin plus other antibacterial agents for the treatment of extremely drug-resistant Acinetobacter baumannii bloodstream infections. Eur J Clin Microbiol Infect Dis 33:1311. doi:10.1007/s10096-014-2070-6
178. Li J, Nation RL, Owen RJ, Wong S, Spelman D, Franklin C (2007) Antibiograms of multidrug-resistant clinical Acinetobacter baumannii: promising therapeutic options for treatment of infection with colistin-resistant strains. Clin Infect Dis 45(5):594–598. doi:10.1086/520658
179. Bulitta JB, Li J, Poudyal A, Yu HH, Owen RJ, Tsuji BT, Nation RL, Forrest A (2009) Quantifying synergy of colistin combinations against MDR Gram-negatives by mechanism-based models (abstract A1-573, p. 41). Paper presented at the In: Abstracts of the 49th Annual Interscience Conference of Antimicrobial Agents and Chemotherapy (ICAAC), San Francisco, CA, September 12–15, 2009
180. Pachon-Ibanez ME, Docobo-Perez F, Lopez-Rojas R, Dominguez-Herrera J, Jimenez-Mejias ME, Garcia-Curiel A, Pichardo C, Jimenez L, Pachon J (2010) Efficacy of rifampin and its combinations with imipenem, sulbactam, and colistin in experimental models of infection caused by imipenem-resistant Acinetobacter baumannii. Antimicrob Agents Chemother 54(3):1165–1172. doi:10.1128/AAC.00367-09
181. Pantopoulou A, Giamarellos-Bourboulis EJ, Raftogannis M, Tsaganos T, Dontas I, Koutoukas P, Baziaka F, Giamarellou H, Perrea D (2007) Colistin offers prolonged survival in experimental infection by multidrug-resistant Acinetobacter baumannii: the significance of co-administration of rifampicin. Int J Antimicrob Agents 29(1):51–55. doi:10.1016/j.ijantimicag.2006.09.009
182. Cirioni O, Ghiselli R, Silvestri C, Kamysz W, Orlando F, Mocchegiani F, Di Matteo F, Riva A, Lukasiak J, Scalise G, Saba V, Giacometti A (2007) Efficacy of tachyplesin III, colistin, and imipenem against a multiresistant Pseudomonas aeruginosa strain. Antimicrob Agents Chemother 51(6):2005–2010. doi:10.1128/AAC.01576-06
183. Michail G, Labrou M, Pitiriga V, Manousaka S, Sakellaridis N, Tsakris A, Pournaras S (2013) Activity of tigecycline in combination with colistin, meropenem, rifampin, or gentamicin against KPC-producing Enterobacteriaceae in a murine thigh infection model. Antimicrob Agents Chemother 57(12):6028–6033. doi:10.1128/AAC.00891-13

184. Demiraslan H, Dinc G, Ahmed SS, Elmali F, Metan G, Alp E, Doganay M (2014) Carbapenem-resistant Klebsiella pneumoniae sepsis in corticosteroid receipt mice: tigecycline or colistin monotherapy versus tigecycline/colistin combination. J Chemother 26:276. doi:10.1179/1973947813Y.0000000143
185. Mutlu Yilmaz E, Sunbul M, Aksoy A, Yilmaz H, Guney AK, Guvenc T (2012) Efficacy of tigecycline/colistin combination in a pneumonia model caused by extensively drug-resistant Acinetobacter baumannii. Int J Antimicrob Agents 40(4):332–336. doi:10.1016/j.ijantimicag.2012.06.003
186. Corvec S, Furustrand Tafin U, Betrisey B, Borens O, Trampuz A (2013) Activities of fosfomycin, tigecycline, colistin, and gentamicin against extended-spectrum-beta-lactamase-producing Escherichia coli in a foreign-body infection model. Antimicrob Agents Chemother 57(3):1421–1427. doi:10.1128/AAC.01718-12
187. Montero A, Ariza J, Corbella X, Domenech A, Cabellos C, Ayats J, Tubau F, Borraz C, Gudiol F (2004) Antibiotic combinations for serious infections caused by carbapenem-resistant Acinetobacter baumannii in a mouse pneumonia model. J Antimicrob Chemother 54(6):1085–1091. doi:10.1093/jac/dkh485
188. Cappelletty DM, Rybak MJ (1996) Comparison of methodologies for synergism testing of drug combinations against resistant strains of Pseudomonas aeruginosa. Antimicrob Agents Chemother 40(3):677–683
189. Tan TY, Ng LS, Tan E, Huang G (2007) In vitro effect of minocycline and colistin combinations on imipenem-resistant Acinetobacter baumannii clinical isolates. J Antimicrob Chemother 60(2):421–423. doi:10.1093/jac/dkm178
190. Souli M, Rekatsina PD, Chryssouli Z, Galani I, Giamarellou H, Kanellakopoulou K (2009) Does the activity of the combination of imipenem and colistin in vitro exceed the problem of resistance in metallo-beta-lactamase-producing Klebsiella pneumoniae isolates? Antimicrob Agents Chemother 53(5):2133–2135. doi:10.1128/AAC.01271-08
191. Principe L, Capone A, Mazzarelli A, D'Arezzo S, Bordi E, Di Caro A, Petrosillo N (2013) In vitro activity of doripenem in combination with various antimicrobials against multidrug-resistant Acinetobacter baumannii: possible options for the treatment of complicated infection. Microb Drug Resist 19(5):407–414. doi:10.1089/mdr.2012.0250
192. Tangden T, Hickman RA, Forsberg P, Lagerback P, Giske CG, Cars O (2014) Evaluation of double- and triple-antibiotic combinations for VIM- and NDM-producing Klebsiella pneumoniae by in vitro time-kill experiments. Antimicrob Agents Chemother 58(3):1757–1762. doi:10.1128/AAC.00741-13
193. Gaibani P, Lombardo D, Lewis RE, Mercuri M, Bonora S, Landini MP, Ambretti S (2014) In vitro activity and post-antibiotic effects of colistin in combination with other antimicrobials against colistin-resistant KPC-producing Klebsiella pneumoniae bloodstream isolates. J Antimicrob Chemother 69:1856. doi:10.1093/jac/dku065
194. Oleksiuk LM, Nguyen MH, Press EG, Updike CL, O'Hara JA, Doi Y, Clancy CJ, Shields RK (2014) In vitro responses of Acinetobacter baumannii to two- and three-drug combinations following exposure to colistin and doripenem. Antimicrob Agents Chemother 58(2):1195–1199. doi:10.1128/AAC.01779-13
195. Tripodi MF, Durante-Mangoni E, Fortunato R, Utili R, Zarrilli R (2007) Comparative activities of colistin, rifampicin, imipenem and sulbactam/ampicillin alone or in combination against epidemic multidrug-resistant Acinetobacter baumannii isolates producing OXA-58 carbapenemases. Int J Antimicrob Agents 30(6):537–540. doi:10.1016/j.ijantimicag.2007.07.007
196. Nastro M, Rodriguez CH, Monge R, Zintgraff J, Neira L, Rebollo M, Vay C, Famiglietti A (2014) Activity of the colistin-rifampicin combination against colistin-resistant, carbapenemase-producing Gram-negative bacteria. J Chemother 26:211. doi:10.1179/1973947813Y.0000000136
197. Sun HY, Shields RK, Cacciarelli TV, Muder RR, Singh N (2010) A novel combination regimen for the treatment of refractory bacteremia due to multidrug-resistant Pseudomonas aeruginosa in a liver transplant recipient. Transpl Infect Dis 12(6):555–560. doi:10.1111/j.1399-3062.2010.00543.x
198. Betts JW, Phee LM, Hornsey M, Woodford N, Wareham DW (2014) In vitro and in vivo activity of tigecycline/colistin combination therapies against carbapenem resistant Enterobacteriaceae. Antimicrob Agents Chemother 58:3541. doi:10.1128/AAC.02449-14
199. Souli M, Galani I, Boukovalas S, Gourgoulis MG, Chryssouli Z, Kanellakopoulou K, Panagea T, Giamarellou H (2011) In vitro interactions of antimicrobial combinations with fosfomycin against KPC-2-producing Klebsiella pneumoniae and protection of resistance development. Antimicrob Agents

Chemother 55(5):2395–2397. doi:10.1128/AAC.01086-10
200. Lora-Tamayo J, Murillo O, Bergen PJ, Nation RL, Poudyal A, Luo X, Yu HY, Ariza J, Li J (2014) Activity of colistin combined with doripenem at clinically relevant concentrations against multidrug-resistant Pseudomonas aeruginosa in an in vitro dynamic biofilm model. J Antimicrob Chemother 69:2434. doi:10.1093/jac/dku151
201. Clancy CJ, Chen L, Hong JH, Cheng S, Hao B, Shields RK, Farrell AN, Doi Y, Zhao Y, Perlin DS, Kreiswirth BN, Nguyen MH (2013) Mutations of the ompK36 porin gene and promoter impact responses of sequence type 258, KPC-2-producing Klebsiella pneumoniae strains to doripenem and doripenem-colistin. Antimicrob Agents Chemother 57(11):5258–5265. doi:10.1128/AAC.01069-13
202. Falagas ME, Rafailidis PI, Kasiakou SK, Hatzopoulou P, Michalopoulos A (2006) Effectiveness and nephrotoxicity of colistin monotherapy vs. colistin-meropenem combination therapy for multidrug-resistant Gram-negative bacterial infections. Clin Microbiol Infect 12(12):1227–1230. doi:10.1111/j.1469-0691.2006.01559.x
203. Falagas ME, Rafailidis PI, Ioannidou E, Alexiou VG, Matthaiou DK, Karageorgopoulos DE, Kapaskelis A, Nikita D, Michalopoulos A (2010) Colistin therapy for microbiologically documented multidrug-resistant Gram-negative bacterial infections: a retrospective cohort study of 258 patients. Int J Antimicrob Agents 35(2):194–199. doi:10.1016/j.ijantimicag.2009.10.005
204. Hirsch EB, Tam VH (2010) Detection and treatment options for Klebsiella pneumoniae carbapenemases (KPCs): an emerging cause of multidrug-resistant infection. J Antimicrob Chemother 65(6):1119–1125. doi:10.1093/jac/dkq108
205. Lee JY, Song JH, Ko KS (2011) Identification of nonclonal Pseudomonas aeruginosa isolates with reduced colistin susceptibility in Korea. Microb Drug Resist 17(2):299–304. doi:10.1089/mdr.2010.0145
206. Queenan AM, Pillar CM, Deane J, Sahm DF, Lynch AS, Flamm RK, Peterson J, Davies TA (2012) Multidrug resistance among Acinetobacter spp. in the USA and activity profile of key agents: results from CAPITAL Surveillance 2010. Diagn Microbiol Infect Dis 73(3):267–270. doi:10.1016/j.diagmicrobio.2012.04.002
207. Jones RN, Guzman-Blanco M, Gales AC, Gallegos B, Castro AL, Martino MD, Vega S, Zurita J, Cepparulo M, Castanheira M (2013) Susceptibility rates in Latin American nations: report from a regional resistance surveillance program (2011). Braz J Infect Dis 17(6):672–681. doi:10.1016/j.bjid.2013.07.002

Chapter 11

Vancomycin Pharmacodynamics: Optimal vs. Controversial

Ben M. Lomaestro

Abstract

After more than 55 years of use vancomycin still remains a viable agent primarily in the treatment of *Staphylococcus aureus* infections, but not without controversy. Issues of rising MICs ("MIC creep"), increased treatment failure, recommendations for more aggressive dosing, and an associated increased incidence of vancomycin-associated renal dysfunction have reinforced the importance of pharmacokinetic dosing services and antimicrobial stewardship initiatives to optimize safe and effective administration. This chapter addresses recent literature regarding optimal pharmacodynamic vancomycin administration to improve efficacy, minimize toxicity, adjust for specific patient populations, address caveats in the interpretation of MICs and creatinine clearance calculations, and compare various dosing methods. Although we are unlikely to see randomized controlled trials for many of these concerns, there remain unmet opportunities for new research.

Key words Vancomycin, Area under the curve (AUC) and AUC_{0-24}/MIC, Creatinine clearance, Minimum inhibitory concentration (MIC), Pediatrics, Obesity, Bayesian analysis, Linear regression, Nephrotoxicity, MRSA

1 Introduction and Brief History

Worsening outcomes in patients treated with vancomycin for invasive methicillin-resistant *S. aureus* (MRSA) infections such as pneumonia and bacteremia has led to a reassessment of its dosing and monitoring. Vancomycin is known to have slow bactericidal activity (particularly at high inoculum) and be associated with the emergence of resistant isolates and "MIC creep" among susceptible strains [1]. Efficacy may also be adversely impacted by limited penetration into important sites of infection such as bone, epithelial lining fluid and cerebral spinal fluid (CSF). Yet a recent review by Van Hal and Fowler [2] concluded that vancomycin remains the standard of care for most infections caused by MRSA despite elusive optimal dosing targets, concerns for increased mortality when the MRSA MIC is greater than 1.0 mg/L, issues with MIC testing methodology, aggressive dosing leading to more nephrotoxicity, and the availability of alternatives.

John C. Rotschafer et al. (eds.), *Antibiotic Pharmacodynamics*, Methods in Pharmacology and Toxicology,
DOI 10.1007/978-1-4939-3323-5_11,

In 2009, the vancomycin consensus guidelines attempted to standardize the administration and monitoring of vancomycin in adult patients with infections caused by *Staphylococcus aureus* [3] (recommendations summarized in Table 1). A ratio of the 24 h area under the concentration–time curve (AUC_{0-24}) to the minimum inhibitory concentration (MIC) of 400 was recommended to optimize efficacy with little mention of pharmacokinetic or pharmacodynamic alteration for specific disease states. Monitoring serum trough concentrations were proposed as a surrogate to more cumbersome AUC_{0-24}/MIC calculation. Pre-dose trough concentrations under steady-state conditions (defined as prior to the fourth dose) were recommended. The guidelines proposed a target steady-state trough of 15–20 mg/L for serious infections (defined as osteomyelitis, meningitis, endocarditis, bacteremia, or pneumonia) when the MIC is ≤1 mg/L for most adult patients with normal renal function. Maintenance dosing with 15–20 mg/kg of actual body weight (ABW) every 8–12 h after consideration of a 25–30 mg/kg loading dose was recommended. For mild to moderate infections, maintaining a trough ≥10 mg/L was suggested to diminish development of resistance. Peak serum concentrations were not advised due to a lack of data to suggest correlation with either efficacy or adverse reactions. Other pathogens such as methicillin-susceptible *S. aureus* or enterococcus and patient populations such as those who were obese, pediatric patients, those on dialysis or with augmented renal clearance were briefly mentioned if at all. The 2011 MRSA guidelines also endorsed maintenance vancomycin dosing of 15–20 mg/kg every 8–12 h based on ABW and adjusted for renal function with an added caveat to not exceed 2 g per dose [1]. A loading dose of 25 mg/kg was also to be considered in serious infections. Severe skin infections were added as an additional serious infection indication [1]. The MRSA guidelines suggested that more traditional (less intensive) dosing in adult patients with less serum concentration monitoring may be adequate for less severe infections when there is a good clinical response [1].

There are still several challenges in defining optimal therapy of vancomycin and mixed acceptance of the evidence incorporated into the guidelines. Dosing and monitoring practices since the 2009 vancomycin guidelines were evaluated in a questionnaire of 163 participants of the Making a Difference in Infectious Diseases Pharmacotherapy (MAD-ID) research network representing academic and nonacademic hospitals as well as rural and urban settings [4]. A relative lack of compliance with several recommendations identified several concerns in need of clarification and future research. Inconsistent application of the guidelines was noted for appropriate timing of trough values, initial loading doses, and use of ABW.

Table 1
Recommendations from the 2009 Vancomycin Monitoring Guidelines [3]

1. Therapeutic drug monitoring parameters
• Trough serum vancomycin concentrations recommended as the most accurate and practical monitoring parameter to assess efficacy.
• Troughs should be obtained at steady-state (approximately after the fourth dose).
• Serum vancomycin trough concentrations should be maintained above 10 mg/L to avoid development of resistance.
• Pathogens with an MIC of 1 mg/L, the minimum trough concentration should be at least 15 mg/L to approximate an AUC_{0-24}/MIC of 400.
• For serious infections (bacteremia, endocarditis, osteomyelitis, meningitis, hospital-acquired pneumonia) caused by *S. aureus* serum trough concentrations of 15–20 mg/L are recommended.
2. Dosing regimen
• 15–20 mg/kg ABW administered every 8–12 h is recommended for most patients with normal renal function when the MIC is ≤1 mg/L.
• In patients with normal renal function, an AUC_{0-24}/MIC target of >400 is not achievable with conventional dosing when the MIC is ≥2 mg/L.
• In seriously ill patients a loading dose of 25–30 mg/kg ABW can be used to rapidly attain target trough serum concentrations.
• Continuous infusion was not thought to offer advantages over intermittent dosing.
3. Monitoring for nephrotoxicity and ototoxicity
• A minimum of 2 or 3 consecutive documented increases in serum creatinine concentrations (defined as an increase of 0.5 mg/dL or a >50 % increase from baseline, whichever is greater) after several days of vancomycin therapy.
• Routine monitoring for ototoxicity was not recommended for vancomycin monotherapy but should be considered if concurrent ototoxic agents such as aminoglycosides are administered.
4. Criteria and frequency of monitoring
• Peak concentration monitoring was not recommended.
• Trough monitoring was recommended especially for aggressive dosing to attain troughs of 15–20 mg/L and in patients at high risk for nephrotoxicity.
• Monitoring was also recommended for patients with unstable renal function or courses lasting >3–5 days.
• Frequent monitoring prior to steady-state was not recommended for short courses or regimens targeted to troughs below 15 mg/L.
• All patients on >3–5 day courses of vancomycin should have at least one steady-state trough concentration obtained no earlier than following the fourth dose and repeated as deemed clinically appropriate.
• The limited data, at the time, to support sustained trough concentrations of 15–20 mg/L was noted. Once weekly monitoring was recommended for hemodynamically stable patients and more frequently for hemodynamically unstable patients.

(continued)

Table 1 (continued)

5. Additional recommendations from the 2011 MRSA guidelines [1].
• Severe skin and skin structure infections (necrotizing fasciitis for example) were added as serious infections.
• Also recommended 15–20 mg/kg ABW every 8–12 h but with a maximum dose of 2 g
• Also recommended consideration of a 25–30 mg/kg loading dose with a prolonged infusion time to minimize the potential for red man syndrome and possible anaphylaxis.
• Reminded clinicians that for most skin and skin structure infections in nonobese patients with normal renal function, 1 g every 12 h is sufficient and trough monitoring is not required.
• Pediatric dosing of 15 mg/kg/dose every 6 h was recommended for serious or invasive disease.
• The efficacy and safety of vancomycin trough concentrations of 15–20 mg/L in children was noted to require additional study but was recommended to be considered in patients with serious infections.

2 Pharmacokinetics

2.1 Overview

Vancomycin is a large molecule with a molecular weight of ~1450 Da [5]. It is not appreciably absorbed by the oral route [1]. Its pharmacokinetic profile is best explained by a 2 or 3 compartment model with a volume of distribution of 0.4–1.0 L/kg within a larger reported range of 0.26–1.25 L/kg [1, 3, 5–9]. In patients with normal renal function, the alpha-distribution phase ranges from 30 min to 1 h and the beta-elimination half-life from 6 to 12 h [1, 3]. The prolonged distribution phase can be a potential source of error when interpreting peak concentrations or fitting to a one compartment model [9]. Clearance of vancomycin is approximately 70–80 % of creatinine clearance which is the approximate amount of drug thought to be cleared by the kidneys [10, 11].

Tissue penetration is highly variable and dependent upon the degree of inflammation [1]. Distribution can be permeability-rate-limited and/or affected by blood flow, tissue-partition coefficients, and/or tissue volume [12]. There is a decreased penetration into sequestered compartments of important sites of infection such as epithelial lining fluid (ELF) and cerebral spinal fluid (CSF) [13]. With uninflamed meninges, CSF concentrations of vancomycin range from 0 to 4 mg/L versus 6.4–11.1 mg/L in inflamed meninges [3]. Investigators have found an ELF concentration of approximately 2 mg/L achieved with vancomycin serum concentrations of 15 mg/L, while others found a vancomycin exposure in ELF relative to plasma (mean AUC_{ELF}/ AUC_{plasma} penetration ratio) of 0.675 [13, 14]. The guidelines noted concentrations in lung tissue to range from 5 to 41 % of serum vancomycin concentrations [3]. Penetration into skin tissue is lower in diabetic patients and may not be reflected in serum concentration targets [3]. As discussed below, since vancomycin is about 55 % protein bound and has about 50 % of serum concentration penetration into the ELF, a serum target AUC_{0-24}/MIC ratio of ≥400 could be suboptimal in the treatment for MRSA pneumonia when the MIC exceeds 1 mg/L [13, 14].

2.2 Creatinine Clearance Calculations to Determine Dosing Interval

Dosing interval calculation involves estimating the length of time required after dosing to achieve either a target trough or desired exposure (AUC) prior to redosing [6]. Because vancomycin is predominantly eliminated through the kidney, this is based on renal function estimates and assumption that its renal clearance will be related to creatinine clearance [6]. Equations such as Cockcroft–Gault, Modification of Diet in Renal Disease (MDRD), and Chronic Kidney Disease Epidemiology Collaboration (CKD-EPI) are used to provide estimations of glomerular filtration or creatinine clearance with varying result. For example, MDRD and CKD-EPI have been found to significantly overestimate creatinine clearance (compared to measured or Cockcroft–Gault values) in elderly individuals frequently resulting in higher calculated dosing regimens [15]. Use of total body weight or adjusted body weight in the Cockcroft–Gault equation for morbidly obese patients has been found to overestimate creatinine clearance [16]. Augmented renal clearance in critically ill patients secondary to increased cardiac output and copious fluid administration during a systemic inflammatory response is another population in which the utility of dosing based on creatinine clearance calculation may be limited and result in underdosing [17, 18]. The treatment duration of vancomycin may also affect clearance. Prolonged vancomycin regimens (>4 weeks) have been associated with reduced vancomycin systemic clearance despite an unchanged creatinine clearance [19]. The data highlight the need to closely monitor vancomycin concentrations and population-specific pharmacodynamics in place of exclusively relying on traditional metrics assessing renal function.

3 Pharmacodynamics

3.1 Introduction to Basic Principles

Vancomycin is a slowly bactericidal antibiotic whose activity is adversely affected by increasing bacterial inoculum [3]. It exhibits time-dependent (concentration independent) killing, but since it also has a post-antibiotic effect, AUC/MIC is accepted as the most accurate pharmacodynamic predictor [3, 20]. This was initially proposed by Ebert et al. [20], in a neutropenic mouse thigh model where AUC_{0-24}/MIC was the best predictor as T>MIC did not correlate with bacterial killing.

3.1.1 Issues with the MIC

The Clinical Laboratory and Standards Institute reduced the minimum inhibitory concentration breakpoint of *S. aureus* to vancomycin from 4 to 2 mg/L in 2006 due to concerns of reduced vancomycin efficacy [2]. The IDSA MRSA treatment guidelines published in 2011 supported the current breakpoints and more aggressive dosing for severe infections [1]. Expert comment noted for isolates with a vancomycin MIC < 2.0 mg/L, the patient's clinical response should dictate continued use of vancomycin independent of the MIC result [1].

If AUC/MIC is the pharmacodynamic predictor of vancomycin efficacy, precise determination of the MIC is of utmost importance. An AUC_{0-24}/MIC ratio ≥ 400 is difficult to achieve when the MIC is greater than 1 mg/L (discussed below). MIC determination is subject to method-dependent variation with up to a one-fold dilution difference between commonly used methods of broth microdilution, Etest, and automated systems [21, 22]. This difference can have significant impact upon target attainment if not adjusted for testing method and can make generalization about success or failure based on an MIC (in the absence of clinical context) difficult [23]. The reference method for vancomycin MIC is broth microdilution (BMD) but many laboratories use less labor-intensive methods such as Etest, disc diffusion, and commercial assays such as Vitek-2, Phoenix, or Microscan [23]. It is important for clinicians to know which method is used to determine the MIC.

The central vancomycin MIC tendency (including increases sometimes referred to as an MIC "creep" for *S. aureus* populations) is an unstable phenomenon due to multiple factors including clonal replacement, antibiotic exposure, different testing, and whether isolates are tested at the time of isolation or after prolonged storage [2, 23]. The issue of MIC creep has prompted clinicians to use higher intensity vancomycin regimens. The tendency for increasingly higher MICs to vancomycin over time has also been observed for MSSA [24].

The influence of vancomycin's MIC upon outcome may also be favorably affected by co-administered antibiotics. Vancomycin plus a beta-lactam is more likely to achieve bacterial eradication in patients with MRSA bacteremia than vancomycin [25]. These combinations may be more effective than vancomycin monotherapy due to either enhanced vancomycin interaction with cell wall precursors, other alteration of the MRSA cell wall, or enhancement of beta-lactam activity [25].

In any case, the MIC affects the likelihood of target attainment and has been identified as an important predictor of vancomycin efficacy as discussed below.

3.1.2 Importance of the MIC and Treatment Outcome

Does a higher, yet susceptible vancomycin MIC impact clinical outcome? Van Hal et al. [26] conducted a meta-analysis on the impact of high vancomycin MICs (≥1.5 mg/L) upon outcomes of *S. aureus* infected patients. Despite issues of retrospective design, differing definitions of treatment failure and MIC testing, the preponderance of data demonstrate an association between high-MIC but susceptible vancomycin *S. aureus* infections and poorer outcomes independent of MIC methodology or site of infection. This was postulated to be due to the MIC as a biomarker for pathogen-specific factors responsible for worse outcomes, the presence of hVISA, or the suboptimal pharmacodynamic dosing of vancomycin. An exposure–nephrotoxicity relationship with higher troughs (≥15 mg/L) and a prolonged duration of therapy was associated with increased risk of nephrotoxicity relative to lower (<15 mg/L) troughs. The authors recommend performing Etest MICs on all MRSA bacteremia isolates and use of alternative agents if the MIC is ≥2.0 mg/L. Most of the literature relating MIC > 1.0 mg/L to vancomycin treatment failure has referenced Etest MICs. Soriano et al. [27] found Etest vancomycin MIC > 1 mg/L to be associated with higher MRSA bacteremia mortality and recommended aggressive empiric vancomycin dosing targeting troughs to ≥20 mg/L pending MIC results. Haque et al. [28] investigated the relationship of vancomycin MIC to 28 day all cause mortality in patients with MRSA hospital-, ventilator-, or health care-associated pneumonia and also observed increased 28 day mortality to be a function of vancomycin MIC even with values within the susceptible range. They recommended caution when treating similar patients when the vancomycin MIC is >1 mg/L.

Holmes et al. [21] confirmed an association between higher vancomycin MIC and mortality in patients with *S. aureus* bacteremia (MSSA or MRSA) but it was *not* related to specific antibiotic treatment. Other investigators have found vancomycin MIC > 1.5–2.0 mg/L *not* to have a significant impact on mortality when analyzing MRSA bacteremia [29–31]. Wang et al. [32] found high MIC and also hVISA phenotype *not* to be associated with higher mortality but both were associated with persistent MRSA bacteremia Comorbidities, high-risk sources, severity of sepsis, increasing age, presence of devices, presence of devices, ICU residence and other host or organism characteristics may be more important predictors of treatment failure. Han et al. [31] found reduced vancomycin susceptibility (defined as an Etest MIC > 1.0 mg/L) to be associated with increased 30 day mortality in patients with MSSA bacteremia but not with MRSA bacteremia. The authors speculate this may be in part due to lower virulence and fitness of MRSA strains vs. MSSA. A multicenter cohort study of 532 MSSA and MRSA bacteremic patients found vancomycin MIC was associated with mortality but in vancomycin-treated ***and*** in patients who never received vancomycin [21]. The data suggested factors other than antibiotic choice may be the primary determinants of patient outcome and/or higher vancomycin MIC may be a marker for an organism not likely to respond well to any antibiotic.

3.2 AUC_{0-24}/MIC as a Pharmacodynamic Target

Moise et al. [33] identified an AUC_{0-24}/MIC ratio of >345 to have the highest correlation with clinical success in 70 patients with *S. aureus* respiratory tract infections. Later, Moise-Broder et al. [34]

used classification and regression tree (CART) analysis to identify an AUC_{0-24}/MIC ratio ≥ 400 to be associated with improvement in clinical response in 108 mostly elderly patients with vancomycin-treated *S. aureus* pneumonia. The odds of a successful clinical response were approximately sevenfold greater in patients who achieved an AUC_{0-24}/MIC of ≥ 350 and a greater chance of bacteriologic eradication was predicted for an AUC_{0-24}/MIC of ≥ 400. The AUC was calculated based on vancomycin dosing and creatinine clearance: AUC = total vancomycin mg dose over 24 h/{(Clcr in mL per min × 0.79) + 15.4} × 0.06. In patients who achieved an AUC_{0-24}/MIC ratio of 400 or more, the median time to bacterial eradication was 10 days vs. >30 days for patients with an $AUC_{0-24}/MIC < 400$. Broth microdilution (BMD) was used to determine MICs. Subsequently, this AUC_{0-24}/MIC target was adopted by the 2009 vancomycin consensus guidelines and others to best predict vancomycin efficacy [3, 5, 35–37]. Whether this pharmacodynamic target pertains to all types of infections or those involving hVISA or *agr* dysfunction is controversial. As previously mentioned, a fixed AUC_{0-24}/MIC ratio of 400 based on serum concentrations may not account for variability in concentrations at target sites of infection. More aggressive dosing to achieve a fixed target of AUC_{0-24}/MIC ratio > 400 may also carry a higher risk of toxicity [2, 11].

For pathogens with an MIC of 1 mg/L, 1 g of vancomycin every 12 h will provide an AUC_{0-24}/MIC of approximately 250 in a patient with an ABW of 80 kg and normal renal function [3]. Because it can be difficult to obtain multiple serum concentrations, the 2009 guidelines recommended monitoring steady state trough concentrations (approximately after the fourth dose) as a surrogate to AUC calculation for monitoring target attainment [3]. Optimal trough concentrations and their use as a reliable surrogate for AUC calculation have been questioned. Jeffres et al. [38] found no evidence that troughs of 15–20 mg/L or specific AUC_{0-24} improved survival or hospital outcomes in the treatment of 102 patients with MRSA pneumonia over a 6.5 year period. However, optimal AUC_{0-24}/MIC was not calculated due to a lack of MIC testing. Time to targeted serum vancomycin concentration attainment was not measured but may also be a critical factor in patient outcome. Hermsen et al. [39] did not find statistically significant differences in outcome for 55 patients being treated for deep-seated MRSA infection with higher (≥15 mg/L) vs. lower vancomycin trough concentrations. Nephrotoxicity *was* consistently higher with vancomycin troughs ≥15 mg/L. Ackerman et al. [40] investigated vancomycin troughs from 604 treatment courses in 560 patients with either suspected or documented gram-positive infection in patients with burns <20 % of total body surface area. Data were stratified by trough concentration of <5, 5–10, and >10 mg/L to determine the relationship between response and trough concentration. Using analysis of variance, no relationship was found for the 3 trough strata and outcome, suggesting no real benefit from higher trough concentrations. The greatest risk of nephrotoxicity occurred with prolonged duration of therapy.

3.3 Impact of MIC and Target Attainment on Outcome and Toxicity

Hidayat et al. [41] evaluated 95 patients with MRSA bacteremia and/or pneumonia for clinical response, nephrotoxic incidence and infection-related mortality of high dose vancomycin (trough ≥15 mg/L). Aggressive vancomycin dosing produced an 85 % response rate when the MIC was ≤1 mg/L but only 62 % when the MIC was 1.5 or 2 mg/L. In addition, nephrotoxicity occurred only in the high trough group (11/63, 12 %) and was significantly predicted by administration of other concurrent nephrotoxic agents. The authors recommended use of combination therapy or alternative agents when the vancomycin MIC is 2 mg/L. Lodise et al. [42] evaluated 92 adult patients with MRSA bacteremia and also found an increased probability of treatment failure when the MIC is ≥1.5 mg/L using CART analysis. Patients with an MIC ≥ 1.5 mg/L had a 2.4-fold higher risk of treatment failure than counterparts with an MIC ≤ 1.0 mg/L. A body weight of >112 kg was found to be an independent variable associated with treatment failure. Patel et al. [43] performed a 9999 subject Monte Carlo simulation using a previously published 2 compartment model of 37 patients to identify the probability of achieving an AUC_{72-96}/MIC of ≥400 and trough of 15–20 mg/L with a variety of MICs and dosing regimens ranging from 1 to 4 g/day. Their analysis found the likelihood of achieving target AUC_{0-24}/MIC values to be inversely related to creatinine clearance and vancomycin MIC across a range of dosing regimens. Further, if the MIC is 2 mg/L, a 4 g/day regimen was predicted to be only 57 % effective in reaching the target AUC with a projected 35 % risk of nephrotoxicity. Trough levels of 15–20 mg/L were not always needed to achieve an AUC_{0-24}/MIC ≥ 400 if the MIC was ≤1 mg/L, did not consistently result in AUC_{0-24}/MIC ratios of ≥400 with an MIC of 2 mg/L, and patients with augmented renal function were less likely to achieve target attainment. (summarized in Table 2) The authors summed up their view of vancomycin dosing and target attainment in the title "We can't get there from here."

Kullar et al. [44] found vancomycin guideline recommended trough values of 15–20 mg/L to be associated with significantly lower failure rates compared with troughs of <10 or 10–14.9 mg/L in a retrospective investigation of 320 adult patients with MRSA bacteremia (Table 3). Patients failing therapy had lower AUC_{0-24}/MIC ratios and higher MIC Etest values. Independent predictors of vancomycin failure were endocarditis, nosocomial-acquired bacteremia, initial vancomycin trough <15 mg/L and vancomycin MIC > 1 mg/L by Etest. CART analysis identified vancomycin AUC_{0-24}/MIC ratios of <421 as having a significantly higher rate of failure compared with higher ratios ($p = 0.038$).

An association with treatment failure was found using Etest MICs but not broth microdilution, again pointing out differences in MIC testing methodology.

Kullar et al. [45] demonstrated 15 % improvement in outcomes and decreased duration of vancomycin therapy with aggressive dosing per the 2009 guidelines targeted to attain serum trough concentrations of 15–20 mg/L within a median of 2 days. Two hundred patients with documented complicated MRSA bacteremia were dosed with more aggressive guideline-compliant regimens and compared to a cohort dosed with a less aggressive traditional regimen depending on time period of the study. Patients in the pre-guideline period had lower success rates with vancomycin than the post-period (45 % vs. 60 %, $p=0.034$) and a longer median duration of vancomycin therapy (13 days vs. 8.5 days, $p<0.001$). The failure rate was still high in the aggressively dosed group, but only about 10 % of patients received a loading dose which could have affected outcome. Nephrotoxicity was numerically but not significantly higher in the more aggressively dosed cohort (18 % vs. 15 %, $p=0.85$). Higher doses of vancomycin were associated with a 15 % improvement in outcomes and decreased duration of therapy. The authors concluded that targeting serum trough concentrations of 15–20 mg/L improved outcome in patients with MRSA bacteremia.

3.4 Is the AUC_{0-24}/MIC Target always 400?

Holmes et al. [46] analyzed trough levels and vancomycin AUC_{0-24}/MIC values in 182 patients with *S. aureus* bacteremia. The median trough level was 19.5 mg/L within the first 96 h. The AUC_{0-24}/MIC ratio varied significantly by MIC testing method with a median of 436.1 for broth microdilution (BMD) compared to an Etest MIC calculated AUC median of 271.5 ($p<0.001$). An AUC_{0-24}/MIC ratio of ≥400 using BMD was not associated with lower mortality. However, a breakpoint AUC_{0-24}/MIC of >375 for 30 day all-cause mortality using BMD MICs was found using CART analysis ($p=0.043$). There was no association

Table 2
Impact of vancomycin trough concentrations and outcomes in patients with MRSA bacteremia

Characteristics $n=308$	Vancomycin failure n (%)	P vs. reference category	Nephrotoxicity n (%)	P vs. reference category
Trough <10 mg/L ($n=70$)	46 (65.7 %)	0.001	10/65 (15.4 %)	0.682
10–14.9 mg/L ($n=90$)	52 (57.8 %)	0.016	13/76 (17.1 %)	0.476
15–20 mg/L ($n=86$)	34 (39.5 %)	Reference value	10/77 (13.0 %)	Reference value
20 mg/L ($n=62$)	31 (50 %)	0.206	17/62 (27.4 %)	0.032

Adapted from Kullar et al. (Ref. [44])

Table 3
Probability of pharmacodynamic target attainment and nephrotoxicity

	AUC_{0-24}/MIC ratio ≥ 400			Nephrotoxic event	
MIC value	0.5 mg/L (%)	1.0 mg/L (%)	2.0 mg/L (%)	Non-ICU (%)	ICU (%)
500 mg IV q12h	57	15	0.7	3	10
1 g IV q12h	90	57	15	6	16
1.5 g q12h	97	79	38	9	25
2.0 g IV q12h	98	90	57	14	34

Adapted from Patel N. et al. (Ref. [43])

between achieving a vancomycin AUC_{0-24}/MIC of ≥400 or >373 and secondary endpoints of reduction in attributable mortality, persistent bacteremia, or recurrent bacteremia. There was moderate correlation between the measured trough concentrations and calculated AUC ($r = 0.246$, $p = 0.002$). The authors concluded an $AUC_{0-24}/MIC > 373$ within 96 h was associated with reduced mortality and the MIC test method had significant impact on vancomycin AUC_{0-24}/MIC estimation. Differences in Cockcroft–Gault or MDRD creatinine clearance calculation resulted in little influence on vancomycin AUC but the equivalent recommended target AUC_{0-24}/MIC when testing by Etest was 226 rather than 400.

Gawronski et al. [47] found a greater than 2.5-fold increase in time to microbiologic clearance in 59 patients with MRSA bacteremia and associated osteomyelitis if unable to achieve a vancomycin breakpoint AUC_{0-24}/MIC of >293 identified by CART analysis. In multivariate analysis, AUC_{0-24}/MIC was the only independent predictor of time to bacterial clearance. All patients were initially treated with 15 mg/kg per dose ABW to a maximum of 2 g per dose. No patients received loading doses. Only 39 % of patients were able to have the infection source removed. MICs were determined by two different methods (Etest and Microscan) during differing periods of study. Only 9 % of patients were able to achieve an optimal AUC_{0-24}/MIC target if the isolate MIC was >1 mg/L. Trough concentrations poorly correlated with AUC_{0-24}/MIC.

Brown et al. [48] using CART analysis found a lower AUC_{0-24}/MIC breakpoint of <211 to be associated with a fourfold increase in attributable mortality in patients with complicated MRSA bacteremia ($n = 32$) or infective endocarditis ($n = 18$). Of interest, hVISA and *agr* dysfunction were not related to increasing mortality risk.

Few institutions actually measure AUC and there are several caveats to the assumption that a vancomycin trough is always a good surrogate for the AUC [11, 49]. Optimal trough concentrations and adequate correlation to an AUC_{0-24}/MIC target is dependent on the MIC and pharmacokinetic parameters of a given patient [11]. The optimal AUC_{0-24}/MIC may not always be a fixed ratio depending on source of infection, MIC testing methodology or other factors.

3.5 Other Patient Populations and Concerns

3.5.1 Pediatrics

Adult pharmacodynamic targets for vancomycin troughs may not be applicable to pediatric populations. Analysis of 702 pediatric patients with 1660 vancomycin serum concentrations (who are commonly dosed every 6 h) found an AUC_{0-24}/MIC of approximately 400 corresponded to a trough of roughly 8–9 mg/L for regimens 60–70 mg/kg/day in 75 % of patients [50]. Higher doses were more likely to be required in patients between 1 and 2 years of age and those with serum creatinine falling between 0.2 and 0.4 mg/dL. Target attainment was dependent on the MIC distribution of the hospitals involved. The authors recommended to monitor AUC in pediatrics with MIC ratio calculation if possible. Dosing based only on trough levels would potentially lead to unnecessary increases in drug exposure in 25–35 % of pediatric subjects who had already achieved a target AUC_{0-24}/MIC. Frymoyer et al. [51] used a population pharmacokinetic modeling and software (NONMEM version 7.3, ICON Development Solutions, Ellicott City, MD) to simulate the pharmacokinetic profiles in 5000 pediatric patients and compare three different pharmacokinetic models. In contrast to adults, the trough predictive of >90 % of children achieving AUC_{0-24}/MIC > 400 ranged from 7 to 10 mg/L. Using a daily dose of 60 mg/kg/day divided every 8 h, the trough predictive of an AUC_{0-24}/MIC > 400 was 6–8 mg/L. Results were highly dependent on the MIC. Their data also suggests troughs of 15–20 mg/L to achieve an AUC_{0-24}/MIC > 400 are likely unnecessary in the typical child.

Dosing metrics used in regimen calculation may also be evolving. Body surface area based dosing may be more likely than weight based dosing to achieve target AUC values in children and young adults. Camaione et al. [52] found body surface area based dosing to be more accurate than weight-based dosing of vancomycin in children using a one-compartment pharmacokinetic model to determine maximum a posteriori probability (MAP)-Bayesian pharmacokinetic parameter estimates and to evaluate relationships of body size descriptors. Vancomycin clearance was a nonlinear function of weight and a linear-proportionate function of BSA whereas the central compartment volume of distribution was linear-proportionate to weight. AUC_{0-24} achieved with weight based dosing of 60–70 mg/kg/day varied with patient weight but isometric AUC_{0-24} was predicted with BSA. Confirmatory studies are needed.

3.5.2 Obesity

Dosing of vancomycin in obese patients remains controversial. The 2009 vancomycin consensus guidelines recommended dosing on ABW [3]. Dosing based on ABW may not be correct if the central compartment volume of distribution for vancomycin does not increase proportionally with weight as this may put morbidly obese patients at risk for toxicity when dosed by ABW. Blouin et al. [53], Bauer et al. [54], and Vance-Bryan et al. [55] found vancomycin clearance to be greater and volume of distribution to be smaller in morbidly obese patients than in their nonobese counterparts with a stronger correlation between clearance and total body weight rather than lean body weight. Recent review by Grace [7] noted alteration in volume of distribution, increased circulating proteins (resulting in altered free serum concentration) and increased blood flow secondary to increased cardiac output and blood volume results in increased vancomycin clearance in obese patients. He concluded vancomycin volume of distribution correlates best with total body weight and not ideal body weight.

Reynolds et al. [56] found 15 mg/kg every 8–12 h ABW produced a trough of >20 mg/L 55 % of the in 64 patients compared 18 % of 74 patients dosed with a newer protocol of 10 mg/kg every 12 h or 15 mg/kg every 24 h. Patients in both groups were ≥100 kg with normal renal function. The authors concluded obese patients should receive a smaller mg/kg dosage than nonobese patients. Rushing and Ambrose [57] found the lesser of ideal body weight (IBW) or total body weight (TBW) and Leong et al. [58] found adjusted body weight (ABW (kg) = IBW + 0.4 (TBW-IBW)) to best correlate with vancomycin clearance. Lodise et al. [42, 59] identified a body weight >100 kg as a risk factor for vancomycin-associated renal dysfunction.

The controversy regarding dosing based on ABW in morbidly obese patients has led some clinicians to either "cap" vancomycin loading and maintenance doses or give multiple loading doses of 2 or 3 g.

3.5.3 Loading Doses

The 2009 vancomycin guidelines recommended consideration of a loading dose of 25–30 mg/kg for complicated infections and 20–25 mg/kg for mild-moderate infections [3]. Loading doses theoretically allow a more rapid attainment of therapeutic concentrations. A loading dose of 25 mg/kg was found to be safe in 28 ICU patients who achieved 1 h post infusion levels of 26.4 ± 9.3 mg/L (mean ± SD) [60]. DeRyke and Alexander [11], recommended a loading dose targeted to achieve a peak concentration of 30–40 mg/L using the equation dose = Cp × Vd where Vd = 0.83 L/kg (based on ABW) if CrCl is <60 mL/min and Vd = 0.57 L/kg (based on ABW) if CrCl is 60 mL/min or greater.

Denetclaw et al. [61] proposed a divided loading dose policy for critically ill patient to rapidly attain targeted trough concentrations of 15–20 mg/L for severe infections. Initial dosing of 15 mg/kg ABW every 6 h in patients with normal renal function (not to exceed 4 g per day or 1.5 g per dose initially) resulted in 62 of 79 patients (90 %) achieving therapeutic concentrations 12–24 h after initiation of therapy. For morbidly obese patients with normal renal function, the lesser of 20 mg/kg IBW or 1.5 g per dose was recommended and/or more frequent dosing to achieve target concentrations within 3 doses.

Utilization of a loading dose is most important in seriously infected patients and those with renal dysfunction for whom steady state would occur only after an extended time period [6, 11].

3.5.4 Continuous Infusion

Continuous infusion to a vancomycin steady state level of 20–25 mg/L appears to be effective and result in similar AUC/MIC as optimal intermittent therapy [62]. Pea et al. [63] proposed 2 dosing nomograms to target a steady-state concentration of 15 or 20 mg/L in critically ill patients with borderline susceptible MICs. Each involves administration of a 15 mg/kg loading dose but maintenance dosing with initiation of a continuous infusion based on the assumption of a significant relationship between Cl_{vanco} and Cl_{creat}. The formula for the continuous infusion rate was: grams per 24 h = [0.029 × Cl_{creat} (mL/min) + 0.94] × target Css × (24/1000).

Meta-analysis of mostly observational studies has concluded there is a lower risk of nephrotoxicity (RR 0.6, 95 % CI 0.4–0.9, $p = 0.02$) but no difference in mortality with continuous vancomycin infusion vs. intermittent regimens [62]. This may infer nephrotoxicity is related to higher peak concentrations since steady state targets with continuous infusion are similar to (or higher than) targeted troughs with intermittent administration. However, other reviews have concluded there is inconsistent and insufficient evidence of significant difference in nephrotoxicity or efficacy between the methods of administration [64, 65]. The 2009 vancomycin consensus guidelines did not advocate the need for continuous infusion of vancomycin [3]. More recent data seems to confirm no obvious harm but insufficient advantage to continuous infusion regimens.

3.5.5 Augmented Renal Clearance

Vancomycin monitoring involves assessment of renal *dysfunction* and intervention to decrease dosing and/or prolong frequency. Less appreciated are patients with substantially ***augmented*** renal elimination of drugs such as vancomycin especially among critically ill patients throughout their first week in the ICU. Udy et al. [35] identified 65.1 % of ICU patients to have augmented renal clearance during this time period. These patients may require more aggressive dosing initially and a loading dose may be important to achieve pharmacodynamics targets. The authors remind clinicians to assess "renal function" and not just "renal injury" and caution that calculated creatinine clearance as a descriptor of renal drug elimination in this population can be inaccurate.[3201] This group may also benefit from a loading dose. Aubron et al. [66] investigated 48 critically ill patients and noted a lower percentage of patients with a trough in the desired range during the first 24 h of therapy occurred when a loading dose was not given. Truong et al. [67] found implementation of a 2 g vancomycin loading dose policy in intensive care patients to improve attainment of therapeutic concentrations (15–20 mg/L) to 33 % from 13 % ($p=0.08$) with mean trough concentrations increased from 9.8 ± 6.6 mg/L to 14.9 ± 6.3 mg/L ($p=0.01$). They noted this population can have an increase in capillary permeability as a response to sepsis which can increase vancomycin's distribution volume. Edema, pleural effusion, ascites, and fluid resuscitation may also increase the volume of distribution and result in a drop in serum concentration without adequate loading and maintenance dosing. They also note that the hyperdynamic state of sepsis and burn patients leads to increased cardiac output and blood flow that can increase elimination of vancomycin.

4 Clinical Application of Pharmacodynamic Data

4.1 Therapeutic Drug Monitoring

The focus on AUC and MIC for initial empiric dosing suggests a clearance-based rather than weight-based strategy through calculating the daily dose by multiplying a patient's estimated vancomycin clearance by the desired AUC_{0-24} [6]. Weight is accounted for through estimation of creatinine clearance via Cockcroft–Gault [6]. This method predicts the average steady-state serum concentration [6]. A variation of this relationship to quickly estimate vancomycin AUC_{0-24} by dividing total vancomycin dose (mg) per 24 h by the vancomycin clearance in liters per hour [11]. Accepting the clearance of vancomycin is approximately 70–80 % of the creatinine clearance, this correction must be made prior to the calculation.

It is possible that AUC calculation can be performed relatively easily with minimal serum concentrations required. Neely et al. [49] used 3 independent data sets from 47 healthy volunteers and previously published patient pharmacokinetic analysis (with Pmetrics nonparametric population modeling package version 1.1.1 for R reversion) to compare AUCs estimated from models derived from "trough only" and "peak–trough" versions of the full data set to test the relationship between trough and AUC. Data sets comprised a total of 569 vancomycin concentrations and a wide range of dosing and estimated creatinine clearance values. The model was based on richly sampled vancomycin data used as a Bayesian prior. Simulation in adults with normal renal function achieving a therapeutic AUC_{0-24} of *greater than* 400 mg·h/L suggested approximately 50–60 % will have a trough *less than* 15 mg/L which could result in an unneeded increase in dosing. However, the data also demonstrated trough-only data could be used to generate reliable AUC estimates. In contrast, the peak and trough concentration data analysis was worse at predicting a true vancomycin AUC. Even in an ideal population of adults with normal renal function, AUC values varied up to 30-fold between patients with a high degree of variability in peak and trough values as well. Trough concentrations were a very poor surrogate for AUC estimation and overall vancomycin exposure, underestimating the true AUC by about 25 %. Of simulated patients with a trough >20 mg/L, about 25–55 % had an $AUC_{0-24} \geq 700$ mg · h/L, depending on the dose. The authors propose that AUC-guided dosing is more precise and can now be easily calculated with available computer programs such as Best Dose (freely available at the Laboratory of Applied Pharmacokinetics and Bioinformatics website at www.lapk.org).

AUC measurement may be more accurate than using serum trough concentrations as a surrogate marker. Further, AUC calculation by computer software may be less cumbersome than calculation methods of decades past.

4.2 Methods of Monitoring Vancomycin

4.2.1 Linear Regression Analysis

Linear regression analysis fits serum concentrations to individual patient models and assumes a one-compartment model [68]. These methods use serum concentration data around a dosing interval and do not account for other factors such as changing renal function [68]. The lack of population data and necessity to have two concentrations can be a limitation.

4.2.2 Population Methods

Vancomycin dosing is based on population pharmacokinetic parameters (called an a priori dosing method) without using individual patient pharmacokinetic results [68]. Several nomograms have been developed to empirically dose vancomycin in such a manner. Assumptions include linear pharmacokinetics, strong correlation between drug clearance and creatinine clearance, and dosing weight (ideal vs. actual) [68]. Only one nomogram targets the recommended trough concentrations of 15–20 mg/L and has been validated in a select group of patients [69].

Several nomograms were published decades ago at a time when troughs were targeted to 5–10 mg/L. Since it is the dose that defines the difference between peak and trough, the shortest practical dosing interval with the smallest dose would tend to yield the higher trough and achieve a higher likelihood of the trough being >15 mg/L [6]. AUC_{0-24} calculated as the daily dose divided by the clearance and targeted to an average concentration of 15 mg/L was proposed over 30 years ago by Moellering et al. [71] and Rodvold et al. [70] The Moellering et al. [71] nomogram was based on a pharmacokinetic analysis of 22 patients targeting a mean steady-state concentration of 15 mg/L and recommended 30 mg/kg/day in divided doses which would be 2 g daily in a 70 kg individual with normal renal function. The Rodvold et al. [70] dosing chart was developed from data in 37 adult patients and used measured creatinine clearance which explained only 59 % of the variance in vancomycin clearance pointing out how essential it is to monitor serum concentrations. Matzke et al. [8] developed a nomogram based on 57 patients, a one-compartment model and CrCl as determined by the Cockcroft–Gault equation (using ABW) in 56 patients. An initial dose of 25 mg/kg was followed by 19 mg/kg at a frequency determined by the nomogram. The target serum concentrations were a peak of 30 mg/L and a trough of 7.5 mg/L.

Rybak and Boike [72] compared the Matzke and Moellering nomograms and found the former to be more accurate. Murphy et al. [73] compared the ability of seven methods including those by Matzke and Rodvold to predict measured concentrations in 189 patients and found Matzke to have the higher precision and less bias. However, none of the nomograms were sufficiently reliable to replace monitoring vancomycin serum concentrations. Karam et al. [74] attempted to minimize monitoring of vancomycin by comparing traditional peak and trough pharmacokinetics to trough-only values utilized in a vancomycin dosing chart with regimens provided for 9 ranges of CrCl and 13 ranges of body weight targeting troughs of 5–20 mg/L. No differences were noted with respect to clinical efficacy or toxicity but a considerable cost savings was noted due to fewer levels ordered with the use of the nomogram.

More recently recommendations for more aggressive dosing have resulted in new and revised nomograms. In 2011, Kullar et al. [69] published an updated nomogram somewhat similar to that of Karam et al. [74], in that ABW and estimated creatinine clearance were used to determine dose and frequency. However, the new nomogram was refined to achieve a trough of 15–20 mg/L and an AUC_{0-24}/MIC of ≥400. When tested in 200 patients, it achieved a trough target on the first measurement in 58 % of patients and subsequently in 77 % of patients. If the acceptable trough range were expanded to 12–22 mg/L, 80 % would have achieved the targets.

Golenia et al. [75] used ABW and MDRD to develop a nomogram in intensive care unit patients noting differences with renal clearance in this population (discussed above). The nomogram resulted in 42 % of patients ($n = 60$) attaining troughs between 15 and 20 mg/L compared with 19 % pre-implementation patients ($n = 57$) ($p = 0.0099$). Benefits may have been limited by capping loading doses at 2.25 g for patients ≥90 kg and maintenance doses at a maximum of 2.0 g every 8 h for patients with eGFR > 60 mL/min/1.73 m^2 and ≥60 kg.

It is important to ensure an individual patient matches the population for which a nomogram was developed and clinicians remember nomograms assume pharmacokinetic parameters are stable which may not be the case in severely ill patients [68]. Nomograms do not replace clinical judgment and adjustments may be best made based on clinical response and therapeutic drug monitoring [69].

4.2.3 Bayesian Analysis

Modern Bayesian modeling algorithms incorporate both population pharmacokinetic parameters (a priori) and patient specific data (*a posteriori*) estimates of clearance and distribution to individualize dosing [76]. It is possible to predict starting doses using patient demographic data to define patient-specific parameters and value estimates [10, 18]. A major advantage is timeliness since maintenance regimen predictions can be made from software using first-dose concentrations whereas guidelines usually recommend levels at steady-state [76]. However, non-steady-state concentrations provide less than optimal information in Bayesian prediction of future steady-state concentrations [77]. An early example of this method was published by Rodvold et al. [78], using the Abbott Pharmacokinetic System computer program and two-compartment population parameter model data derived from 45 patients to accurately individualize vancomycin dosing with just two measured concentrations. Precision was improved when a set of peak and trough vancomycin concentrations were obtained at steady-state and used to individualize patient pharmacokinetic parameter estimates.

Bayesian models can be used to adjust dosing after a drug concentration is obtained but less accurately predict pharmacokinetics of patients whose parameters lie outside of the 95th percentile, and they are most accurate when the appropriate patient population has been characterized in the model [10, 61]. Nunn et al. [76] investigated the accuracy of MM-USC*Pack program (Jelliffe R, University of Southern California, 2008, version 12.10) comparing the predicted concentrations to observed concentrations in 77 patients (204 concentrations) prescribed vancomycin over a 6-week period. The program uses a Bayesian algorithm with a two compartment population model to update pharmacokinetic parameters with newly available patient data as it becomes available. The most common dosing regimen was 1 g every 12 h which resulted in initial trough concentrations <10 mg/L in 58.4 % of patients and therapeutic concentrations (10–20 mg/L) in 33.8 %. The software predictions in this heterogeneous cohort of patients demonstrated little systemic bias (−3.1 %) but only moderate precision (median prediction error) of 23 %. Predictions with this program have been notably poorer in severely ill, obese (BMI > 35 kg/m^2) or in patients with unstable renal function [66, 76]. Hurst et al. [10] used an earlier version of the same software (USC*PACK PC collection, University of Southern California) based on data from 12 cardiac outpatients receiving single doses of vancomycin for dental procedures and found a lower bias than other Bayesian algorithms. Seven acutely ill patients with suspected staphylococcal infection were also studied with regimens targeted to troughs of <15 mg/L and peaks of 35–50 mg/L. The Bayesian method did outperform one-compartment linear regression in prediction of future vancomycin concentrations.

5 Toxicity and Adverse Reactions

Impurities in early formulations of vancomycin were thought accountable for many of its adverse reactions with little potential for ototoxicity or nephrotoxicity from current formulations unless co-administered with other nephrotoxins or by very aggressive vancomycin dosing [3]. The most important concentration-dependent adverse event associated with vancomycin administration is renal dysfunction. Vancomycin-associated renal dysfunction has been reported to temporally occur in 2–28 % of patients prescribed the antibiotic [79]. Vancomycin is thought to be an oxidative stressor in the renal proximal tubule, can cause toxicity in the medullary region, and may also rarely cause interstitial nephritis [3]. Uncertainty remains over the causality of vancomycin in most associated renal dysfunction cases or whether concurrent nephrotoxins and an underlying incidence of MRSA-infection-associated renal dysfunction increases risk [2]. The vancomycin consensus guidelines did note there were insufficient data to support the safety of the higher recommended vancomycin trough concentrations over a prolonged treatment duration [3]. The guidelines did try to standardize the definition of nephrotoxicity as multiple (at least 2 or 3 consecutive) high serum creatinines which increase by at least 0.5 mg/dL or ≥50 % from baseline (whichever is greater) documented after several days of vancomycin administration and in the absence of alternative explanation [3]. Data related to vancomycin-associated renal dysfunction is plagued by different definitions and metrics to define renal dysfunction.

Lodise et al. [59] retrospectively examined the relationship between vancomycin dosing and rate of nephrotoxicity. Linezolid usage was included as a comparator. Patients receiving ≥4 g/day had a threefold higher chance of developing nephrotoxicity (34.9 %) than patients receiving <4 g/day (10.9 %) or linezolid (6.7 %). Multivariate analysis confirmed the relationship between dosage and nephrotoxicity and also identified weight ≥101.4 kg, estimated Clcr of ≤86.6 mL/min and ICU residence as independent risk factors for nephrotoxicity. The same group found initial troughs >15 mg/L (within 96 h of therapy initiation) and steady-state AUC_{0-24} values ≥1300 mg·h/L to be independent predictors of nephrotoxicity even after correcting for confounders [80].

In addition to the use of AUC calculation as a pharmacodynamic target, an AUC_{0-24} of >700–1300 mg·h/L has been proposed as an alternative marker for increased risk of vancomycin-associated renal dysfunction to trough concentrations [3, 49, 80, 81]. Other risk factors identified in literature reviews for vancomycin-associated renal dysfunction include: doses exceeding 4 g/day, concurrent administration of nephrotoxins, prolonged duration of therapy, residence in intensive care units, higher acuity scores, and weight greater than 100 kg [3, 79, 82]. Systematic review and meta-analysis of vancomycin-associated renal dysfunction identified an exposure–nephrotoxicity relationship and concluded the probability increases as a function of increasing trough concentration and duration of therapy [82]. In rats, high doses of vancomycin (350 mg/kg twice daily for 4 days) are associated with increased nephrotoxicity risk [83]. This may imply high peak concentrations in humans with excessive maintenance or loading doses as an additional risk factor.

Ototoxicity is a dose dependent adverse effect of vancomycin evaluated in recent years by Forouzesh et al. [84] A review of 89 patients with baseline audiograms and audiograms performed after an average of 27 days of vancomycin therapy showed a 12 % rate of high-frequency hearing loss with a trend in univariate analysis to higher incidence with advancing age. However, only one patient received more than 2 g of vancomycin per day and others have questioned the findings and methodology. A review of older data noted ototoxicity to occur with a reported frequency of 1–9 % and to be associated with serum vancomycin concentrations >40 mg/L [3].

6 Summary

Optimal dosing of vancomycin has led to more aggressive regimens and more frequent temporally associated renal dysfunction. Interpretation of vancomycin troughs and their relationship to AUC, variation in MIC results due to testing methodology, caveats to calculated creatinine clearances and glomerular filtration rates, different methods to calculate regimens, and issues with different patient populations all complicate optimal dosing. The 2009 vancomycin guidelines identified AUC_{0-24}/MIC as the best pharmacodynamic predictor. With the current widespread use and access to powerful computers it may now be possible and practical to reexamine software programs envisioned decades ago to more accurately identify optimal vancomycin dosing regimens instead of using surrogate markers such as serum vancomycin troughs. After over 55 years of use, there is still room for improvement and a sustained commitment to the monitoring of vancomycin regimens.

References

1. Liu C, Bayer A, Cosgrove SE et al (2011) Clinical practice guidelines by the Infectious Diseases Society of America for the treatment of methicillin-resistant *Staphylococcus aureus* infections in adults and children. Clin Infect Dis 52:e18–e55
2. Tenover FC, Moellering RC Jr (2007) The rationale for revising the Clinical and Laboratory Standards institute vancomycin minimal inhibitory concentration interpretive criteria for *Staphylococcus aureus*. Clin Infect Dis 44:1208–1215

3. Rybak M, Lomaestro B, Rotschafer JC, Moellering R et al (2009) Therapeutic monitoring of vancomycin in adult patients: a consensus review of the American Society of Health-System Pharmacists, the Infectious Diseases Society of America, and the Society of Infectious Diseases Pharmacists. Am J Health Syst Pharm 66:82–98
4. Davis SL, Scheetz MH, Bosso JA et al (2013) Adherence to the 2009 consensus guidelines for vancomycin dosing and monitoring practices: a cross-sectional survey of U.S. Hospitals. Pharmacotherapy 33:1250–1263
5. Rybak MJ (2006) The pharmacokinetic and pharmacodynamic properties of vancomycin. Clin Infect Dis 42:S35–S39
6. Brown JL, Lalla CE, Masselink A (2013) AUC versus peak-trough dosing of vancomycin: applying new pharmacokinetic paradigms to an old drug. Ther Drug Monit 35:443–449
7. Grace E (2012) Altered vancomycin pharmacokinetics in obese and morbidly obese patients: what we have learned over the past 30 years. J Antimicrob Chemother 67:1305–1310
8. Matzke GR, McGory RW, Halstenson CE et al (1984) 1984. Pharmacokinetics of vancomycin in patients with various degrees of renal function. Antimicrob Agents Chemother 25:433–437
9. Rotschafer JC, Crossley K, Zaske DE et al (1982) Antimicrob Agents Chemother 22:391–394
10. Hurst AK, Yoshinaga MA, Mitani GH et al (1990) Application of a Bayesian method to monitor and adjust vancomycin dosage regimens. Antimicrob Agents Chemother 34: 1165–1171
11. DeRyke CA, Alexander DP (2009) Optimizing vancomycin dosing through pharmacodynamic assessment targeting area under the concentration-time curve/minimum inhibitory concentration. Hosp Pharm 44:751–765
12. Lim HS, Chong YP, Noh YH et al (2014) Exploration of optimal dosing regimens of vancomycin in patients infected with methicillin-resistant Staphylococcus aureus by modeling and simulation. Clin Pharmacol Ther 39:196. doi:10.1111/jcpt.12123
13. Scheetz MH, Wunderink RG, Postelnick MJ et al (2006) Potential impact of vancomycin pulmonary distribution on treatment outcomes in patients with methicillin-resistant *Staphylococcus aureus* pneumonia. Pharmacotherapy 26:539–550
14. Lodise TP, Drusano GL, Butterfield JM et al (2011) Penetration of vancomycin into epithelial lining fluid in healthy volunteers. Antimicrob Agents Chemother 35:5507–5511
15. Dowling TC, Wang ES, Ferrucci L et al (2013) Glomerular filtration rate equations overestimate creatinine clearance in older individuals enrolled in the Baltimore longitudinal study on aging: impact on renal drug dosing. Pharmacotherapy 33:912–921
16. Demirovic JA, Barton Pai A, Pai MP (2009) Estimation of creatinine clearance in morbidly obese patients. Am J Health Syst Pharm 66:642–648
17. Baptista JP, Sousa E, Martins PJ et al (2012) Augmented renal clearance in septic patients and implications for vancomycin optimization. Int J Antimicrob Agents 39:420–423
18. Ocampos-Martinez E, Penaccini L, Scolletta S et al (2012) Determinants of early inadequate vancomycin concentrations during continuous infusion in septic patients. Int J Antimicrob Agents 39:332–337
19. Nakayama H, Echizen H, Tanaka M et al (2008) Reduced vancomycin clearance despite unchanged creatinine clearance in patients treated with vancomycin for longer than 4 weeks. Ther Drug Monit 30:103–107
20. Ebert S, Leggert J, Vogelman B (1987) In vivo cidal activity and pharmacokinetic parameters for vancomycin against methicillin-susceptible and -resistant S. aureus (abstract 439). In: Program and abstracts of the 27th Interscience Conference on Antimicrobial Agents and Chemotherapy (New York). American Society of Microbiology, Washington, DC, p 173
21. Holmes NE, Turnidge JD, Munckhof WJ et al (2011) Antibiotic choice may not explain poorer outcomes in patients with *Staphylococcus aureus* bacteremia and high vancomycin minimum inhibitory concentrations. J Infect Dis 204:340–347
22. Holmes NE, Johnson PDR, Howden BP (2012) Relationship between vancomycin-resistant *Staphylococcus aureus*, vancomycin-intermediate *S. aureus*, high vancomycin MIC, and outcome in serious *S. aureus* infections. J Clin Microbiol 50:2548–2552
23. Edwards B, Milne K, Lawes T et al (2012) Is vancomycin MIC "Creep" method dependent? Analysis of methicillin-resistant Staphylococcus aureus susceptibility trends in blood isolates from North East Scotland from 2006 to 2010. J Clin Microbiol 50:318–325
24. Wang G, Hindler JF, Ward KW et al (2006) Increased vancomycin MIC for Staphylococcus aureus clinical isolates from a university hospital during a 5-year period. J Clin Microbiol 44:3883–3886
25. Dillworth TJ, Ibrahim O, Hall P et al (2014) B-lactams enhance vancomycin activity against methicillin-resistant Staphylococcus aureus

bacteremia compared to vancomycin alone. Antimicrob Agents Chemother 58:102–109
26. Van Hal SJ, Lodise TP, Paterson DL (2012) The clinical significance of vancomycin minimum inhibitory concentration in *Staphylococcus aureus* infections: a systematic review and meta-analysis. Clin Infect Dis 54:755–771
27. Soriano A, Marco F, Martinez JA et al (2008) Influence of vancomycin minimum inhibitory concentration on the treatment of methicillin resistant Staphylococcus aureus bacteremia. Clin Infect Dis 46:193–200
28. Haque NZ, Zuniga LC, Peyrani P et al (2010) Relationship of vancomycin minimum inhibitory concentration to mortality in patients with methicillin-resistant Staphylococcus aureus hospital-acquired, ventilator-associated, or health-care-associated pneumonia. Chest 138:1356–1362
29. Gasch O, Camoez M, Dominguez MA et al (2013) Predictive factors for mortality in patients with methicillin-resistant *Staphylococcus aureus* bloodstream infections: impact on outcome of host, microorganism and therapy. Clin Microbiol Infect 19:1049–1057
30. Honda H, Doern CD, Michael-Dunne W et al (2011) The impact of vancomycin susceptibility on treatment outcomes among patients with methicillin-resistant *Staphylococcus aureus* bacteremia. BMC Infect Dis 11:335
31. Han JH, Mascitti KB, Edelstein PH et al (2012) Effect of reduced vancomycin susceptibility on clinical and economic outcomes in *Staphylococcus aureus* bacteremia. Antimicrob Agents Chemother 56:5164–5170
32. Wang JL, Lai CH, Lin HH et al (2013) High vancomycin minimum inhibitory concentrations with heteroresistant vancomycin-intermediate Staphylococcus aureus in methicillin-resistant *S. aureus* bacteraemia patients. Int J Antimicrob Agents 42:390–394
33. Moise PA, Forrest A, Bhavnani SM et al (2000) Area under the inhibitory curve and a pneumonia scoring system for predicting outcomes of vancomycin therapy for respiratory infections by *Staphylococcus aureus*. Am J Health Syst Pharm 57(suppl 2):S4–S9
34. Moise-Broder PA, Forrest A, Birmingham MC et al (2004) Pharmacodynamics of vancomycin and other antimicrobials in patients with *Staphylococcus aureus* lower respiratory tract infections. Clin Pharmacokinet 43:925–942
35. Udy AA, Baptista JP, Lim NL et al (2014) Augmented renal clearance in the ICU: results of a multicenter observational study of renal function in critically ill patients with normal plasma creatinine clearance. Crit Care Med 42:520–527
36. Craig WA (1998) Pharmacokinetic/pharmacodynamic parameters: rationale for antibacterial dosing of mice and men. Clin Infect Dis 26:1–12
37. Craig WA (2003) Basic pharmacodynamics of antibacterials with clinical applications to the use of beta-lactams, glycopeptides, and linezolid. Infect Dis Clin North Am 17:479–501
38. Jeffres MN, Isakow W, Doherty JA et al (2006) Predictors of mortality for methicillin-resistant *Staphylococcus aureus* health-care-associated pneumonia: specific evaluation of vancomycin pharmacokinetic indices. Chest 130:947–955
39. Hermsen ED, Handon M, Sankaranarayanan J et al (2010) Clinical outcomes and nephrotoxicity associated with vancomycin trough concentrations during treatment of deep-seated infections. Expert Opin Drug Saf 9:9–14
40. Ackerman BH, Guilday RE, Reigart CL et al (2013) Evaluation of the relationship between elevated vancomycin trough concentrations and increased efficacy and/or toxicity. J Burn Care Res 34:e1–e9
41. Hidayat LK, Hsu DI, Quist R et al (2006) High-dose vancomycin therapy for methicillin-resistant *Staphylococcus aureus* infections. Arch Intern Med 166:2138–2144
42. Lodise TP, Graves J, Evans A et al (2008) Relationship between vancomycin MIC and failure among patients with methicillin-resistant *Staphylococcus aureus* bacteremia treated with vancomycin. Antimicrob Agents Chemother 52:3315–3320
43. Patel P, Pai MP, Rodvold KA et al (2011) Vancomycin: we can't get there from here. Clin Infect Dis 52:969–974
44. Kullar R, Davis SL, Levine DP et al (2011) Impact of vancomycin exposure on outcomes in patients with methicillin-resistant *Staphylococcus aureus* bacteremia: support for consensus guidelines suggested targets. Clin Infect Dis 52:975–981
45. Kullar R, Davis SL, Taylor TN et al (2013) Effects of targeting higher vancomycin trough levels on clinical outcomes and costs in a matched patient cohort. Pharmacotherapy 32:195–201
46. Holmes NE, Turnidge JD, Munckhot WJ et al (2013) Vancomycin AUC/MIC ratio and 30-day mortality in patients with *Staphylococcus aureus* bacteremia. Antimicrob Agents Chemother 57:1654–1663
47. Gawronski KM, Goff DA, Brown J et al (2013) A stewardship program's retrospective evaluation of vancomycin AUC24/MIC and time to microbiological clearance in patients with methicillin-resistant *Staphylococcus aureus* bacteremia and osteomyelitis. Clin Ther 35:772–779

48. Brown J, Brown K, Forrest A (2012) Vancomycin AUC24/MIC ratio in patients with complicated bacteremia and infective endocarditis due to methicillin-resistant *Staphylococcus aureus* and its association with attributable mortality during hospitalization. Antimicrob Agents Chemother 56:634–638
49. Neely MN, Youn G, Jones B et al (2014) Are vancomycin trough concentrations adequate for optimal dosing? Antimicrob Agents Chemother 58:309–316
50. Le J, Bradley JS, Murray W et al (2013) Improved vancomycin dosing in children using area under the curve exposure. Pediatr Infect Dis J 32:e155–e163
51. Frymoyer A, Guglielmo J, Hersh AL (2013) Desired vancomycin trough serum concentrations for treating invasive methicillin-resistant Staphylococcal infections. Pediatr Infect Dis J 32:1077–1079
52. Camaione L, Elliott K, Mitchell-Van Steele A et al (2013) Vancomycin dosing in children and young adults: back to the drawing board. Pharmacotherapy 33:1278–1287
53. Blouin RA, Bauer LA, Miller DD et al (1982) Vancomycin pharmacokinetics in normal and morbidly obese subjects. Antimicrob Agents Chemother 4:575–580
54. Bauer LA, Black DJ, Lill JS (1998) Vancomycin dosing in morbidly obese patients. Eur J Clin Pharmacol 8:621–625
55. Vance-Bryan K, Guay DR, Gilliand SS et al (1993) Effect of obesity on vancomycin pharmacokinetic parameters as determined by using a Bayesian forecasting technique. Antimicrob Agents Chemother 3:436–440
56. Reynolds DC, Waite LH, Alexander DP et al (2012) Performance of a vancomycin dosage regimen developed for obese patients. Am J Health Syst Pharm 69:944–950
57. Rushing TA, Ambrose PJ (2001) Clinical application and evaluation of vancomycin dosing in adults. J Pharm Technol 17:33–38
58. Leong JVB, Boro MS, Winter ME (2011) Determining vancomycin clearance in an overweight and obese population. Am J Health Syst Pharm 68:599–603
59. Lodise TP, Lomaestro B, Graves J et al (2008) Larger vancomycin doses (> 4 grams/day) are associated with increased incidence of nephrotoxicity. Antimicrob Agents Chemother 52:1330–1336
60. Wang JT, Fang CT, Chen YC et al (2001) Necessity of a loading dose when using vancomycin in critically ill patients. J Antimicrob Chemother 47:246
61. Denetclaw TH, Dowling TC, Steinke D (2013) Performance of a divided-load intravenous vancomycin dosing strategy for critically ill patients. Ann Pharmacother 47:1611–1617
62. Cataldo MA, Tacconelli E, Grilli E et al (2012) Continuous versus intermittent infusion of vancomycin for the treatment of Gram-positive infections: systematic review and meta-analysis. J Antimicrob Chemother 67:17–24
63. Pea F, Furlanut M, Negri C et al (2009) Prospectively validated dosing nomograms for maximizing the pharmacodynamics of vancomycin administered by continuous infusion in critically ill patients. Antimicrob Agents Chemother 53:1863–1867
64. DiMondi VP, Rafferty K (2013) Review of continuous-infusion vancomycin. Ann Pharmacother 47:219–227
65. Man SS, Carr RR, Ensom MHH (2010) Comparison of continuous and intermittent IV infusion of vancomycin: systematic review. Can J Hosp Pharm 63:373–381
66. Aubron C, Corallo CE, Nunn MO et al (2011) Evaluation of the accuracy of a pharmacokinetic dosing program in predicting serum vancomycin concentrations in critically ill patients. Ann Pharmacother 45:1193–1198
67. Truong J, Levkovich BJ, Padiglione AA (2012) Simple approach to improving vancomycin dosing in intensive care: a standardized loading dose results in earlier therapeutic levels. Intern Med J 42:23–29
68. Avent ML, Vaska VL, Rogers BA et al (2013) Vancomycin therapeutics and monitoring: a contemporary approach. Intern Med J 43:110–119
69. Kullar R, Leonard SN, Davis SL et al (2011) Validation of the effectiveness of a vancomycin nomogram in achieving target trough concentrations of 15-20 mg/L suggested by the vancomycin consensus guidelines. Pharmacotherapy 31:441–448
70. Rodvold KA, Blum RA, Fischer JH et al (1988) Vancomycin pharmacokinetics in patients with various degrees of renal function. Antimicrob Agents Chemother 32:848–852
71. Moellering RC, Krogstad DJ, Greenblatt DJ (1981) Vancomycin therapy in patients with impaired renal function: a nomogram for dosage. Ann Intern Med 94:343–346
72. Rybak MJ, Boike SC (1986) Individualized adjustment of vancomycin dosage: comparison with two dosage nomograms. Drug Intell Clin Pharm 20:64–68
73. Murphy JE, Gillespie DE, Bateman CV (2006) Predictability of vancomycin trough concentrations using seven approaches for estimating pharmacokinetic parameters. Am J Health Syst Pharm 63:2365–2370
74. Karam CM, McKinnon PS, Neuhauser MN et al (1999) Outcome assessment of minimizing

vancomycin monitoring and dosing adjustments. Pharmacotherapy 19:257–266

75. Golenia BS, Levine AR, Moawad IM et al (2013) Evaluation of a vancomycin dosing nomogram based on the modification of diet in renal disease equation in intensive care unit patients. J Crit Care 28:710–716
76. Nunn MO, Corallo CE, Aubron C et al (2011) Vancomycin dosing: assessment of time to therapeutic concentration and predictive accuracy of pharmacokinetic modeling software. Ann Pharmacother 45:757–763
77. Rodvold KA, Rotschafer JC, Gilliland SS et al (1994) Bayesian forecasting of serum vancomycin concentrations with non-steady-state sampling strategies. Ther Drug Monit 16:37–41
78. Rodvold KA, Pyrka RD, Garrison M et al (1989) Evaluation of a two-compartment Bayesian forecasting program for predicting vancomycin concentrations. Ther Drug Monit 11:269–275
79. Wong-Beringer A, Joo J, Tse E et al (2011) Vancomycin-associated nephrotoxicity: a critical appraisal of risk with high dose therapy. Int J Antimicrob Agents 2:95–101
80. Lodise TP, Patel N, Lomaestro BM et al (2009) Relationship between initial vancomycin concentration-time profile and nephrotoxicity among hospitalized patients. Clin Infect Dis 49:507–514
81. Suzuki Y, Kawasaki K, Sato Y et al (2012) Is peak concentration needed in therapeutic drug monitoring of vancomycin? A pharmacokinetic-pharmacodynamic analysis in patients with methicillin—resistant *Staphylococcus aureus* pneumonia. Chemotherapy 58:308–312
82. Van Hal SJ, Paterson DL, Lodise TP (2013) Systematic review and meta-analysis of vancomycin-induced nephrotoxicity associated with dosing schedules that maintain troughs between 15 and 20 mg per liter. Antimicrob Agents Chemother 57:734–744
83. Aronoff GR, Sloan RS, Dinwiddie CB et al (1981) Effects of vancomycin on renal function in rats. Antimicrob Agents Chemother 19:306–308
84. Forouzesh A, Moise PA, Sakoulas G (2009) Vancomycin ototoxicity: a reevaluation in an era of increasing doses. Antimicrob Agents Chemother 53:483–486

Chapter 12

Pharmacodynamics of Lipoglycopeptides

Eric Wenzler, Siyun Liao, and Keith A. Rodvold

Abstract

Telavancin, dalbavancin, and oritavancin are lipoglycopeptide anti-infective agents with a broad in vitro spectrum against gram-positive microorganisms, including methicillin-resistant *Staphylococcus aureus* (MRSA). The research and development programs of these agents have been challenging and have resulted in the generation of various pharmacokinetic and pharmacodynamic data over the past 10–15 years. All of the lipoglycopeptide agents exhibit concentration-dependent bactericidal activity with the ratio of unbound area-under-the-curve to minimum inhibitory concentration (*f*AUC/MIC) best predicting antibacterial efficacy in vitro and in vivo. The pharmacokinetic and exposure-response characteristics support the recommended once-daily dosing regimen for telavancin, a two-dose regimen for dalbavancin (1000 mg followed 1 week later by a 500 mg dose) and a novel single-dose regimen for oritavancin (1200 mg). Further research and clinical experiences with these lipoglycopeptide agents are needed in order to expand their use to other types of invasive infections caused by MRSA.

Key words Lipoglycopeptide, Telavancin, Dalbavancin, Oritavancin, Methicillin-resistant *Staphylococcus aureus* (MRSA)

1 Overview

Several antibiotics from the lipoglycopeptide class have recently become available for treatment of serious infections caused by gram-positive microorganisms, including resistant phenotypes of *Staphylococcus aureus* [1, 2]. Each of these agents differs from vancomycin by having unique pharmacokinetic (PK) and pharmacodynamic (PD) properties that allow for alternative dosing schemes.

Telavancin, the first available lipoglycopeptide, has demonstrated rapid, potent, concentration-dependent bactericidal activity against multiple gram-positive pathogens, including resistant phenotypes of methicillin-resistant *S. aureus* (MRSA). Its dual mechanism of action contributes to its demonstrated superiority compared to other glycopeptides and lipopeptides in various in vitro PD and animal models. The PK of telavancin supports the convenient once-daily dosing; however, the increased adverse effects observed in clinical trials, particularly nephrotoxicity, limit

John C. Rotschafer et al. (eds.), *Antibiotic Pharmacodynamics*, Methods in Pharmacology and Toxicology, DOI 10.1007/978-1-4939-3323-5_12, © Springer Science+Business Media New York 2016

its use to specific patient populations. The primary urinary excretion requires that dosage adjustments be made for renal dysfunction and a dearth of data exists on the PKs of telavancin during any type of dialysis. Furthermore, despite the promising outcomes seen in both skin and soft tissue infection and pneumonia trials, the observation of increased mortality in patients with moderate to severe renal impairment will continue to place limits on the use of telavancin for the treatment of serious gram-positive infections, especially MRSA.

Dalbavancin exhibits linear PK with steep dose–response curves and a long terminal elimination half-life. Its activity is concentration-dependent and the ratio of the area under the concentration–time curve to minimum inhibitory concentration (AUC/MIC) has been shown to be the PK/PD index associated with optimal antibacterial efficacy in vitro. The mechanism of action is similar to other glycopeptides and therefore it does not retain activity against *vanA* phenotypes of enterococcus. Synergy was demonstrated with one agent, oxacillin, and intrinsic or acquired resistant to dalbavancin has not been demonstrated to date. In 2014, the US Food and Drug Administration (FDA) approved dalbavancin for the treatment of adult patients with acute bacterial skin and structure infections (ABSSSI) caused by susceptible isolates of gram-positive microorganisms. The PK and exposure-response analysis supported the recommended two-dose intravenous regimen of dalbavancin 1000 mg followed 1 week later by a 500 mg dose. Dosage adjustment is required for patients with creatinine clearance (CrCl) <30 mL/min and not receiving regularly scheduled hemodialysis. Dalbavancin has been proven to be efficacious across a range of clinical syndromes, primarily in animal models, including endocarditis and pneumonia. Dalbavancin was well tolerated throughout clinical trials and observed adverse events were mild and infrequent.

Oritavancin exhibits multi-exponential linear PK best described by a three-compartment model. Its concentration-dependent bactericidal activity and extremely long terminal half-life makes it ideal for single-dose dosing schemes, which have shown clinical efficacy in PD and animal models as well as clinical trials. Its multiple mechanisms of action allow it to maintain potent bactericidal activity against difficult to treat pathogens including MRSA, vancomycin-intermediate *S. aureus* (VISA), vancomycin-resistant *S. aureus* (VRSA), and vancomycin-resistant *Enterococcus* (VRE) while other agents may be ineffective. The current FDA-approved indication of oritavancin is for the treatment of adult patients with ABSSSI caused by susceptible isolates of gram-positive microorganisms. The PK and PD data supported the recommended single-dose regimen of oritavancin 1200 mg administered by intravenous infusion over 3 h in adult patients. The minimal renal and fecal elimination do not warrant dosage adjustments, even with dialysis, and alterations in clearance due to body weight and antibacterial activity due to protein binding can be overcome by increasing dosages. Oritavancin has proven to be efficacious across a broad range of clinical syndromes in in vitro, animal, and clinical models including endocarditis, meningitis, and pneumonia. Synergy has been demonstrated with several antimicrobials including gentamicin and linezolid, importantly against simulated high-inoculum infections. Observed adverse events were mild and infrequent, and intrinsic or acquired resistance has not been demonstrated during clinical studies with oritavancin.

2 Telavancin

Telavancin, (TD-6424), is a semisynthetic derivative of vancomycin with a hydrophobic decylaminoethyl moiety attached to the vancosamine sugar, classifying it as a lipoglycopeptide [1, 3]. This lipophilic side chain improves the affinity for the D-Ala-D-Ala target site and is responsible for the activity of telavancin against methicillin-resistant *Staphylococcus aureus* (MRSA) and VanB enterococci. Common to the newer lipoglycopeptides, telavancin's lipophilic side chains help anchor the molecule to the cell membrane, concentrating the drug at the site of action and dramatically increasing its potency while leading to membrane destabilization and loss of membrane potential [4]. This dual mechanism of action provides ten times the inhibition of transglycosylation and synthesis of peptidoglycan compared to vancomycin and is the primary reason for telavancin's rapid bactericidal activity. Telavancin has potent activity against *Streptococcus pneumoniae* and staphylococci including VISA, with limited activity against VRSA. Telavancin displays poor activity against VanA VRE but modest activity against VanB VRE [1–4]. Telavancin was initially approved by FDA in 2009 for the treatment of complicated skin and skin structure infections (cSSSI) [3, 5]. Issues at a manufacturing site and a change in commercialization partnerships subsequently led to the lack of product supply of telavancin [3]. In 2013, a new manufacturer was established and reliable distribution of telavancin was reestablished. At that same time, FDA approved the indication for the treatment of adults with hospital-acquired bacterial pneumonia (HABP) or ventilator-associated bacterial pneumonia (VABP) caused by susceptible isolates of *S. aureus* when alternative treatment agents are not suitable [3]. The European Medicines Agency authorized marketing of telavancin for nosocomial pneumonia, including VABP, in March 2014.

2.1 Pharmacokinetics of Telavancin

In healthy adult volunteers, total exposure to telavancin increases proportionally with dose with a maximum (C_{max}) and minimum plasma concentrations (C_{min}) of 186 and 16 mg/L for the 15 mg/kg

Table 1
Summary of telavancin pharmacokinetics at steady state

	Telavancin 7.5 mg/kg			Telavancin 15 mg/kg		
Parameter	Male (*n*=23)	Female (*n*=16)	All (*n*=39)	Male (*n*=22)	Female (*n*=12)	All (*n*=34)
C_{max} (mg/L)	87±14.5	88.2±10	87.5±12.8	188±27	183±28	186±27
AUC_{0-24} (mg·h/L)	608±104	585±86	599±96	1330±171	1194±229	1282±201
$t_{1/2}$ (h)	6.1±0.6	5.8±0.6	6±0.6	7.9±1.2	6.8±1.3	7.5±1.3
CL (mL/h/kg)	13±4.5	13.1±1.8	13±3.6	11.5±1.6	12.9±2.1	12±1.9
V_{ss} (mL/kg)	116±40	106±13	111±32	122±16	114±10.5	119±14
CL_R (mL/h/kg)	7.9±3.1	8.8±4.9	8.3±3.9	7.9±2.5	10.2±6.3	8.7±4.3
Urinary recovery (% dose)						
Telavancin	62.9±23.5	66.7±33.2	64.4±27.5	68.6±19.3	77.3±37.6	71.7±27
THRX-651540[a]	5.84±1.3	6.14±2.57	5.96±1.9	3.19±1.75	3.61±0.97	3.34±1.52

Data are presented as mean±SD

C_{max} maximum plasma concentration, AUC_{0-24} 24-hour area under the plasma concentration–time curve, $t_{1/2}$ elimination half-life, *CL* clearance, V_{ss} apparent volume of distribution at steady-state, CL_R renal clearance

[a]Primary metabolite

dose and 88 and 6 mg/L for the 7.5 mg/kg, respectively. The AUC is also approximately twofold higher at 1282 (15 mg/kg dose) compared to 599 mg·h/L (7.5 mg/kg dose). Steady-state PK parameters and urinary excretion stratified by gender can be found in Table 1 [6]. Plasma concentrations of the inactive primary metabolite of telavancin (THRX-651540) are minimal at approximately 2 %. Approximately 82.3 % of telavancin is excreted in the urine after 48 h with negligible fecal excretion at 0.7 %. Interestingly, the mean half-life of the total radioactivity is over 13-fold longer than the mean half-life of telavancin potentially resulting from emanation from tissues or low CL of other minor unidentified metabolites or impurities [7]. PK parameters on day one were not significantly different from those on day 7 indicating a lack of accumulation. Median trough bactericidal titers of telavancin against MRSA on day 7 were 16, 24, and 32 after 7.5, 12.5, and 15 mg/kg doses, respectively [8]. These respective titers were 128, 256, and ≥512 against *S. pneumoniae*. This serum bactericidal activity is not affected by renal dysfunction. Telavancin is approximately 93 % bound to albumin [9].

A population PK model has been developed from patients in phase 2 and 3 trials with cSSSI and HABP treated with telavancin

Table 2
Population pharmacokinetic estimated parameters for patients with cSSSI and HABP stratified by degree of renal impairment[a]

Patients with cSSSI				
Parameter	No renal impairment (n=575)	Mild renal impairment (n=122)	Moderate renal impairment (n=36)	Severe renal impairment (n=16)
V_{ss} (L)	11.87±3.47	13.06±3.95	14.17±3.45	14.89±4.44
CL (L/h)	1.22±0.32	1±0.24	0.82±0.223	0.59±0.15
V_1 (L)	5.28±2.41	6.43±2.81	7.57±2.53	8.62±4.02
Patients with HABP				
Parameter	No renal impairment (n=271)	Mild renal impairment (n=88)	Moderate renal impairment (n=48)	Severe renal impairment (n=26)
V_{ss} (L)	11.47±6.78	14.11±5.23	13.68±3.61	15.64±3.76
CL (L/h)	1.1±0.35	1.03±0.26	0.91±0.24	0.64±0.22
V_1 (L)	5.74±5.7	7.17±4.07	6.77±2.11	8.19±2.53

Data are presented as mean±SD

V_{ss} apparent volume of distribution at steady-state, *CL* clearance, V_1 apparent volume of distribution in the central compartment

[a]Degree of renal impairment was classified as follows: severe, CrCl of <30 mL/min and including patients on dialysis; moderate, CrCl of <50 mL/min to ≥30 mL/min; mild, CrCl of <80 mL/min to ≥50 mL/min; none, CrCl of ≥80 mL/min

[10]. A two-compartment open model fit the plasma concentration–time data and was adequate to evaluate the potential contribution of covariates. The final population PK models included approximately 8912 plasma telavancin concentrations from 710 patients and 236 subjects without infection. The estimated PK parameters from the final model in patients with cSSSI and HABP and stratified by degree of renal impairment are shown in Table 2. Overall, the population PK estimates for infected patients and non-infected subjects were similar and consistent to the results from Phase 1 clinical studies. The CL of telavancin was highly correlated with CrCl and to a lesser degree, body weight. In patients with cSSSI, CL was approximately 10 % higher in males than in females and the AUC was about 11 % higher in patients ≥75 years of age. The median AUC was 34 % higher in obese patients (body mass index [BMI] ≥35 kg/m^2) despite a 50 % increase in dose while median CL was 24 % higher. In patients with HABP, AUC decreased by 6 % in patients ≥75 years of age and increased only 18 % in obese while CL was 27 % higher. The linear relationship between weight and CL of telavancin supported dosing on a mg/kg

bases, evidenced by the modest increases in exposure and CL in obese patients despite increases in absolute doses. The population PK analysis provided further support for the approved product package insert and dosing recommendations based body weight and renal function.

2.1.1 Special Populations

Age and hepatic impairment do not have an effect on the PKs of telavancin [11, 12] and it does not induce or inhibit CYP3A [13].

PKs of telavancin were studied in subjects on hemodialysis given a 7.5 mg/kg dose 2–4 h before a standard 4-h hemodialysis session [14]. The mean PK parameters were different between subjects with normal renal function compare to those on hemodialysis, including total C_{max} of 70.6 versus 52.1 mg/L, $AUC_{0-\infty}$ of 568 versus 1147 mg · h/L, CL of 14 versus 7 mL/h/kg, volume of distribution at steady-state (V_{ss}) of 0.139 versus 0.189 L/kg, and elimination half-life of 8.1 versus 19.7 h. No differences were observed in protein binding (approximately 87 %) between the groups. Although there are no specific dosing recommendations provided for patients on intermittent hemodialysis in the package insert for telavancin, these data help support the 10 mg/kg every 48 h dosing regimen given to patients on dialysis in the phase III studies.

Additionally, the previously described population PK model was used to simulate telavancin concentration–time profiles and to evaluate the ability to achieve PD targets of interest in patients with renal dysfunction [15]. Concentration–time profiles were simulated for 10 mg/kg daily in individuals with CrCl >50 mL/min, 7.5 mg/kg daily for individuals with CrCl 30–50 mL/min, and 10 mg/kg every 48 h for CrCl <30 mL/min. The AUC_{0-Tau} values were relatively similar across the three dosing regimens and at least 93 % of subjects achieved the PD target (AUC/MIC of 219) for MIC values up to 2 mg/L. The percentage of subjects with severe renal impairment achieving an AUC/MIC of 219 with an MIC of 2 mg/L was 89.3 % for the 24-h AUC (AUC_{0-24}) and 23.6 % for the second 24-h AUC (AUC_{24-48}), respectively. This analysis helped solidify the renal dose adjustments suggested by Monte Carlo simulations performed from phase I study data and confirmed the lack of difference in exposure profiles of telavancin across varying degrees of renal impairment.

Telavancin is available as an intravenous preparation formulated with hydroxy propyl-β-cyclodextrin to enhance solubility, a renally eliminated solubilizer known to cause adverse effects if accumulation occurs. Telavancin is highly protein bound (93 %) and has a large molecular weight (1792 Da) suggesting its removal by extracorporeal circuits would be minimal; however, its small apparent V (0.15 L/kg) and primary renal elimination may lead to significant dialytic CL. The mean total CL of telavancin during continuous renal replacement therapy is equal to that in healthy volunteers (12–18 mL/min) given 7.5 mg/kg up to ultrafiltration or dialysate rates of 3 L/h [16]. At rates of 6 L/h, the CL exceeds that of healthy subjects. These data suggest that telavancin may be removed by both continuous hemofiltration and hemodialysis particularly when high ultrafiltration or dialysate flow rates are used. Hydroxy propyl-β-cyclodextrin transmembrane CL approached ultrafiltration or dialysate flow rates and would not likely accumulate in patients receiving continuous renal replacement therapy [16]. This work suggests that dose and/or frequency increases of telavancin may be needed in patients receiving continuous renal replacement therapy with high ultrafiltration or dialysate flow rates.

2.1.2 Disposition and Penetration

The mean C_{max} and time to C_{max} (T_{max}) of telavancin in blister fluid after administration of 7.5 mg/kg daily for 3 days was 16 mg/L and occurred at 9.3 h [17]. The mean AUC at steady state was 241 mg · h/L and the elimination half-life was 6.91 h. Over the dosing interval, the ratio of the AUC in blister fluid to that in plasma was 40.3 %. The derived total (AUC/MIC) and unbound AUC/MIC (*f*AUC/MIC) using an MIC of 0.5 to *S. aureus* in blister fluid were 482 and 24.1, respectively.

The pulmonary penetration of telavancin was evaluated in healthy subjects. The mean concentration in ELF (3.7 mg/L) peaked 8 h after the start of the last infusion and the trough concentration in ELF (0.9 mg/L) remaining above the MIC_{90} value for MRSA (0.5 mg/L) at 24 h after multiple doses of 10 mg/kg [18]. The C_{max} observed in alveolar macrophages (AM) was substantially higher at 45 mg/L at 12 h and 42 mg/L at 24 h after multiple doses of telavancin. The ratio of ELF and AM C_{max} to the estimated unbound C_{max} in plasma were 32 and 388 %, respectively. The estimated AUC_{0-24} in ELF using the linear-trapezoidal rule was 47.4 mg · h/L compared to 785 mg · h/L for total plasma concentrations. The estimated penetration of telavancin over the dosing interval based on ratio of AUC_{0-24} in ELF to unbound AUC_{0-24} (*f*AUC) in plasma was 60.4 %. A second analysis of this data using population PK modeling and Monte Carlo simulation reported respective mean and median AUC_{0-24} values of telavancin in pulmonary epithelial lining fluid (ELF) were 74.75 and 53.74 mg · h/L, with the median penetration ratio of AUC in ELF to *f*AUC in plasma of 73 % [19]. The mean parameter vector from the population model for ELF penetration was 66 %. The results of both analyses indicate the telavancin penetrates reasonably well into the ELF compared to plasma, with AUC_{0-24} values in the ELF able to achieve the estimated $fAUC_{0-24}/MIC$ target ratio of 78 for *S. aureus* isolates with an MIC <1 mg/L. Pulmonary surfactant had no effect on the in vitro activity of telavancin against *S. pneumoniae* or MRSA. These data also suggest that telavancin penetrates relatively well into the ELF and extensively into alveolar macrophages and the activity is not hindered by pulmonary surfactant.

Telavancin has been shown to be extremely potent against extracellular methicillin-susceptible *S. aureus* (MSSA) and MRSA, achieving bactericidal activity at the 1× MIC value at 18 h and at C_{max} at 2–10 h [20, 21]. Telavancin caused complete eradication at C_{max} within 6–24 h and a 4.5 log reduction against VISA and VRSA. Interestingly, no gross membrane destabilization of macrophages was detected in the model indicating that the intracellular bactericidal effect of telavancin were unlikely to result from direct contact of extracellular telavancin with phagocytized *S. aureus*. A concentration–effect curve was clearly demonstrated for intraphagocytic *S. aureus* and telavancin is known to penetrate alveolar macrophages; therefore, further analyses is required to delineate this mechanism. Also of note was the persistence of viable intracellular bacteria even after exposure to concentrations of telavancin at 1000× MIC for 24 h, a phenomenon not unique to telavancin. The potent intracellular and extracellular activity of telavancin against *S. aureus* observed in this study indicate that telavancin may be effective at decreasing persistence and recurrence, two common features of serious staphylococcal infections.

2.2 Pharmacodynamics of Telavancin

2.2.1 In Vitro Models

The activity of telavancin has been evaluated in numerous different in vitro models. It has been shown to have rapidly bactericidal, concentration-dependent activity against Gram positive pathogens, including those with reduced glycopeptide susceptibility [22]. Telavancin has displayed in vitro synergy with multiple other agents including nafcillin, meropenem, imipenem, ceftriaxone, rifampin, and gentamicin against MSSA, MRSA and heteroresistant vancomycin-intermediate *S. aureus* (hVISA) [23, 24]. Telavancin has also demonstrated activity against VISA and VRSA at 4 and 8× the MIC. The presence of human serum (albumin) causes a twofold increase in the static MIC but does not affect the cidality in dynamic assays. This may be due to a weaker protein binding affinity than predicted by experiments or a lack of effect on the membrane destabilization mechanism of telavancin [25, 26].

Telavancin has previously been shown to be more active than vancomycin against *Clostridium difficile* with an MIC_{90} of 0.25 mg/L compared to 1 mg/L for vancomycin. To further investigate the potential utility of telavancin in the treatment of *C. difficile* infection, time-kill studies were performed for telavancin and compared to vancomycin and metronidazole against five strains of *C. difficile* [27]. Overall, vancomycin achieved a greater $\log_{10}$ reduction in colony forming units (CFU/mL) at 24 h than telavancin against all strains tested except for the ATCC strain in which they were comparable. Metronidazole was more bactericidal than both telavancin and vancomycin at all concentrations except against one strain where regrowth occurred at 2 and 4 times the MIC.

In an in vitro PD model examining the activity of telavancin against MSSA, MRSA, VISA, vancomycin-susceptible enterococci

(VSE), and VRE, the bactericidal concentration was explored along with dose-ranging studies to establish the *f*AUC/MIC associated with efficacy [28, 29]. The 90 % maximum antibacterial effect occurred at *f*AUC/MIC of >40 for vancomycin-susceptible *S. aureus* strains compared to a *f*AUC/MIC of 6 for a 2 log reduction against VISA. Against enterococci, doses were simulated from 9 to 14 mg/kg and the 90 % maximum antibacterial effect occurred at a *f*AUC/MIC >70. Given the unbound drug AUC of approximately 50–100 mg·h/L observed in healthy volunteers given 10 mg/kg of telavancin, antibacterial efficacy for staphylococci and enterococci could be reasonably expected up to MICs of 1 mg/L.

Finally, in an in vitro PD model examined the activity of telavancin alone and in combination with gentamicin or rifampin against various phenotypes of *S. aureus* in simulated endocardial vegetations against MSSA, MRSA, VISA, and hVISA strains [30]. Telavancin achieved ≥2-log reduction in CFU/g against all strains at the end of the experiment (96 h) and was bactericidal against hVISA and VISA at 64 h. When combined with rifampin or gentamicin, the time to achieve bactericidal activity was shortened by 20–40 h against MRSA although the extent of killing was only significantly improved against MSSA. The combination of telavancin and gentamicin tested against hVISA and VISA demonstrated rapid bactericidal effect by 27 h and log reduction below the detectable limit by 48 h. Telavancin combined with rifampin did not demonstrate enhanced killing.

2.2.2 Animal Models

The demonstrated concentration-dependent, rapidly bactericidal activity of telavancin of in vitro models has translated well into in vivo animal models. In the mouse neutropenic thigh and subcutaneous infection models using strains of MSSA, MRSA, methicillin-resistant *Staphylococcus epidermidis* (MRSE), methicillin-susceptible *S. epidermidis* (MSSE), penicillin-resistant *S. pneumoniae* (PRSP), penicillin-susceptible *S. pneumoniae* (PSSP), and VRE, the total daily dose of telavancin was directly proportional to the total decrease in bacterial load while the frequency of dosing did not affect decrease in CFU/g [31]. When total drug concentrations were examined, AUC/MIC and time above the MIC were equal predictors of antibacterial efficacy while AUC/MIC was the best predictor when unbound drug concentrations were used ($R^2 = 0.83$). This study confirms that the in vivo efficacy of telavancin is driven by total drug exposure (AUC/MIC) and that once-daily dosing is the preferred regimen for optimal efficacy.

In a neutropenic mouse bacteremia model, telavancin has demonstrated potent activity against MRSA, hVISA and VISA [32–34]. In all studies, blood and spleen bacterial titers were reduced significantly with the majority of mice surviving to the end of the observation period.

Telavancin has also been shown to significantly reduce vegetation titers of MRSA and VISA in rabbit endocarditis models, including isolates that were daptomycin-nonsusceptible [35–37].

With regards to pneumonia, telavancin has again demonstrated significant reductions in bacterial titers and improved clinical outcomes when tested against MSSA, MRSA, hVISA and VISA. Telavancin achieved a significantly greater reduction in bacterial burden than its comparator agents, nafcillin and linezolid, in an MSSA pneumonia model [38], whereas the proportion of survivors was 19/22 (86 %) compared to 3/22 (14 %) for the control group after 14 days in an MRSA immunocompromised model [39, 40].

In a rabbit meningitis model, telavancin reached a C_{max} in cerebrospinal fluid (CSF) of 3.8 mg/L at 8 h post-dose compared to 0.13 mg/L in uninfected controls [41]. The C_{max} and AUC in CSF relative to plasma were 3 and 2 % for infected animals. Telavancin was rapidly bactericidal against PRSP and the CSF of 6/10 rabbits were sterilized. Against MSSA, telavancin produced a 4.32 log CFU/mL reduction and also sterilized 6/10 rabbits. Despite the low level of penetration into inflamed meninges, telavancin was efficacious as monotherapy against PRSP and MSSA meningitis. Given the MIC of 2 mg/L to MSSA, higher doses of telavancin may be warranted for staphylococcal meningitis.

Telavancin has also demonstrated low levels of penetration into bone albeit with improved clinical outcomes over control groups [42]. The concentration of telavancin in infected rabbit left tibial bone matrix was 0.27 μg/g compared to 0.25 μg/g in uninfected right tibias. At 56 days post-infection, 3/15 (20 %) rabbits treated with telavancin had MRSA-positive tibial cultures compared to 9/15 (60 %) rabbits in the control group.

The bactericidal activity of telavancin has also translated into improved efficacy in foreign body infection models [43]. In one study, the rate of both device colonization and infection with MRSA were both significantly lower with doses of telavancin ≥15 mg/kg (doses of 30 and 45 mg/kg). The respective rate of colonization and infection were 6/54 (11 %) and 5/54 (9 %) at the dose of 30 mg/kg, 6/54 (11 %) and 6/54 (11 %) for the dose of 45 mg/kg, and 21/54 (39 %) and 19/54 (35 %) with the 15 mg/kg dose. All (48/48) control devices were both colonized and infected along with 52 % of the rabbits given vancomycin.

2.3 Telavancin Clinical Trials: Proof of Pharmacokinetic-Pharmacodynamic Concepts

Telavancin has been under clinical investigation in human trials since the early 2000s and therefore has a wealth of data in several different disease states [1, 2]. In patients with cSSSI due to gram-positive bacteria, the FAST 1 and 2 trials were randomize, double-blind phase 2 trials comparing telavancin to standard of therapy [44, 45]. In FAST 1, cure rates were 92 % for telavancin and 96 % for standard therapy ($p = 0.53$). In patients with MRSA at baseline, cure was achieved in 82 and 69 % of the telavancin and standard therapy groups, respectively [44]. In FAST 2, the clinically evaluable population cure rates were 96 % for telavancin and 94 % for standard therapy [45]. In the microbiologically evaluable population of patients infected with MRSA the cure rates were 96 % for telavancin and 90 % for standard therapy. Telavancin achieved a significantly higher rate of MRSA eradication in the microbiologically evaluable group at the test-of-cure visit ($p = 0.04$).

The ATLAS I and II studies were two phase 3 randomized trials in patients with cSSSI in which telavancin was compared to vancomycin [46]. The overall cure rate in the clinically evaluable and all treated patients in the telavancin and vancomycin arms were 88.3 % versus 87.1 % and 76.5 % versus 74.2 %, with no significant differences between the groups or between the individual studies. Of the 579 clinically evaluable patients with MRSA at baseline, there were no differences in the cure rates between telavancin and vancomycin (90.6 % versus 84.4 %). The overall therapeutic response rate, including the number of patients who were cured and had a pathogen eradicated at the test-of-cure visit, was also similar between telavancin and vancomycin (88.6 % versus 86.2 %).

The ATTAIN trials were also two methodologically identical, randomized, double-blind, comparator-controlled, parallel-group phase III clinical trials designed to assess the efficacy and safety of telavancin compared to vancomycin in the treatment of hospital-acquired pneumonia due to gram-positive pathogens, particularly MRSA [47]. The cure rates in the pooled all-treatment population were 58.9 % for telavancin and 59.5 % for vancomycin compared to 82.4 and 80.7 % for the clinically evaluable population. The only statistically significant difference in outcomes was seen in patients in the microbiologically evaluable population at the test-of-cure visit with monomicrobial *S. aureus* pneumonia with a vancomycin MIC ≥1 mg/L; the cure rate for telavancin was 87.1 % compared to 74.3 % for vancomycin ($p = 0.03$).

A *post hoc* analysis of survival at 28 days from the ATTAIN trials demonstrated similar survival rates of 76 % for telavancin and 77 % for vancomycin [48, 49]. For patients with CrCl values ≥50 mL/min survival rates were similar at 84 and 81 % for telavancin and vancomycin, respectively, while lower survival rates were observed for patients in the telavancin group with CrCl values <50 mL/min, although not statistically significantly lower. Survival rates were 59 % versus 70 % and 47 % versus 61 % for telavancin versus vancomycin in patients with CrCl values <50 mL/min and <30 mL/min, respectively [48]. A second *post hoc* analysis excluding patients with CrCl <30 mL/min showed no differences in survival [49].

Finally, in a phase II trial comparing telavancin to standard therapy for uncomplicated *S. aureus* bacteremia, cure rates were similar between the groups in the clinically evaluable population at 88 and 89 % for telavancin and standard treatment, respectively [50]. Microbiological eradication was achieved at the test-of-cure visit for 88 % of patients in the telavancin group compared to 78 % of standard therapy patients. Telavancin is currently under investigation for the treatment of *S. aureus* bacteremia in a multicenter phase III trial [3].

3 Dalbavancin

Dalbavancin is a novel parenteral, semisynthetic, long-acting lipoglycopeptide [1]. Its mechanism of action is similar to other glycopeptides, via binding to the terminal D-alanyl-D-alanine pentapeptide chain of nascent peptidoglycan, while the monoamide substituent at the peptide carboxy group is responsible for the increased potency against staphylococci, particularly coagulase-negative staphylococci [1, 51]. Its structure and spectrum of activity most closely resemble that of teicoplanin; however, it has greater potency against many gram-positive organisms including anaerobes [1, 52]. Dalbavancin has demonstrated potent activity against clinically relevant aerobic and anaerobic gram-positive organisms, including methicillin-resistant staphylococci, penicillin-resistant *Streptococcus pneumoniae*, and certain vancomycin-resistant enterococci (*vanB* phenotypes) [1, 53].

3.1 Pharmacokinetics of Dalbavancin

The PKs of dalbavancin have been explored in healthy volunteers, renally impaired subjects, and hepatically impaired subjects. The C_{max} of dalbavancin is achieved immediately following the end of the infusion with an apparent V_{ss} of 8–12 L [54, 55]. Plasma concentrations increase in a linear dose-dependent manner and the protein binding is approximately 93 %. Maximum tissue concentrations are approximately 300 mg/L and are observed within 24 h after dose administration [56, 57]. Dalbavancin is not a substrate, inhibitor nor inducer of hepatic CYP450 isoenzymes. It is eliminated through renal and nonrenal routes primarily as intact drug. The clearance in healthy volunteers is estimated to be 0.04 L/h with a half-life of approximately 8 days [57, 58]. The PK parameters of dalbavancin after single and multiple escalating doses are shown in Table 3.

Importantly, hepatic and renal dysfunction has demonstrated minimal effects on the concentration and exposure [54, 56, 59]. A minor metabolite of dalbavancin, hydroxyl-dalbavancin, has been found in human urine while significant amounts have not been found in plasma. Approximately 35 % of the parent drug is excreted in the urine while 8–12 % of dalbavancin is excreted as hydroxyl-dalbavancin [1, 7]. Approximately 20 % of the parent drug is excreted in human feces and approximately 70 % of the administered parent dose has been accounted for in collected excreta through day 70. In a mass balance study in rats, by day 14 only the kidneys, liver, brown fat, skin, and skeletal muscle retained >1 % of the initial radiolabeled dose and <5 % of total radioactivity was retained in the entire carcass at 70 days after dosing of dalbavancin [56].

Table 3
Pharmacokinetic parameters of dalbavancin in healthy subjects

Parameters following a single intravenous infusion							
Dose (mg)	C_{max} *(mg/L)*	AUC_{0-24} *(mg·h/L)*	*CL (L/h)*	V_{ss} *(L)*	$t_{1/2}$ *(h)*		
140	39.7 ± 1.64	3251 ± 86.5	0.043 ± 0.001	10.9 ± 0.206	189 ± 3.59		
220	65.3 ± 14.8	4955 ± 562	0.045 ± 0.005	11.3 ± 1.34	188 ± 17.3		
350	96.1 ± 6.95	8094 ± 1186	0.044 ± 0.007	10.7 ± 2.34	181 ± 16.2		
500	153 ± 36.4	12451 ± 2001	0.041 ± 0.006	8.58 ± 1.23	159 ± 4.99		
630	190 ± 59	14758 ± 4024	0.045 ± 0.011	10.5 ± 3.2	172 ± 16.1		
840	243 ± 11.2	22225 ± 1136	0.038 ± 0.002	7.75 ± 0.56	152 ± 5.47		
1120	325 ± 41.1	25790 ± 2447	0.044 ± 0.004	8.49 ± 1.05	149 ± 3.60		
Parameters following multiple infusions							
Dose (LD/daily MD, mg)	C_{max} *(mg/L)*	C_{max} *(mg/L)*	C_{min} *(mg/L)*	C_{min} *(mg/L)*	AUC_{0-24} *(mg·h/L)*	*CL (L/h)*	$t_{1/2}$ *(h)*
	Day 1	Day 7	Day 1	Day 7	Day 7	Day 7	Day 7
300/30	57.3 ± 8.11	29.6 ± 5.20	14.4 ± 4.03	22.7 ± 3.49	597 ± 75.7	0.051 ± 0.007	191 ± 14.2
400/40	77.6 ± 11.8	42.3 ± 7.51	21.6 ± 0.57	30.9 ± 3.18	825 ± 6.3	0.049 ± 0.005	184 ± 17.2
600/60	115 ± 7.81	67.7 ± 2.12	30.2 ± 3.41	47.1 ± 2.59	1221 ± 77.3	0.049 ± 0.003	198 ± 18.7
800/80	131 ± 31.2	67.7 ± 2.12	36.5 ± 7.25	54 ± 0.71	1371 ± 36.7	0.058 ± 0.002	198 ± 13.7
1000/100	180 ± 25	98.9 ± 18.8	57.2 ± 7.75	77.7 ± 12.3	1997 ± 310	0.051 ± 0.007	189 ± 11.8

Data are presented as mean ± SD

LD loading dose, *MD* maintenance dose, C_{max} maximum plasma concentration, AUC_{0-24} 24-h area under the plasma concentration–time curve, *CL* clearance, V_{ss} apparent volume of distribution at steady-state, $t_{1/2}$ elimination half-life, C_{min} minimum plasma concentration

The mean AUC over 7 days in blister fluid was 6438 mg·h/L and mean penetration into blister fluid was approximately 60 % following a single 1000 mg dose of dalbavancin [60]. Concentrations of dalbavancin in blister fluid remained well above the MIC_{90} for *S. aureus* and streptococci through day 7 in all subjects, supporting its use for patients with acute bacterial skin and skin structure infections.

The serum bactericidal activity of dalbavancin against MRSA ranged from 0.5 to 4 mg/L and remained measurable for 7 days after administration for all patients receiving ≥500 mg of dalbavancin [54, 57]. All samples in which the plasma concentration of dalbavancin exceeded 20 mg/L had detectable bactericidal activity upon twofold or greater dilution. The results of this study provided the basis for a once-weekly dosing regimen that would provide plasma concentrations with adequate and sustained bactericidal activity against *S. aureus*. PK simulations indicated that this could be achieved with a single 1000 mg dose for the first 7 days followed by a 500 mg dose on day 8 to maintain therapeutic concentrations out to 14 days. In the phase 1 dose escalation study, both these doses were tolerated well by healthy volunteers [57].

A population PK model has also been developed from patients enrolled in the phase 2 and 3 trials of dalbavancin [61]. A two compartment model with first-order elimination best fit the data. The apparent V_{ss} derived from the model was 15.7 L and the mean terminal half-life was 8.5 days. When the impact of covariates was examined, a BSA >2.25 m^2 resulted in a 34 % decrease in C_{max} but did not affect CL. A simulated CrCl of 20–50 mL/min did not affect C_{max} but did decrease CL by approximately 21 %. Low BSA and low CrCl resulted in 30 % higher C_{max} and 27 % lower clearance. Although these values were statistically significant, they were all within 20–30 % of an average weight patient with normal CrCl. The CL of dalbavancin was influenced by BSA and CrCl while a linear relationship existed between BSA and apparent volume of distribution in the central compartment (*Vc*).

Overall, the PKs of dalbavancin are predictable and consistent with dose proportionality, exhibited low interindividual variability, and have been found to be similar between patients and healthy subjects [62]. After a single 1000 mg dose in healthy subjects, the mean PK parameter values (coefficient of variation) for dalbavancin were C_{max} of 287 mg/L (13.9 %), AUC_{0-24} of 3185 mg·h/L (12.8 %), AUC_{0-168} of 11,160 mg·h/L (41.1 %), CL of 0.0513 L/h (46.8 %), and terminal $t_{1/2}$ of 346 h (16.5 %). In patients receiving the recommended two-dose regimen of dalbavancin for the treatment of ABSSSI, mean plasma concentrations of dalbavancin were 30.4 mg/L immediately before the second dose and 21.2 mg/L 12 days after the second dose. These observed plasma concentrations of dalbavancin are similar to values observed in healthy volunteers.

3.1.1 Renal and Hepatic Impairment

Findings from three phase I studies that investigated the safety and PKs in patients with varying degrees of renal or hepatic dysfunction have been reported [59]. Patients with moderate renal impairment had an approximate 50 % increase in $AUC_{0-\infty}$ compared to normal controls, although the mean AUC through day 7 was only 23 % higher. The C_{max} of dalbavancin was also increased by 30 % in patients with moderate renal impairment. CL and V_{ss} of dalbavancin decreased by 35 and 21 %, respectively, as renal impairment increased. Mean terminal half-life with moderate renal impairment ranged from 389 to 432 h, but overall mean terminal elimination half-life remained relatively unchanged across groups as well as the fraction of urinary excretion. For patients with severe renal impairment, plasma concentration–time profiles were similar to normal controls up to 7 days after dalbavancin administration but increased after day 7. Patients with severe renal impairment had a 100 % increase in $AUC_{0-\infty}$, but only a 16 % increase through day 7. C_{max} was similar, even in patients with severe impairment who received the 1000 mg dose. The CL of dalbavancin was reduced by half and the terminal half-life was slightly longer. In dialysis-dependent patients, concentration–time profiles were similar to normal controls through day 7 and measurable dalbavancin concentrations were not found in the dialysate. Compared to normal subjects, C_{max} was not increased; however, $AUC_{0-\infty}$ was 62 and 28 % higher when dalbavancin was dosed before and after dialysis, respectively.

For patients with hepatic impairment, those with moderate and severe impairment had a 27–36 % decrease in AUC and an 18–29 % increase in C_{max}. CL increased by up to 58 % while V_{ss} increased up to 30 %. Terminal half-life remained unchanged [59].

The minimal changes in exposure in patients with renal impairment through the first 7–14 days is likely due to the fact that 7-day AUC and 14-day AUC accounted for only 1/3 and 1/2 of the total $AUC_{0-\infty}$ given the long half-life of dalbavancin [59]. When these data are taken into account, dosage adjustment is not needed for patients with mild renal impairment and may not be necessary for patients with moderate renal impairment. Patients with severe renal impairment had a marked increase in exposure that likely requires dose adjustment. With the intent of matching concentrations and exposures during the 14 treatment period with the two-dose intravenous regimen, PK simulations were carried out in participants with severe renal impairment who do not receive dialysis, including investigating various doses of dalbavancin. Based on these simulations, a dose of 750 mg of dalbavancin followed 1 week later by 375 mg of dalbavancin was suggested for treatment for patients with a CrCl <30 mL/min. This dosage regimen maintains concentrations above 20 mg/L and matches the treatment exposures observed for subjects with normal renal function. Although a slight decrease in dalbavancin exposure and an increase in CL and V_{ss} were evident for patients with moderate or severe hepatic insufficiency, the values overlapped with the range noted for healthy subjects. Notably, the mean concentrations of dalbavancin were maintained above 20 mg/L throughout the 14-day treatment period in all groups of hepatically impaired patients. When these data are taken into consideration, no adjustment of dalbavancin dosage is required for patients with any degree of hepatic impairment [59].

3.1.2 Intermittent and Continuous Renal Replacement

Despite large molecular size (1817 Da), high degree of protein binding (93 %), and minimal renal elimination of dalbavancin, Vilay and colleagues assessed the transmembrane clearance of dalbavancin with in vitro renal replacement therapy models [63]. When the CL of dalbavancin by continuous renal replacement therapy (CRRT) was added to the nonrenal clearance observed from healthy subjects in order to estimate the total CL of drug during CRRT, the standard dosing scheme of dalbavancin (1000 mg followed by 500 mg on day 7) was adequate for dialysate rates up to 1 L/h. For dialysate rates of ≥2 L/h with a polysulfone filter, a dose increase should be considered as extracorporeal clearance exceeded 30 % of total CL, translating to a total CL during CRRT exceeding that of total CL in healthy subjects. At a dialysate rate of 6 L/h, the half-life of dalbavancin would also be shortened from 7 to 8 days to approximately 4 days [63]. This finding could have important ramifications for dalbavancin dosing in critically ill patients on CRRT. Of note, this study only reported transmembrane CL and not the contribution of drug adsorption to extracorporeal CL.

3.2 Pharmacodynamics of Dalbavancin

3.2.1 In Vitro Models

Dalbavancin has exhibited rapid bactericidal activity against multiple phenotypes of *S. aureus*, including those with reduced glycopeptide susceptibility, at clinically relevant unbound drug plasma concentrations [64]. The time to 99.9 % reduction in CFU/mL ranged from 24 to 48 h while the AUC_{24}/MIC required for a static and 2-log reduction effect was 36–100 and 214–331, respectively. Simulated unbound concentrations of dalbavancin produced marked but non-concentration dependent killing of multiple strains of *S. aureus* and $fAUC_{24}$/MIC was related to efficacy up to 240 h.

The activity of dalbavancin in combination with several other antimicrobials has been evaluated in vitro [65]. Antimicrobials tested against ten staphylococci, enterococci, and streptococci isolates included oxacillin, gentamicin, clindamycin, levofloxacin, rifampin, vancomycin, quinupristin/dalfopristin, linezolid, and daptomycin. Synergy was only present in 5.6 % of tests, all with the combination of dalbavancin and oxacillin. After dalbavancin and oxacillin, the combinations of dalbavancin and gentamicin and dalbavancin and vancomycin were equally effective, producing partial synergy or additive effects against 9 bacterial strains. The least active combination was dalbavancin plus linezolid. No antagonistic interactions were observed with any combination.

3.2.2 Animal Models

In vivo animal studies of dalbavancin have demonstrated that increasing the dosing interval resulted in a shifting of the dose–response curve to the left, indicating greater killing effect when large doses were given infrequently [66]. When correlating the PK/PD indices with CFU/mL reduction, the AUC_{24}/MIC resulted in the strongest correlation (R^2 = 77 %) for *S. aureus* while C_{max} was the strongest (R^2 = 78 %) for *S. pneumoniae.* T > MIC was a poor fit (R^2 < 10 %) for both organisms. The mean (±SD) AUC_{24}/MIC required for static and 2-log killing effect against *S. pneumoniae* and *S. aureus* were 7.2 ± 4.52 and 16.6 ± 12.3 and 160 ± 67 and 266 ± 88, respectively, when dalbavancin was dosed every 72 h. The dose–response curves were steep and the AUC_{24}/MIC associated with 1 and 2-log killing were not appreciably higher than those required to achieve a static effect. In addition, when dalbavancin was dosed every 72 h versus every 24 h, the 24-h AUC/MICs associated with killing and stasis were 1.3- to 2.4-fold lower, supporting the larger, infrequent dosing regimens. When the effect of neutrophils on the activity of dalbavancin was examined by using nonneutropenic and neutropenic mice, the doses required to achieve the same endpoints were 1.7- to 2.1-fold lower for the nonneutropenic mice, although these differences were not statistically significant.

To determine the impact of site of infection, the dose–response curves were compared for the thigh and lung *S. pneumoniae* murine infection models [66]. The dose–response curves were nearly identical for these two models, suggesting that the PDs target is independent of the infection site, at least for *S. pneumoniae.* Given that dalbavancin serum exposure following a single 1000 mg dose produces a *f*AUC of more than 1500 mg · h/L, current dosing regimens of dalbavancin would exceed the necessary targets for both organisms studied.

Dalbavancin has exhibited excellent activity in an MRSA rabbit endocarditis model and was not influenced by the reduced susceptibility to other glycopeptides [67], while a single dose of dalbavancin was able to sterilize the lungs of rats with penicillin-resistant *S. pneumoniae* pneumonia [68].

At high concentrations (32 × MIC), dalbavancin is bactericidal against both logarithmic and stationary-phase MRSA. In a foreign body infection model, only dalbavancin at 60 and 80 mg/kg prevented planktonic bacterial growth while combination with rifampin produced a bactericidal effect for all dosing regimens of dalbavancin [69]. Complete elimination of implant-adherent staphylococci was not achieved with any dalbavancin dose tested. The combination of dalbavancin with rifampin achieved cure rates of 25–36 %, which was similar to rifampin alone (33 %). Rifampin did not enhance the activity of dalbavancin, although dalbavancin did prevent the emergence of rifampin resistance. Dalbavancin monotherapy achieved only a static effect against planktonic MRSA in the cage fluid and showed no eradication for adherent MRSA at any dose. Addition of rifampin did not increase killing in either environment.

Concentrations of dalbavancin in the bone marrow of rabbits at 15.14 μg/g were more than threefold higher than plasma concentrations at 72 h and remained constant at 12.02 μg/g between 12 and 336 h after an intravenous dose of 20 mg/kg [^{14}C] dalbavancin [70]. The resulting penetration into bone, bone marrow, and nucleus pulposus compared to plasma was 63, 248, and 12 %, respectively. Penetration into the synovial space and compact bone was 21 and 5 %, respectively, with concentrations at 12 h of 6.56 and 1.56 μg/g, respectively. Overall, total drug concentrations were maintained above the MICs for key pathogens for up to 168 h in all tissues studied except compact bone.

These in vitro and animal models assess the amount of total drug needed for activity and the PK/PD index associated with efficacy, including a bactericidal effect against *S. aureus*. When coupled with PK data and simulations, these results provide support of the proposed human dose and schedule to be studied in proof of concept trials.

3.3 Dalbavancin Clinical Trials: Proof of Pharmacokinetic-Pharmacodynamic Concepts

Clinical trials with dalbavancin have been ongoing since 1999 and five different sponsors have been involved with the development of this agent [71, 72]. A New Drug Application (NDA) was filed with FDA in 2004 based on clinical trial data for the indication of cSSSI [71, 72] but was subsequently withdrawn. A second NDA for the indication of ABSSSI was approved and was based on data from over 1200 subjects treated with dalbavancin in during earlier phase 1, 2 or 3 studies plus the two recent multinational, double-blind, double-dummy phase 3 noninferiority clinical trials (DISCOVERY 1 and 2) [71–75].

Clinical trials in patients with skin and soft-tissue infections and cSSSI initially provided initial evidence of effectiveness of a two-dose regimen of dalbavancin compared to vancomycin. Importantly, clinical response rates were lower when dalbavancin was given as a single intravenous dose of 1100 mg compared to the two dose dalbavancin regimen (1000 mg dose followed by 500 mg on day 8) [73]. The two-dose dalbavancin group had a 32 and 18 % higher clinical success rate when compared to the single-dose dalbavancin group and standard therapy (vancomycin), respectively. The two-dose group also had a 34 and 21 % higher microbiological success rate when compared to the single-dose and standard therapy groups, respectively. There were no laboratory abnormalities observed and dalbavancin was well tolerated overall.

The initial phase 3 noninferiority registration trials of patients with cSSSI (VER001-09), dalbavancin intravenous regimen of

1000 mg followed 1 week later by a 500 mg dose demonstrated noninferiority to either twice-daily linezolid alone or initial vancomycin with step-down to oral linezolid [71, 72, 74]. When the results of the two trials were pooled, 79.7 % versus 79.8 % of patients achieved a successful outcome at 48–72 h in the dalbavancin and vancomycin-linezolid groups, respectively.

The two recent multinational phase 3 clinical trials established the effectiveness and safety of intravenous dalbavancin (1000 mg on day 1 and 500 mg on day 8) in patients with ABSSSI compared to vancomycin (at least 3 days of intravenous vancomycin with an option to switch to oral linezolid for a 10- to 14-day treatment course) [71, 75]. The early clinical response rates for the pooled analysis of the intent-to-treat population were 79.7 and 79.8 % for dalbavancin and vancomycin-linezolid regimens, respectively. Similarly, the end-of-treatment clinical response rates were 90.7 and 92.1 %, respectively. Adverse events observed with dalbavancin were transient and mild to moderate intensity.

These studies indicate that for the treatment of cSSSI or ABSSSI, the efficacy of intravenous dalbavancin administered as 1000 mg followed by 500 mg 1 week later is noninferior to comparator treatment regimens for both early time endpoints and investigator-assessed clinical success of therapy.

4 Oritavancin

Oritavancin, (LY333328), is a second-generation semisynthetic lipoglycopeptide antimicrobial agent [1, 2]. Oritavancin possesses multiple mechanisms of action including inhibition of transglycosylation, binding to the pentaglycyl bridging segment in peptidoglycan, and disruption of the cell membrane resulting in rapid depolarization and concentration-dependent cell death [1, 76]. These multiple mechanisms of action confer rapid killing versus actively growing, stationary phase, and biofilm-producing gram-positive bacteria including those resistant to vancomycin and daptomycin [76]. Oritavancin has demonstrated potent in vitro activity against a wide spectrum of gram-positive bacteria commonly associated with serious infections; including methicillin-susceptible and -resistant *Staphylococcus aureus* (MRSA), vancomycin-susceptible and -resistant enterococci (VRE; *Enterococcus faecium and Enterococcus faecalis*), *Streptococcus pyogenes*, and penicillin-susceptible and -resistant *Streptococcus pneumoniae* [1, 76].

4.1 Pharmacokinetics of Oritavancin

The chemical structure of oritavancin gives rise to its unique PK properties, particularly its lengthy terminal half-life [1, 77]. These unique properties have been evaluated in several healthy volunteer phase I PK studies over a range of doses. In an open-label dose-escalation study in nine healthy volunteers aged 21–55 years with normal body weight, oritavancin was administered in eight stepwise doses of 0.02–0.5 mg/kg. Serial plasma levels were obtained after the start of the infusion along with 24 h urine and fecal collections. After non-compartmental analysis, oritavancin plasma concentrations declined in a multi-exponential manner over the 2 week sampling period. The median C_{max} for the 0.5 mg/kg group was 6.5 mg/L, which declined to less than 10 % of C_{max} within the first 24 h. The median AUC for the 0.5 mg/kg dose group was 68.3 mg·h/L. C_{max} and $AUC_{0\text{-}Tau}$ increased proportionally to the dose, suggesting the PKs of oritavancin are linear over the dose range studied. The median plasma terminal half-life was 207.3 h while the mean renal clearance was 0.457 mL/min. Fecal concentrations were undetectable for the majority of subjects and less than 5 % of the drug was recovered in the urine over 7 days.

Oritavancin displays linear PKs best described by a 3-compartment model with terminal half-lives of 2.4, 18, and 360 h for the α, β, and γ phases, respectively [77]. The long terminal half-life ($t_{1/2\gamma}$) suggests that drug accumulation can occur after administration of multiple-dose regimens and that alternative dosage regimen such as a single-dose may be feasible.

Oritavancin has no active metabolites and shows high retention and slow clearance from tissues in reticuloendothelial systems and accumulation of the administered dose in the liver (59–64 %), kidney (2.7 %), spleen (1.8 %), and lung (1.7 %). Oritavancin exhibited >80 % protein binding throughout various species including human (87.5 %), mouse (85.3 %), rat (>80 %), and dog (97.1 %) [78]. Albumin is the protein responsible for the majority of serum oritavancin binding [78].

Table 4 displays the mean PK parameters for a pooled population model of 560 subjects and 6336 oritavancin plasma concentrations from 12 clinical phase 1, 2, and 3 studies from either healthy subjects or infected patients with complicated skin and skin structure infections or *S. aureus* bacteremia [79]. The CL of oritavancin appeared to be effected by body weight, with CL increasing in a linear fashion up to 80 kg of total body weight and resulting in a lower AUC_{24} in subjects given 200 mg daily for 3 days who had a total body weight >110 kg. The magnitude of this relationship was such that the population predicted CL would be expected to increase by 53 % over a body weight range of 80–200 kg. Increasing the dose to 300 mg normalized the $AUC_{0\text{–}24}$ similarly to those with total body weight of ≤110 kg. Age did not seem to affect CL or C_{max} as dose-normalized C_{max} did not increase in elderly subjects.

Patients with available plasma concentration–time data from the two pivotal Phase 3 trials (SOLO I and II) and from the previously described population PK model above were used to evaluate patient-specific covariates and drug variability of patients with

Table 4
Summary of oritavancin pharmacokinetic parameter estimates

Parameter	Phase 1 (n=200)		Phase 2/3 (n=360)	
C_{max} (mg/L)[a]	35.7 ± 9.09	34.5 (20.4–80)	28.5 ± 12.2	25.9 (10.9–131)
C_{min} (mg/L)[a]	4.11 ± 1.80	3.65 (1.23–10.2)	1.99 ± 1.10	1.74 (0.54–9.81)
AUC_{0-24} (mg·h/L)[a]	252 ± 78.6	240 (104–614)	146 ± 63.7	133 (42.2–618)
CL (L/h)	0.351 ± 0.11	0.350 (0.12–0.70)	0.601 ± 0.20	0.584 (0.17–1.45)
V_c (L)	5.19 ± 1.27	5.04 (2.37–13.8)	7.10 ± 2.46	6.79 (1.17–18.3)
$t_{1/2}\alpha$ (h)	2.56 ± 0.65	2.48 (1.23–4.78)	2.04 ± 0.44	2.04 (0.91–4.08)
$t_{1/2}\beta$ (h)	27 ± 11.5	25.4 (9.38–99.6)	31.2 ± 11.4	29.2 (8.37–86.3)
$t_{1/2}\gamma$ (h)	318 ± 59.1	314 (191–584)	393 ± 73.5	394 (142–602)

Data presented as mean ± SD or as median (range)
C_{max}, maximum plasma concentration, C_{min}, minimum plasma concentration, AUC_{0-24} 24-h area under the plasma concentration–time curve, CL clearance, V_c apparent volume of distribution of central compartment, $t_{1/2}$ half-life of the alpha (α), beta (β), and gamma (γ) phases
[a]AUC_{24}, C_{max}, C_{min} have been normalized to a dose of 200 mg for subjects ≤110 kg and to 300 mg for those ≥110 kg

ABSSSI [80]. The analysis included 297 patients with a total of 1337 plasma oritavancin concentrations, with 90 % of patients having 4 or 5 plasma concentrations available. After a single intravenous 1200 mg dose of oritavancin infused over 3 h, the mean PK parameter values (coefficient of variation) were C_{max} of 138 mg/L (23.0 %), AUC_{0-72} of 1530 mg·h/L (36.9 %), $AUC_{0-\infty}$ of 2800 mg·h/L (28.6 %), CL of 0.445 L/h (27.2 %), V_{ss} of 97.8 L (56.4 %), $t_{1/2}\alpha$ of 2.29 h (49.8 %), $t_{1/2}\beta$ of 13.4 h (10.5 %), and $t_{1/2}\gamma$ of 245 h (14.9 %). Although covariate analysis revealed statistically significant relationships between patient height and interindividual variability in CL, and between age and interindividual variability in V_c; neither tended to impact oritavancin exposure in the patient population studied. This population PK analysis support the recommendations that dosage adjustments are not required in patients treated for ABSSSI with renal impairment (CrCl >29 mL/min) or mild to moderate hepatic impairment, and that patient covariates such as age, body size, BMI, race, gender, or diabetes status had no significant influence on measurements of oritavancin exposure (C_{max} or AUC values).

4.1.1 Plasma and Skin Blister Fluid

Through its development as an antimicrobial designed to treat complicated skin and skin structure infections, the extracellular blister fluid concentrations of oritavancin were explored after various dosages [81]. Mean C_{max} of oritavancin were observed at 1 and 10 h in plasma and blister fluid, respectively. The plasma concentration at these time points was approximately eightfold higher than in blister fluid (46.2 mg/L versus 5.85 mg/L). Oritavancin concentrations were undetectable in blister fluid 100–150 h after the last dose while total drug oritavancin exposure in interstitial fluids was approximately 19 % of that in plasma, regardless of dosing regimen. In this study, mean free-drug plasma concentrations associated with the two dosing regimens exceed the MIC_{90} for *Staphylococcus aureus* for ≥92 % of the dosing interval.

4.1.2 Lung penetration and Intracellular Activity

Despite its large size and molecular weight, oritavancin has been shown to penetrate well into human pulmonary ELF and AM [82]. In 30 healthy adult subjects receiving oritavancin 800 mg daily for 5 days, the AUC_{0-24} of oritavancin in ELF and AM was 106 and 3297 mg · h/L, respectively. Oritavancin distributed slowly into and out of both the ELF and AM and concentrations were maintained above the MIC for most gram-positive pathogens out to 24 h. These findings support that oritavancin 800 mg once daily provide a significant exposure in ELF and AM after 5 days of dosing.

The extensive intracellular concentration of oritavancin causes deposition of concentric lamellar structures and other materials [83]. This deposition is consistent with a mixed-lipid storage disorder and has been postulated to inhibit macrophage microbicidal function, a phagocytic effector function necessary for host defense against microbial pathogens such as *S. aureus* and *Acinetobacter baumannii* [84]. Cells incubated with carbon-labeled oritavancin have demonstrated intracellular concentrations that were 200-fold above extracellular concentrations at 24 h. Despite this accumulation, killing of *S. aureus* by oritavancin-loaded macrophages was substantially enhanced by approximately 75 % when compared to control macrophages. These data suggest that the accumulation of lipoglycopeptides in macrophages does not correspond with dysfunction in macrophage killing of microbes, and oritavancin in particular may enhance this function against *S. aureus* [83].

Small-colony variants (SCVs) demonstrate an ability to invade and persist in phagocytic and nonphagocytic cells and are a well-recognized phenomenon of serious infections due to *S. aureus* [84]. The treatment of these SCVs requires antibiotics with the ability to act intracellularly and have activity against SCVs. The results of several studies indicate that oritavancin may be able to eradicate intracellular SCVs more effectively than its comparators (vancomcyin, daptomycin, gentamicin, rifampin, and moxifloxacin) and may offer promising activity against these forms of intracellular infections at clinically relevant concentrations [84]. Detailed evaluation of the intracellular activity of oritavancin against variant strains of *S. aureus* has also been conducted [85–88].

4.1.3 Clearance by Dialysis

Despite the minimal renal elimination, large size, extensive volume of distribution, and high degree of protein binding of oritavancin, Kumar and colleagues examined the in vitro CL of oritavancin from human blood via low-flux, high-flux, and CRRT dialyzers [89]. Overall, the mean dialytic clearances of oritavancin were below zero for all dialyzers tested except for Optiflux F160NR which was 0.34 ± 18.8 mL/min. The concentration of oritavancin in the dialysate was undetectable at all sampling points for all dialyzers. The results of this study indicate that no adjustments to oritavancin dosing schemes are needed for patients undergoing any type of dialysis tested. Of note, the ultrafiltration rate was intentionally minimized in this study, limiting the ability to extrapolate these findings to hemodialysis and CRRT procedures involving positive ultrafiltration rates and more rapid blood and dialysate flow rates.

4.2 Pharmacodynamics of Oritavancin

Although oritavancin was originally designated as a candidate for clinical development by Eli Lilly in 1994, it was felt that the long terminal half-life beginning at plasma concentrations ≤4 mg/L was too low to exert efficient antimicrobial efficacy for staphylococci and enterococci with MICs up to 4 mg/L. It was proposed that increasing the dose above the initial 200 and 300 mg originally studied in patients could increase these concentrations and contribute to improved antimicrobial efficacy. Also, it was not until the mid-2000s before the propensity of oritavancin to adhere to the plastic tubes used for broth microdilution tests was appreciated. Once polysorbate 80 was added, the MICs to staphylococci and enterococci were reduced approximately 16- to 32-fold [1, 90].

4.2.1 In Vitro Models

In contrast to other glycopeptides, oritavancin possesses rapid, concentration-dependent antibacterial efficacy supported by the results of a range of in vitro microbiological evaluations [1, 91–93]. Oritavancin has displayed potent activity against *S. aureus* and vancomycin-resistant *E. faecium,* although eightfold higher concentrations were required to achieve the same degree of microbial killing against VRE as compared to MRSA. The post-antibiotic effect of oritavancin was determined to be concentration dependent at 7.68 and 4.25 h for MRSA and VRE, respectively. Synergism was consistently observed with gentamicin, regardless of the dosing schedule, and significantly improved the bacterial killing compared to oritavancin alone [91–93].

Oritavancin has also displayed excellent activity against multidrug-resistant strains of *S. aureus,* including hVISA, VISA, and VRSA, and *S. pneumonia.* The in vitro activity of oritavancin appears to be hampered by the addition of albumin, although this appears to be concentration dependent [94, 95]. Oritavancin has demonstrated improved magnitude and duration of bacterial killing against hVISA when compared to its bactericidal comparators, including daptomycin [96]. These results suggest that oritavancin could be an effective choice for the treatment of staphylococcal infections regardless of the resistance phenotype with minimum bactericidal concentration (MBC) and MIC values between 16 and

64 with the addition of polysorbate-80 [90]. Additionally, oritavancin is active against both MRSA and VRSA biofilms, likely due to its ability to alter membrane integrity and target the septum of *S. aureus* cells to prevent biofilm formation [97].

4.2.2 Animal Models

The results of in vivo animal model data have correlated well with the efficacy of oritavancin seen with in vitro models. Against *S. aureus*, the PK-PD index best determining in vivo efficacy in a neutropenic mouse-thigh model was the C_{max} ($r^2 = 96$ %) followed by time above the MIC (%Time > MIC) and the AUC/MIC ($r^2 = 83$ and 77 %, respectively) [98]. This concentration-dependent activity allows for improved efficacy when oritavancin is administered large, infrequent doses [99, 100]. Oritavancin has demonstrated equal bactericidal activity as oxacillin in an MSSA endocarditis model, with lower relapse rates at 3 days after treatment [101].

In a rabbit model of both susceptible and VanA and VanB phenotypes of *E. faecalis*, only oritavancin reduced CFUs per gram of vegetation when compared to control vegetations amongst vancomycin and teicoplanin [102]. The greatest efficacy was observed when daily oritavancin was combined with twice-daily gentamicin, although the mean reduction in inoculum was modest at 1.5 logs even for the susceptible strain [103]. There are no data to date on oritavancin performance in endocarditis models of *E. faecium*, although in rats with a central venous catheter-associated infection model due to VanA positive *E. faecium* a 75 % reduction in rats with infected catheters was observed when compared to controls [104].

Oritavancin has been shown to bind to lung surfactant, albeit to a much lower extent than daptomycin. The oritavancin MIC against *S. pneumoniae* ATCC 6303 increased eightfold when exposed to 5 % surfactant. In contrast, the oritavancin MIC against *S. aureus* ATCC 29213 increased 16-fold when exposed to 5 % surfactant (from 0.06 to 1 mg/L), which would be difficult to overcome with a single intravenous dose of 1200 mg [105, 106]. Oritavancin has demonstrated improved efficacy in both MSSA and MRSA pneumonia models in relation to its comparators [107].

In a standard rabbit pneumococcal meningitis model, the penetration of oritavancin into the CSF was about 2–5 %, with mean C_{max} in CSF for doses of 2.5, 10, and 40 mg/kg of 0.54, 0.76, and 1.36 mg/L, respectively. This would allow for treatment of pneumococcal meningitis and potentially coagulase-negative staphylococci given the low MIC ranges, while data on *S. aureus* are lacking [108]. Other animal models have also evaluated oritavancin as oral therapy for *Clostridium difficile* colitis and activity against *Bacillus anthracis* [109].

These models are fundamental in establishing the optimal dosing regimen of oritavancin in humans. Given the long plasma half-life of oritavancin, a fixed-dose strategy would result in a prolonged time to steady-state exposure. In clinical practice the primary goal is to have the greatest drug exposure early in therapy in order to maximize PK-PD parameters and clinical outcomes. This would favor a single dose regimen of oritavancin, a regimen that has been validated by both animal and clinical models.

4.2.3 Staphylococcus aureus *Bacteremia*

Early phase clinical studies in humans have also investigated the activity of oritavancin in patients with uncomplicated *S. aureus* bacteremia who received 10–14 days of either sequential doses of oritavancin (5, 6.5, 8, and 10 mg/kg) every 24 h or a control treatment (vancomycin or a beta-lactam) [110]. The mean AUC_{24}/MIC, C_{max}/MIC, %Time > MIC, and unbound concentration %T > MIC (*f*T > MIC) on day one for all dosing exposures were 219.4, 39.3, 96.2, and 28.2, respectively. Doses of 5–10 mg/kg/day resulted in AUC_{0-24} values of 144.5–1478.5 μg·h/mL, respectively. Successful microbiological and clinical responses occurred in 85 and 78 % of patients, respectively. Using classification and regression tree (CART) analysis, a breakpoint was identified for *f*T > MIC at 22 %. There was a lack of relationship between %Time > MIC and microbiological or clinical response, which was not surprising given that the majority of patients achieved 100 % %Time > MIC due to the prolonged half-life and low MIC values. The assessment of oritavancin PKs based on these phase 2 data from bacteremic patients was consistent with a previous evaluation based on data from healthy volunteers and those with skin and soft tissue infections. Both analysis confirmed the multicompartmental characteristics of the plasma concentration–time profile and linear PKs of oritavancin.

4.3 Oritavancin Clinical Trials: Proof of Pharmacokinetic-Pharmacodynamic Concepts

Clinical trials with oritavancin have been ongoing since 1990s and four different sponsors have been involved with the development of this agent [111]. The recent phase 2 and 3 in human registration trials have provided a proof-of-concept for the single 1200 mg dose regimen of oritavancin as compared to smaller, more frequent doses that were evaluated in earlier clinical trials and phase 2 SIMPLIFI study [111–114]. Compared to 7–10 days of vancomycin, a single 1200 mg intravenous dose of oritavancin was noninferior for patients with ABSSSI in two, large phase 3 clinical trials (SOLO I and II) [113, 114]. Efficacy outcomes were also similar when stratified by pathogen, including MRSA, and the overall frequency of adverse events was low, with nausea being more common in the oritavancin group. Efficacy rates for oritavancin did not differ from vancomycin in SOLO I when analyzed according to body-mass index or the presence or absence of diabetes [113]. The majority (98.3 %) of treatment failures were due a lack of post-therapy evaluation. In the second phase 3 trial (SOLO II) in adults with ABSSSI [114], oritavancin had a lower response rate at the primary endpoint than vancomycin (81 % versus 89.9 %) in patients with a major cutaneous abscess. The primary reasons for failure in this study was at the early clinical evaluation were the presence of fever or missing temperature data. The efficacy outcome for the primary endpoint was also lower for patients with streptococci, diabetes, and subcutaneous abscesses at baseline who received oritavancin. A single-dose regimen for ABSSSI that resulted in early and sustained clinical response has the potential to reduce complications associated with multiple intravenous administrations, improve treatment adherence, and reduce utilization of health care resources [115].

References

1. Zhanel GG, Calic D, Schweizer F et al (2010) New lipoglycopeptides: a comparative review of dalbavancin, oritavancin, and telavancin. Drugs 70:859–886
2. Rodvold KA, McConeghy KW (2014) Methicillin-resistant *Staphylococcus aureus* therapy: past, present, and future. Clin Infect Dis 58(Suppl 1):S20–S27
3. Wenzler E, Rodvold KA (2015) Telavancin: the long and winding road from discovery to Food and Drug Administration approvals and future directions. Clin Infect Dis 61(Suppl S2):S38–S47
4. Higgins DL, Chang R, Debabov DV et al (2005) Telavancin, a multifunctional lipoglycopeptide, disrupts both cell wall synthesis and cell membrane integrity in methicillin-resistant *Staphylococcus aureus*. Antimicrob Agents Chemother 49:1127–1134
5. Chang MH, Kish TD, Fung HB (2010) Telavancin: a lipoglycopeptide antimicrobial for the treatment of complicated skin and skin structure infections caused by gram-positive bacteria in adults. Clin Ther 32:2160–2185
6. Wong SL, Barriere SL, Kitt MM, Goldberg MR (2008) Multiple-dose pharmacokinetics of intravenous telavancin in healthy male and female subjects. J Antimicrob Chemother 62:780–783
7. Shaw JP, Cheong J, Goldberg MR, Kitt MM (2010) Mass balance and pharmacokinetics of [^{14}C]telavancin following intravenous administration to healthy male volunteers. Antimicrob Agents Chemother 54:3365–3371
8. Barriere SL, Farrell DJ, Rhomberg PR, Jones RN (2014) Serum inhibitory and bactericidal activity of telavancin in non-infected subjects with severe renal impairment or end-stage renal disease. Diagn Microbiol Infect Dis 80:327–329
9. Shaw JP, Seroogy J, Kaniga K, Higgins DL, Kitt M, Barriere S (2005) Pharmacokinetics, serum inhibitory and bactericidal activity, and safety of telavancin in healthy subjects. Antimicrob Agents Chemother 49:195–201
10. Samara E, Shaw JP, Barriere SL, Wong SL, Worboys P (2012) Population pharmacokinetics of telavancin in healthy subjects and patients with infections. Antimicrob Agents Chemother 56:2067–2073
11. Goldberg MR, Wong SL, Shaw JP, Kitt MM, Barriere SL (2010) Single-dose pharmacokinetics and tolerability of telavancin in elderly men and women. Pharmacotherapy 30:806–811
12. Goldberg MR, Wong SL, Shaw JP, Kitt MM, Barriere SL (2010) Lack of effect of moderate hepatic impairment on the pharmacokinetics of telavancin. Pharmacotherapy 30:35–42
13. Wong SL, Sorgel F, Kinzig M, Goldberg MR, Kitt MM, Barriere SL (2009) Lack of pharmacokinetic drug interactions following concomitant administration of telavancin with aztreonam or piperacillin/tazobactam in healthy participants. J Clin Pharmacol 49:816–823
14. Duchin K, Shaw J, Seroogy J, Barriere S, Novack R (2005) Effect of hemodialysis on single dose pharmacokinetics (PK) of telavancin (TLV) [poster]. Proceedings of the 15th European congress of clinical microbiology and infectious diseases, Copenhagen, Denmark. [P897]
15. Lodise TP, Butterfield JM, Hegde SS, Samara E, Barriere SL (2012) Telavancin pharmacokinetics and pharmacodynamics in patients with complicated skin and skin structure infections and various degrees of renal function. Antimicrob Agents Chemother 56: 2062–2066
16. Patel JH, Churchwell MD, Seroogy JD, Barriere SL, Grio M, Mueller B (2009) Telavancin and hydroxy propyl-beta-cyclodextrin clearance during continuous renal replacement therapy: an in vitro study. Int J Artif Organs 32:745–751

17. Sun HK, Duchin K, Nightingale CH, Shaw JP, Seroogy J, Nicolau DP (2006) Tissue penetration of telavancin after intravenous administration in healthy subjects. Antimicrob Agents Chemother 50:788–790
18. Gotfried MH, Shaw JP, Benton BM et al (2008) Intrapulmonary distribution of intravenous telavancin in healthy subjects and effect of pulmonary surfactant on in vitro activities of telavancin and other antibiotics. Antimicrob Agents Chemother 52:92–97
19. Lodise TP Jr, Gotfried M, Barriere S, Drusano GL (2008) Telavancin penetration into human epithelial lining fluid determined by population pharmacokinetic modeling and Monte Carlo simulation. Antimicrob Agents Chemother 52:2300–2304
20. Barcia-Macay M, Lemaire S, Mingeot-Leclercq MP, Tulkens PM, Van Bambeke F (2006) Evaluation of the extracellular and intracellular activities (human THP-1 macrophages) of telavancin versus vancomycin against methi cil lin-susceptible, methicillin-resistant, van comy cin-intermediate and vancomycin-resistant Staphylococcus aureus. J Antimicrob Chemother 58:1177–1184
21. Barcia-Macay M, Mouaden F, Mingeot-Leclercq MP, Tulkens PM, Van Bambeke F (2008) Cellular pharmacokinetics of telavancin, a novel lipoglycopeptide antibiotic, and analysis of lysosomal changes in cultured eukaryotic cells (J774 mouse macrophages and rat embryonic fibroblasts). J Antimicrob Chemother 61:1288–1294
22. Marconescu P, Graviss EA, Musher DM (2012) Rates of killing of methicillin-resistant Staphylococcus aureus by ceftaroline, daptomycin, and telavancin compared to that of vancomycin. Scand J Infect Dis 44:620–622
23. Leonard SN, Supple ME, Gandhi RG, Patel MD (2013) Comparative activities of telavancin combined with nafcillin, imipenem, and gentamicin against *Staphylococcus aureus*. Antimicrob Agents Chemother 57: 2678–2683
24. Leonard SN, Szeto YG, Zolotarev M, Grigoryan IV (2011) Comparative in vitro activity of telavancin, vancomycin and linezolid against heterogeneously vancomycin-intermediate *Staphylococcus aureus* (hVISA). Int J Antimicrob Agents 37:558–561
25. Leuthner KD, Cheung CM, Rybak MJ (2006) Comparative activity of the new lipoglycopeptide telavancin in the presence and absence of serum against 50 glycopeptide non-susceptible staphylococci and three vancomycin-resistant *Staphylococcus aureus*. J Antimicrob Chemother 58:338–343
26. Odenholt I, Lowdin E, Cars O (2007) Pharmacodynamic effects of telavancin against methicillin-resistant and methicillin-susceptible *Staphylococcus aureus* strains in the presence of human albumin or serum and in an in vitro kinetic model. Antimicrob Agents Chemother 51:3311–3316
27. Goldstein EJ, Citron DM, Tyrrell KL, Warren YA (2010) Bactericidal activity of telavancin, vancomycin and metronidazole against *Clostridium difficile*. Anaerobe 16:220–222
28. MacGowan AP, Noel AR, Tomaselli S, Elliott HC, Bowker KE (2011) Pharmacodynamics of telavancin studied in an in vitro pharmacokinetic model of infection. Antimicrob Agents Chemother 55:867–873
29. Lubenko IY, Strukova EV, Smirnova MV et al (2008) Telavancin and vancomycin pharmacodynamics with *Staphylococcus aureus* in an in vitro dynamic model. J Antimicrob Chemother 62:1065–1069
30. Leonard SN, Vidaillac C, Rybak MJ (2009) Activity of telavancin against *Staphylococcus aureus* strains with various vancomycin susceptibilities in an in vitro pharmacokinetic/pharmacodynamic model with simulated endocardial vegetations. Antimicrob Agents Chemother 53:2928–2933
31. Hegde SS, Reyes N, Wiens T et al (2004) Pharmacodynamics of telavancin (TD-6424), a novel bactericidal agent, against gram-positive bacteria. Antimicrob Agents Chemother 48:3043–3050
32. Reyes N, Skinner R, Benton BM et al (2006) Efficacy of telavancin in a murine model of bacteraemia induced by methicillin-resistant *Staphylococcus aureus*. J Antimicrob Chemother 58:462–465
33. Hegde SS, Skinner R, Lewis SR, Krause KM, Blais J, Benton BM (2010) Activity of telavancin against heterogeneous vancomycin-intermediate *Staphylococcus aureus* (hVISA) in vitro and in an in vivo mouse model of bacteraemia. J Antimicrob Chemother 65:725–728
34. Hegde SS, Difuntorum S, Skinner R, Trumbull J, Krause KM (2009) Efficacy of telavancin against glycopeptide-intermediate *Staphylococcus aureus* in the neutropenic mouse bacteraemia model. J Antimicrob Chemother 63:763–766
35. Madrigal AG, Basuino L, Chambers HF (2005) Efficacy of telavancin in a rabbit model of aortic valve endocarditis due to methicillin-resistant *Staphylococcus aureus* or vancomycin-intermediate *Staphylococcus aureus*. Antimicrob Agents Chemother 49:3163–3165
36. Miro JM, Garcia-de-la-Maria C, Armero Y et al (2007) Efficacy of telavancin in the

treatment of experimental endocarditis due to glycopeptide-intermediate *Staphylococcus aureus*. Antimicrob Agents Chemother 51:2373–2377

37. Xiong YQ, Hady WA, Bayer AS, Chen L, Kreiswirth BN, Yang SJ (2012) Telavancin in therapy of experimental aortic valve endocarditis in rabbits due to daptomycin-nonsusceptible methicillin-resistant *Staphylococcus aureus*. Antimicrob Agents Chemother 56:5528–5533
38. Hegde SS, Reyes N, Skinner R, Difuntorum S (2008) Efficacy of telavancin in a murine model of pneumonia induced by methicillin-susceptible *Staphylococcus aureus*. J Antimicrob Chemother 61:169–172
39. Reyes N, Skinner R, Kaniga K et al (2005) Efficacy of telavancin (TD-6424), a rapidly bactericidal lipoglycopeptide with multiple mechanisms of action, in a murine model of pneumonia induced by methicillin-resistant *Staphylococcus aureus*. Antimicrob Agents Chemother 49:4344–4346
40. Crandon JL, Kuti JL, Nicolau DP (2010) Comparative efficacies of human simulated exposures of telavancin and vancomycin against methicillin-resistant *Staphylococcus aureus* with a range of vancomycin MICs in a murine pneumonia model. Antimicrob Agents Chemother 54:5115–5119
41. Stucki A, Gerber P, Acosta F, Cottagnoud M, Cottagnoud P (2006) Efficacy of telavancin against penicillin-resistant pneumococci and *Staphylococcus aureus* in a rabbit meningitis model and determination of kinetic parameters. Antimicrob Agents Chemother 50:770–773
42. Yin LY, Calhoun JH, Thomas TS, Wirtz ED (2009) Efficacy of telavancin in the treatment of methicillin-resistant *Staphylococcus aureus* osteomyelitis: studies with a rabbit model. The J Antimicrob Chemother 63:357–360
43. Darouiche RO, Mansouri MD, Schneidkraut MJ (2009) Comparative efficacies of telavancin and vancomycin in preventing device-associated colonization and infection by *Staphylococcus aureus* in rabbits. Antimicrob Agents Chemother 53:2626–2628
44. Stryjewski ME, O'Riordan WD, Lau WK et al (2005) Telavancin versus standard therapy for treatment of complicated skin and soft-tissue infections due to gram-positive bacteria. Clin Infect Dis 40:1601–1607
45. Stryjewski ME, Chu VH, O'Riordan WD et al (2006) Telavancin versus standard therapy for treatment of complicated skin and skin structure infections caused by gram-positive bacteria: FAST 2 study. Antimicrob Agents Chemother 50:862–867
46. Stryjewski ME, Graham DR, Wilson SE et al (2008) Telavancin versus vancomycin for the treatment of complicated skin and skin-structure infections caused by gram-positive organisms. Clin Infect Dis 46:1683–1693
47. Rubinstein E, Lalani T, Corey GR et al (2011) Telavancin versus vancomycin for hospital-acquired pneumonia due to gram-positive pathogens. Clin Infect Dis 52:31–40
48. Corey GR, Kollef MH, Shorr AF et al (2014) Telavancin for hospital-acquired pneumonia: clinical response and 28-day survival. Antimicrob Agents Chemother 58:2030–2037
49. Torres A, Rubinstein E, Corey GR, Stryjewski ME, Barriere SL (2014) Analysis of phase 3 telavancin nosocomial pneumonia data excluding patients with severe renal impairment and acute renal failure. J Antimicrob Chemother 69:1119–1126
50. Stryjewski ME, Lentnek A, O'Riordan W et al (2014) A randomized phase 2 trial of telavancin versus standard therapy in patients with uncomplicated Staphylococcus aureus bacteremia: the ASSURE study. BMC Infect Dis 14:289
51. Malabarba A, Goldstein BP (2005) Origin, structure, and activity in vitro and in vivo of dalbavancin. J Antimicrob Chemother 55(Suppl 2):ii15–ii20
52. Jones RN, Sader HS, Flamm RK (2013) Update of dalbavancin spectrum and potency in the USA: report from the SENTRY Antimicrobial Surveillance Program (2011). Diagn Microbiol Infect Dis 75:304–307
53. Fritsche TR, Rennie RP, Goldstein BP, Jones RN (2006) Comparison of dalbavancin MIC values determined by Etest (AB BIODISK) and reference dilution methods using gram-positive organisms. J Clin Microbiol 44:2988–2990
54. Dorr MB, Jabes D, Cavaleri M et al (2005) Human pharmacokinetics and rationale for once-weekly dosing of dalbavancin, a semi-synthetic glycopeptide. J Antimicrob Chemother 55(Suppl 2):ii25–ii30
55. Dowell JA, Goldstein BP, Buckwalter M, Stogniew M, Damle B (2008) Pharmacokinetic-pharmacodynamic modeling of dalbavancin, a novel glycopeptide antibiotic. J Clin Pharmacol 48:1063–1068
56. Cavaleri M, Riva S, Valagussa A et al (2005) Pharmacokinetics and excretion of dalbavancin in the rat. J Antimicrob Chemother 55(Suppl 2):ii31–ii35
57. Leighton A, Gottlieb AB, Dorr MB et al (2004) Tolerability, pharmacokinetics, and serum bactericidal activity of intravenous dalbavancin in healthy volunteers. Antimicrob Agents Chemother 48:940–945

58. White RJ, Brown GL, Cavelero M et al (2000) Glycopeptide: phase 1 single- and multiple-dose placebo controlled intravenous safety, pharmacokinetic and pharmacodynamic study in healthy subjects. 40th Interscience Conference on Antimicrobial Agents and Chemotherapy. Toronto, ON, 17-20 September (Abstract 682)
59. Marbury T, Dowell JA, Seltzer E, Buckwalter M (2009) Pharmacokinetics of dalbavancin in patients with renal or hepatic impairment. J Clin Pharmacol 49:465–476
60. Nicolau DP, Sun HK, Seltzer E, Buckwalter M, Dowell JA (2007) Pharmacokinetics of dalbavancin in plasma and skin blister fluid. J Antimicrob Chemother 60:681–684
61. Buckwalter M, Dowell JA (2005) Population pharmacokinetic analysis of dalbavancin, a novel lipoglycopeptide. J Clin Pharmacol 45:1279–1287
62. Dalvance (dalbancin) Prescribing Information. Durata Therapeutic U.S. Limited, May 2014. http://www.accessdata.fda.gov/drugsatfda_docs/label/2014/021883s000lbl.pdf
63. Vilay AM, Shah KH, Churchwell MD, Patel JH, DePestel DD, Mueller BA (2010) Modeled dalbavancin transmembrane clearance during intermittent and continuous renal replacement therapies. Blood Purif 30:37–43
64. Bowker KE, Noel AR, MacGowan AP (2006) Pharmacodynamics of dalbavancin studied in an in vitro pharmacokinetic system. J Antimicrob Chemother 58:802–805
65. Johnson DM, Fritsche TR, Sader HS, Jones RN (2006) Evaluation of dalbavancin in combination with nine antimicrobial agents to detect enhanced or antagonistic interactions. Int J Antimicrob Agents 27:557–560
66. Andes D, Craig WA (2007) In vivo pharmacodynamic activity of the glycopeptide dalbavancin. Antimicrob Agents Chemother 51:1633–1642
67. Lefort A, Pavie J, Garry L, Chau F, Fantin B (2004) Activities of dalbavancin in vitro and in a rabbit model of experimental endocarditis due to *Staphylococcus aureus* with or without reduced susceptibility to vancomycin and teicoplanin. Antimicrob Agents Chemother 48:1061–1064
68. Candiani G, Abbondi M, Borgonovi M, Romano G, Parenti F (1999) In-vitro and in-vivo antibacterial activity of BI 397, a new semi-synthetic glycopeptide antibiotic. J Antimicrob Chemother 44:179–192
69. Baldoni D, Furustrand Tafin U, Aeppli S et al (2013) Activity of dalbavancin, alone and in combination with rifampicin, against meticillin-resistant *Staphylococcus aureus* in a foreign-body infection model. Int J Antimicrob Agents 42:220–225
70. Solon EG, Dowell JA, Lee J, King SP, Damle BD (2007) Distribution of radioactivity in bone and related structures following administration of [14C]dalbavancin to New Zealand white rabbits. Antimicrob Agents Chemother 51:3008–3010
71. Scott LJ (2015) Dalbavancin: a review in acute bacterial skin and skin structure infections. Drugs 75:1281–1291
72. Anderson VR, Keating GM (2008) Dalbavancin. Drugs 68:639–648
73. Seltzer E, Dorr MB, Goldstein BP et al (2003) Once-weekly dalbavancin versus standard-of-care antimicrobial regimens for treatment of skin and soft-tissue infections. Clin Infect Dis 37:1298–1303
74. Jauregui LE, Babazadeh S, Seltzer E et al (2005) Randomized, double-blind comparison of once-weekly dalbavancin versus twice-daily linezolid therapy for the treatment of complicated skin and skin structure infections. Clin Infect Dis 41:1407–1415
75. Boucher HW, Wilcox MD, Talbot GH et al (2014) Once-weekly dalbavancin versus daily conventional therapy for skin therapy. N Engl J Med 370:2169–2178
76. Zhanel GG, Schweizer F, Karlowsky JA (2012) Oritavancin: mechanism of action. Clin Infect Dis 54(Suppl 3):S214–S219
77. Bhavnani SM, Owen JS, Loutit JS, Porter SB, Ambrose PG (2004) Pharmacokinetics, safety, and tolerability of ascending single intravenous doses of oritavancin administered to healthy human subjects. Diagn Microbiol Infect Dis 50:95–102
78. Arhin FF, Belley A, McKay G et al (2010) Assessment of oritavancin serum protein binding across species. Antimicrob Agents Chemother 54:3481–3483
79. Rubino CM, Van Wart SA, Bhavnani SM, Ambrose PG, McCollam JS, Forrest A (2009) Oritavancin population pharmacokinetics in healthy subjects and patients with complicated skin and skin structure infections or bacteremia. Antimicrob Agents Chemother 53:4422–4428
80. Rubino CM, Bhavnani SM, Moeck G, Bellibas SE, Ambrose PG (2015) Population pharmacokinetic analysis for a single 1,200-millgram dose of oritavancin using data from two pivotal phase 3 clinical trials. Antimicrob Agents Chemother 59:3365–3372
81. Fetterly GJ, Ong CM, Bhavnani SM et al (2005) Pharmacokinetics of oritavancin in plasma and skin blister fluid following administration of a 200-milligram dose for 3 days or a single 800-milligram dose. Antimicrob Agents Chemother 49:148–152

82. Rodvold KA, Gotfried MH, Loutit JS, Porter SB (2004) Plasma and intrapulmonary concentrations of oritavancin and vancomycin in normal healthy adults [abstract O256]. In: 14th European conference of clinical microbiology and infectious diseases. Prague, Czech Republic
83. Van Bambeke F, Saffran J, Mingeot-Leclercq MP, Tulkens PM (2005) Mixed-lipid storage disorder induced in macrophages and fibroblasts by oritavancin (LY333328), a new glycopeptide antibiotic with exceptional cellular accumulation. Antimicrob Agents Chemother 49:1695–1700
84. Baquir B, Lemaire S, Van Bambeke F, Tulkens PM, Lin L, Spellberg B (2012) Macrophage killing of bacterial and fungal pathogens is not inhibited by intense intracellular accumulation of the lipoglycopeptide antibiotic oritavancin. Clin Infect Dis 54(Suppl 3):S229–S232
85. Garcia LG, Lemaire S, Kahl BC et al (2012) Pharmacodynamic evaluation of the activity of antibiotics against hemin- and menadione-dependent small-colony variants of *Staphylococcus aureus* in models of extracellular (broth) and intracellular (THP-1 monocytes) infections. Antimicrob Agents Chemother 56:3700–3711
86. Garcia LG, Lemaire S, Kahl BC et al (2012) Influence of the protein kinase C activator phorbol myristate acetate on the intracellular activity of antibiotics against hemin- and menadione-auxotrophic small-colony variant mutants of *Staphylococcus aureus* and their wild-type parental strain in human THP-1 cells. Antimicrob Agents Chemother 56:6166–6174
87. Nguyen HA, Denis O, Vergison A et al (2009) Intracellular activity of antibiotics in a model of human THP-1 macrophages infected by a *Staphylococcus aureus* small-colony variant strain isolated from a cystic fibrosis patient: pharmacodynamic evaluation and comparison with isogenic normal-phenotype and revertant strains. Antimicrob Agents Chemother 53:1434–1442
88. Nguyen HA, Denis O, Vergison A, Tulkens PM, Struelens MJ, Van Bambeke F (2009) Intracellular activity of antibiotics in a model of human THP-1 macrophages infected by a Staphylococcus aureus small-colony variant strain isolated from a cystic fibrosis patient: study of antibiotic combinations. Antimicrob Agents Chemother 53:1443–1449
89. Kumar A, Mann HJ, Keshtgarpour M et al (2011) In vitro characterization of oritavancin clearance from human blood by low-flux, high-flux, and continuous renal replacement therapy dialyzers. Int J Artif Organs 34: 1067–1074
90. McKay GA, Beaulieu S, Arhin FF et al (2009) Time-kill kinetics of oritavancin and comparator agents against *Staphylococcus aureus*, *Enterococcus faecalis* and *Enterococcus faecium*. J Antimicrob Chemother 63:1191–1199
91. Lin G, Pankuch G, Appelbaum P, Kosowska-Shick K (2014) Antistaphylococcal activity of oritavancin and its synergistic effect in combination with other antimicrobial agents. Antimicrob Agents Chemother 58: 6251–6254
92. Mercier RC, Houlihan HH, Rybak MJ (1997) Pharmacodynamic evaluation of a new glycopeptide, LY333328, and in vitro activity against *Staphylococcus aureus* and *Enterococcus faecium*. Antimicrob Agents Chemother 41:1307–1312
93. Zelenitsky SA, Booker B, Laing N, Karlowsky JA, Hoban DJ, Zhanel GG (1999) Synergy of an investigational glycopeptide, LY333328, with once-daily gentamicin against vancomycin-resistant *Enterococcus faecium* in a multiple-dose, in vitro pharmacodynamic model. Antimicrob Agents Chemother 43:592–597
94. Aeschlimann JR, Allen GP, Hershberger E, Rybak MJ (2000) Activities of LY333328 and vancomycin administered alone or in combination with gentamicin against three strains of vancomycin-intermediate *Staphylococcus aureus* in an in vitro pharmacodynamic infection model. Antimicrob Agents Chemother 44:2991–2998
95. Coyle EA, Rybak MJ (2001) Activity of oritavancin (LY333328), an investigational glycopeptide, compared to that of vancomycin against multidrug-resistant *Streptococcus pneumoniae* in an in vitro pharmacodynamic model. Antimicrob Agents Chemother 45:706–709
96. Belley A, Arhin FF, Sarmiento I, Deng H, Rose W, Moeck G (2013) Pharmacodynamics of a simulated single 1,200-milligram dose of oritavancin in an in vitro pharmacokinetic/pharmacodynamic model of methicillin-resistant *Staphylococcus aureus* infection. Antimicrob Agents Chemother 57:205–211
97. Belley A, Neesham-Grenon E, McKay G et al (2009) Oritavancin kills stationary-phase and biofilm *Staphylococcus aureus* cells in vitro. Antimicrob Agents Chemother 53:918–925
98. Boylan CJ, Campanale K, Iversen PW, Phillips DL, Zeckel ML, Parr TR Jr (2003) Pharmacodynamics of oritavancin (LY333328) in a neutropenic-mouse thigh model of *Staphylococcus aureus* infection. Antimicrob Agents Chemother 47:1700–1706
99. Knudsen JD, Raber S, Leggett J, Fuursted K, Espersen F, Fridmodt-Moller N (1997) Comparison of effect of LY333328 with

teicoplanin and vancomycin against pneumococci in mouse peritonitis model [abstract F-10]. In: 37th Interscience conference on antimicrobial agents and chemotherapy. American Society for Microbiology, Washington, DC
100. Kaatz GW, Seo SM, Aeschlimann JR, Houlihan HH, Mercier RC, Rybak MJ (1998) Efficacy of LY333328 against experimental methicillin-resistant *Staphylococcus aureus* endocarditis. Antimicrob Agents Chemother 42:981–983
101. Xiong YQ, Yin L, Hady WA et al. (2008) Efficacy of oritavancin (ORI), a lipoglycopeptide antibiotic, in a rat Staphylococcal aureus endocarditis (IE) model: microbiological and bioluminescent assessments [abstract B-1011]. In: 48th Interscience conference on antimicrobial agents and chemotherapy/ Infectious Diseases Society of America 46th annual meeting. American Society for Microbiology, Washington, DC
102. Saleh-Mghir A, Lefort A, Petegnief Y et al (1999) Activity and diffusion of LY333328 in experimental endocarditis due to vancomycin-resistant *Enterococcus faecalis*. Antimicrob Agents Chemother 43:115–120
103. Lefort A, Saleh-Mghir A, Garry L, Carbon C, Fantin B (2000) Activity of LY333328 combined with gentamicin in vitro and in rabbit experimental endocarditis due to vancomycin-susceptible or -resistant *Enterococcus faecalis*. Antimicrob Agents Chemother 44:3017–3021
104. Rupp ME, Fey PD, Longo GM (2001) Effect of LY333328 against vancomycin-resistant *Enterococcus faecium* in a rat central venous catheter-associated infection model. J Antimicrob Chemother 47:705–707
105. Craig W, Andes D (2004) Activity of oritavancin (O) versus vancomycin (V)in the neutropenic murine thigh- and lung-infection models [abstractA-1863]. In: 44th Interscience conference on antimicrobial agents and chemotherapy. American Society for Microbiology, Washington, DC
106. Lehoux D, McKay GA, Fadhil I et al (2007) Efficacy of oritavancin in a mouse model of *Streptococcus pneumoniae* pneumonia [abstract P-1781]. In: 17th European conference of clinical microbiology and infectious diseases. Munich, Germany
107. Ostiguy V, Fadhil I, Malouin M et al (2009) Efficacy of oritavancin in the rat haematogenous pneumonia model [abstract P1028]. In: 19th European congress of clinical microbiology and infectious diseases. Helsinki, Finland
108. Gerber J, Smirnov A, Wellmer A et al (2001) Activity of LY333328 in experimental meningitis caused by a *Streptococcus pneumoniae* strain susceptible to penicillin. Antimicrob Agents Chemother 45:2169–2172
109. Ambrose PG, Drusano GL, Craig WA (2012) In vivo activity of oritavancin in animal infection models and rationale for a new dosing regimen in humans. Clin Infect Dis 54(Suppl 3):S220–S228
110. Bhavnani SM, Passarell JA, Owen JS, Loutit JS, Porter SB, Ambrose PG (2006) Pharmacokinetic-pharmacodynamic relationships describing the efficacy of oritavancin in patients with *Staphylococcus aureus* bacteremia. Antimicrob Agents Chemother 50:994–1000
111. Markham A (2014) Oritavancin: first global approval. Drugs 74:1823–1828
112. Dunbar LM, Milata J, McClure T, Wasilewski MM, Team SS (2011) Comparison of the efficacy and safety of oritavancin front-loaded dosing regimens to daily dosing: an analysis of the SIMPLIFI trial. Antimicrob Agents Chemother 55:3476–3484
113. Corey GR, Kabler H, Mehra P et al (2014) Single-dose oritavancin in the treatment of acute bacterial skin infections. N Engl J Med 370:2180–2190
114. Corey GRGS, Jiang H et al (2014) Single-dose oritavancin compared to 7-10 days of vancomycin in the treatment of gram-positive acute bacterial skin and skin structure infections; the SOLO II non-inferiority study. Clin Infect Dis 60:254–262
115. Tice A (2012) Oritavancin: a new opportunity for outpatient therapy of serious infections. Clin Infect Dis 54(Suppl 3):S239–43

Chapter 13

Pharmacodynamics of Daptomycin

Eric Wenzler, Siyun Liao, and Keith A. Rodvold

Abstract

The pharmacokinetics and pharmacodynamics of daptomycin have been extensively explored in a host of in vitro models, multiple different patient populations, and clinical studies. Daptomycin exhibits concentration-dependent bactericidal activity with the ratio of unbound area-under-the-curve to minimum inhibitory concentration (*f*AUC/MIC) best predicting antibacterial efficacy in vitro. The large body of evidence suggests that higher doses (e.g., 8–10 mg/kg) of daptomycin are more effective and equally safe and should be used for specific pathogens (i.e., methicillin-resistant *Staphylococcus aureus*, *Enterococcus*) and in certain patient scenarios (i.e., critically ill, bacteremia, endocarditis). The emergence of resistance to daptomycin during therapy and clinical failure in serious infections brings its efficacy as monotherapy into question while the ease of administration, dosing schedule, and lack of nephrotoxicity continues to drive its use until more reliable therapeutic alternatives for gram-positive infections are established.

Key words Lipopeptide, Daptomycin, Methicillin-resistant *Staphylococcus aureus* (MRSA)

1 Overview

Daptomycin is a novel cyclic lipopeptide antibiotic with a unique mechanism of action. Daptomycin has been shown to cause calcium-dependent disruption of the electrochemical gradient of the gram-positive cell membrane leading to an efflux of potassium from the cell. This efflux in turn inhibits the transport of cell wall amino acids, formation of sugar-peptide precursors and shutting down biosynthesis of the cell wall peptidoglycan but does not directly cause cell lysis [1, 2]. In vitro, daptomycin demonstrates a rapid concentration-dependent bactericidal activity against most clinically relevant gram-positive pathogenic bacteria, including *Staphylococcus aureus* and enterococci, including isolates resistant to methicillin, vancomycin, and linezolid [3, 4].

Daptomycin is the first approved member of an old class of antibiotics, the cyclic lipopeptides. It was originally discovered by the Eli Lilly Company in the 1980s and designated LY146032, dapcin, or cidecin in early years [5]. Daptomycin showed promise in 19 phase I and 2 phase II trials involving more than 370 subjects

John C. Rotschafer et al. (eds.), *Antibiotic Pharmacodynamics*, Methods in Pharmacology and Toxicology,
DOI 10.1007/978-1-4939-3323-5_13, © Springer Science+Business Media New York 2016

in the 1980s and early 1990s, although unexpected treatment failures occurred in patients with bacteremia and endocarditis [5–8]. These failures were attributed to inadequate dosing of the drug (i.e., 2 mg/kg every 24 h and 3 mg/kg every 12 h), but unacceptably high incidences of myalgias and muscle weakness were seen when the daptomycin was dosed every 12 h. Unsatisfied with these results, Eli Lilly abandoned the drug which was subsequently acquired by Cubist Pharmaceuticals in 1997. New findings with once-daily dosing in animal studies and the increasing emergence of bacterial resistance among gram-positive species, specifically methicillin-resistant *S. aureus* (MRSA), contributed to the reassessment of the benefit/risk ratio of daptomycin. Following successful phase III studies for the treatment of complicated skin and skin structure infections (cSSSI) at 4 mg/kg intravenously (IV) once daily, daptomycin was approved by the US Food and Drug Administration (FDA) in November 2003 under the trade name Cubicin®. Subsequently, the completion a randomized, controlled, multicenter, open-label study supported the May 2006 FDA approval of daptomycin for the treatment of patients with *S. aureus* bloodstream infections (bacteremia), including those with right-sided infective endocarditis, at an IV dose of 6 mg/kg once daily. Intravenous dosage regimens up to 12 mg/kg once daily have been used off-label successively for the treatment of life-threatening and/or highly resistant gram-positive infections, including bacteremia and endocarditis, without evidence of significant toxicity.

2 Pharmacokinetics

Daptomycin displays linear pharmacokinetics (PK) after single and multiple IV doses up to 12 mg/kg [9–12]. Plasma concentration–time profile of daptomycin is best described by a two-compartment open model with first-order elimination. In healthy volunteers, the predicted maximum concentrations (C_{max}) after a single 2-min injection and 30-min infusion of 6 mg/kg of daptomycin were 86.6 and 76.4 mg/L, respectively [12]. The area under the curve (AUC) and C_{max} increased proportionally to dose on day 1 and day 7 in the multiple dose regimen, while clearance (CL), volume of distribution (Vd), and elimination half-life remained unchanged. At doses of 8 mg/kg, the mean C_{max} was approximately 2.2 times higher compared to the 4 mg/kg, indicating 20 % nonlinearity at dose levels above 6 mg/kg. At 4, 6, and 8 mg/kg, the median trough daptomycin concentrations (C_{min}) were 6.37, 9.13, and 15.3 mg/L, respectively.

Daptomycin has a mean apparent Vd of approximately 0.1 L/kg and is highly protein bound ranging between 92 and 96.4 %.

Protein binding is linear over a range of daptomycin concentrations between 1.2 and 31 mg/L. Interestingly, daptomycin has shown limited binding to albumin or alpha-1-acid glycoprotein individually, but is extensive binding once combined. Initial pharmacokinetic studies suggested that the distribution phase of daptomycin was not complete until 4–6 h after administration [9].

Renal excretion is the major pathway of elimination for daptomycin. Urinary excretion ranges from 34 to 68 % over 24 h. Renal elimination does not appear to be dose-dependent and remains linear in patient with renal impairment. The mean elimination half-life ranges between 8 and 9 h. Steady-state is reached by day 3 independent of dose. The accumulation factor observed at steady-state in this trial was 1.2, indicating that the same total daily dose given every 12 h is associated with a 42 % higher daily exposure and could explain the decreased incidence of adverse effects when daptomycin is given once daily [9].

The PK and tolerability of daptomycin have been explored up to 12 mg/kg in healthy volunteers (Table 1) [11]. The $AUC_{0-\infty}$ increased proportionally to the dose at all dosing levels, with a mean $AUC_{0-\infty}$ of approximately 1200 µg·h/mL on day four for the 12 mg/kg dose. Pharmacokinetic parameters at dose levels of 10 mg/kg and 12 mg/kg were similar after days 4 and 14 of daily dosing. No serious adverse events and no myalgia were reported by any subject. The most common adverse event was headache and creatinine phosphokinase (CPK) values were within normal limits for all subjects in all groups. Considered together, this study indicates that daptomycin offers consistent and linear pharmacokinetics with minimal accumulation after multiple doses and is well tolerated at doses up to 12 mg/kg once daily for 14 days.

A population PK model was established for daptomycin using data from phase 1, 2, and 3 clinical studies involving 282 adult subjects and 3325 plasma concentrations [4]. Table 2 summarizes the pharmacokinetic parameters stratified by estimated creatinine clearance (CrCl) for a single dose of daptomycin 4 mg/kg. The estimated median parameter values (and interindividual variabilities) for the entire study population included CL of 0.688 L/h (52.1 %), volume of the central compartment of 4.8 L (60.6 %), volume of the peripheral compartment of 3.6 L (31.9 %), and intercompartmental CL was 3.6 L/h (74.4 %).

The apparent steady-state volume of distribution (V_{ss}) for a healthy subject with a median body weight of 75 kg was estimated to be 7.9 L, which increased to 10.8 L in patients with an acute bacterial infection. The median terminal half-life was estimated to be 7.07 h in a normothermic male with normal renal function. The median value for the elimination half-life increased to 10.36 h for a male subject with a CrCl of 40 mL/min and to 20.68 h for a male subject receiving dialysis. This population analysis indicates

Table 1
Pharmacokinetics of daptomycin on day 1 and day 4 (steady-state)

Dose	C_{max} (mg/L)		AUC[a] (mg·h/L)		CL (mL/h/kg)		V (L/kg)		$t_{1/2}$ (hours)	
(mg/kg)	Day 1	Day 4	Day 1	Day 4	Day 1	Day 4	Day 1	Day 4	Day 1	Day 4
6	95.7 (31.8 %)	93.9 (6.4 %)	729.8 (32.2 %)	631.8 (12.3 %)	9.9 (12.5 %)	9.1 (16.9 %)	0.106 (13.3 %)	0.101 (7.1 %)	7.5 (10.9 %)	7.9 (12.8 %)
8	106.2 (20.0 %)	123.3 (13.0 %)	773.2 (20.3 %)	858.2 (24.9 %)	10.1 (24.0 %)	9.0 (33.0 %)	0.103 (11.8 %)	0.101 (12.8 %)	7.3 (18.4 %)	8.3 (26.1 %)
10	129.7 (11.3 %)	141.1 (17.0 %)	1013.5 (16.2 %)	1038.8 (17.2 %)	9.9 (20.7 %)	8.8 (25.3 %)	0.117 (11.5 %)	0.098 (17.2 %)	8.4 (12.0 %)	7.9 (8.0 %)
12	164.8 (7.4 %)	183.7 (13.6 %)	1269.2 (22.2 %)	1277.4 (19.8 %)	10.0 (23.7 %)	9.0 (30.5 %)	0.111 (13.7 %)	0.098 (18.3 %)	7.8 (12.1 %)	7.7 (13.0 %)

Data are presented as means (coefficient of variation)
Data adapted from Ref. [11]
[a]AUC values are $AUC_{0-\infty}$ for day 1 values and AUC_{0-tau} for day 4 values

Table 2
Summary of pharmacokinetic parameters of daptomycin stratified by estimated CrCl

Parameter	≥80 mL/min (n=165)	<80 to >40 mL/min (n=80)	≤40 mL/min (n=16)	Dialysis (n=21)
CL (L/h)	0.86 (0.41–2.19)	0.64 (0.23–1.64)	0.37 (0.21–0.70)	0.24 (0.17–0.58)
V_{ss} (L)	9.73 (5.10–32.77)	8.75 (3.77–19.24)	10.36 (6.19–34.89)	10.44 (6.84–17.63)
$AUC_{0-\infty}$ (μg·h/mL)	400.8 (160.6–1143.7)	436.5 (151.68–1181)	716.2 (297.72–1677)	1205 (367–1906)
$t_{1/2}$ (h)	8.28 (4.64–48.01)	9.07 (5.17–71.16)	18.96 (8.84–58.83)	29.32 (14.69–41.80)

Data presented as median (range)
Adapted from Ref. [4]

that renal function is the single most important factor contributing to differences in daptomycin clearance. The relationship between rate and extent of extravascular distribution and body weight support the dosing of daptomycin on a mg/kg basis [4].

This initial population PK model has subsequently been updated by increasing the number of subjects ($n=442$) and plasma daptomycin concentrations ($n=4875$) [13]. Simulations were performed to provide dosing recommendations of patients with *S. aureus* bacteremia and severe renal impairment (CrCl <30 mL/min) (see Sect. 2.6). Several other population PK models have been developed and used to determine parameter estimates and/or dosing recommendations for critically ill patients with serious gram-positive infections, and to evaluate the relationship between systemic exposure and elevations in CPK [14–17].

2.1 Infants and Children

The PK of daptomycin have been reported for infants <120 days of age, infants 3 months to 2 years of age, and pediatric patients between 2 and 17 years of age [18–23]. In a group of 20 infants stratified into four categories (gestational age <32 or ≥32 weeks [range: 23–40 weeks]; postnatal age <14 and ≥14 days [range: 1–85 days]) were administered a single dose of daptomycin 6 mg/kg and an average of 4 plasma daptomycin concentrations were obtained from each infant (total of 85 evaluable plasma daptomycin concentrations were collected). The median pharmacokinetic parameter estimates included AUC_{0-24}, Vd, CL and half-life of 262.4 mg·h/L, 0.21 L/kg, 0.021 L/h/kg, and 6.2 h, respectively. The median C_{max} was 25.5 mg/L. No adverse events related to daptomycin were recorded, and no relationship between age and daptomycin clearance or Vd was observed. Interestingly, the median AUC_{0-24} was approximately half of the AUC_{0-24} observed for adults receiving 4 mg/kg for cSSSI (417 mg·h/L), likely owing to the increased clearance observed in this population. Infants <120 days of age may require a higher dosage of daptomycin to achieve exposures estimated to be efficacious in adults [18–20].

Nineteen pediatric patients between 3 and 24 months of age were administered a single-dose of daptomycin of either 4 mg/kg (<13 months of age; $n=14$) or 6 mg/kg (13–24 months of age; $n=5$) [21]. Mean pharmacokinetic parameter estimates observed in pediatric patients 3–6 months ($n=7$) vs. 7–12 months ($n=7$) were similar in value: C_{max} 38.7 vs. 37.1 mg/L; $AUC_{0-\infty}$ 215.0 vs. 219.3 mg·h/L; V_{ss} 127.7 vs. 134.9 mL/kg; CL 19.72 vs. 19.63 mL/h/kg; and half-life 5.10 vs. 5.45 h. Pediatric patients 13–24 months of age received a higher dose of daptomycin resulting in a higher systemic exposure (mean C_{max} was 67.0 mg/L and $AUC_{0-\infty}$ was 281.5 mg·h/L) with similar pharmacokinetic parameters to the lower age groups studied (V_{ss} was 121.7 mL/kg; CL 21.76 mL/h/kg; half-life 4.41 h).

Twenty-two children (2–17 years of age) with suspected or proven gram-positive infections were administered a single-dose of intravenous daptomycin 4 mg/kg and had serial blood sampling for 24 h to determine plasma daptomycin concentrations. The mean AUC_{0-24} values between children 2–6 years vs. 7–11 years vs. 12–17 years were statistically different (215.3 vs. 271.0 vs. 374.4 mg·h/L) and decreased proportionally with decreasing age. The AUC_{0-24} in adolescents (e.g., age 12–17 years) were approximately 1.7 fold higher than in children <6 years of age. In addition, AUC_{0-24} values in adolescents were similar to adult estimates while AUC_{0-24} values were lower in children <12 years of age secondary to an increased clearance of daptomycin in this latter group. The mean CL values between children 2–6 years vs. 7–11 years vs. 12–17 years were statistically different (20.1 vs. 17.0 vs. 11.1 mL/h/kg) and daptomycin CL (and elimination rate constant) were inversely associated with age. The mean C_{max} and V_{ss} values were similar across cohorts and ranged from 43.8 to 50.0 mg/L and 0.11 to 0.13 L/kg, respectively. Of note, age only accounted for 30 % of the interindividual variation observed between children in this study [22]. The pharmacokinetic results from these pediatric studies, along with ongoing clinical trials investigating the safety and efficacy of daptomycin for the treatment of specific gram-positive infections in children, will be useful in further defining dosing recommendations for various pediatric population.

2.2 Geriatric

A single-dose pharmacokinetic study of daptomycin was conducted in young (18–30 years of age; $n=12$) and geriatric (≥75 years; $n=12$) healthy subjects [24]. Following a 4 mg/kg dose of daptomycin, the total $AUC_{0-\infty}$ was 58 % higher in the geriatric group (473.7 vs. 300.6 mg·h/L; $p=0.0001$) while no difference in C_{max} was observed (43.98 vs. 42.32 mg/L). Total CL was also 35 % lower in geriatric subjects (9.86 vs. 15.09 mL/h/kg) with no difference in V_{ss}, while the elimination half-life was approximately 5 h longer (11.85 vs. 6.79 h). Of note, the mean CrCl in the geriatric group was 57.6 mL/min compared to 94.8 mL/min although the mean fraction of daptomycin excreted in the urine was not statistically different (34.3 vs. 42.6 %).

2.3 Obesity

Pai et al. compared the single-dose pharmacokinetics of 4 mg/kg of daptomycin in seven morbidly obese female patients (mean ± SD, body mass index [BMI]: 46.2 ± 5.5 kg/m^2) vs. seven normal-weight, healthy female subjects (mean ± SD, BMI: 21.8 ± 1.9 kg/m^2) [25]. Importantly, glomerular filtration rate (GFR) was determined using radiolabeled sodium iothalamate and estimated fat-free weight using bioelectric impedance. The cohorts were matched for age, sex, race, serum creatinine, and serum albumin. Pharmacokinetic parameters did not differ between the groups, despite total body weight dosing resulting in almost twice the dose in the morbidly obese group. C_{max} and $AUC_{0–24}$ were 60 % higher ($p < 0.001$) in the obese group as a function of the total dose administered, as weight-normalized C_{max} and $AUC_{0–24}$ were not different. The apparent Vd (10.04 vs. 7.69 L) and CL (0.82 vs. 0.73 L/h) were higher in the morbidly obese group, although not statistically significantly. The relationship of Vd and CL to weight was best predicted by total body weight ($r^2 = 0.66$ and 0.30) compared to ideal and fat-free weight, although the correlation was somewhat poor. No significant relationship was noted between daptomycin CL and measure or estimated GFR or CrCl. Estimation of CrCl using the Cockcroft–Gault equation with total body weight (TBW) grossly overestimated true CL among morbidly obese patients and may affect the dosing interval of daptomycin. At the time of this publication, the authors suggested that dosing of daptomycin based on TBW be considered in morbidly obese subjects given the association between Vd and TBW, the fact that C_{max} is dependent on Vd, and that daptomycin is a concentration-dependent antimicrobial agents. Dosing on IBW or fat-free weight may decrease C_{max}, especially in acutely ill patients, while calculating CrCl using the Cockcroft–Gault equation with ideal body weight (IBW) provides a more accurate reflection of GFR in obese subjects. Dvorchik and Damphouse had also shown similar results in a separate study [26].

Since these original publications on the pharmacokinetics of daptomycin in obese subjects, questions on the rationale for TBW-based dosing of daptomycin continue to be raised and several authors have recently suggested a 500 mg or 750 mg fixed-dose approach [15, 17, 27–29]. In addition, clinical outcomes (e.g., clinical and microbiological outcomes, length of stay, mortality, adverse effects) were similar when daptomycin dosing was based on IBW ($n = 48$ patients) vs. actual body weight ($n = 69$ patients) [30]. In obese and critically ill patients, dosing using simplified PK equations and measurement of two plasma daptomycin concentrations to calculate AUC for daptomycin has been recently suggested [31].

2.4 Critically Ill

Two population PK studies in critically ill patients have demonstrated altered disposition of daptomycin. In 58 patients with severe gram-positive infections receiving doses of 4–12 mg/kg, the median values for CL and Vd were 0.80 L/h and 12.29 L (0.19 L/kg), respectively [14]. Observed C_{max} values for 6, 7, and 8 mg/kg doses were lower than expected based on previous pharmacokinetic models (35.9, 47.1, and 76.9 mg/L), likely due to the 23 % increase in Vd observed in this patient population. These results indicate that these patients may require a higher daily dose depending on the severity of infection and clinical condition of the patient.

Population pharmacokinetics and clinical outcomes were determined in a cohort of 50 critically ill patients with MRSA bacteremia [15]. Thirty-two patients received 6 mg/kg of daptomycin and 18 patients received 8 mg/kg for a median duration of 16 days. The median CL and apparent V of the central compartment (V_c) were 0.845 L/h and 11.1 L, respectively. A subpopulation of 13 patients demonstrated augmented CL of daptomycin, evidenced by CL values of ≥1.36 L/h. These patients also demonstrated significantly lower C_{max} and AUC values despite receipt of comparable doses of daptomycin to other patients studied. Cumulative fraction of response (CFR) was >90 % for nearly all targets (e.g., AUC_{0-24}/MIC ratio of ≥579, ≥666, ≥753) with the 8 and 10 mg/kg/day (and 750 or 1000 mg) dose but not the 6 mg/kg/day (or 500 mg) dose for patients with sepsis. All weight-based and fixed-dose regimens provided CFR >90 % for patients without sepsis. The dosage regimens of 8 mg/kg/day and 750 mg were also associated with a low probability (0.78 and 1.26 %, respectively) of C_{min} values ≥24.3 mg/L (an exposure threshold linked to skeletal muscle toxicity [17]). In summary, daptomycin exposures were lower in critically ill patients with sepsis primarily related to MRSA bacteremia when treated with standard doses and these patients likely requires dosage increases to ≥8 mg/kg/day (or ≥750 mg/day). Therapeutic drug monitoring and individualizing daptomycin dosing by calculating a target AUC/MIC ratio has also been suggested [14, 28, 29, 31].

Pharmacokinetics of daptomycin were evaluated in 29 adult cancer patients with neutropenic fever [32]. Compared to reported PK parameters of healthy subjects, the V_{ss} (mean ± SD: 0.18 ± 0.05 L/kg) of daptomycin was markedly increased in patients with febrile neutropenia. Clearance (15.51 ± 5.65 mL/h/kg) was also increased contributing to a lower observed C_{max} (48.92 ± 12.63 mg/L) and $AUC_{0-\infty}$ (427.3 ± 135.7 mg·h/L). An initial intravenous daptomycin dosage of 6 mg/kg every 24 h was recommended for neutropenic cancer patients.

A PK study was conducted in nine patients with thermal burn injury who received a single dose of 6 mg/kg of daptomycin [33]. Patients enrolled had completed initial fluid resuscitation, were ≥7 days after burn injury, and had total body surface area burns ranging from 18 to 50 %. Compared to literature reported PK parameters of daptomycin in healthy subjects, burn patients had significantly lower mean C_{max} (53.5 mg/L; 44 % reduction) and $AUC_{0-\infty}$ (388 mg·h/L; 47 % reduction) values and significantly higher mean Vd (0.18 L/kg; 64 % increase) and CL (17.5 mL/h/kg; 77 % increase). Protein binding was also significantly lower at 86.5 %. The authors recommended that a daptomycin dose of 10–12 mg/kg/day be considered in burn patients in order to provide similar drug exposures as observed in healthy subjects receiving 6 mg/kg/day.

2.5 Meningitis

Although daptomycin has been traditionally regarded as having poor central nervous system penetration, case reports have demonstrated clinical success with daptomycin in meningitis despite low or undetectable cerebrospinal fluid (CSF) concentrations [34–41]. In patients with external CSF shunts, mean serum concentrations at 0.5, 6, 12, and 24 h post-infusion were 93.7, 43.3, 27.0, and 13.8 mg/L, respectively. In comparison, the respective mean CSF concentrations were 0.126, 0.461, 0.442, and 0.221 mg/L. Mean AUC_{0-24} values in serum and CSF were 906 and 8.3 mg·h/L, which corresponds to a mean CSF-to-serum penetration ratio of 8 % (11.5 % after correcting for protein binding) [42]. A similar CSF-to-serum penetration ratio (range: 9–11 %) for daptomycin has been reported for rabbits [43].

2.6 Dialysis and Renal Replacement Therapy

The original population PK model for daptomycin has been recently updated to further consider dosing recommendations for patients with *S. aureus* bacteremia and severe renal impairment (CrCl <30 mL/min) [13]. The final PK model, along with reference efficacy exposure range and safety threshold, was used in simulations to support a dosage recommendation of 6 mg/kg every 48 h for patients with *S. aureus* bacteremia and CrCl <30 mL/min, or receiving hemodialysis (HD) or continuous ambulatory peritoneal dialysis (CAPD). These recommendations refer only to outpatient dialysis and should not be extended to patients undergoing continuous renal replacement therapy (CRRT) or extended dialysis while in the intensive care unit. Dosing with 4 mg/kg every 48 h was considered inferior in patients with severe renal impairment or on HD or CAPD, and is no longer recommended for the treatment of *S. aureus* bacteremia or infective endocarditis.

2.6.1 Continuous Ambulatory Peritoneal Dialysis (CAPD)

The pharmacokinetics of daptomycin after IV administration of 6 mg/kg was examined in eight patients undergoing CAPD in order to determine the penetration of daptomycin into the peritoneal cavity and identify optimal CAPD dosing schemes using population PK modeling and Monte Carlo simulations [44]. The dialysate concentration at the end of an exchange was between 2 and 6 mg/L for most patients. Compared to patients administered daptomycin for *S. aureus* endocarditis, CL was markedly reduced (0.96 L/h) while Vd remained similar (6.56 L). In the Monte Carlo simulations for both the 4 and 6 mg/kg, AUC_{0-72} was similar to values from patients in the endocarditis study. The mean AUC in the peritoneal cavity to AUC in plasma ratio was 0.058 and CAPD patients did not have a higher probability of a C_{min} ≥24.3 mg/L. These results indicate that daptomycin at 4 or 6 mg/kg every 48 h is an appropriate dosage to treat non-peritoneal infections in patients on CAPD. Given that less than 6 % of the total AUC observed in plasma was recovered in the peritoneal cavity, intravenous daptomycin is likely inappropriate for treating peritoneal infections [44–47].

Benziger and colleagues reported the plasma pharmacokinetics of single and multiple doses of daptomycin 6 mg/kg administered every 48 h before CAPD in eight noninfected adult subjects [48]. The mean apparent V_{ss} (0.12 and 0.12 L/kg), CL (249 and 233 mL/h), fraction unbound (0.13 and 0.12), and half-life (25.8 and 26.7 h) of daptomycin were similar after the first and third doses (days 1 and 5), respectively. The respective mean (±SD) C_{max} and $AUC_{0–48}$ after the first dose (75.2 ± 15.6 mg/L and 1354 ± 333 mg·h/L) increased to 93.9 ± 21.9 mg/L and 2016 ± 581 mg h/L following the third dose. Mean trough concentrations before and 48 h after the third dose of daptomycin were 19.5 and 20.7 mg/L, respectively. Accumulation ratio was estimated to be 1.49 by day 5 of therapy. These observations lend support to the dosage regimen of 6 mg/kg every 48 h for patients undergoing CAPD.

2.6.2 Hemodialysis (HD)

Three studies have reported pharmacokinetic data with daptomycin during HD [48–50]. Benziger and colleagues also reported single- and multiple-dose plasma pharmacokinetics of daptomycin in five noninfected adult subjects undergoing high-flux HD [48]. Daptomycin was dosed 6 mg/kg after each HD during a 48–48–72-h weekly dialysis schedule. The mean parameter values on days 1 and 5 (first and third dose) included an apparent V_{ss} (0.13 and 0.17 L/kg), CL (253 and 270 mL/h), fraction unbound (0.11 and 0.11), and half-life (28.0 and 35.9 h). The respective mean (±SD) C_{max} and $AUC_{0–48}$ after the first dose (69.0 ± 11.0 mg/L and 1318 ± 235 mg·h/L) increased to 81.6 ± 13.4 mg/L and 1813 ± 316 mg·h/L following the third dose. Mean trough concentrations before and 72 h after the third dose of daptomycin were 13.1 and 15.3 mg/L, respectively. Accumulation ratio was estimated to be 1.39 by day 5 of therapy. During high-flux HD on day 5, pre-dialysis plasma concentrations decreased from 21.4 to 13.1 mg/L post-dialysis (approximately 39 % of daptomycin was removed).

Salama and coinvestigators reported single-dose pharmacokinetics of daptomycin in six healthy end-stage renal disease patients on chronic HD [49]. Six subjects received 6 mg/kg of daptomycin after their usual HD session ended and blood samples were obtained before, during and after their next regular hemodialysis session. The second hemodialysis session was fixed at 4 h in length. The mean C_{max} was 61.1 mg/L, $AUC_{0–\infty}$ was 2168 mg·h/L, CL was 3.4 mL/min, Vd was 0.08 L/kg, and a half-life of 19.4 h during the interval between dialysis sessions. The elimination rate constant and half-life while undergoing dialysis were 0.20 h^{-1} and 3.77 h, respectively. Daptomycin concentrations 1 h post-dialysis differed by only 0.9 mg/L when compared to concentrations at the end of dialysis, indicating minimal rebound. Serum concentrations of daptomycin were reduced approximately 51.7 % during a 4 h hemodialysis session. Based on PK modeling and simulations, adequate daptomycin concentrations were likely to be maintained through the 44 and 68 h interdialytic period when 6 mg/kg is given post-HD. Also, higher doses of daptomycin may not be necessary to account for the 68 h interdialytic period despite the recommended every 48 h dosing interval for hemodialysis patients [49, 50].

Twelve adult patients received daptomycin 6 mg/kg and had 26 blood samples collected over 72 h, including before, during, and after HD [51]. Mean (±SD) PK parameters from population PK analysis included Vc of 4.77 ± 1.08 L and nondialytic CL of 0.25 ± 0.06 L/h. The mean (±SD) CL during HD was 0.87 L/h, which was similar to the mean CL value observed in non-HD patients with *S. aureus* bacteremia and endocarditis.

Dosing regimens were evaluated using a series of Monte Carlo simulations that have a low probability of a C_{min} ≥24.3 mg/L and AUC distribution values that closely approximates doses of 4 and 6 mg/kg every 24 h in non-HD patients with *S. aureus* bacteremia and endocarditis.

The results from all of these HD studies were pooled together and used in a pharmacokinetic and pharmacodynamics analysis of 26 patients on thrice-weekly hemodialysis [52]. Monte Carlo simulations were performed to identify dosing schemes that would have a low probability of a C_{min} ≥24.3 mg/L and provide AUC distribution values similar to those associated with dosing regimens of 4 and 6 mg/kg every 24 h in non-HD patients (based PK parameters from the *S. aureus* bacteremia–endocarditis study). Daily AUC values were similar to patients with endocarditis when daptomycin was administered post-HD, but not before or during, with a 48-h interdialytic period. With a 72 h interdialytic period, even post-HD administration of 4 or 6 mg/kg resulted in AUC_{48-72} values roughly half of those with *S. aureus* bacteremia–endocarditis. Evaluation of 12 mg/kg post-HD dosing resulted in AUC values comparable to those achieved in patients with *S. aureus* however with a high probability of C_{min} exceeding the 24.3 mg/L toxicity threshold (19.1 %). Therefore, intra- or post-HD doses of 4 or 6 mg/kg of daptomycin was recommended for patients on thrice-weekly HD prior to a 48-h interdialytic period. Intra- or post-HD doses should be increased to 6 or 9 mg/kg for patients on thrice-weekly HD prior to a 72-h interdialytic period. Increased CPK monitoring may also be warranted in these patients due to the potential increase in probability of exceeding toxic C_{min}.

2.6.3 Continuous Renal Replacement Therapy (CRRT)

Continuous renal replacement therapy (CRRT) is a dialysis modality used to treat critically ill patients in the intensive care unit who develop acute kidney injury. Some of the most commonly applied modalities are continuous venovenous hemofiltration (CVVH), continuous venovenous hemodialysis (CVVHD), and continuous venovenous hemodiafiltration (CVVHDF). In addition, sustained low-efficiency dialysis (SLED) or slow low efficiency daily dialysis (SLEDD) has also been used because of higher solute clearance and decreased supply costs compared to conventional CRRT. Limited data are available describing the impact of SLED on daptomycin disposition.

Based on in vitro models, CL of daptomycin during CRRT was comparable or exceeded renal CL of daptomycin from healthy volunteers (9.3–10.5 mL/min) [53, 54]. Filter type, dialysate flow, and ultrafiltration will impact amount of drug removal and variation in CL. The mean sieving coefficient in whole blood over time was 0.40 and did not change based on daptomycin concentration while mean CL from the blood circuit was 19.8 mL/min. Approximately 20 % of the initial daptomycin dose was lost to adsorption. These experimental findings suggest that increased or more frequent doses of daptomycin may be needed in critically ill patients receiving CRRT.

Two reports have described the effect of SLED on daptomycin CL [55, 56]. A case report demonstrated that a 12-h SLED session resulted in a higher CL (0.92 vs. 0.24 L/h) and shorter elimination half-life (9.49 vs. 29.32 h) of daptomycin compared to intermittent HD. Similar results were reported for 10 critically ill patients receiving g a single dose of daptomycin 6 mg/kg 8 h before SLED. The mean (±SD) CL during SLED was 1.03 ± 0.29 L/h and the elimination half-lives during and off SLED were 8.0 ± 1.8 and 27.7 ± 4.3 h, respectively. The average total amount of daptomycin removed during SLED 116 mg or 23 % of the administered dose. However, a 31 % increase (rebound) in plasma daptomycin concentrations occurred with 30 min after the end of SLED. A dosage regimen of daptomycin 6 mg/kg once daily (vs. every 48 h for HD or CAPD) has been recommended for patients undergoing SLED.

Several studies have evaluated the pharmacokinetics of daptomycin in critically ill patients undergoing CRRT, most commonly with either CVVHD or CVVHDF [57–64]. Findings from these studies suggest that daptomycin may need to be given every 24 h or at higher doses administered every 48 h in order to achieve effective concentrations in critically ill patients on CRRT. It is important to note that none of the studies to date have examined clinical outcomes in these patients and the AUC/MIC or C_{max}/MIC ratio most associated with efficacy in vivo has not been well established. Even so, given the increased Vd, fraction unbound and transmembrane clearance of daptomycin during CRRT, daptomycin doses ≥6 mg/kg once-daily or ≥8 mg/kg administered every 48 h are likely to be efficacious and avoid toxicity in this patient population.

2.7 Disposition and Penetration

The mean concentration of daptomycin into the inflammatory exudate from induced blisters was 9.4 and 14.5 mg/L at 1 and 2 h respectively [65]. The C_{max} was 27.6 mg/L and occurred at 3.7 h after a 4 mg/kg dose of daptomycin. The mean half-life and AUC_{0-24} in blister fluid were 17.3 h and 318.2 mg h/L, respectively. The penetration of daptomycin into blister fluid was estimated to be 68.4 % based ratio of AUC_{0-24} for inflammatory exudate and plasma.

An in vivo microdialysis study describes the pharmacokinetic profile of daptomycin in the interstitial fluid of soft tissues and compares the degree of penetration between healthy and diabetic subjects [66]. Six subjects in each group were evenly matched and recruited receive a single 4 mg/kg dose of daptomycin. The mean in vivo recovery levels for daptomycin in subcutaneous tissue were 34 and 31 % for diabetic and healthy volunteers, respectively. The C_{max} in tissue occurred within 2 h of the dose and was approximately 4 mg/L. Tissue concentrations remained ≥1 mg/L for both groups up to 12 h after dosing. The mean $AUC_{0-\infty}$ and half-life values were greater in the diabetic subjects (45.1 mg·h/L and 12.4 h) compared healthy subjects (33.5 mg·h/L and 8.8 h), although not meaningfully different. The percent tissue penetration for diabetic subjects was 93 % compared to 73 % for healthy subjects. Mean C_{min} values in tissue were 0.59 and 0.39 for diabetics and healthy subjects, respectively, allowing for 100 % time over the MIC for common skin and soft tissue pathogens with daptomycin MICs of ≤0.25 mg/L.

Daptomycin has also demonstrated excellent penetration into synovial fluid and long bone [67, 68]. The mean daptomycin concentration in synovial fluid, thigh bone, and shin bone were 21.6, 3.3, and 3.4 mg/L, respectively [67]. Comparing these to plasma samples, the median penetration into synovial fluid, thigh bone, and shin bone was 54, 9.5, and 8.2 %. All samples were collected approximately 7 h after a single daptomycin dose of 8 mg/kg. All concentrations were maintained above 1 mg/L at all sampling times, indicating that daptomycin may be useful in the management of osteoarticular infections due to gram-positive pathogens, including *S. aureus.*

Complete equilibration between unbound concentrations of daptomycin in plasma, soft tissues, and bone was observed at approximately 2 h in diabetic patients with bacterial food infection [69]. The mean penetration in healthy tissue, inflamed subcutaneous adipose tissue, and bone were 154, 106, and 117 %, respectively, following once daily dosing of daptomycin 6 mg/kg for at least four consecutive days based the ratios of unbound AUC_{0-24} of site and plasma concentrations.

Two case reports have reported concentrations of daptomycin in valve tissue and vegetation in patients with bacterial endocarditis [70]. In a 61-year-old man with a mitro-aortic native valve,

Streptococcus oralis endocarditis, daptomycin concentrations were 8.6 and 30.8 μg/g in aortic and mitral values, respectively, and 26 μg/g in the mitral vegetation, following multiple daily doses of daptomycin 700 mg (9.7 mg/kg). In a 69-year-old man with an aortic, porcine prosthetic valve, *Staphylococcus epidermitis* endocarditis, daptomycin concentrations were 53.1 and 18.1 μg/g, respectively, of tissues in the prosthetic aortic valve and perivalvular tissue, following daily doses of daptomycin 500 mg (7.1 mg/kg). These data, along with the plasma concentration–time profile of daptomycin in patients undergoing pulmonary bypass surgery [71], provide pharmacokinetic and tissue penetration information in patients with endocarditis and may need to undergo cardiothoracic surgery.

Pericardial fluid and intravitreal concentrations of daptomycin have been reported in a 53-year-old woman with MRSA bacteremia, pericarditis, and endophthalmitis [72]. At approximately 42 h following a single dose of daptomycin 1000 mg, concentrations in serum, pericardial fluid, and vitreous humor were 44.01, 27.79, and 12.43 mg/L, respectively. The percentage of penetration compared to serum concentration was 63 and 28 % for pericardial fluid and vitreous, respectively.

3 Pharmacodynamics

3.1 In Vitro Models

Daptomycin has been extensively evaluated in various in vitro studies. Importantly, the addition of calcium to laboratory media is essential when testing daptomycin in vitro [73, 74]. Additionally, albumin has been shown to increase the MIC values of daptomycin much like the other lipoglycopeptides with minimal effect on the degree of bacterial killing in dynamic models [74].

Daptomycin has demonstrated rapid and pronounced bactericidal activity against a plethora of gram-positive pathogens, including MRSA, vancomycin-intermediate *S. aureus* (VISA) and vancomycin-resistant enterococci (VRE). The PD validity of the once-daily dosing approach has also been confirmed in vitro. The dose requirement to achieve 80 % maximal activity was 3 mg/kg against MRSA, correlating to an unbound AUC (*f*AUC) and AUC of 26 and 370 mg·h/L, respectively [75]. In all studies, the activity of daptomycin is more pronounced against *S. aureus* than against enterococci.

In Monte Carlo simulations, the probability of target attainment (PTA) and cumulative fraction of response (CFR) for an AUC_{0-24}/MIC of 666 was calculated from daptomycin doses of 4, 6, 8, 10, and 12 mg/kg/day [76]. The PTA was ≥99 % for all doses studied up to an MIC of 0.5 mg/L, while only doses ≥8 mg/kg achieved this for an MIC of 1 mg/L. The CFR >90 % were achieved for doses ≥8 mg/kg for *Enterococcus faecalis* and all

Staphylococcus and *Streptococcus* spp. tested, while even the 12 mg/kg dosing regimen achieved a CFR of just 17 % against *Enterococcus faecium*. This analysis suggests that the Clinical Laboratory and Standards Institute (CLSI) breakpoint for *Enterococcus* spp. should be lowered to 1 mg/L to avoid treatment failures due to inability to achieve PK/PD targets when enterococcal isolates are reported as susceptible.

Multiple in vitro studies have confirmed this need for higher doses of daptomycin (≥8 mg/kg) when attempting to treat *E. faecium* [77]. Combination studies have been completed, although the addition of rifampin and/or gentamicin has shown no additional benefit over daptomycin alone when treating *E. faecium* [78]. Interestingly, the combination of daptomycin and β-lactams like ceftriaxone and ertapenem have shown significant synergy in vitro against enterococci [79] Minimum resistance-prevention exposures were AUC/MIC ratios of 781 and 1562 for *E. faecium* and *E. faecalis*, respectively [80].

Importantly, in vivo studies have demonstrated that *S. aureus* isolates previously exposed to vancomycin have lower response rates to daptomycin and often produce heteroresistant isolates even without previous daptomycin exposure [81]. Alternative anti-MRSA agents other than daptomycin may be warranted in patients with serious *S. aureus* infections with previous exposure to vancomycin. In contrast to enterococci, the addition of gentamicin has been shown to reduce the time to 99.9 % kill in vitro. Daptomycin also does not appear to lose overall killing efficiency at high inoculums [82]. Increasing the dose to 10 mg/kg has provided little increases in activity against daptomycin nonsusceptible strains with MIC values of 2–4 mg/L [83, 84].

3.2 Animal Models

The animal models exploring the activity of daptomycin have demonstrated much of the same results as the in vitro studies, particularly with regard to the differential killing of *S. aureus* and *E. faecium*. In the neutropenic murine thigh infection model, the 24-h AUC/MIC best correlated with efficacy ($R^2=86$ %), followed by C_{max}/MIC ($R^2=83$ %) and Time > MIC ($R^2=8$ %) [85]. In animals, daptomycin displayed a post-antibiotic effect of 5 and 10 h for *S. aureus* and *S. pneumoniae*, respectively.

At least three other pharmacodynamic studies of daptomycin in the neutropenic murine thigh model have been published [86–88], all supporting the conclusion that AUC_{0-24}/MIC is the pharmacodynamic index linked to efficacy and therefore once-daily dosing should be used (Fig. 1). These results support once-daily dosing of daptomycin to target pathogen-specific AUC values best associated with efficacy.

Animal models of meningitis show similar results to the previous studies, i.e., low overall penetration (5 %) with adequate bactericidal activity able to sterilize the CSF of most tested animals [89, 90].

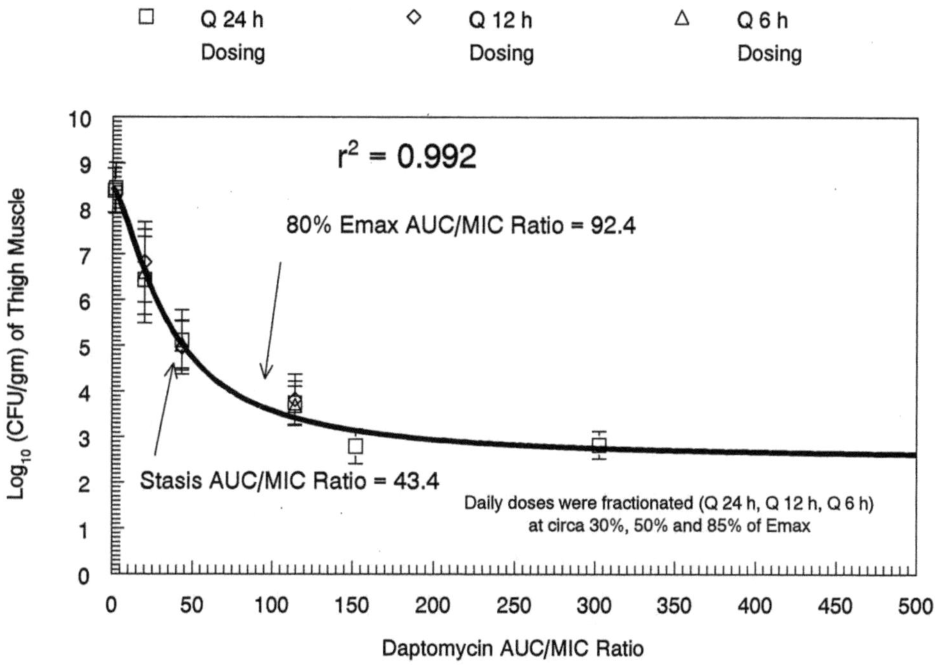

Fig. 1 Relationship between the 24-h AUC/MIC ratio of daptomycin and $\log_{10}$ CFU of *S. aureus* per gram of thigh muscle (mean ± 1 SD) when the total daily dose of daptomycin is given as one dose in 24 h, two equally divided doses every 12 h, or four equally divided doses every 6 h. Reproduced with permission from Ref. [86]

Daptomycin has displayed conflicting results in animal models of enterococcal endocarditis, with some authors suggesting that monotherapy should not be used due to the low rates of vegetation sterilization [91–93].

In vitro foreign body models using the rat tissue cage model with MSSA have demonstrated synergy and improved activity when daptomycin was administered with oxacillin even when compared to high-dose daptomycin monotherapy and combination of daptomycin and rifampin [94]. In contrast, the combination of daptomycin and rifampin was the most effective treatment for MRSA in the same model [95].

3.3 Monte Carlo Simulations

In order to attempt to link PK-PD parameters to predict in vivo efficacy, several Monte Carlo simulations have been completed for daptomycin [96–99]. Daptomycin at doses of 4 and 6 mg/kg/day were incorporated into 5000-subject simulation, using at a fixed weight of 80 kg, a range of CrCl of 50–120 mL/min, and a target $fAUC_{0-24}/MIC$ >40. Daptomycin achieved a CFR ≥90 % against all methicillin-susceptible *S. aureus* (MSSA) and MRSA isolates at both dosing regimens regardless of patient location (intensive care unit [ICU] vs. non-ICU) and specimen source (respiratory or blood vs. other sites) [97].

Simulations have also been performed for 10,000-subject assigned true body weight and CrCl values from a log-normal distribution [97]. Patients with CrCl <30 mL/min were excluded. Concentration–time profiles were calculated for doses of 6, 8, 10, and 12 mg/kg for 14 days. The probability of toxicity was assessed as the probability of a final trough concentration (C_{min}) ≥24.3 mg/L at 336 h. Bacteriostatic and bactericidal AUC_{0-24}/MIC targets were 388–537 and 788–1460, respectively. Doses of 6 mg/kg/day achieved bacteriostatic targets for all strains at an MIC of 0.5 mg/L, but only 75 % of strains at an MIC of 1 mg/L. For strains with an MIC of 2 mg/L, PTA for bacteriostatic targets was poor, ranging from 0.08 to 7.37 %. Doses of 8 mg/kg achieved static targets against all strains with an MIC ≤1 mg/L. Bactericidal targets were reached for 75 % of strains at an MIC of 0.5 mg/L. At 10 mg/kg/day, all stasis targets were again achieved only up to MIC of ≤1 mg/L and bactericidal targets were achieved for all strains at MIC 0.5 mg/L. Finally, at the highest dose of 12 mg/kg/day static targets were achieved in 75 % strains at MIC 2 mg/L and bactericidal targets for only 75 % strains at MIC of 1 mg/L. The probability of toxicity increased 5.35-fold (range: 3.3–17.7 %) when doses were increased from 6 to 12 mg/kg. This study demonstrates that bacteriostatic target AUC_{0-24}/MIC ratios were achieved in all strains with MIC levels at or below the CLSI breakpoint of 1 mg/L with an 11.3 % probability of toxicity.

Bactericidal therapy is often preferred in serious, high inoculum infections but was only achieved in 25 % strains tested at the highest dose of 12 mg/kg with susceptible MICs [97–99]. These analyses also consistently demonstrate a lower PTA and CFR with daptomycin against enterococci, especially *E. faecium* [76].

3.4 Daptomycin Exposure and Elevation Creatinine Phosphokinase Levels

PD modeling, classification and regression tree (CART) analysis, and Monte Carlo simulations were used to evaluate the relationship between PK exposure parameters and the probability of creatinine phosphokinase (CPK) elevation. The dataset consisted of 108 patients being treated for *S. aureus* bacteremia, with or without endocarditis, and receiving intravenous daptomycin 6 mg/kg once daily. Six patients (5.56 %) demonstrated a predefined CPK elevation. A plasma trough concentration (C_{min}) of daptomycin ≥24.3 mg/L was significantly associated with a CPK elevation (Fig. 2). The predicted probability of CPK elevation at a daily dose of 4, 6, 8, 10, and 12 mg/kg were 3.73, 6.92, 10.7, 15.3, and 19.5 %, respectively. The predicted probabilities of CPK elevations associated with musculoskeletal adverse events (i.e., muscle weakness and pain) at the same daily doses were 1.24, 2.31, 3.57, 5.11, and 8.49 %, respectively. These associations should be use to evaluate the risk and benefit of various dosing regimens with daptomycin.

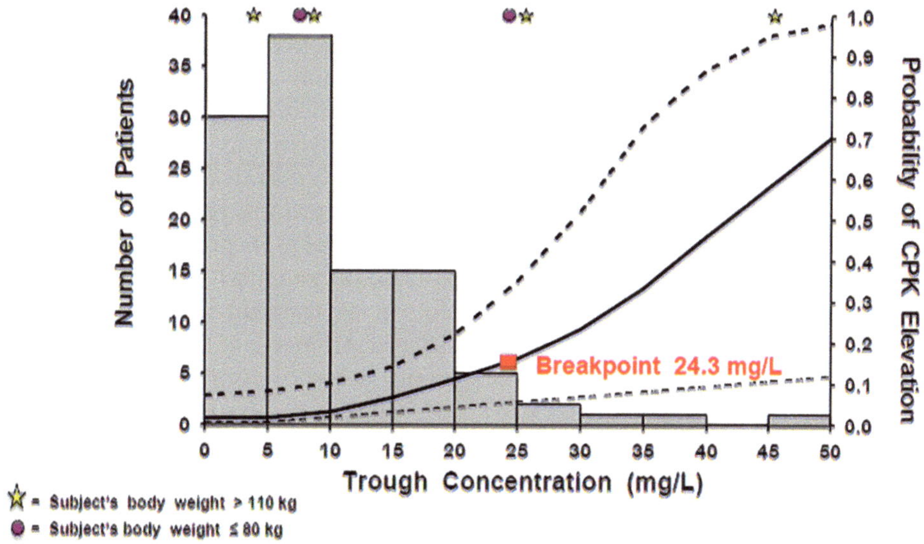

Fig. 2 Relationship between trough concentration of oritavancin (C_{min}) and the probability of creatine phosphokinase (CPK) elevation (*solid line*) and 95 % confidence interval (*dashed lines*) for the 108 patients who received intravenous daptomycin 6 mg/kg once-daily. *Shaded bars* are the distribution of the number of patients. Adapted from Ref. [17]

4 Clinical Trials: Proof of Pharmacokinetic-Pharmacodynamic Concepts

The efficacy and safety of daptomycin at 4 mg/kg every 24 h for 7–14 days was compared with conventional antibiotics in two randomized, international clinical trials involving 1092 patients with cSSSI [100]. Among 902 clinically evaluable patients, success rates were 83.4 and 84.2 % for the daptomycin and comparator-treated groups, respectively. The majority of patients (63 %) treated successfully with daptomycin required only 4–7 days of therapy compared to 33 % of comparators. Relapse or recurrence was observed at the poststudy visit in 4.2 and 5.5 % of the daptomycin and comparator groups, respectively. Clinical success rates in the microbiologically evaluable population by infecting organism were lowest for patients with *E. faecalis* (73 %). No emergence of resistance isolates was observed, including in patients who failed therapy.

Since these clinical trials, several trials have examined the clinical efficacy of daptomycin in specific patient populations and infections. Daptomycin and standard therapy has been evaluated as first-line treatment for cSSSI in elderly patients in an open-label, randomized phase IIIb trial and showed 89 % clinical success at the test-of-cure visit compared to 83.3 % for daptomycin and comparator-treated patients, respectively [101]. In Japanese patients with SSSI caused by MRSA, the efficacy of daptomycin at 4 mg/kg/day was similar to vancomycin although the authors suggest a trend toward a lower clinical success rate as daptomycin MICs increased [102]. No difference in clinical success rates was observed between daptomycin and vancomycin in patients with cellulitis and erysipelas [103]. When high-dose (10 mg/kg/day), short-course (4 days) of daptomycin was evaluated against standard therapy for cSSSI, clinical success rates were 75 and 87.5 % for the daptomycin and comparator groups, respectively (Confidence Interval [CI]: −27.9 to 2.9) [104]. In post-hoc analyses of this study, some subgroups (i.e., outpatients) performed better with the high-dose, short-course daptomycin therapy. Finally, a randomized, controlled trial of daptomycin at 6 or 8 mg/kg and standard therapy for patients with osteomyelitis associated with prosthetic devices [105]. Clinical success rates at the test-of-cure visit were 58.3–60.9 % for daptomycin and 38.1 % for the comparator. Microbiological success rates were 50–52.2 % for daptomycin and 38.1 % for the comparator.

The effectiveness of 6 mg/kg of daptomycin and an anti-staphylococcal penicillin or vancomycin plus initial low-dose gentamicin was evaluated in 236 patients with *S. aureus* bacteremia with or without endocarditis [106]. The primary end point was treatment success 42 days after the end of therapy. A successful outcome was documented in 44.2 and 41.7 % of patients in the daptomycin and standard therapy groups, respectively (CI: −10.2 to 15.1). Daptomycin was noninferior to standard therapy overall, and in subgroups of patients with complicated bacteremia, right-sided endocarditis, and MRSA. Microbiological failure was more common in the daptomycin group (19 vs. 11 patients, $p = 0.17$) and daptomycin-resistant isolates emerged in this population during the study. Therapy failed in all nine patients with left-sided endocarditis caused by MRSA. The respective median time to clear MRSA and MSSA bacteremia was 8 and 9 days for the daptomycin group and 4 and 3 days for the comparator groups. Treatment failures in the daptomycin group were more often attributed to persistent or relapsing *S. aureus* infection while failure of standard therapy seemed to be associated with adverse events. Of note, the clinical success rate demonstrated in this study was lower than previous studies likely due to the strict definition for success. Patients who did not have repeat blood cultures drawn at the test of cure visit were considered failures, even without signs and symptoms of infection. The authors conclude that daptomycin given at 6 mg/kg/day is noninferior to standard therapy for the treatment of bacteremia and right-sided endocarditis due to MSSA or MRSA. Further data is needed to support the use of daptomycin in left-sided endocarditis.

Carugati and colleagues evaluated the efficacy of high-dose daptomycin in patients with left-sided endocarditis as part of a prospective study from the international collaboration on endocarditis [107]. This cohort included 1112 cases of left sided endocarditis due to *S. aureus*, coagulase-negative staphylococci, and *E. faecalis* treated with daptomycin or standard therapy. The primary outcome was in-hospital mortality. Only 29 patients were included in the daptomycin group and these patients had significantly higher prevalence of previous episodes of endocarditis. The median daptomycin dose was 9.2 mg/kg/day and most of these patients (67 %) had already failed a previous antibiotic regimen. In-hospital and 6-month mortality did not differ between the groups and was not associated with daptomycin therapy in log-binomial analysis. Daptomycin given for MRSA endocarditis was associated with a decreased duration of bacteremia (1 vs. 5 days, $p<0.01$) and shorter length of stay (33 vs. 64.5 days, $p=0.04$) in this cohort. Adverse events were mild and uncommon.

Kullar and colleagues examined the efficacy and safety of ≥8 mg/kg of daptomycin in patients with suspected or confirmed staphylococcal or enterococcal endocarditis in a multicenter observational study [108]. Seventy patients were included, 47.1 % with right-sided endocarditis and 50 % with left-sided endocarditis. The majority of these patients (93 %) received daptomycin as salvage therapy and 84.4 % had MRSA bacteremia. The median dose used was 9.8 mg/kg and 89.1 % of patients cleared their blood cultures. No patients required discontinuation due to adverse events and 85.9 % achieved a clinical success. Six patients with MRSA developed nonsusceptibility to daptomycin, despite being treated with high-dose therapy.

In vitro data has suggested synergy between daptomycin and β-lactams, especially ceftaroline Daptomycin plus ceftaroline was used as salvage in 26 cases of refractory staphylococcal bacteremia at 10 medical centers [109]. The majority ($n=20$) of cases were due to MRSA, with the remaining cases cause by VISA, MSSA, and methicillin-resistant coagulase negative staphylococci (2 cases for each pathogen). Patients were bacteremic for a median of 10 days prior to switching to daptomycin–ceftaroline. Blood cultures were reported negative in a median of 2 days after starting combination therapy. In vitro studies on the clinical isolates demonstrated synergy and enhanced MRSA killing by cathelicidin and neutrophils. The combination of daptomycin and ceftaroline (or other β-lactams) may be an effective therapeutic option in cases of refractory staphylococcal bacteremia and may have benefits beyond synergy.

Daptomycin has experienced extensive clinical use for various types of infections caused by gram-positive bacteria. Although daptomycin penetrates into the lung, daptomycin is not effective for the treatment of community-acquired bacterial pneumonia [110] and is not recommended for the treatment of pulmonary infections. Daptomycin has been shown to interact with pulmonary surfactant in vitro that results in an inhibition of the antibacterial activity [111].

References

1. Allen NE, Alborn WE Jr, Hobbs JN Jr (1991) Inhibition of membrane potential-dependent amino acid transport by daptomycin. Antimicrob Agents Chemother 35(12): 2639–2642
2. Straus SK, Hancock RE (2006) Mode of action of the new antibiotic for Gram-positive pathogens daptomycin: comparison with cationic antimicrobial peptides and lipopeptides. Biochim Biophys Acta 1758(9):1215–1223
3. Fuchs PC, Barry AL, Brown SD (2002) In vitro bactericidal activity of daptomycin against staphylococci. J Antimicrob Chemother 49(3):467–470
4. Dvorchik B, Arbeit RD, Chung J, Liu S, Knebel W, Kastrissios H (2004) Population pharmacokinetics of daptomycin. Antimicrob Agents Chemother 48(8):2799–2807
5. Tally FP, DeBruin MF (2000) Development of daptomycin for gram-positive infections. J Antimicrob Chemother 46(4):523–526
6. Garrison MW, Rotschafer JC, Crossley KB (1989) Suboptimal effect of daptomycin in the treatment of bacteremias. South Med J 82(11):1414–1415
7. Garrison MW, Vance-Bryan K, Larson TA, Toscano JP, Rotschafer JC (1990) Assessment of effects of protein binding on daptomycin and vancomycin killing of *Staphylococcus aureus* by using an in vitro pharmacodynamic model. Antimicrob Agents Chemother 34(10):1925–1931
8. Rybak MJ, Bailey EM, Lamp KC, Kaatz GW (1992) Pharmacokinetics and bactericidal rates of daptomycin and vancomycin in intravenous drug abusers being treated for gram-positive endocarditis and bacteremia. Antimicrob Agents Chemother 36(5):1109–1114
9. Woodworth JR, Nyhart EH Jr, Brier GL, Wolny JD, Black HR (1992) Single-dose pharmacokinetics and antibacterial activity of daptomycin, a new lipopeptide antibiotic, in healthy volunteers. Antimicrob Agents Chemother 36(2):318–325
10. Dvorchik BH, Brazier D, DeBruin MF, Arbeit RD (2003) Daptomycin pharmacokinetics and safety following administration of escalating doses once daily to healthy subjects. Antimicrob Agents Chemother 47(4):1318–1323
11. Benvenuto M, Benziger DP, Yankelev S, Vigliani G (2006) Pharmacokinetics and tolerability of daptomycin at doses up to 12 milligrams per kilogram of body weight once daily in healthy volunteers. Antimicrob Agents Chemother 50(10):3245–3249
12. Chakraborty A, Roy S, Loeffler J, Chaves RL (2009) Comparison of the pharmacokinetics, safety and tolerability of daptomycin in healthy adult volunteers following intravenous administration by 30 min infusion or 2 min injection. J Antimicrob Chemother 64(1):151–158
13. Chaves RL, Chakraborty A, Benziger D, Tannenbaum S (2014) Clinical and pharmacokinetic considerations for the use of daptomycin in patients with *Staphylococcus aureus* bacteremia and severe renal impairment. J Antimicrob Chemother 69:200–210
14. Di Paolo A, Tascini C, Polillo M, Gemignani G, Nielsen EI, Bocci G, Karlsson MO, Menichetti F, Danesi R (2013) Population pharmacokinetics of daptomycin in patients affected by severe Gram-positive infections. Int J Antimicrob Agents 42(3):250–255
15. Falcone M, Russo A, Venditti M, Novelli A, Pai MP (2013) Considerations for higher doses of daptomycin in critically ill patients with methicillin-resistant *Staphylococcus aureus* bacteremia. Clin Infect Dis 57(11):1568–1576
16. Soon RL, Turner SJ, Forrest A, Tsuji BT, Brown J (2013) Pharmacokinetic/pharmacodynamic evluation of the efficacy and safety of daptomycin against *Staphylococcus aureus*. Int J Antimicrob Agnets 42:53–58
17. Bhavnani SM, Rubino CM, Ambrose PG, Drusano GL (2010) Daptomycin exposure and the probability of elevations in the creatinine phosphokinase level: data from a randomized trial of patients with bacteremia and endocarditis. Clin Infect Dis 50:1568–1574
18. Cohen-Wolkowiez M, Watt KM, Hornik CP, Benjamin DK Jr, Smith PB (2012) Pharmacokinetics and tolerability of single-dose daptomycin in young infants. Pediatr Infect Dis J 31(9):935–937
19. Cohen-Wolkowiez M, Smith PB, Benjamin DK Jr, Fowler VG Jr, Wade KC (2008) Daptomycin use in infants: report of two cases with peak and trough drug concentrations. J Perinatol 28(3):233–234
20. Antachopoulos C, Iosifidis E, Sarafidis K, Bazoti F, Gikas E, Katragkou A, Drossou-Agakidou V, Roilides E (2012) Serum levels of daptomycin in pediatric patients. Infection 40(4):367–371
21. Bradley JS, Benziger D, Bokesch P, Jacobs R (2014) Single-dose pharmacokinetics of daptomycin in pediatric patients 3-24 months of age. Pediatri Infect Dis J 33(9):936–939
22. Abdel-Rahman SM, Benziger DP, Jacobs RF, Jafri HS, Hong EF, Kearns GL (2008)

Single-dose pharmacokinetics of daptomycin in children with suspected or proved gram-positive infections. Pediatr Infect Dis J 27(4): 330–334

23. Abdel-Rahman SM, Chandorkar G, Akins RL, Bradley JS, Jacobs RF, Donovan J, Benziger DP (2011) Single-dose pharmacokinetics and tolerability of daptomycin 8 to 10 mg/kg in children aged 2 to 6 years with suspected or proved Gram-positive infections. Pediatr Infect Dis J 30(8):712–714
24. Dvorchik B, Damphousse D (2004) Single-dose pharmacokinetics of daptomycin in young and geriatric volunteers. J Clin Pharmacol 44(6):612–620
25. Pai MP, Norenberg JP, Anderson T, Goade DW, Rodvold KA, Telepak RA, Merceier R-C (2007) Influence of morbid obesity on the single-dose pharmacokinetics of daptomycin. Antimicrob Agents Chemother 51(8):2741–2747
26. Dvorchik BH, Damphousse D (2005) The pharmacokinetics of daptomycin in moderately obese, morbidly obese, and matched nonobese subjects. J Clin Pharmacol 45(1):48–56
27. Pai MP (2012) Drug dosing based on weight and body surface area: mathematical assumptions and limitations of obese adults. Pharmacotherapy 32:856–868
28. Di Paolo A, Polillo M, Tascini C, Lewis R, Menichetti F, Danesi R (2014) Different recommendations for daptomycin dosing over time in patients with severe infections. Clin Infect Dis 58(12):1788–1789
29. Falcone M, Russo A, Venditti M, Novelli A, Pai MP. Reply to Di Paolo et al (2014) Clin Infect Dis 58(12):1789–1790
30. Ng JK, Schulz LT, Rose WE, Fox BC, Andes DR, Buhr KA, Fish JT (2014) Daptomycin dosing based on ideal body weight versus actual body weight: comparison of clinical outcomes. Antimicrob Agents Chemother 58:88–93
31. Pai MP, Russo A, Novelli A, Venditti M, Flacone M (2014) Simplified equations using two concentrations to calculate area under the curve for antimicrobials with concentration-dependent pharmacodynamics: daptomycin as a motivating example. Antimicrob Agents Chemother 58(6):3162–3167
32. Bubalo JS, Munar MY, Cherala G, Hayes-Lattin B, Maziarz R (2009) Daptomycin pharmacokinetics in adult oncology patients with neutropenic fever. Antimicrob Agents Chemother 53(2):428–434
33. Mohr JF 3rd, Ostrosky-Zeichner L, Wainright DJ, Parks DH, Hollenbeck TC, Ericsson CD (2008) Pharmacokinetic evaluation of single-dose intravenous daptomycin in patients with thermal burn injury. Antimicrob Agents Chemother 52(5):1891–1893
34. Erritouni M, Ktaich N, Rahal JJ et al (2012) Use of daptomycin for the treatment of methicillin-resistant coagulase-negative staphylococcal ventriculitis. Case Rep Med 2012:593578
35. Wahby KA, Alangaden GJ (2012) Daptomycin failure in a neutropenic leukemia patient with *Staphylococcus aureus* meningitis. Leuk Lymphoma 53(8):1610–1612
36. Kelesidis T, Humphries R, Ward K, Lewinski MA, Yang OO (2011) Combination therapy with daptomycin, linezolid, and rifampin as treatment option for MRSA meningitis and bacteremia. Diagn Microbiol Infect Dis 71(3):286–290
37. Le J, Bookstaver PB, Rudisill CN, Hashem MG, Igbal R, James CL, Sakoulas G (2010) Treatment of meningitis caused by vancomycin-resistant *Enterococcus faecium*: high-dose and combination daptomycin therapy. Ann Pharmacother 44(12):2001–2006
38. Riser MS, Bland CM, Rudisill CN, Bookstaver PB (2010) Cerebrospinal fluid penetration of high-dose daptomycin in suspected *Staphylococcus aureus* meningitis. Ann Pharmacother 44(11):1832–1835
39. Jaspan HB, Brothers AW, Campbell AJ, McGuire JK, Browd SR, Manley TJ, Park D, Weissman SJ (2010) Multidrug-resistant *Enterococcus faecium* meningitis in a toddler: characterization of the organism and successful treatment with intraventricular daptomycin and intravenous tigecycline. Pediatr Infect Dis J 29(4):379–381
40. Lee DH, Palermo B, Chowdhury M (2008) Successful treatment of methicillin-resistant *Staphylococcus aureus* meningitis with daptomycin. Clin Infect Dis 47(4):588–590
41. Taglietti F, Campanile F, Capone A et al (2012) Daptomycin efficacy in the central nervous system of a patient with disseminated methicillin-resistant *Staphylococcus aureus* infection: a case report. J Med Case Rep 6:264
42. Kullar R, Chin JN, Edwards DJ, Parker D, Coplin WM, Rybak MJ (2011) Pharmacokinetics of single-dose daptomycin in patients with suspected or confirmed neurological infections. Antimicrob Agents Chemother 55(7):3505–3509
43. Vivas M, Force E, Garrigos C et al (2014) Experimental study of the efficacy of daptomycin for the treatment of cephalosporin-resistant pneumococcal meningitis. J Antimicrob Chemother 69(11):3020–3026

44. Cardone KE, Lodise TP, Patel N, Hoy CD, Meola S, Manley HJ, Drusano GL, Grabe DW (2011) Pharmacokinetics and pharmacodynamics of intravenous daptomycin during continuous ambulatory peritoneal dialysis. Clin J Am Soc Nephrol 6(5):1081–1088
45. Goedecke VA, Clajus C, Burkhardt O, Martens-Lobenhoffer J, Bode-Boger SM, Kielstein JT, Hiss M (2009) Pharmacokinetics and dialysate levels of daptomycin given intravenously in a peritoneal dialysis patient. Scand J Infect Dis 41(2):155–157
46. Bahte SK, Bertram A, Burkhardt O, Martens-Lebenhoffer J, Goedecke V, Bode-Boger SM, Hiss M, Kielstein JT (2010) Therapeutic serum concentrations of daptomycin after intraperitoneal administration in a patient with peritoneal dialysis-associated peritonitis. J Antimicro Chemother 65(6):1312–1314
47. Huen SC, Hall I, Topal J, Mahnensmith RL, Brewster UC, Abu-Alfa AK (2009) Successful use of intraperitoneal daptomycin in the treatment of vancomycin-resistant Enterococcus peritonitis. Am J Kidney Dis 54(3):538–541
48. Benziger DP, Pertel PE, Donovan J, Yankelev S, Schwab RJ, Swan SK, Cannon C (2011) Pharmacokinetics and safety of multiple doses of daptomycin 6 mg/kg in noninfected adults undergoing hemodialysis or continuous ambulatory peritoneal dialysis. Clin Nephrol 75(1):63–69
49. Salama NN, Segal JH, Churchwell MD, Patel JH, Gao L, Heung M, Mueller BA (2010) Single-dose daptomycin pharmacokinetics in chronic haemodialysis patients. Nephrol Dial Transplant 25(4):1279–1284
50. Salama NN, Segal JH, Churchwell MD, Patel JH, Gao L, Heung M, Mueller BA (2009) Intradialytic administration of daptomycin in end stage renal disease patients on hemodialysis. Clin J Am Soc Nephrol 4(7):1190–1194
51. Patel N, Cardone K, Grabe DW, Meola S, Hoy C, Manely H, Drusano GL, Lodise TP (2011) Use of pharmacokinetic and pharmacodynamic principles to determine optimal administration of daptomycin in patients receiving standardized thrice-weekly hemodialysis. Antimicrob Agents Chemother 55(4):1677–1683
52. Butterfield JM, Mueller BA, Patel N, Cardone KE, Grabe DW, Salama NN, Lodise TP (2013) Daptomycin pharmacokinetics and pharmacodynamics in a pooled sample of patients receiving thrice-weekly hemodialysis. Antimicrob Agents Chemother 57(2):864–872
53. Churchwell MD, Pasko DA, Mueller BA (2006) Daptomycin clearance during modelled continuous renal replacement therapy. Blood Purif 24:548–554
54. Wagner CC, Steiner I, Zeitlinger M (2009) Daptomycin elimination by CVVH in vitro: evaluation of factors influencing sieving and membrane adsorption. Int J Clin Pharmacol Ther 47(3):178–186
55. Burkhardt O, Joukhadar C, Traunmuller F, Hadem J, Welte T, Kielstein JT (2008) Elimination of daptomycin in a patient with acute renal failure undergoing extended daily dialysis. J Antimicrob Chemother 61:224–225
56. Kielstein JT, Engbers C, Bode-Boeger SM, Martens-Lobenhoffer J, Haller H, Joukhadar C, Traunmuller F, Kritsch W, Hafer C, Burkhardt O (2010) Dosing of daptomycin in intensive care unit patients with acute kidney injury undergoing extended dialysis: a pharmacokinetic study. Nephrol Dial Transplant 25:1537–1541
57. Khadzhynov D, Slowinski T, Lieker I, Spies C, Puhlmann B, Konig T, Uhrig A, Eggers K, Neumayer H-H, Traunmuller F, Joukhader C, Peters H (2011) Plasma pharmacokinetics of daptomycin in critically ill patients with renal failure and undergoing CVVHD. Int J Clin Pharmacol Ther 49(11):656–665
58. Vilay AM, Grio M, DePestel DD, Sowinski KM, Gao L, Heung M, Salama NN, Mueller BA (2011) Daptomycin pharmacokinetics in critically ill patients receiving continuous venovenous hemodialysis. Crit Care Med 39(1):19–25
59. Rudiger A, Rentsch K, Maggiorini M, Corti N (2011) Daptomycin pharmacokinetics in critically ill patients receiving continuous venovenous hemodialysis (Letter). Crit Care Med 39(5):1243–1244
60. Vilay AM, DePestel DD, Mueller BA (2011) Daptomycin pharmacokinetics in critically ill patients receiving continuous venovenous hemodialysis (Letter). Crit Care Med 39(5):1244–1245
61. Wenisch JM, Meyer B, Fuhrmann V, Saria K, Zuba C, Dittrich P, Thalhammer F (2012) Multiple-dose pharmacokinetics of daptomycin during continuous venovenous haemodiafiltration. J Antimicrob Chemother 67(4):977–983
62. Preiswerk B, Rudiger A, Fehr J, Corti N (2013) Experience with daptomycin daily dosing in ICU patients undergoing continuous renal replacement therapy. Infection 41:533–537
63. Corti N, Rudiger A, Chiesa A, Marti I, Jetter A, Rentsch K, Muller D, Bechir M, Maggiorini

M (2013) Pharmacokinetics of daily daptomycin in critically ill patients undergoing continuous renal replacement therapy. Chemotherapy 59(2):143–151

64. Falcone M, Russo A, Cassetta MI, Lappa A, Tritapepe L, Fallani S, Vullo V, Venditti M, Novelli A (2012) Daptomycin serum levels in critical patients undergoing continuous renal replacement. J Chemother 24:253–256
65. Wise R, Gee T, Andrews JM, Dvorchik B, Marshall G (2002) Pharmacokinetics and inflammatory fluid penetration of intravenous daptomycin in volunteers. Antimicrob Agents Chemother 46(1):31–33
66. Kim A, Suecof LA, Sutherland CA, Gao L, Kuti JL, Nicolau DP (2008) In vivo microdialysis study of the penetration of daptomycin into soft tissues in diabetic versus healthy volunteers. Antimicrob Agents Chemother 52(11):3941–3946
67. Montange D, Berthier F, Leclerc G, Serre A, Jeunet L, Berard M, Muret P, Vettoretti L, Leroy J, Hoen B, Chirouze C et al (2014) Penetration of daptomycin into bone and synovial fluid in joint replacement. Antimicrob Agents Chemother 58(7):3991–3996
68. Ritchie ND, Lovering AM, Seaton RA (2010) Daptomycin in synovial fluid during treatment of methicillin-resistant *Staphylococcus aureus* septic arthritis. J Antimicrob Chemother 65(6):1314–1315
69. Traunmuller F, Schintler MV, Metzler J, Spendel S, Mauric O, Popovic M, Konz KH, Scharnagi E, Joukhader C (2010) Soft tissue and bone penetration abilities of daptomycin in diabetic patients with bacterial foot infections. J Antimicrob Chemother 65(6):1252–1257
70. Tascini C, Di Paolo A, Poletti R, Flammini S, Emdin M, Ciullo I, Tagliaferri E, Moter A, Menichetti F (2013) Daptomycin concentrations in valve tissue and vegetation in patients with bacterial endocarditis. Antimicrob Agents Chemother 57(1):601–602
71. Nguyen MH, Eells SJ, Tan J, Sheth CT, Omari B, Flores M, Wang J, Miller LG (2011) Prospective, open-label investigations of the pharmacokinetics of daptomycin during cardiopulmonary bypass surgery. Antimicrob Agents Chemother 55(6):2499–2505
72. Sheridan KR, Potoski BA, Shields RK, Nau GJ (2010) Presence of adequate intravitreal concentrations of daptomycin after systemic intravenous administration in a patient with endogenous endophthalmitis. Pharmacotherapy 30(12):1247–1251
73. Hanberger H, Nilsson LE, Maller R, Isaksson B (1991) Pharmacodynamics of daptomycin and vancomycin on *Enterococcus faecalis* and *Staphylococcus aureus* demonstrated by studies of initial killing and postantibiotic effect and influence of Ca2+ and albumin on these drugs. Antimicrob Agents Chemother 35(9):1710–1716
74. Cha R, Rybak MJ (2004) Influence of protein binding under controlled conditions on the bactericidal activity of daptomycin in an in vitro pharmacodynamic model. J Antimicrob Chemother 54(1):259–262
75. Cha R, Grucz RG Jr, Rybak MJ (2003) Daptomycin dose-effect relationship against resistant gram-positive organisms. Antimicrob Agents Chemother 47(5):1598–1603
76. Asin E, Isla A, Canut A, Rodriguez GA (2012) Comparison of antimicrobial pharmacokinetic/pharmacodynamic breakpoints with EUCAST and CLSI clinical breakpoints for Gram-positive bacteria. Int J Antimicrob Agents 40(4):313–322
77. Hall AD, Steed ME, Arias CA, Murray BE, Rybak MJ (2012) Evaluation of standard- and high-dose daptomycin versus linezolid against vancomycin-resistant *Enterococcus* isolates in an in vitro pharmacokinetic/pharmacodynamic model with simulated endocardial vegetations. Antimicrob Agents Chemother 56(6):3174–3180
78. Luther MK, Arvanitis M, Mylonakis E, LaPlante KL (2014) Activity of daptomycin or linezolid in combination with rifampin or gentamicin against biofilm-forming *Enterococcus faecalis* or *E. faecium* in an in vitro pharmacodynamic model using simulated endocardial vegetations and an in vivo survival assay using *Galleria mellonella* larvae. Antimicrob Agents Chemother 58(8):4612–4620
79. Hall Snyder A, Werth BJ, Barber KE, Sakoulas G, Rybak MJ (2014) Evaluation of the novel combination of daptomycin plus ceftriaxone against vancomycin-resistant enterococci in an in vitro pharmacokinetic/pharmacodynamic simulated endocardial vegetation model. J Antimicrob Chemother 69(8):2148–2154
80. Werth BJ, Steed ME, Ireland CE et al (2014) Defining daptomycin resistance prevention exposures in vancomycin resistant *Enterococcus* (VRE) *faecium* and *E. faecalis*. Antimicrob Agents Chemother 58(9):5253–5261
81. Bhalodi AA, Hagihara M, Nicolau DP, Kuti JL (2014) In vitro pharmacodynamics of human simulated exposures of ceftaroline and daptomycin against MRSA, hVISA, and VISA with and without prior vancomycin exposure. Antimicrob Agents Chemother 58(2): 672–677

82. LaPlante KL, Rybak MJ (2004) Impact of high-inoculum *Staphylococcus aureus* on the activities of nafcillin, vancomycin, linezolid, and daptomycin, alone and in combination with gentamicin, in an in vitro pharmacodynamic model. Antimicrob Agents Chemother 48(12):4665–4672
83. Rose WE, Leonard SN, Rybak MJ (2008) Evaluation of daptomycin pharmacodynamics and resistance at various dosage regimens against *Staphylococcus aureus* isolates with reduced susceptibilities to daptomycin in an in vitro pharmacodynamic model with simulated endocardial vegetations. Antimicrob Agents Chemother 52(9):3061–3067
84. Steed M, Vidaillac C, Rybak MJ (2011) Evaluation of ceftaroline activity versus daptomycin (DAP) against DAP-nonsusceptible methicillin-resistant *Staphylococcus aureus* strains in an in vitro pharmacokinetic/pharmacodynamic model. Antimicrob Agents Chemother 55(7):3522–3526
85. Safdar N, Andes D, Craig WA (2004) In vivo pharmacodynamic activity of daptomycin. Antimicrob Agents Chemother 48(1):63–68
86. Louie A, Kaw P, Liu W, Jumbe N, Miller MH, Drusano GL (2001) Pharmacodynamics of daptomycin in a murine thigh model of *Staphylococcus aureus* infection. Antimicrob Agents Chemother 45(3):845–851
87. Dandekar PK, Tessier PR, Williams P, Nightingale CH, Nicolau DP (2003) Pharmacodynamic profile of daptomycin against Enterococcus species and methicillin-resistant *Staphylococcus aureus* in a murine thigh infection model. J Antimicrob Chemother 52(3):405–411
88. Dandekar PK, Tessier PR, Williams P, Zhang C, Nightingale CH, Nicolau DP (2004) Determination of the pharmacodynamic profile of daptomycin against *Streptococcus pneumoniae* isolates with varying susceptibility to penicillin in a murine thigh infection model. Chemotherapy 50(1):11–16
89. Gerber P, Stucki A, Acosta F, Cottagnoud M, Cottagnoud P (2006) Daptomycin is more efficacious than vancomycin against a methicillin-susceptible *Staphylococcus aureus* in experimental meningitis. J Antimicrob Chemother 57(4):720–723
90. Cottagnoud P, Pfister M, Acosta F et al (2004) Daptomycin is highly efficacious against penicillin-resistant and penicillin- and quinolone-resistant pneumococci in experimental meningitis. Antimicrob Agents Chemother 48(10):3928–3933
91. Ramos MC, Grayson ML, Eliopoulos GM, Bayer AS (1992) Comparison of daptomycin, vancomycin, and ampicillin-gentamicin for treatment of experimental endocarditis caused by penicillin-resistant enterococci. Antimicrob Agents Chemother 36(9):1864–1869
92. Bush LM, Boscia JA, Kaye D (1988) Daptomycin (LY146032) treatment of experimental enterococcal endocarditis. Antimicrob Agents Chemother 32(6):877–881
93. Kennedy S, Chambers HF (1989) Daptomycin (LY146032) for prevention and treatment of experimental aortic valve endocarditis in rabbits. Antimicrob Agents Chemother 33(9):1522–1525
94. El Haj C, Murillo O, Ribera A et al (2014) Comparative efficacies of cloxacillin-daptomycin and the standard cloxacillin-rifampin therapies against an experimental foreign-body infection by methicillin-susceptible *Staphylococcus aureus*. Antimicrob Agents Chemother 58(9):5576–5580
95. Garrigos C, Murillo O, Lora-Tamayo J et al (2012) Efficacy of daptomycin-cloxacillin combination in experimental foreign-body infection due to methicillin-resistant *Staphylococcus aureus*. Antimicrob Agents Chemother 56(7):3806–3811
96. Housman ST, Sutherland CA, Nicolau DP (2014) Pharmacodynamic profile of commonly utilised parenteral therapies against meticillin-susceptible and meticillin-resistant *Staphylococcus aureus* collected from US hospitals. Int J Antimicrob Agents
97. Soon RL, Turner SJ, Forrest A, Tsuji BT, Brown J (2013) Pharmacokinetic/pharmacodynamic evaluation of the efficacy and safety of daptomycin against *Staphylococcus aureus*. Int J Antimicrob Agents 42(1):53–58
98. Canut A, Isla A, Betriu C, Gascon AR (2012) Pharmacokinetic-pharmacodynamic evaluation of daptomycin, tigecycline, and linezolid versus vancomycin for the treatment of MRSA infections in four western European countries. Eur J Clin Microbiol Infect Dis 31(9):2227–2235
99. Salem AH, Zhanel GG, Ibrahim SA, Noreddin AM (2014) Monte Carlo simulation analysis of ceftobiprole, dalbavancin, daptomycin, tigecycline, linezolid and vancomycin pharmacodynamics against intensive care unit-isolated methicillin-resistant *Staphylococcus aureus*. Clin Exp Pharmacol Physiol 41(6):437–443
100. Arbeit RD, Maki D, Tally FP, Campanaro E, Eisenstein BI (2004) The safety and efficacy of daptomycin for the treatment of complicated skin and skin-structure infections. Clin Infect Dis 38(12):1673–1681

101. Konychev A, Heep M, Moritz RK et al (2013) Safety and efficacy of daptomycin as first-line treatment for complicated skin and soft tissue infections in elderly patients: an open-label, multicentre, randomized phase IIIb trial. Drugs Aging 30(10):829–836
102. Aikawa N, Kusachi S, Mikamo H et al (2013) Efficacy and safety of intravenous daptomycin in Japanese patients with skin and soft tissue infections. J Infect Chemother 19(3):447–455
103. Pertel PE, Eisenstein BI, Link AS et al (2009) The efficacy and safety of daptomycin vs. vancomycin for the treatment of cellulitis and erysipelas. Int J Clin Pract 63(3):368–375
104. Katz DE, Lindfield KC, Steenbergen JN et al (2008) A pilot study of high-dose short duration daptomycin for the treatment of patients with complicated skin and skin structure infections caused by gram-positive bacteria. Int J Clin Pract 62(9):1455–1464
105. Byren I, Rege S, Campanaro E et al (2012) Randomized controlled trial of the safety and efficacy of daptomycin versus standard-of-care therapy for management of patients with osteomyelitis associated with prosthetic devices undergoing two-stage revision arthroplasty. Antimicrob Agents Chemother 56(11):5626–5632
106. Fowler VG Jr, Boucher HW, Corey GR et al (2006) Daptomycin versus standard therapy for bacteremia and endocarditis caused by *Staphylococcus aureus*. N Engl J Med 355(7):653–665
107. Carugati M, Bayer AS, Miro JM et al (2013) High-dose daptomycin therapy for left-sided infective endocarditis: a prospective study from the international collaboration on endocarditis. Antimicrob Agents Chemother 57(12):6213–6222
108. Kullar R, Casapao AM, Davis SL et al (2013) A multicentre evaluation of the effectiveness and safety of high-dose daptomycin for the treatment of infective endocarditis. J Antimicrob Chemother 68(12):2921–2926
109. Sakoulas G, Moise PA, Casapao AM et al (2014) Antimicrobial salvage therapy for persistent staphylococcal bacteremia using daptomycin plus ceftaroline. Clin Ther 36(10):1317–1333
110. Pertel PE, Bernardo P, Fogarty C et al (2008) Effects of prior effective therapy on the efficacy of daptomycin and ceftriaxone for the treatment of community-acquired pneumonia. Clin Infect Dis 46:1142–1151
111. Silverman JA, Mortin LI, Vanpraagh AD et al (2003) Correlation of daptomycin bactericidal activity and membrane depolarization in Staphylococcus aureus. Antimicrob Agents Chemother 47:2538–2544

Chapter 14

Pharmacodynamics of Macrolides, Azalides, and Ketolides

Wonhee So and David P. Nicolau

Abstract

Macrolides and azalides have been widely utilized in clinical practice. With the increased use of these agents over the past two decades an accompanied increase in bacterial resistance as defined by laboratory based criteria has been observed. As a result, new derivatives have been introduced or are under development to overcome this emerging resistance. As the chemical structure of the macrolides progressed to the azalides and then ketolides, convenient once-daily oral dosing regimens and enhanced antibacterial activity over the earlier generation macrolides contributed to their widespread use for the treatment of community-acquired respiratory tract infections. As a result of the high penetration into respiratory tract tissues/fluids, the post antibiotic effect, uptake into white blood cells, and their immunomodulatory properties as well as their pharmacodynamic profile, the newer generation macrolides and azalides continue to be used in clinical practice with a high level of treatment success. Despite escalating macrolide resistance in target pathogens, the commercial withdrawal of telithromycin due to drug-related toxicities has tempered the development of new ketolides. The aims of this chapter are to provide principles to understand pharmacokinetic and pharmacodynamic properties of these agents and to provide insights supporting the application of this knowledge in clinical practice.

Key words Macrolides, Azalides and ketolides, Pharmacokinetic and pharmacodynamics, Community-acquired respiratory infection

1 History and Chemistry

Erythromycin, the first macrolide utilized in clinical practice, was introduced into the market in 1952 [1]. It has been used for decades to treat a variety of infections involving the respiratory tract, skin and soft tissues, genital tract as well as being considered as useful alternative therapy in the penicillin allergic patient [2]. However, several shortcomings, including instability in acidic media, gastrointestinal intolerance, and a short serum half-life, have limited its use and led to the development of synthetic macrolides such as dirithromycin and clarithromycin in 1990s. Furthermore, introduction of a nitrogen atom to the 14-membered macrolide ring yielded 15-membered ring, which was named azalide; and azithromycin, the first azalide, became available in the market in 1990s (Fig. 1) [1, 2].

John C. Rotschafer et al. (eds.), *Antibiotic Pharmacodynamics*, Methods in Pharmacology and Toxicology,
DOI 10.1007/978-1-4939-3323-5_14, © Springer Science+Business Media New York 2016

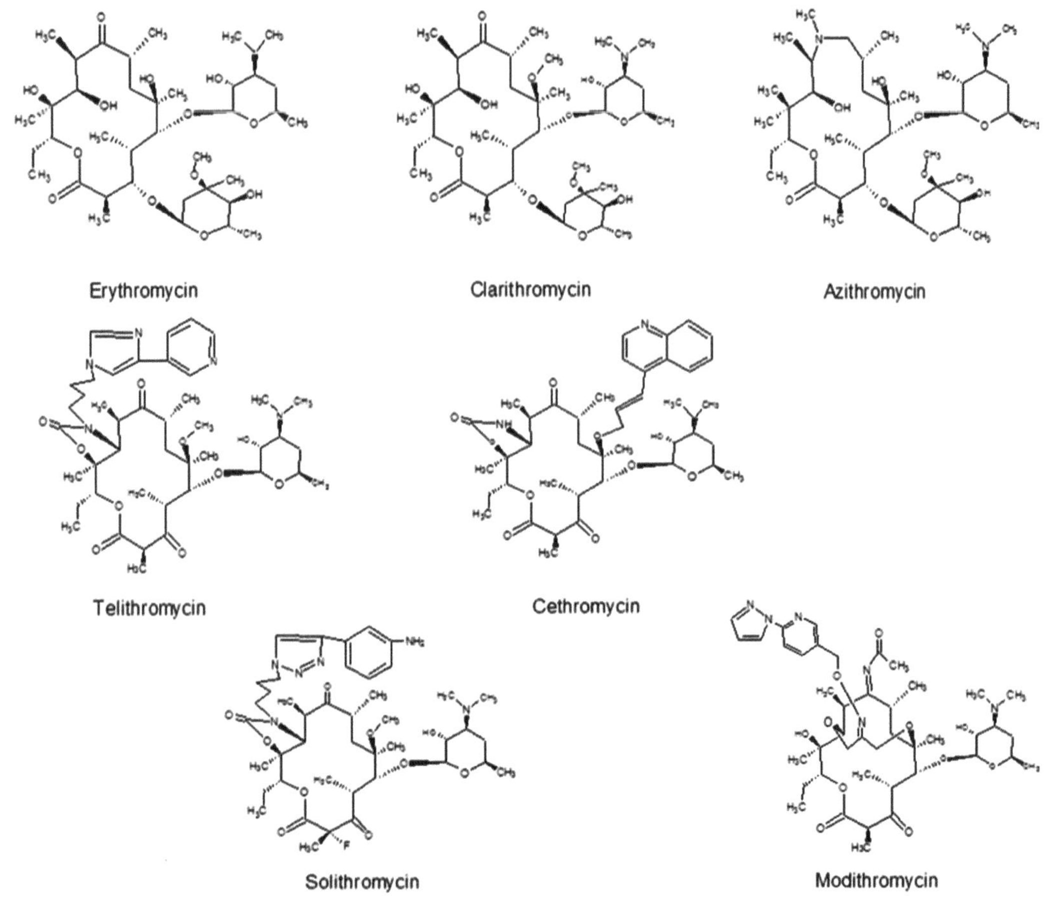

Fig. 1 Chemical structures of macrolides, azalides, and ketolides

Major advantages of these newer macrolides and azithromycin compared to erythromycin include broadened antibacterial coverage, improved pharmacokinetic characteristics, stability to acidity, and high gastrointestinal tolerability. However, widespread usage of macrolides and azithromycin has promoted the emergence of resistance against these agents over the last two decades [3], which in turn accelerated the research for newer derivatives. Ketolides were developed to overcome macrolide resistance, and the first clinically available ketolide, telithromycin entered the market in 2004. Ketolides are 14-membered semisynthetic derivatives of erythromycin A [4], which is characterized by the replacement of the neutral L-cladinose sugar at the third position of the ring with a 3-keto functional group and the addition of a heteroaryl-alkyl side chain attached to the macrocyclic ring (Fig. 1). The attachment of heteroaryl-alkyl side chain to the macrocyclic ring allows an additional binding to the ribosome and significantly enhances their affinity for the ribosomes [5]. The absence of cladinose also prevents ketolides from acting as inducers of macrolide-lincosamide-streptograminB (MLSB) resistance [5]. Additionally, this structural modification accounts for improved pharmacokinetic properties of ketolides including acid stability and higher lipophilicity when compared with 14-membered macrolides [6]. However, in 2007, FDA made a decision to restrict telithromycin's use to CAP and dropped other indications such as treatment of acute sinusitis and acute exacerbation of chronic bronchitis due to concerns with its serious toxicities from post-marketing reports [7]. Severe and irreversible, in some cases, fatal hepatotoxicity as well as other safety issues such as life-threatening respiratory failure in patients with myasthenia gravis, visual disturbances, loss of consciousness, and QTc prolongation have tempered its use in clinical practice [5, 8, 9].

While the etiology of telithromycin's hepatotoxicity or whether it is a class effect is not known [10], there are three other ketolides that progressed to the clinical trials for CAP: cethromycin (ABT-773) which completed phase III; solithromycin (CEM-101) in phase III; and modithromycin (EDP-420) in phase II trials in Japan [11]. The development of cethromycin began in 1997 and a New Drug Application was submitted to FDA in 2008 seeking its approval for the treatment of CAP. However, FDA's Anti-Infective Drugs Advisory Committee denied its approval pending more evidences for its efficacy in the treatment of CAP in 2009 while it was voted in favor of the safety profile [12]. Modithromycin, a novel bicyclolide possesses a C6,11-bridged ether of a 14-membered macrolide ring containing a pyrazole-pyridine side chain at the bridged-linker [13]. Solithromycin was synthesized by introducing a different type of heteroaryl-alkyl side chain from telithromycin, i.e., 11,12-carbamate-butyl-[1–3]-triazolyl-aminophenyl side chain, and by adding a fluorine atom to C2 of the macrocyclic lactone ring [14].

2 Mechanism of Action for Antibacterial Activity

All agents in these classes exert their antibacterial activities by blocking RNA-dependent protein synthesis within 50S subunit of bacterial ribosomes [5]. Macrolides and ketolides prevent the formation of functional 50S subunits by inhibiting the assembly of several ribosomal proteins and two ribosomal RNA (rRNA) molecules (5S and 23S) [15, 16]. More importantly, macrolides bind to the peptidyl transferase loop in domain V and to hairpin 35 in domain II of the 23S ribosomal RNA (rRNA) in the 50S subunit [17]. These two regions are thought to be folded closely together in the 23S rRNA tertiary structure and form a binding pocket for macrolides, azalides, and ketolides. Binding to peptidyl transferase loop blocks the translocation of the peptidyl transfer RNA (tRNA) from the amino acid site to the polypeptide site [18]. Ketolides were synthesized from erythromycin A by replacing cladinose with a keto-group at C3 and adding a flexible, heteroaryl-alkyl side chain attached to the macrocyclic ring. Extension of heteroaryl-alkyl side chain contributed to enhanced affinity to ribosomal domain II as well as IV and the lack of cladinose reduced the recognition by the *mef* efflux pump [14, 19]. These unique characteristics of ketolides translate to their improved antibacterial activity and susceptibility to resistance. Solithromycin's fluorine at the C2 position of the 14-membered macrocyclic ring improves its capacity to bind to the Erm-methylated ribosomes [14]. Also, solithromycin's heteroaryl-alkyl side chain with the aminophenyl moiety demonstrated stronger interaction with A752 compared with telithromycin [14].

3 In Vitro Antibacterial Spectrum and Potency

In vitro minimal inhibitory concentration (MIC) testing does not account for the active metabolites of antibacterials and may underestimate the activity of antibacterials such as clarithromycin when considering its potency against *Haemophilus influenzae* (*H. influenzae*) [2]. Moreover, the MIC does not account for the pharmacokinetic and pharmacodynamic properties of an antibacterial such as tissue distribution, intracellular half-life and post antibiotic effect (PAE); thus, in vivo efficacy at the site of infection may not always be predicted relatively to MIC for the macrolides, azalides, and ketolides [2].

The MIC_{50} and MIC_{90} of macrolides, azalides, and ketolides from various surveillance studies are compiled in Tables 1 and 2 [20–31]. Erythromycin, when first developed, had good activity against common community-acquired respiratory pathogens such as streptococci and atypical bacteria. Azithromycin is intrinsically more potent against gram-negative pathogens such as *H. influenzae* and *Moraxella catarrhalis* (*M. catarrhalis*) compared to erythromycin and clarithromycin, but less potent against *Streptococcus pneumoniae* (*S. pneumoniae*) compared to macrolides. Since the extensive usage of macrolides and azalides during the last two decades resulted in significant increase in the resistance rates among gram-positive cocci including the development of multidrug-resistant *Streptococcus pneumoniae* (MDRSP) worldwide [20, 21], in vitro ketolides activities were evaluated based on an enhanced mechanism of action for the compound class. Macrolide resistance are predominantly due to two mechanisms: (1) structural modification of the ribosomal target site by methylation mediated primarily by *erm*(B) and (2) efflux pumps mediated by *mef*(A) [27]. The first mechanism by *erm*(B) confers high-level (MIC_{90} ≥64 mg/L) resistance and is shared by macrolide, lincosamides, and streptogramins since

Table 1
In vitro activity of macrolides, azalides, and ketolides against gram-positive organisms

Organism	Antibacterial agent	MIC (mg/L) MIC50	MIC90	Range	References	Isolates collection
Streptococcus pneumoniae	Erythromycin	≤0.06	256	≤0.06 to ≥256	[26]	2003–2004, US
	Clarithromycin	≤0.03	128	≤0.03 to ≥256	[26]	2003–2004, US
	Azithromycin	0.12	256	≤0.03 to ≥256	[26]	2003–2004, US
	Telithromycin	≤0.25	0.5	≤0.015 to ≥4	[20]	2009, US/Europe
	Cethromycin	0.008	0.06	≤0.004–16	[27]	1994–2000, North America
	Solithromycin	≤0.03	0.12	≤0.03–1	[20]	2009, US/Europe
	Modithromycin	≤0.063	0.125	≤0.063–0.5	[21]	2006, Japan
Streptococcus pyogenes	Erythromycin	≤0.063	16	≤0.063 to >64	[21]	2006, Japan
	Clarithromycin	≤0.063	8	≤0.063 to >64	[21]	2006, Japan
	Azithromycin	≤0.063	8	≤0.063 to >64	[21]	2006, Japan
	Telithromycin	≤0.063	0.5	≤0.063 to >8	[21]	2006, Japan
	Solithromycin	0.015	0.06	0.008–0.25	[30]	2012–2013, North America
	Modithromycin	≤0.063	0.125	≤0.063–0.25	[21]	2006, Japan
Staphylococcus aureus (methicillin-susceptible)	Erythromycin	0.5	>2	≤0.25 to >2	[20]	2009, US/Europe
	Clarithromycin	0.25	>64	≤0.063 to >64	[21]	2006, Japan
	Azithromycin	0.5	>64	0.25 to >64	[21]	2006, Japan
	Telithromycin	≤0.25	≤0.25	≤0.25 to >2	[20]	2009, US/Europe
	Cethromycin				[25]	2003, Italy
	Solithromycin	0.06	0.06	≤0.03 to >4	[20]	2009, US/Europe
	Modithromycin	0.125	0.125	≤0.063 to >64	[21]	2006, Japan
Staphylococcus aureus (methicillin-resistant)	Erythromycin	>2	>2	≤0.25 to >2	[20]	2009, US/Europe
	Telithromycin	≤0.25	>2	≤0.25 to >2	[20]	2009, US/Europe
	Solithromycin	0.06	>4	≤0.03 to >4	[20]	2009, US/Europe
Enterococcus faecalis	Erythromycin	>2	>2	≤0.25 to >2	[20]	2009, US/Europe
	Telithromycin	≤0.25	>2	≤0.25 to >2	[20]	2009, US/Europe
	Solithromycin	0.06	2	≤0.03 to >4	[20]	2009, US/Europe
Enterococcus faecium	Erythromycin	>2	>2	≤0.25 to >2	[20]	2009, US/Europe
	Telithromycin	>2	>2	≤0.25 to >2	[20]	2009, US/Europe
	Solithromycin	2	4	≤0.03 to >4	[20]	2009, US/Europe

Table 2
In vitro activity of macrolides, azalides, and ketolides against gram-negative and atypical organisms

Organism	Antibacterial agent	MIC (mg/L) MIC50	MIC90	Range	References	Isolates Collection
Haemophilus influenzae β-lactamase positive	Erythromycin	8	16	2–16	[22]	1999–2000, US
	Clarithromycin	8	16	2 to >32	[20]	2009, US/Europe
	Azithromycin	1	4	≤0.5 to >4	[20]	2009, US/Europe
	Telithromycin	2	4	0.5 to >8	[20]	2009, US/Europe
	Cethromycin	4	4	1–8	[22]	1999–2000, US
	Solithromycin	1	2	0.12 to >16	[20]	2009, US/Europe
	Modithromycin[a]	4	8	1–16	[21]	2006, Japan
Haemophilus. influenzae β-lactamase negative	Erythromycin	8	16	2 to >16	[22]	1999–2000, US
	Clarithromycin	8	16	≤0.25 to >32	[20]	2009, US/Europe
	Azithromycin	1	2	≤0.5 to >4	[20]	2009, US/Europe
	Telithromycin	2	4	0.12 to >8	[20]	2009, US/Europe
	Cethromycin	4	4	1–8	[22]	1999–2000, US
	Solithromycin	1	2	0.12 to >16	[20]	2009, US/Europe
	Modithromycin[a]	4	8	1–16	[21]	2006, Japan
Moraxella catarrhalis	Erythromycin	0.12	0.25	≤0.06–0.5	[20]	2009, US/Europe
	Clarithromycin	≤0.25	≤0.25	0.25–0.5	[22]	1999–2000, US
	Azithromycin	0.125	0.125	0.06–0.25	[22]	1999–2000, US
	Telithromycin	0.12	0.25	≤0.06–0.25	[20]	2009, US/Europe
	Cethromycin	0.125	0.25	0.125–0.5	[22]	1999–2000, US
	Solithromycin	0.06	0.12	≤0.008–0.25	[20]	2009, US/Europe
	Modithromycin	≤0.25	0.5	≤0.063–1	[21]	2006, Japan
Legionella pneumophila	Erythromycin	0.25	1	0.125–2	[21]	2006, Japan
	Clarithromycin	0.031	0.063	0.016–0.125	[21]	2006, Japan
	Azithromycin	0.125	1	0.063–2	[21]	2006, Japan
	Telithromycin	0.125	0.125	0.031–0.25	[21]	2006, Japan
	Solithromycin[b]	≤0.015	0.031	≤0.015–0.063	[28]	1980–2011, Canada
	Modithromycin	0.031	0.031	0.016–0.25	[21]	2006, Japan

Mycoplasma pneumoniae	Erythromycin	≤0.001	≤0.004	≤0.001–0.016	[23]	1987–1999, US
	Clarithromycin	≤0.001	≤0.001	≤0.001–0.004	[23]	1987–1999, US
	Azithromycin	≤0.001	≤0.001	≤0.001	[23]	1987–1999, US
	Telithromycin	<0.001	0.001	<0.001 to ≥32	[29]	1992–2006, US
	Cethromycin	≤0.001	≤0.001	≤0.001–0.016	[23]	1987–1999, US
	Solithromycin	<0.001	<0.001	<0.001–0.5	[29]	1992–2006, US
Chlamydophila pneumoniae	Erythromycin	0.125	0.25	0.015–0.25	[24]	US/Japan
	Clarithromycin	0.06	0.06	0.015–0.06	[31]	US/Japan
	Azithromycin	0.125	0.125	0.015–0.125	[31]	US/Japan
	Telithromycin	0.06	0.06	0.015–0.25	[31]	US/Japan
	Solithromycin	0.25	0.25	0.25–1.0	[31]	US/Japan

[a]β-lactamase positive and negative combined
[b]Serogroup 1 only

these antibacterials target the same site of action in 50S subunit of bacterial ribosomes. *Erm* expression is either constitutive ($cMLS_B$) or inducible ($iMLS_B$), which means the presence of an inducing antibacterial is required for enzyme production [32]. *Mef*(A) gene encodes the efflux pump and does not affect the lincosamide or streptogramins. Contrary to *erm*(B), it results in low-level (MIC_{90} 4 mg/L) macrolide resistance [3]. Structural modification of ketolides allowed them to remain active against macrolide- and azalide-resistant streptococci. However, telithromycin has intrinsically low activity against *H. influenzae*, which is attributed to intrinsic efflux pumps acting in synergy with slow penetration through the bacterial outer membrane [33]. From PROTEKT (Prospective Resistant Organism Tracking and Epidemiology for the Ketolide Telithromycin) US study [26], telithromycin demonstrated potent in vitro activity against *S. pneumoniae* isolates including *erm*(B) plus *mef*(A) macrolide-resistant strains. Even though telithromycin still remained active with MIC_{90} of 0.06 against *Streptococcus pyogenes* (*S. pyogenes*) in 2004–2005, its resistance to *S. pyogenes* had increased from 1.2 % in 2002–2003 ($n = 2165$) to 4.7 % in 2004–2005 ($n = 2333$) [34]. Ketolides' resistance in *S. pyogenes* has been investigated in relation to methylation mediated by *erm* genes; isolates with fully dimethylated A2058 mediated by *erm*(B) showed highest MIC while the strains with monomethylated rRNA remained susceptible to ketolides [35]. Also, telithromycin exhibited higher MIC against $cMLS_B$-resistant streptococci than against the strains with $iMLS_B$ resistance [36]. Cethromycin showed increased potency against methicillin-susceptible *Staphylococcus aureus* (MSSA), *S. pneumoniae*, *Enterococcus faecalis (E. faecalis)*, and *M. catarrhalis* compared with erythromycin, clarithromycin, and azithromycin [25]. It was not active against either *Enterococcus faecium* or methicillin-resistant *Staphylococcus aureus* (MRSA). Solithromycin demonstrated more potent activity against gram-positive (*S. pneumoniae*, *β-hemolytic streptococci, viridans group streptococci*, MSSA, and *E. faecalis*) and gram-negative organisms (*H. influenzae* and *M. catarrhalis*) compared with telithromycin [20]. While its MIC_{50} was 0.12 mg/L for all 45 hospital-acquired and 30 community-acquired MRSA isolates, MIC_{90} was >16 mg/L consistent with other macrolides and ketolides [37]. Its potency against *H. influenzae* was comparable to azithromycin [20]. Modithromycin displayed comparable potency to telithromycin against gram-positives (*S. pneumoniae*, *S. pyogenes*, MSSA), but reduced potency against *H. influenzae* compared to telithromycin or azithromycin [13, 21]. All agents in macrolides, azalides, and ketolides classes have potent in vitro activity against atypical respiratory pathogens such as *Legionella pneumophila*, *Mycoplasma pneumoniae*, and *Chlamydophila pneumoniae*.

4 Pharmacokinetics

Erythromycin salts/esters show variable bioavailability depending on the formulations and are affected by food since acid degrades erythromycin base and stearate while it increases the absorption of ethylsuccinate [38]. Structural modification to clarithromycin, azithromycin, and ketolides overcomes the instability to acidity and poor bioavailability of erythromycin, which allows their dosages to be administered without regards to meals. The pharmacokinetic parameters after a single and multiple doses of erythromycin base, clarithromycin, azithromycin, and ketolides are summarized in Tables 3 and 4, respectively [3, 38–40]. The peak serum concentration of azithromycin is lower than that of the comparable doses of clarithromycin or telithromycin, but it has higher tissue concentration as reflected in the large volume of distribution. Clarithromycin, azithromycin, and ketolides also have a prolonged terminal half-life compared to erythromycin. Clarithromycin is metabolized to an active metabolite, 14-hydroxyclarithromycin. Large doses of clarithromycin yields nonlinear increases in terminal half-life as the metabolic pathway becomes saturated [2].

All ketolides and macrolides demonstrate dose-dependent plasma protein binding (PPB); PPB decreases with increasing concentrations as the binding sites of plasma proteins become saturated [41, 42]. In a murine model, telithromycin's PPB ranged from 94.6 to 69.8 % for serum concentrations of 2–25 mg/L, while in human it was reported to be approximately 90 % [43].

Table 3
Pharmacokinetic parameters in plasma after a single oral dose

Drug	Dose (mg)	C_{max} (mg/L)	AUC_{24} (mg·h/L)	$t_{1/2\beta}$ (h)	CL (L/h)	V_d (L)	References
Erythromycin base	500	0.3–0.9	8	2–3			[38]
Clarithromycin	500	1.8	12.4	3.7	21.9	117.0	[3]
14-Hydroxy metabolite of clarithromycin	[a]	0.6	5.7	4–7			[38]
Azithromycin	500	0.3	2.6	55.5	40	3083.3	[3]
Telithromycin	800	1.9	8.3	7.16–13	50.9	530.2	[3]
Cethromycin	150	0.3	1.6	5.7	54.5	450	[3]
Solithromycin	400	0.6	4.8	4.8			[39]
Modithromycin	400	0.5	8.1	17.4			[40]

AUC_{24} area under the concentration–time curve from time zero to 24 h, *CL* apparent total body clearance, C_{max} maximum plasma concentration, $t_{1/2\beta}$ terminal elimination half-life, V_d apparent volume of distribution
[a]After 500 mg of clarithromycin

Table 4
Pharmacokinetic parameters in plasma after multiple oral doses

Drug	Dose (mg)	C_{max} (mg/L)	AUC_{∞} (mg h/L)	$t_{1/2\beta}$ (h)	CL (L/h)	V_d (L)	References
Clarithromycin	500 mg bid × 4 days	2.9	20.8	4.8	13.2	91.8	[3]
Azithromycin	500 mg × 1, then 250 mg qd × 4 days	0.23	15.9	66.1	11.1	1114.5	[3]
Telithromycin	800 mg qd × 7 days	2.27	12.6	9.8	28.7	512.4	[3]
Cethromycin	300 mg qd × 5 days	0.5	3.23	4.94	107.4	769	[3]
Solithromycin	400 mg qd × 7 days	1.09	13.27[a]	7.47			[39]
Modithromycin	400 mg × 1, then 200 mg qd × 2 days	5.1	15.1	17.7			[40]

AUC_{∞} area under the concentration–time curve from time zero to infinity, *bid* twice daily, *CL* apparent total body clearance, C_{max} = maximum plasma concentration, *qd* once daily, $t_{1/2\beta}$ terminal elimination half-life, V_d apparent volume of distribution
[a]Reported as AUC during the dosing interval of 24 h

PPB of clarithromycin is reported to be approximately 70 % of serum concentration [38].

The longer half-life of these drugs is also a result of their extensive tissue penetration [44]; macrolides, azalides, and ketolides are lipophilic and penetrate extensively into mammalian tissue, especially pulmonary tissue. The active metabolite of clarithromycin, 14-hydroxyclarithromycin also penetrates well into pulmonary tissue but to a lesser degree than the parent compound [44]. Azithromycin has particularly slow elimination, which is presumed to be due to the slow efflux of azithromycin from the cellular compartment into extracellular fluid [45]. Therefore, the long half-life of azithromycin is really an estimate of the half-life of tissue elimination [46]. The high degree of penetration into epithelial lining fluid of these agents adds to their clinical effectiveness against extracellular respiratory pathogens, such as *S. pneumoniae*, *H. influenzae*, and *M. catarrhalis*. Additionally, their penetration into alveolar macrophages (AM) provides an advantage as treatment options for infections caused by intracellular organisms such as *Chlamydophila pneumoniae* and *Legionella sp.* Concentrations of macrolides, azalides, and ketolides in plasma, epithelial lining fluid (ELF) and alveolar macrophage (AM) are summarized in Table 5 [41, 47–53]. Like in healthy subjects, the ELF and AM concentrations derived from patients who underwent diagnostic bronchoscopy were approximately 10-times and 100-times higher than in the plasma (Table 5). Compared to azithromycin's ELF concentration of 0.9 [52] or 2.18 mg/L [48] which were lower than MIC_{90} of 256 mg/L against *S. pneumoniae*, all four ketolides achieved

Table 5
Concentrations in plasma, ELF, and AM in healthy subjects and patients undergoing diagnostic bronchoscopy[a]

	Dose	C_{max} (T_{max}), plasma (mg/L)	C_{max} (T_{max}), ELF (mg/L)	C_{max} (T_{max}), AM (mg/L)	References
Erythromycin	250 mg qid × 9 doses	0.7 (4 h)	0.8 (4 h)	0.8 (12 h)	[47]
Clarithromycin	500 mg bid × 5 days	2.0 (4 h)	34.5 (4 h)	480 (4 h)	[48]
Azithromycin	500 mg × 1, then 250 mg qd × 4 days	0.09 (8 h)	2.18 (8 h)	57.2 (8 h)	[48]
		0.1 (4 h)[a]	0.9 (12 h)[a]	205.2 (24 h)[a]	[52]
Telithromycin	800 mg qd × 5 days	1.14 (2 h)	5.5 (2 h)	81 (8 h)	[49]
		1.09 (2 h)[a]	3.91 (2 h)[a]	65.96 (12 h)[a]	[53]
Cethromycin	300 mg qd × 5 days	0.38 (4 h)	2.7 (4 h)	55.4 (6 h)	[41]
Solithromycin	400 mg qd × 5 days	0.730 (3 h)	7.58 (3 h)	101.7 (6 h)	[50]
Modithromycin	400 mg × 1 dose	0.646 (2 h)	16.7 (2 h)	176 (12 h)	[51]

ELF epithelial lining fluid, *AM* alveolar macrophages, *CL* apparent total body clearance, C_{max} maximum concentration, T_{max} time between the last dose and sampling time, *qd* once daily, *bid* twice daily, *qid* four times daily, $t_{1/2\beta}$ = terminal elimination half-life, V_d apparent volume of distribution
[a]Data from patients undergoing diagnostic bronchoscopy

higher ELF concentrations and they were well above their respective MIC_{90} against *S. pneumoniae* (Tables 1 and 5). On the other hand, clarithromycin, azithromycin, and all ketolides achieved AM concentrations well above the MIC_{90} against intracellular organisms (Tables 2 and 5). Even though the mechanisms behind high concentrations of these agents in ELF and AM have not been fully elucidated, the cellular antibacterial uptake and back-release has been suggested [50]; neutrophilic granulocytes, macrophages, and connective tissue cells such as fibroblasts are believed to serve as reservoirs for these agents. There is also a report about MDR1 transporters on alveolar epithelial cells as well as the high uptake by the AMs via active transport mechanisms being responsible for the increased disposition of clarithromycin and azithromycin from blood into ELF [54].

5 Pharmacodynamics

5.1 Discussion of Pharmacodynamic Targets of Class

Antibacterial activity has been described to be dependent on the concentration, time of exposure, or a product of the two. When both of the factors impact antibacterial activity, the effectiveness is considered to be driven by the overall exposure (i.e., the area under the concentration–time curve, AUC). Thus commonly used pharmacodynamic parameters to predict antibacterial efficacy are the ratio of maximum concentration to MIC (C_{max}/

MIC), the percent of the time during which concentrations are above the MIC (%T > MIC), as well as the ratio of the AUC over MIC (AUC/MIC) [44]. While certain antibacterial activity can be predominantly predicted by one pharmacodynamic parameter, there are cases where antibacterial activity is closely correlated to more than one parameter since these parameters are highly interdependent. Whether bacterial killing is concentration dependent or concentration independent, the relatively long, persistent PAE of macrolides, azalides, and ketolides often renders the AUC/MIC to be most predictive of their efficacy as long as dosing intervals are 24 h or less [55].

5.2 Concentrations at the Infection Site

Typically drug concentrations in blood are used to determine the pharmacodynamic parameters that best predict antibacterial effects. However, the use of drug concentrations in blood is only reasonable if the blood concentration is a proper surrogate for drug concentration at the site of infection. Drug concentrations at the site of infections can be much different than the free drug concentrations in plasma depending on the ratio of surface area of the capillary bed to volume of the tissue compartment, special anatomic barriers such as blood–brain barrier, and the physiochemical characteristic of the drug [56]. As noted in Table 5, the macrolides, azalides, and ketolides penetrate extensively into target extracellular and intracellular sites of the respiratory tract. Therefore, the pharmacodynamic parameters derived from the actual site of infection, i.e., ELF and AM, may predict the antibacterial activity of these agents for respiratory tract infections more accurately than the parameters derived from blood concentrations [55]. Moreover, blood concentrations appear to be poorly predictive of the intracellular concentrations which are necessary for the treatment of intracellular pathogens [56].

5.3 Role of White Blood Cells

The ability of white blood cells to transport macrolides, azalides, and ketolides may contribute to their efficacy despite relatively low plasma concentration [55]. In vitro studies have shown that azithromycin concentrates 500-folds in human neutrophils and migrate toward a bacterial stimulus and release the active drug [57, 58]. Double-layer plates were made by pouring a layer of chemotaxis agarose into tissue culture plates and then adding a thin layer of trypticase soy agar [58]. Neutrophils were incubated with antibiotic for 1 h, then were allowed to migrate under the agar toward a chemoattractant well containing formyl-methionine-leucine-phenylalanine for 3 h. Then, *Streptococcus pyogenes* was plated on top of the agar and grown overnight. When the polymorphonuclear neutrophils (PMN) migration and the zones of inhibition of bacterial growth were measured, neutrophils migrated 2.51 ± 0.16 mm toward the chemoattractant well and 1.48 ± 0.12 mm toward the control well; migration was not significantly influenced by any of the antibiotics used. However, for PMN incubated with azithromycin (3 pg/ml), an agent highly concentrated inside phagocytes, a large degree of inhibition which was significantly greater in the direction of chemoattractant than in the direction of medium (3.47 ± 0.30 versus 1.89 ± 0.25 mm; $P < 0.001$) was observed, indicating that bioactive azithromycin was released by neutrophils after migration. Ketolides were also shown to accumulate in PMN, and it was suggested that despite varying chemical structure, all erythromycin A derivatives have a transmembrane transport system in common [59]. In vivo studies also supported these observations [60]. After administering 50 mg/kg of oral azithromycin treatment, 0.05 μg of azithromycin was found in peritoneal fluids of mice 20 h later. Following caseinate-induced PMN infiltration, the azithromycin concentration in peritoneal cavity increased by sixfold to 0.32 μg. Therefore, it was concluded that the uptake, transport and later release of azithromycin by neutrophils may contribute to the delivery of active drug to sites of infection.

5.4 Post Antibiotic Effect (PAE)

PAE is a term to describe the prolonged bacterial growth inhibition of antibacterials after the short exposure against the damaged but viable organisms under the influence of host immune system [61]. PAE has been characterized for macrolides, azalides, and ketolides [61–66]; the duration of this effect varies depending on the drug, isolates, concentration and duration of exposure (Table 6). For example, azithromycin has exhibited longer in vitro PAEs against *H. influenzae* than against *S. pneumoniae* [61]. While macrolides have shown time-dependent bacterial killing [18], prolonged PAE makes their efficacy rely less on time, but more on AUC once their maximum concentrations exceed the MIC [56]. On the other hand, azithromycin and ketolides exhibit concentration-dependent bactericidal action and prolonged PAE [46]. Both the bactericidal action and duration of PAE for these drugs are concentration-dependent.

Table 6
Post antibiotic effects (hours) of macrolides, azalides, and ketolides

	S. pneumoniae	*S. pyogenes*	*H. influenzae*	References
Erythromycin	10	0.5		[62]
Clarithromycin	2.9	4.8	5.1	[61]
Azithromycin	4.7	4.1	8.0	[61]
Telithromycin	1.9	3.4	1.2	[65]
Cethromycin	2.3–6		2.7–9.1	[64]
Solithromycin	3.0	6.1	3.2	[65]

5.5 Immunomodulatory/Anti-Inflammatory Effects

In addition to their antibacterial activity, macrolides, azalides, and ketolides possess immunomodulatory effect, which adds more beneficial effects on infectious and/or noninfectious inflammatory respiratory conditions [67]. Multiple mechanisms were identified for their anti-inflammatory effect: inhibition of pro-inflammatory cytokine production such as CXCL8 (interleukin-8) and tumor necrosis factor-α (TNF-α) [68]; inhibition of a neutrophil chemotactic mediator, leukotriene B_4 [69]; reduction in mucus secretion in the airways [70]; and inhibition of pro-inflammatory transcription factors such as nuclear factor-κB (NF-κB) [67, 71, 72], just to name a few. Solithromycin appears to exert superior anti-inflammatory effect via NF-κB inhibition compared to erythromycin, clarithromycin, azithromycin, and telithromycin [67].

5.6 Pharmacodynamic Driver and Required Magnitudes

Erythromycin has been categorized as time-dependent agent by most investigators [44, 73]. When used in murine thigh infection model, erythromycin showed a trend for increased survival with multiple-dosing regimen compared to a single dose regimen of the same daily dose with significantly higher survival when the concentrations sustained above MIC for a longer period of time [73]. The minimum amount of time that is required for optimal efficacy varied, but it was suggested that 50 % T > MIC should be sufficient in immunocompetent patients [44]. For clarithromycin, the interdependence among the pharmacodynamic parameters seems more apparent than other macrolides or ketolides [44]. Some investigators found it to be time-dependent agent for its antibacterial efficacy [74] while others observed its concentration-dependent antibacterial effect [73]. Furthermore, some positioned the clarithromycin in between erythromycin and azithromycin [75], possessing elements of both concentration dependence and independence.

Tessier et al. assessed the pharmacodynamic profile of clarithromycin in a neutropenic murine pneumonia model against *S. pneumoniae* with various susceptibility profiles [76]. They found that %T > MIC, AUC/MIC, and C_{max}/MIC are all closely correlated to bacterial killing and survival ($P < 0.001$). Efficacy for bacteriostatic effect was detected at approximately 50 % T > MIC, AUC_{0-24}/MIC of 40, and C_{max}/MIC of 7 while 90 % T > MIC, AUC_{0-24}/MIC of 200, and C_{max}/MIC of 12 were more consistent with bactericidal effects. As a result of parameter interdependency, the authors concluded that AUC/MIC is the most reasonable predictor of antibacterial efficacy for clarithromycin since it incorporates both T > MIC and C_{max}/MIC.

In contrast to erythromycin or clarithromycin, AUC/MIC is considered to be the most predictive pharmacodynamic parameter of azithromycin's antibacterial efficacy [74, 77]. Some investigators speculated that azithromycin's prolonged PAE reduces its dependence on the extent of time for which it should remain above the MIC [61].

Telithromycin has shown a greater dependence on concentration rather than time [78]. In an in vitro time-kill study, Boswell et al. showed concentration-dependent efficacy of telithromycin against *S. aureus, S. pneumoniae, S. pyogenes, E. faecalis, E. faecium, and H. influenzae* in both time-kill curves and PAE profiles [78]. In an in vivo neutropenic murine thigh model using *S. pneumoniae* isolates with telithromycin MIC $\leq$ 0.5 mg/L, *f*AUC/MIC in serum was predictive of its antibacterial activity ($r^2 = 0.86$); *f*AUC/MIC of 200 was required for bacteriostatic effect and >1000 for 95 % of the maximum antibacterial effects (ED_{95}) [42]. fC_{max}/MIC was also predictive of reduction in bacterial density ($r^2 = 0.84$) while %T > MIC had relatively poor goodness of fit ($r^2 = 0.61$) compared to other parameters. Similarly to telithromycin, cethromycin (ABT-773) has demonstrated concentration-dependent bacterial killing. In a neutropenic murine pneumonia model, bactericidal activity of cethromycin against *S. pneumoniae* was evaluated [79]. All three pharmacodynamic parameters (i.e., %T > MIC, AUC/MIC, C_{max}/MIC) were significantly correlated with changes in $\log_{10}$ CFU. However, both fC_{max}/MIC and *f*AUC/MIC had better correlation when the goodness of fit was assessed with the E_{max} model (both $r^2 = 0.81$) compared to %*f*T > MIC ($r^2 = 0.61$). The authors identified an approximate *f*AUC/MIC of 50 or fC_{max}/MIC of 1 for bacteriostatic target and *f*AUC/MIC of 1000 or fC_{max}/MIC of 100 for maximal bactericidal activity. When the similar model was used to compare the pharmacodynamic parameters in immunocompetent versus neutropenic mice, the *f*AUC/MIC ratios required for bacteriostatic effect were 8 and 20 for immunocompetent versus neutropenic mice, respectively [80]. For bactericidal activity, *f*AUC/MIC ratios of 32 and 129 were required for immunocompetent and neutropenic mice, respectively [80]. Like in other ketolides, *f*AUC/MIC was the key pharmacodynamic driver for modithromycin regardless of phenotypic or genotypic profile to macrolides and penicillin when evaluated in a neutropenic pneumococcal murine pneumonia model [81]. The *f*AUC/MIC required for stasis and 1 log CFU reduction in bacterial density were 4–53 and 9–69, respectively.

5.7 Pharmacokinetic and Pharmacodynamic (PK/PD) Application

Pneumococcal resistance to macrolides as defined by laboratory criteria has increased rapidly over the past two decades in parallel with their wide utilization in clinical practice. Despite these recognized resistance trends, the macrolides and azalides still appear to provide high rates of clinical cure in the setting of community-acquired respiratory tract infections. The disparity between in vitro resistance and in vivo efficacy has been a topic of discussion for some time in the pneumonia patient since the mortality rate has remained constant despite the drastic increase in antimicrobial resistance rates [82]. For example, in pneumococcal pneumonia, a mortality rate of 13 % was reported from 1952 to 1962 when there was no drug-resistant *S. pneumoniae* (DRSP) [83] and remained similar at 12 % from 1995 to 1997 despite a prevalence of 18 % DRSP [82, 84]. Macrolide treatment failures in bacteremic pneumococcal pneumonia has been reported, but whether macrolide resistance in and of itself accounts for these failures is unknown since mortality has been well recognized in patient with pneumococcus that is fully susceptible to antimicrobials [85].

The clinical success observed with the macrolides and azalides in the face of resistance may in part be due to the complex pharmacodynamic profile of these agents. Since these agents penetrate extensively into target extracellular and intracellular sites of the respiratory tract and the breakpoints for susceptibility have historically been based on serum concentrations, discordance between these in vitro and in vivo efficacy profiles is not unexpected [86]. While the pharmacodynamic parameters derived from the actual site of infection (i.e., ELF and AM) may be a better predictor of the probability of a successful outcome, pharmacokinetic studies to determine the ELF and AM concentration–time profile require an invasive sampling strategy and are therefore difficult to conduct in patients. Moreover, when interpreting ELF concentrations, one needs to consider that the concentrations in ELF are greatly influenced by the study design, sample collection timing, analytical methods, and mathematical modeling [87].

In an attempt to better understand the implications of in vitro resistance when considering concentrations at the site of infections, investigators have attempted to use ex vivo modeling systems simulating humanized exposures in target tissues or fluids. Using an in vitro pharmacodynamic model, Zhanel et al. simulated the serum, ELF, and middle ear fluid concentration profiles of azithromycin at a dose of 500 mg by mouth on day 1 and 250 mg on day 2 [88]. With macrolide-susceptible (azithromycin MIC 0.06 mg/L) *S. pneumoniae*, 100 % *f*T > MIC and $fAUC_{0\text{-}24}$/MIC of 36.7 were reached in serum and 100 % *f*T > MIC and $fAUC_{0\text{-}24}$/MIC of 153 were reached in ELF and middle ear fluid. In all three sites, bacterial density decreased by ≥4 log10 CFU/ml at 24 and 48 h compared to 0 h. However, against azithromycin-resistant *S. pneumoniae* (MIC 2 mg/L), azithromycin showed no bacterial growth inhibition at resultant 0 % *f*T > MIC and $fAUC_{0\text{-}24}$/MIC of ≤1.1 in serum, whereas 0 % *f*T > MIC and $fAUC_{0\text{-}24}$/MIC of 4.6 in ELF and middle ear fluid led to bacteriostatic effect (decrease in bacterial density of 0.2–0.5 $\log_{10}$ CFU/ml at 24 h). Namely, in the absence of functional immune system of the host or the immunomodulatory effects of the compound on the host pneumococcus, this in vitro pharmacodynamic model failed to show the antibacterial effect corresponding to achieved tissue concentrations against the isolate with low-level resistance (MIC=2 mg/L).

In direct contrast to these in vitro observations the same author reported a poor correlation between azithromycin resistance as determined by the current breakpoints and clinical outcome in patients treated with azithromycin for community-acquired respiratory tract infections caused by azithromycin-susceptible or -resistant *S. pneumoniae* [89]. In patients with CAP or acute bacterial exacerbations of chronic bronchitis, there were no differences in cure rates when low-level or high-level azithromycin resistance was considered. On the other hand, in patients with acute bacterial sinusitis and acute otitis media, azithromycin resistance in *S. pneumoniae* resulted in statistically significant increase in clinical failure, although cure rates were not different for patients infected with low-level or high-level resistant isolates. Moreover, the authors reported that at the observed azithromycin resistance rate of nearly 30 %, an additional 3.1 clinical failures per 100 patients would be predicted as a consequence of the compound's phenotypic resistance profile. Once again, the lack of a consistent association between the absolute azalide resistance rate in *S. pneumoniae* and clinical failure in this immunocompetent patient population is related to the composite effects of azithromycin's unique PK/PD properties including the high concentration in ELF/AM, PAE and immunomodulatory activity.

While the utilization of animal infection models has provided great insight into the pharmacodynamic profile of a wide range of antimicrobial agents, as a result of the complex pharmacodynamic profile of the macrolides, azalides, and ketolides, discordance has been observed regarding the required exposure to drive microbiologic and clinical cures between species. For example, when PK/PD were evaluated in patients with CAP who received 800 mg daily dose of telithromycin, the microbiological breakpoint for increased probability of successful outcome was AUC/MIC ratio of ≥3.375 [90], which was much lower than the targets derived from the animal model [42]. Although the reasons for the difference in the identified targets between the animal model and the clinical CAP patients are likely multifactorial, the difference in the concentrations of telithromycin between that of blood and the site of infection for man and mouse, host immune competency and immunomodulatory effects are likely contributors.

These data provide insights into the complexity of the host–bug–drug interactions commonly encountered during the assessment of efficacy among the macrolides, azalides, and ketolides when considering data derived from in vitro experiments (i.e., MIC testing, in vitro pharmacodynamic modeling), in vivo models of infection and patient derived sources.

6 Notes

When considering the utilization of the macrolides, azalides, and ketolides in the setting of infection, an understanding of the local resistance profile of the agent of interest is an important factor in optimizing the probability of success. Of note, in addition to the susceptibility or resistance determination provided by the clinical laboratory, insights into the magnitude of resistance may be garnered by evaluating the susceptibility profile of clindamycin when available as resistance to both clindamycin and macrolides infers high-level macrolide resistance via the *erm*B mediated mechanism [91]. Similar to observations with other antimicrobial classes, factors that can affect macrolide-resistance include previous macrolide use, recent hospitalization and exposure to various health care setting such as a nursing home or day care.

The aim of this review was to provide the current level of understanding into the pharmacodynamic profile of the macrolides, azalides, and ketolides as determined using a variety of in vitro and in vivo experimental techniques. While these data provide great insight into the pharmacodynamic drivers of efficacy for any given compound, these same experiments provide awareness regarding the complexity of the host–bug–drug relationship as it pertains to these agents. More specifically, these studies highlight the challenges when interpreting the required magnitude of pharmacodynamic exposure to ensure good clinical and microbiologic outcomes from in vitro or in vivo modeling experiments to that in man. As a result of this complex pharmacodynamic profile, the impact of host immune competency and the immunomodulatory properties of these agents, discordance between in vitro resistance as defined in the laboratory and good clinical outcomes is likely to continue as newer agents are developed.

References

1. Mutak S (2007) Azalides from azithromycin to new azalide derivatives. J Antibiot 60(2):85–122
2. Zuckerman JM, Qamar F, Bono BR (2011) Review of macrolides (Azithromycin, Clarithromycin), ketolids (telithromycin) and glycylcyclines (tigecycline). Med Clin N Am 95:761–791
3. Zeitlinger M, Wagner CC, Heinisch B (2009) Ketolides – the modern relatives of macrolides: the pharmacokinetic perspective. Clin Pharmacokinet 48(1):23–38
4. Agouidas C, Denis A, Auger JM et al (1998) Synthesis and antibacterial activity of ketolides (6-O-methyl-3-oxoerythromycin derivatives): a new class of antibacterials highly potent against macrolide-resistant and -susceptible respiratory pathogens. J Med Chem 41(21):4080–4100
5. Van Bambeke F, Harms JM, Van Laethem Y et al (2008) Ketolides: pharmacological profile and rational positioning in the treatment of respiratory tract infections. Expert Opin Pharmacother 9(2):267–283
6. Douthwaite S, Champney WS (2001) Structures of ketolides and macrolides determine their mode of interaction with the ribosomal target site. J Antimicrob Chemother 48(Suppl T1):1–8
7. Sanofi-Aventis (2007) Ketek® (telithromycin) dear healthcare professional letter. http://www.fda.gov/downloads/safety/medwatch/safetyinformation/safetyalertsforhumanmedicalproducts/ucm154544.pdfSanofi. Accessed 10 Dec 2013
8. Clay KD, Hanson JS, Pope SD et al (2006) Brief communication: severe hepatotoxicity of telithromycin: three case reports and literature review. Ann Intern Med 144:415–420
9. Sanofi-Aventis-US (2010) Prescribing information. http://products.sanofi.us/ketek/ketek.html. Accessed 10 Dec 2013
10. Georgopapadakou NH (2014) The wobbly status of ketolides: where do we stand? Expert Opin Investig Drugs 23(10):1313–1319
11. Clinicaltrials.gov

12. Mansour H, Chahine EB, Karaoui LR et al (2013) Cethromycin: a new ketolide antibiotic. Ann Pharmacother 47:368–379
13. Sato T, Kawai Y, Matsuda H et al (2011) In vitro and in vivo antibacterial activity of modithromycin against streptococci and Haemophilus influenzae. J Antimicrob Chemother 66(7):1547–1554
14. Llano-Sotelo B, Dunkle J, Klepacki D et al (2010) Binding and action of CEM-101, a new fluoroketolide antibiotic that inhibits protein synthesis. Antimicrob Agents Chemother 54:4961–4970
15. Ban N, Nissen P, Hansen J et al (2000) The complete atomic structure of the large ribosomal subunit at 2.4 A resolution. Science 289(5481):905–920
16. Rodgers W, Frazier AD, Champney WS (2013) Solithromycin inhibition of protein synthesis and ribosome biogenesis in Staphylococcus aureus, Streptococcus pneumoniae, and Haemophilus influenzae. Antimicrob Agents Chemother 57:1632–1637
17. Hansen LH, Mauvais P, Douthwaite S (1999) The macrolide-ketolide antibiotic binding site is formed by structures in domains II and V of 23S ribosomal RNA. Mol Microbiol 31(2):623–631
18. Jain S, Bishai W, Nightingale CH (2007) Macrolide, azalide, and ketolide. In: Nightingale CH, Ambrose PG, Drusano GL et al (eds) Antimicrobial pharmacodynamics in theory and clinical practice, 2nd edn. pp. 217–230, New York, NY
19. Xiong L, Shah S, Mauvais P et al (1999) A ketolide resistance mutation in domain II of 23S rRNA reveals the proximity of hairpin 35 to the peptidyl transferase centre. Mol Microbiol 31:633–639
20. Farrell DJ, Castanheira M, Sader HS et al (2010) The in vitro evaluation of solithromycin (CEM-101) against pathogens isolated in the United States and Europe (2009). J Infect 61:476–483
21. Sato T, Tateda K, Kimura S et al (2011) In vitro antibacterial activity of modithromycin, a novel 6,11-bridged bicyclolide, against respiratory pathogens, including macrolide-resistant gram-positive cocci. Antimicrob Agents Chemother 55:1588–1593
22. Credito KL, Lin G, Pankuch GA et al (2001) Susceptibilities of Haemophilus influenza and Moraxella catarrhalis to ABT-773 compared to their susceptibilities to 11 other agents. Antimicrob Agents Chemother 45:67–72
23. Waites KB, Crabb DM, Duffy LB (2003) In vitro activities of ABT-773 and other antimicrobials against human mycoplasmas. Antimicrob Agents Chemother 47:39–72
24. Roblin PM, Hammerschlag MR (1998) In vitro activity of a new ketolide antibiotic, HMR 3647, against Chlamydia pneumoniae. Antimicrob Agents Chemother 42:1515–1516
25. Bozzolasco M, Debbia EA, Roveta S et al (2004) In vitro activity of ABT773, a new ketolide derivative exhibiting innovative microbiological properties against well-characterised antibiotic resistant pathogens in Italy. Int J Antimicrob Agent 23:11–16
26. Jenkins SG, Brown SD, Farrell DJ et al (2008) Trends in antibacterial resistance among Streptococcus pneumoniae isolated in the USA: update from Protekt US years 1-4. Ann Clin Microbiol Antimicrob 7:1–11
27. Jorgensen JH, Crawford SA, McElmeel ML et al (2004) Activities of cethromycin and telithromycin against recent North American isolates of Streptococcus pneumoniae. Antimicrob Agents Chemother 48:605–607
28. Mallegol J, Fernandes P, Melano RG et al (2014) Antimicrobial activity of solithromycin against clinical isolates of Legionella pneumophila serogroup 1. Antimicrob Agents Chemother 58(2):909–915
29. Waites KB, Crabb DM, Duffy LB (2009) Comparative in vitro susceptibilities of human mycoplasmas and ureaplasmas to a new investigational ketolide, CEM-101. Antimicrob Agents Chemother 53(5):2139–2141
30. Morrissey I, Fernandes P, Lemos B et al (2014) Activity of solithromycin and comparators against Streptococci isolated from respiratory samples collected in 2012-2013 (Abstract No. eP1584). The 24th European Congress of clinical microbiology and infectious diseases, Barcelona, Spain, May 2014.
31. Roblin PM, Kohlhoff SA, Parker C et al (2010) In vitro activity of CEM-101, a new fluoroketolide antibiotic, against Chlamydia trachomatis and Chlamydia (Chlamydophila) pneumoniae. Antimicrob Agents Chemother 54(3):1358–1359
32. Bonnefoy A, Girard AM, Aqouridas C et al (1997) Ketolides lack inducibility properties of MLS(B) resistance phenotype. J Antimicrob Chemother 40(1):85–90
33. Cao Z, Zhong P, Ruan X et al (2004) Ribosome affinity and the prolonged molecular postantibiotic effect of cethromycin (ABT-773) in Haemophilus influenzae. Int J Antimicrob Agents 24:362–368
34. Richter SS, Heilmann KP, Dohrn CL et al (2008) Increasing telithromycin resistance

among Streptococcus pyogenes in Europe. J Antimicrob Chemother 61:603–611

35. Douthwaite S, Jalava J, Jakobsen L (2005) Ketolide resistance in Streptococcus pyogenes correlates with the degree of rRNA dimethylation by ERM. Mol Microbiol 58:613–622
36. Mazzariol A, Koncan R, Vitali LA et al (2007) Activities of 16-membered ring macrolides and telithromycin against different genotypes of erythromycin-susceptible and erythromycin-resistant Streptococcus pyogenes and Streptococcus pneumoniae. J Antimicrob Chemother 59:1171–1176
37. Putnam SD, Sader HS, Farrell DJ et al (2011) Antimicrobial characterization of solithromycin (CEM-101), a novel fluoroketolide: activity against staphylococci and enterococci. Int J Antimicrob Agents 37:39–45
38. Zhanel GG, Dueck M, Hoban DJ et al (2001) Review of macrolides and ketolides focus on respiratory tract infections. Drugs 61(4): 443–498
39. Still JG, Schranz J, Degenhardt TP et al (2011) Pharmacokinetics of Solithromycin (CEM-101) after single or multiple oral doses and effects of food on single-dose bioavailability in healthy adult subjects. Antimicrob Agents Chemother 55(5):1997–2003
40. Jiang LJ, Or YS (2009) Pharmacokinetics of EDP-420 after multiple oral doses in healthy adult volunteers and in a bioequivalence study. Antimicrob Agents Chemother 53(8):3218–3225
41. Conte JE Jr, Golden JA, Kipps J et al (2004) Steady-state plasma and intrapulmonary pharmacokinetics and pharmacodynamics of cethromycin. Antimicrob Agents Chemother 48(9):3508–3515
42. Tessier PR, Mattoes HM, Dandekar PK et al (2005) Pharmacodynamic profile of telithromycin against macrolide- and fluoroquinolone-resistant Streptococcus pneumoniae in a neutropenic mouse thigh model. Antimicrob Agents Chemother 49(1):188–194
43. Gattringer R, Urbauer E, Traunmuller F et al (2004) Pharmacokinetics of telithromycin in plasma and soft tissues after single-dose administration to healthy volunteers. Antimicrob Agents Chemother 48(12):4650–4653
44. Maglio D, Nicolau DP, Nightingale CH (2003) Impact of pharmacodynamics on dosing of macrolides, azalides, and ketolides. Infect Dis Clin N Am 17:563–577
45. Johnson JD, Hand WL, Franis B et al (1980) Antibiotic uptake by alveolar macrophages. J Lab Clin Med 95:429–439
46. Nightingale CH, Mattoes HM (2002) Macrolide, azalide, and ketolide pharmacodynamics. In: Nightingale CH, Murakawa T, Ambrose PG (eds) Antimicrobial pharmacodynamics in theory and clinical practice, 1st edn. pp. 205–220, New York, NY
47. Conte JE Jr, Golden JA, Duncan S et al (1995) Intrapulmonary pharmacokinetics of clarithromycin and of erythromycin. Antimicrob Agents Chemother 39(2):334–338
48. Rodvold KA, Gotfried MH, Danziger LH et al (1997) Intrapulmonary steady-state concentrations of clarithromycin and azithromycin in healthy adult volunteers. Antimicrob Agents Chemother 41(6):1399–1402
49. Muller-Serieys C, Soler P, Cantalloube C et al (2001) Bronchopulmonary disposition of the ketolide telithromycin (HMR3647). Antimicrob Agents Chemother 45(11):3104–3108
50. Rodvold KA, Gotfried MH, Still JG et al (2012) Comparison of plasma, epithelial lining fluid, and alveolar macrophage concentrations of solithromycin (CEM-101) in healthy adult subjects. Antimicrob Agents Chemother 56(10):5076–5081
51. Furuie H, Saisho Y, Yoshikawa T et al (2010) Intrapulmonary pharmacokinetics of S-013420, a novel bicyclolide antibacterial, in healthy Japanese subjects. Antimicrob Agents Chemother 54(2):866–870
52. Capitano B, Mattoes H, Shore E et al (2004) Steady-state intrapulmonary concentrations of moxifloxacin, levofloxacin, and azithromycin in older adults. Chest 125:965–973
53. Ong CT, Dandekar PK, Sutherland C et al (2005) Intrapulmonary concentrations of telithromycin: clinical implications for respiratory tract infections due to Streptococcus pneumoniae. Chemotherapy 51:339–346
54. Togami K, Chono S, Morimoto K (2011) Distribution characteristics of clarithromycin and azithromycin, macrolide antimicrobial agents used for treatment of respiratory infections, in lung epithelial lung fluid and alveolar macrophages. Biopharm Drug Metabol 32:389–397
55. Drusano GL (2005) Infection site concentrations: their therapeutic importance and the macrolide and macrolide-like class of antibiotics. Pharmacotherapy 25:150S–158S
56. Levison ME (2004) Pharmacodynamics of antimicrobial drugs. Infect Dis Clin North Am 18(3):451–465
57. Mandell GL, Coleman E (2001) Uptake, transport, and delivery of antimicrobial agents by human polymorphonuclear neutrophils. Antimicrob Agents Chemother 45(6): 1794–1798
58. Frank MO, Sullivan GW, Carper HT et al (1992) In vitro demonstration of transport and

delivery of antibiotics by polymorphonuclear leukocytes. Antimicrob Agents Chemother 36(12):2584–2588

59. Abdelghaffar H, Vazifeh D, Labro MT (2001) Cellular uptake of two fluoroketolides, HMR 3562 and HMR 3787, by human polymorphonuclear neutrophils in vitro. Antimicrob Agents Chemother 45(10):2798–2806
60. Gladue RP, Bright GM, Isaacson RE et al (1989) In vitro and in vivo uptake of azithromycin by phagocytic cells: possible mechanism of delivery and release at sites of infection. Antimicrob Agents Chemother 33(3):277–282
61. Odenholt-Tornqvist I, Lowdin E, Cars O (1995) Postantibiotic effects and postantibiotic sub-MIC effects of roxithromycin, clarithromycin, and azithromycin on respiratory tract pathogens. Antimicrob Agents Chemother 39(1):221–226
62. Dornbusch K, Olofsson C, Holm S (1999) Postantibiotic effect and postantibiotic sub-mic effect of dirithromycin and erythromycin against respiratory tract pathogenic bacteria. APMIS 107(5):505–513
63. Carbon C (1998) Pharmacodynamics of macrolides, azalides, and streptogramins: effect on extracellular pathogens. Clin Infect Dis 27:28–32
64. Neuhauser MM, Prause JL, Danziger LH et al (2001) Postantibiotic effects of ABT-773 and amoxicillin-clavulanate against Streptococcus pneumoniae and Haemophilus influenzae. Antimicrob Agents Chemother 45(12):3613–3615
65. Woosley LN, Castanheira M, Jones RN (2010) CEM-101 activity against Gram-positive organisms. Antimicrob Agents Chemother 54(5):2182–2187
66. Jacobs MR, Bajaksouzian S, Appelbaum PC (2003) Telithromycin post-antibiotic and post-antibiotic sub-MIC effects for 10 Gram-positive cocci. J Antimicrob Chemother 52:809–812
67. Kobayashi Y, Wada H, Rossios C et al (2013) A novel macrolide solithromycin exerts superior anti-inflammatory effect via NF-κB inhibition. J Pharmacol Exp Ther 345(1):76–84
68. Sakito O, Kadota J, Kohno S et al (1996) Interleukin 1 beta, tumor necrosis factor alpha, and interleukin 8 in bronchoalveolar lavage fluid of patients with diffuse panbronchiolitis: a potential mechanism of macrolide therapy. Respiration 63:42–48
69. Oda H, Kadota J, Kohno S et al (1995) Leukotriene B4 in bronchoalveolar lavage fluid of patients with diffuse panbronchiolitis. Chest 108:116–122
70. Kaneko Y, Yanagihara K, Seki M et al (2003) Long-term efficacy and safety of clarithromycin treatment in patients with diffuse panbronchiolitis. Respir Med 97:844–850
71. Li M, Zhong X, He Z et al (2012) Effect of erythromycin on cigarette-induced histone deacetylase protein expression and nuclear factor-κB activity in human macrophages in vitro. Int Immunopharmacol 12:643–650
72. Leiva M, Ruiz-Bravo A, Moreno E et al (2008) Telithromycin inhibits the production of pro-inflammatory mediators and the activation of NF-kappaB in in vitro-simulated murine cells. FEMS Immunol Med Microbiol 53(3): 343–350
73. Novelli A, Fallani S, Cassetta MI et al (2002) In vivo pharmacodynamic evaluation of clarithromycin in comparison to erythromycin. J Chemother 14(6):584–590
74. Drusano GL, Craig WA (1997) Relevance of pharmacokinetics and pharmacodynamics in the selection of antibiotics for respiratory tract infections. J Chemother 9(Suppl 3):38–44
75. Periti P, Mazzei T (1999) Clarithromycin: pharmacokinetic and pharmacodynamic interrelationships and dosage regimen. J Chemother 11:11–27
76. Tessier PR, Kim MK, Zhou W et al (2002) Pharmacodynamic assessment of clarithromycin in a murine model of pneumococcal pneumonia. Antimicrob Agents Chemother 46:1425–1434
77. Noreddin AM, El-Khatib WF, Aolie J et al (2009) Pharmacodynamic target attainment potential of azithromycin, clarithromycin, and telithromycin in serum and epithelial lining fluid of community-acquired pneumonia patients with penicillin-susceptible, intermediate, and resistant Streptococcus pneumonia. Int J Infect Dis 13(4):483–487
78. Boswell FJ, Andrews JM, Wise R (1998) Pharmacodynamic properties of HMR 3647, a novel ketolide, on respiratory pathogens, enterococci and Bacteroides fragilis demonstrated by studies of time-kill kinetics and post-antibiotics effect. J Antimicrob Chemother 41:149–153
79. Kim MK, Zhou W, Tessier PR et al (2002) Bactericidal effect and pharmacodynamics of cethromycin (ABT-773) in a murine pneumococcal pneumonia model. Antimicrob Agents Chemother 46(10):3185–3192
80. Capitano B, Maglio D, Banevicius MA et al (2003) Bactericidal effect of cethromycin (ABT-773) in an immunocompetent murine pneumococcal pneumonia model. Int J Antimicrob Agents 22:588–593

81. Maglio D, Sun HK, Patel T et al (2014) Pharmacodynamic profiling of modithromycin: assessment in a pneumococcal murine pneumonia model. Int J Antimicrob Agents 43:540–546
82. Bishai W (2002) The in vivo-in vitro paradox in pneumococcal respiratory tract infections. J Antimicrob Chemother 49:433–436
83. Austrian R, Gold J (1964) Pneumococcal bacteremia with especial reference to bacteremic pneumococcal pneumonia. Ann Intern Med 60:759–776
84. Feikin DR, Schuchat A, Kolczak M et al (2000) Mortality from invasive pneumococcal pneumonia in the era of antibiotic resistance, 1995-1997. Am J Public Health 90(2):223–229
85. Yu VL, Chiou CCC, Feldman C et al (2003) An international prospective study of pneumococcal bacteremia: correlation with in vitro resistance, antibiotics administered and clinical outcome. Clin Infect Dis 37:230–237
86. Nuermberger EL, Bishai WR (2003) Significance of macrolide resistance in Streptococcus pneumoniae. J Antimicrob Chemother 52(3):524–525
87. Rodvold KA, George JM, Yoo L (2011) Penetration of anti-infective agents into pulmonary epithelial lining fluid: focus on antibacterial agents. Clin Pharmacokinet 50(10): 637–664
88. Zhanel GG, DeCorby M, Noreddin A et al (2003) Pharmacodynamic activity of azithromycin against macrolide-susceptible and -resistant Streptococcus pneumoniae simulating clinically achievable free serum, epithelial lining fluid and middle ear fluid concentration. J Antimicrob Chemother 52:83–88
89. Zhanel GG, Wolter KD, Calciu C et al (2014) Clinical cure rates in subjects treated with azithromycin for community-acquired respiratory tract infections caused by azithromycin-susceptible or azithromycin-resistant Streptococcus pneumoniae: analysis of phase 3 clinical trial data. J Antimicrob Chemother 69:2835–2840
90. Lodise TP, Preston S, Bhargava V et al (2005) Pharmacodynamics of an 800-mg dose of telithromycin in patients with community-acquired pneumonia caused by extracellular pathogens. Diagn Microbiol Infect Dis 52:45–52
91. Doern GV (2006) Macrolide and ketolide resistance with Streptococcus pneumoniae. Med Clin North Am 90(6):1109–1124

Part III

Pharmacodynamics of Non-Antibacterial Agents

Chapter 15

Antifungal Pharmacokinetics and Pharmacodynamics

William Hope and David R. Andes

Abstract

Antifungal pharmacokinetics and pharmacodynamics (PK–PD) has been used to develop currently available antifungal agents, and further optimize their use for critically ill patients. New experimental models have been developed to enable drug concentration–effect relationships to be characterized. This chapter describes the tools that have been developed and are available for antifungal PK–PD. The PK–PD of currently available antifungal drug classes and agents within those classes are reviewed. As knowledge improves, antifungal PK–PD will become a critical component for the development of new agents.

Key words Pharmacokinetics, Pharmacodynamics, Antifungal, *Aspergillus*, *Candida*, Triazole, Polyene, Echinocandin, PK–PD

1 Introduction

Antifungal PK–PD is a relatively young and rapidly evolving field. The application of modern PK–PD principles to antifungal agents and invasive fungal pathogens has required the development of new experimental models and adaptation of a variety of quantitative techniques. The pharmacology of antifungal agents is invariably complex, which has provided an additional challenge. This chapter reviews current concepts and approaches to antifungal PK–PD and provides an overview of the PK–PD of currently available classes of antifungal agents.

2 Principles of Antifungal Pharmacokinetics and Pharmacodynamics

2.1 Pharmacokinetics

Pharmacokinetics is the study of the time-course of drug concentrations in the body. The serum (or plasma) is the most commonly studied matrix, but drug concentrations in other bodily fluids (e.g., urine, epithelial lining fluid, cerebrospinal fluid, ocular fluids) and tissues (e.g., tissue homogenates) may also be clinically relevant

John C. Rotschafer et al. (eds.), *Antibiotic Pharmacodynamics*, Methods in Pharmacology and Toxicology, DOI 10.1007/978-1-4939-3323-5_15, © Springer Science+Business Media New York 2016

and yield important information related to the disposition of drug. An understanding of drug absorption from the gut (oral bioavailability), disposition, metabolism, and elimination are all relevant for an understanding the time-course of drug concentrations. The use of tissue concentrations may be more informative than plasma, but that does depend on the drug–pathogen combination under consideration. Often (although not invariably), drug concentrations in plasma are predictive of those in tissues. On occasions there may be hysteresis, where there is discordance between the time course of concentrations in the plasma and tissue, in which case measurement of drug concentrations at the site of infection may be more appropriate [1].

Drug concentrations in various matrices can be measured using a variety of methods that include bioassay, high performance liquid chromatography, and mass spectrometry. Each of these methods has strengths and weaknesses. The time course of antifungal agents is then described mathematically. Again, a number of approaches are available, including non-compartmental PK models, compartmental PK models, and population PK models. Each of these approaches differs in terms of simplicity, and the computing power and expertise that are required to solve each problem.

The principal reason for describing the time-course of any compound in a given matrix is to estimate drug exposure that an invading fungal pathogen experiences. Many years of research have demonstrated that the shape of the concentration time curve has an important bearing on the antifungal activity (see below). Information that is contained within the shape is usually condensed into three readily identifiable measures of drug exposure: the peak concentration, the area under the concentration time curve and the time that drug concentrations are above some threshold (which is usually the MIC, see below). These measures of drug exposure are the same as has been employed for antibacterial agents (see review by Drusano [2]).

An additional factor that may be important for a better understanding of PK–PD relationships is the binding of antifungal agents to serum proteins. There is general consensus that only the free non-protein bound drug is pharmacologically active. An estimate of protein binding is important for bridging the findings from PK–PD studies from experimental systems to the clinic. Some studies have systematically measured free concentrations of antifungal agents, although it is more common to adjust the measured total drug concentration using the estimate for overall protein binding.

2.2 In Vitro Drug Potency

The minimum inhibitory concentration has been used for many decades to provide an in vitro measure of antimicrobial potency. These same ideas have been widely applied to antifungal agents and there have been significant efforts to understand the clinical relevance of the MIC. There are a myriad of techniques and approaches to determine the MIC, which include microdilution, Etests, agar dilution, and disk testing. The past decade has seen significant emphasis on the development of standardized techniques that demonstrate an acceptable degree of inter-laboratory reproducibility. There are two leading methodologies that are used for routine clinical care and for regulatory purposes (i.e., Clinical Laboratory Standards Institute (CLSI) and the European Committee on Antifungal Susceptibility Testing (EUCAST) methodology).

One important and frequent misconception is that the absolute value of the MIC has inherent biological significance. The MIC value is influenced by the experimental conditions under which it is determined (e.g., the inoculum, the atmospheric conditions used or the test, the length of incubation). Therefore, at least from a PK–PD perspective the MIC should be viewed as scalar that provides a rank order of the susceptibility of an organism to a given antifungal drug. The biological and clinical validity of an MIC value requires additional datasets (preclinical or clinical; see below in the breakpoint setting section).

Antimicrobial PK–PD differs from other disciplines in that the target for the antimicrobial agents is an organism within an experimental system or patient. This differs from the situation that would ordinarily be present for the study of agents for human cardiovascular or respiratory disease where the target for drug activity is the host itself. The MIC provides a way that drug exposure can be quantified in terms of the invading fungal pathogen rather than the host. Thus, Cmax, AUC, and fraction of the dosing interval that drug concentrations are above some arbitrary concentration are all measures of drug exposure that the host experiences—and certainly may be important in describing and understanding drug-related toxicity. In contrast Cmax:MIC, AUC:MIC, and T > MIC are all measures of drug exposure that the invading fungal pathogen experiences. The ability to transform drug exposure from the host to the invading fungal pathogen is unique to infectious diseases and enables the ability to bridge from experimental systems to the clinic [3].

3 Experimental Models

3.1 *In Vitro* PK–PD Models

A range of in vitro models of invasive fungal infections have been developed. These models have several advantages that include the ability to be performed in laboratories without specialist facilitates, and the ability to control the significant biological variability that is frequently present in laboratory animals and in humans. A disadvantage is related to difficulty in recapitulating some of the pathological events that are typical of advanced invasive disease (e.g., hemorrhagic infarction of the lung that is typical of invasive pulmonary aspergillosis) and that may reasonably have an impact upon exposure response relationships. Some of the models that have been developed include a bilayer of alveolar epithelial cells and pulmonary artery endothelial cells have been shown to be particularly useful to examine the pharmacology of invasive pulmonary aspergillosis treatment [4]. This model has also been valuable in examining novels methods of drug delivery via nebulized or airway route, examining combination antifungal therapy and providing decision support of the setting of in vitro susceptibility breakpoints for voriconazole [5–7].

3.2 Laboratory Animal Models to Investigate PK–PD of Antifungal Agents

The most widely used laboratory animal model is the mouse, but rabbits have also been extensively used to characterize antifungal PK–PD relationships. Both murine and rabbit models of invasive aspergillosis and invasive candidiasis have been developed.

Murine models of invasive candidiasis have been used for many years and used to characterize the majority of antifungal agents that are now clinically available (see, for example [8–10]). Both neutropenic and non-neutropenic models have been developed to reflect the background immunity that is seen in clinical settings. Neutropenia is typically induced and maintained with cyclophosphamide. For some pathogens, such as *Candida glabrata*, further immunosuppression may be required to establish infection (e.g., corticosteroids may also be required) [11].

There have been considerable efforts to develop, characterize and validate laboratory animal models of invasive pulmonary aspergillosis. For many years, a murine tail vein model was used where conidia were injected i.v. The fungal burden in the kidney was determined using quantitative cultures. This model is not a faithful mimic of human disease: humans develop invasive pulmonary disease following inhalation of conidia, and the kidney is generally not a primary site of infection. More recently, conidia have been introduced into the airway via direct instillation (i.e., intranasal inoculation) or via aerosilization (see, for example [12, 13]). An additional obstacle to the development of tenable models of invasive pulmonary aspergillosis has been biomarkers that are both clinically relevant and can be used to estimate the activity of antifungal agents. There have been two biomarkers that have been recently used: galactomannan (from serum) [12] and quantitative PCR to estimate the fungal burden in the lung [14]. Other investigators have also used survival to estimate anti-*Aspergillus* PK–PD relationships [15]. A rabbit model of invasive pulmonary aspergillosis has been extensively used to characterize almost all antifungal agents that are currently available (see, for example [16–19]). A neutropenic model has mostly been used, although a non-neutropenic model has also been developed to mimic invasive disease that is observed in patients in the post engraftment phase of hematopoietic stem cell transplantation (HSCT) [20]. A variety of endpoints have been used in the rabbit model and the size of the lung means that a composite end-points can be used, including fungal burden estimated using quantitative cultures, qPCR, galactomannan, lung weight, infarct score, and survival.

More recently, laboratory animal models of cryptococcal meningitis have been developed. A murine model of disseminated infection following i.v. injection of yeasts has been used to characterize the PK–PD of amphotericin B deoxycholate, liposomal amphotericin B, and flucytosine [21, 22]. A rabbit model in which yeasts are infected intra-cisternally has also been used to characterize various regimens of amphotericin B deoxycholate [23]. The endpoint in the murine model is the fungal burden in the parenchyma, which is clinically relevant since many patients develop encephalitis (cryptococcal meningitis should be more accurately referred to as meningoencephalitis). The primary endpoint in the rabbit is the cryptococcal burden (density) in the CSF, just as it is in patients.

3.3 Experimental Determination of the PK–PD Measure and Magnitude Linked to Efficacy

Traditionally, three PD indices have been used to describe the relationship between drug exposure and the antifungal effect (i.e., the peak:MIC, AUC:MIC, and T > MIC). Antifungal agents tend to exhibit concentration-dependent (e.g., polyenes and echinocandins) or time-dependent activity (e.g., flucytosine). Knowledge regarding the index that best links drug exposure with effect can be used to design appropriate regimens for use in the clinic.

The relevant pharmacodynamic index is determined using dose-fractionation studies. The design of such experiments involves perturbing the total dosage and studying the antifungal fungal effect of different schedules of administration. If the least fractionated regimen has the most antifungal activity, Cmax:MIC is likely to be important. If the most fractionated regimen has the most activity, T > MIC is likely to be important. If the effect is the same regardless of the regimen, then AUC:MIC is likely to be the dynamically linked variable. There are multiple nuances related to the appropriate design of these studies to ensure the "right" result is obtained. Most importantly perhaps is ensuring that the pharmacokinetics have been appropriately and adequately described. Mistakes in the pharmacokinetics can have a profound effect on the pharmacodynamic interpretations that may subsequently be found to be erroneous.

Once the dynamically linked variable has been identified, the next question is the magnitude of the PD index (AUC/MIC, Cmax/MIC, or fraction of the dosing interval T > MIC) that is associated with a suitably high probability of a successful outcome. Decisions about what exactly constitutes a "favorable outcome" or a "high probability" can be difficult to define a priori. The performance of experimental PK–PD models, just like MICs are influenced by the experimental conditions under which they are established. An effect that is seen in one model may not directly translate to a different model constructed under different experimental conditions. Commonly used endpoints for experimental PK–PD models include various orders of logarithmic killing (e.g., 1-log drop in fungal burden, 2-log drop in burden), survival prolongation, and 50 % reduction in a biomarker such as galactomannan. Ultimately, the validity of an endpoint must be cross referenced or validated against a clinical data-set. For disseminated candidiasis, half-maximal maximal effect and echinocandins (stasis) have been successfully used. However, for newer drug classes and for other diseases and experimental models (e.g., invasive aspergillosis), the best outcome measure is often unknown. In this circumstance, investigators typically report a number of endpoints that can be used for current and future analyses.

3.4 Bridging from Experimental Models to the Clinic

When the relevant pharmacodynamic index and the magnitude of that index is known from one or more preclinical studies, the potential implications for patients can be determined. Bridging studies require some knowledge related to the performance of a drug in a patient population of interest. Population pharmacokinetic models are used to summarize the behavior of a drug in a patient population and serve as a mathematical summary of past experiences with that drug. A population pharmacokinetic model provides estimates of measures of central tendency of drug behavior for the population as well as robust estimates of the extent of inter-individual variability [3].

The next stage in the bridging process involves the use of Monte Carlo simulation. Monte Carlo simulation involves the generation of simulated (virtual) patients that are based on the population pharmacokinetic parameter. Each simulated patient then receives a given regimen of the drug and the corresponding drug exposure if calculated. Analysis of each patient in turn enables predictions to made across the simulated population as to the likelihood of success (or otherwise) of the regimen to be tested. The simulations can be performed for a range of MICs and thereby enables the overall efficacy to be estimated [3].

Bridging from experimental studies to the clinic can be used to address a number of problems that includes the identification of optimal regimen (i.e., dosage and schedule of administration) for a patient population as well as providing decision support for the setting of in vitro susceptibility breakpoints. Indeed, EUCAST mandate the use of PK–PD information, and Monte Carlo simulation (if available) in the process of setting breakpoints [24]. Monte Carlo simulation can be used to define regimens for difficult to study populations, such as for pediatric and neonatal patients, and for certain infections where the clinical study of different dosing regimens is simply impractical. For example, studies using the bridging technique of Monte Carlo simulation were performed for neonates and children with hematogenous *Candida* meningoencephalitis (HCME), which is a rare but well recognized and potentially lethal infection, with micafungin and anidulafungin [25, 26]. In both cases, a dosing strategy derived from adults would be expected to lead to suboptimal outcomes in neonates.

4 Polyenes

4.1 Concentration Effect, PD Index and Target

Amphotericin B was discovered nearly 50 years ago. The nephrotoxicity of this agent was initially described in dogs and was related to constriction of renal arterioles. Amphotericin B also causes tubular toxicity, which results in hypokalemia and hyomagnesemia. Amphotericin B-induced renal impairment in patients is associated with prolonged hospitalization and mortality [27].

The toxicity and water insolubility of amphotericin B are the principal reasons a variety of formulations have been developed for clinical use. Widely available formulations include amphotericin B deoxycholate (sometimes called "conventional amphotericin B"), amphotericin B lipid complex (ABLC) and liposomal amphotericin B (LAmB). Amphotericin B colloidal dispersion is available in some centers in the world. Preclinical models of invasive candidiasis suggest that amphotericin B exhibits concentration-dependent antifungal activity. A further feature appears to be a large degree of hysteresis where serum and tissue concentration time profiles are discordant [23]. Persistent concentrations at effect sites, such as the central nervous system, may enable intermittent of abbreviated regimens. The use of such regimens may facilitate ambulatory i.v. therapy and use of parenteral therapy in resource-poor healthcare settings.

Lipid formulations of amphotericin B (LAmB, ABLC, and ABCD) are generally less potent on a mg/kg basis when compared with DAmB. This is because much of the active drug (i.e., amphotericin B) is preferentially complexed with the lipid carrier rather than existing in a free state. The distinct structure of the lipid carriers also has an impact upon the pharmacokinetics of each formulation. There appear to be differences in concentrations that are achieved in the central nervous system and various subcompartments of the lung. For example, LAmB exhibits high serum and CNS concentrations in comparison to other lipid preparations [28]. The relevance of this PK difference was found to be important in a CNS invasive candidiasis model whereby the difference in drug concentration in brain parenchyma was closely related to treatment efficacy in favor of LAmB over the other formulations [28]. Conversely, both ABLC and ABCD achieve much higher concentrations in the intracellular space and in organs of the reticuloendothelial system. In a disseminated candidiasis model, differences in PD potency in the liver, kidney, and lung closely followed the differences in tissue kinetics for each drug in each target organ system [29]. Several animal model and human investigations have demonstrated ABLC attains higher concentrations in the lung relative to other formulations [30].

4.2 Clinical Implications

There are relatively few clinical data that provide an insight into PK–PD relationships for the polyenes. Much of the validation for dosing has been derived over the past two-to-three decades from multiple clinical studies and trials. The advent of lipid formulations provided a hope that the improved therapeutic index that is characteristic of these agents would enable more aggressive dosing and thereby better clinical responses. Unfortunately, this does not appear to be the case. For example, a prospective clinical trial that compared the clinical outcomes of liposomal amphotericin B at 3 versus 10 mg/kg/day did not suggest any benefit of the higher dose [31]. Thus, the drug exposures associated with amphotericin B deoxycholate 1 mg/kg and liposomal amphotericin B 3 mg/kg/day induce near maximal antifungal activity.

An additional feature that is common to all amphotericin B formulations is that the MIC has relatively little predictive value and in general is not used to direct antifungal therapy in the clinic. The MICs for common medically important fungal pathogens cluster tightly and there is rapid transition from no antifungal effect to full antifungal activity over a very narrow concentration range. For these reasons, neither the MIC nor amphotericin B serum concentrations provide useful information to enable individualized antifungal therapy. This limitation is in contrast to flucytosine and the triazoles where both the MIC and serum drug concentrations can be used in the clinic (see below).

5 Flucytosine

5.1 Concentration Effect, PD Index and Target

Several studies have described time-dependent activity of flucytosine against *Candida albicans* [32]. Therefore, fractionated regimens are best used to treat patients with invasive candidiasis. For invasive candidiasis, the fraction of the dosing interval that drug concentrations must be greater than the MIC is approximately 40 % [33]. The corresponding target for cryptococcal meningitis has not been determined in preclinical models. A regimen as low as 25 mg/kg/day (which is two to fourfold lower than currently recommended) is predicted to achieve the pharmacodynamic target against *C. albicans* given the current MIC distribution [34]. Similarly, a preclinical model of cryptococcal meningoencephalitis suggests that a lower dosage of flucytosine could be used in combination with liposomal amphotericin B to achieve near maximal fungicidal activity [22].

5.2 Clinical Implications

There are no clinical data sets that allow for PK–PD analyses for flucytosine. In contrast, toxicodynamic relationships are well established from clinical data. Myelosuppression that is associated with flucytosine therapy is more likely with higher peak drug concentrations (>100 mg/L) [35]. Consequently, fractionated regimens have the dual benefit of maximizing T > MIC and minimizing the peak concentrations that are potentially toxic.

6 Triazoles

6.1 Concentration Effect, PD Index and Target

The triazole class of antifungal agents has been extensively studied in both preclinical models and at the bedside. Dose fractionation studies have consistently suggested that the AUC:MIC is the dynamically linked index that best connects the dosage with the observed effect, although these studies have only been performed in *Candida* [8–10, 36]. An assumption is widely made that the AUC:MIC is also the dynamically linked variable for other fungal pathogens such as *Aspergillus* spp. PK–PD relationships have been defined in preclinical models of *Candida* spp., *Aspergillus fumigatus*, and *Cryptococcus neoformans.* PK–PD studies have been performed with five triazoles currently available for therapy for invasive candidiasis (i.e., fluconazole, itraconazole, voriconazole, posaconazole, isavuconazole). A free drug AUC:MIC of 25–50 appears to be associated with near-maximal antifungal activity for both invasive candidiasis and invasive aspergillosis [8–10, 36, 37].

The pharmacodynamics of the triazoles against *Aspergillus fumigatus* are increasingly understood. A variety of experimental models and study endpoints have been used to estimate these relationships [12, 13, 15, 38]. Clear exposure response relationships have been demonstrated using qPCR, galactomannan and survival as study endpoints. Collectively, these studies have confirmed that the MIC is of both biological and clinical importance, and can therefore be used to guide antifungal therapy in humans.

The pharmacodynamics of fluconazole for cryptococcal meningoencephalitis have been recently described using a murine model of cryptococcal meningoencephalitis [21]. A higher fluconazole AUC:MIC value of approximately 400 was required for stasis, which is higher than is the case for invasive candidiasis and reflects the requirement to drive fluconazole into the central nervous system.

6.2 Clinical Studies

There is a relatively large amount of PK–PD clinical data for fluconazole that is congruent with the conclusions of preclinical PK–PD models. In a study of more than 1000 patients receiving fluconazole for oropharyngeal candidiasis, clinical success was noted in 91–100 % of patients in whom the free drug AUC:MIC was >25; whereas, only 27–35 % had a successful outcome with a free drug

AUC:MIC <25 [39]. These findings are comparable to another study of oropharyngeal candidiasis in which 92 % of patients had a successful outcome with a free drug AUC:MIC > 25, while only 9 were successfully treated with a free drug AUC:MIC <25 [40]. There is a remarkably strong relationship between the AUC:MIC and treatment outcome for patients with invasive candidiasis. A free drug AUC:MIC target of 25–50 is associated with near-maximal survival.

The maximal outcome is associated with a voriconazole trough concentration (Cmin)-to-MIC ratio of approximately 2 [37]. Numerous additional studies suggest that trough concentrations (i.e., independent of MIC) of approximately 1–2 mg/L are associated with improved clinical outcomes for patients with invasive aspergillosis [41]. An increasing number of datasets are available for both itraconazole and posaconazole. For treatment of a variety of invasive fungal diseases (predominantly invasive aspergillosis) a trough concentration of approximately 1 mg/L is generally required and advocated as a target for therapeutic drug monitoring in the clinic. The drug exposure targets for prophylaxis for both itraconazole and posaconazole are approximately 0.5 and 0.7 mg/L, respectively, which is lower than concentrations required for the treatment of established infection [41].

7 Echinocandins

7.1 Concentration Effect, PD Index and Target

The echinocandins are active against the majority of medically important members if the *Candida* genus, although they are less potent against *Candida parapsilosis*. The molecular basis of reduced susceptibility in *Candida parapsilosis* is related to the structure of Fks1 protein, which is the target for all echinocandin agents. Preclinical models suggest the echinocandins (i.e., caspofungin, micafungin, and anidulafungin) all exhibit concentration-dependent antifungal activity [14, 42–44]. The peak:MIC or AUC:MIC consistently provides the best link between echinocandin dosing and the observed effect.

The echinocandins induce a paradoxical antifungal activity, which is purely an in vitro phenomenon. Growth of *Candida* is observed at high drug concentrations. The effect is not universally observed for all echinocandin agents, or *Candida* species/strains. There are no clear in vivo or clinical consequences (i.e., there do not appear to be inferior clinical outcomes with higher echinocandin dosages or drug exposures). The paradoxical effect appears to be related to the induction of stress-response pathways that ultimately lead to a compensatory up-regulation and synthesis of chitin.

The echinocandins are clearly active against *Aspergillus* spp., both in vitro and in experimental models. However, the effect is distinct from that observed against *Candida* in there are concentration-dependent morphological changes in *Aspergillus* without evidence of fungicidal activity or reduction in fungal biomass [14, 45, 46]. The echinocandins induce excessive branching of hyphae, which appear short and dysmorphic [47]. Studies in laboratory animal models of invasive aspergillosis suggest that the echinocandins are clearly active, but do not cause a reduction in fungal burden when estimated using quantitative cultures or other clinically relevant biomarkers (e.g., circulating galactomannan) [48]. The echinocandins do result in survival prolongation, reduced lung weight and fewer pulmonary infarcts in rabbits with invasive pulmonary aspergillosis, and therefore appear to prevent organism mediated pulmonary injury. This protection may be related to the morphological changes that render the organism unable to invade the lung. The dissociation between echinocandin drug concentrations and traditional biomarkers has hampered a deep understanding of the PK–PD relationships of the echinocandins against *Aspergillus* spp.

Preclinical models of invasive candidiasis have provided an insight into the drug exposure targets for the echinocandins against medically important *Candida* species. For *C. albicans* a free drug C_{max}/MIC >1 or AUC/MIC 10–20 is the PD target that is associated with a stasis endpoint [14, 46]. Similar studies with *C. parapsilosis* and *C. glabrata* have suggested that the echinocandin exposure required for stasis is two to threefold lower than for *C. albicans* [46]. Preclinical PK–PD studies that have examined both wild-type susceptible and drug resistant *C. glabrata* clinical isolates with a variety of *Fks* mutations found a comparable AUC:MIC is needed for efficacy [49]. This observation is consistent with PK–PD observations with the triazoles where the MIC explains a large amount of system variance. Nevertheless, there is a complex interplay between the Fks1 genotype, the resultant MIC and the therapeutic response [50]. The echinocandins have a wide therapeutic index and higher dosages can potentially be used to treat (or overcome) a resistance mechanism. On occasions, however, the dosage is simply too high to generate sufficient drug exposure to overcome the resistance mechanism(s), and the mutation must be classified as resistant.

7.2 Clinical Implications

Clinical PD studies with the echinocandins are generally concordant with the findings from preclinical models. For micafungin, a total-drug AUC:MIC > 3000 is associated with near maximal therapeutic outcomes (i.e., 98 % success compared to 84 % in those with an AUC/MIC <3000) [51]. A subgroup analysis based upon *Candida* species suggested patients infected with *C. parapsilosis* have a drug exposure target that is tenfold lower than *Candida albicans*.

8 PK–PD Analysis of Combination Therapy

Combination antifungal therapy remains an areas where there has been a significant amount of preclinical and clinical study. Much of the impetus to combine antifungal agents stems from suboptimal outcomes that can be achieved with agents used alone. Much is made of the concepts of synergy, additivity, and antagonism, and a myriad of definitions (clinical and mathematical) serves to make this area complex and difficult to understand. Perhaps the clearest way to conceive the potential benefits of combining antifungal agents is the way in which maximal antifungal activity can be achieved as rapidly as possible. Prevention of the emergence of drug resistance is not such a clinical problem or concern as is the case in tuberculosis or viral diseases such as HIV.

The best accepted use of combination antifungal therapy is in the treatment of cryptococcal meningitis. Both preclinical and clinical data suggest that the use of a combination of agents generally provides faster and more sustained antifungal activity. The strongest case can be made for combining a polyene (amphotericin B deoxycholate or liposomal amphotericin B) with flucytosine, but the combination of fluconazole and flucytosine is also potentially beneficial.

The suboptimal clinical outcomes resulting from invasive aspergillosis have promoted widespread interest and study for defining combination regimens for this disease. There appears to be general consensus that the combination of a triazole and an echinocandin is beneficial and this idea has been tested in both preclinical models and more recently in a clinical trial [19]. This combination of agents has been explored for the treatment of triazole resistant *Aspergillus* spp. [7]. In general, there appears to be some benefit of combining triazole and echinocandins in this setting, although conclusions depend somewhat on the experimental model that is used, as well as the study endpoint. There has been a longstanding theoretical concern related to the potential for antagonism between the triazoles and polyenes. This has been borne out in at least one well-conducted preclinical model in which the combination of ravuconazole and liposomal amphotericin B appeared to be antagonistic on the basis of a number of well-validated study endpoints [52].

9 Conclusions

Application of PK–PD principles to antifungal drug therapy has provided an increased understanding of drug exposure response relationships. The tools and techniques that have been developed can be further harnessed to improve the use of existing agents, but also address new problems as they arise. A further opportunity is the use of PK–PD to accelerate new compounds and formulations through to the clinic.

References

1. Felton T, Troke PF, Hope WW (2014) Tissue penetration of antifungal agents. Clin Microbiol Rev 27(1):68–88
2. Drusano GL (2004) Antimicrobial pharmacodynamics: critical interactions of 'bug and drug'. Nat Rev Microbiol 2(4):289–300
3. Hope WW, Drusano GL (2009) Antifungal pharmacokinetics and pharmacodynamics: bridging from the bench to bedside. Clin Microbiol Infect 15(7):602–612
4. Hope WW, Kruhlak MJ, Lyman CA et al (2007) Pathogenesis of Aspergillus fumigatus and the kinetics of galactomannan in an in vitro model of early invasive pulmonary aspergillosis: implications for antifungal therapy. J Infect Dis 195(3):455–466
5. Al-Nakeeb Z, Sudan A, Jeans AR et al (2012) Pharmacodynamics of itraconazole against Aspergillus fumigatus in an in vitro model of the human alveolus: perspectives on the treatment of triazole resistant infection and utility of airway administration. Antimicrob Agents Chemother 56(8):4146–4153
6. Jeans AR, Howard SJ, Al-Nakeeb Z et al (2012) Pharmacodynamics of voriconazole in a dynamic in vitro model of invasive pulmonary aspergillosis: implications for in vitro susceptibility breakpoints. J Infect Dis 206(3):442–452
7. Jeans AR, Howard SJ, Al-Nakeeb Z et al (2012) Combination of voriconazole and anidulafungin for treatment of triazole-resistant aspergillus fumigatus in an in vitro model of invasive pulmonary aspergillosis. Antimicrob Agents Chemother 56(10):5180–5185
8. Andes D, Marchillo K, Conklin R et al (2004) Pharmacodynamics of a new triazole, posaconazole, in a murine model of disseminated candidiasis. Antimicrob Agents Chemother 48(1):137–142
9. Andes D, Marchillo K, Stamstad T, Conklin R (2003) In vivo pharmacodynamics of a new triazole, ravuconazole, in a murine candidiasis model. Antimicrob Agents Chemother 47(4):1193–1199
10. Andes D, Marchillo K, Stamstad T, Conklin R (2003) In vivo pharmacokinetics and pharmacodynamics of a new triazole, voriconazole, in a murine candidiasis model. Antimicrob Agents Chemother 47(10):3165–3169
11. Howard SJ, Livermore J, Sharp A et al (2011) Pharmacodynamics of echinocandins against Candida glabrata: requirement for dosage escalation to achieve maximal antifungal activity in neutropenic hosts. Antimicrob Agents Chemother 55(10):4880–4887
12. Howard SJ, Lestner JM, Sharp A et al (2011) Pharmacokinetics and pharmacodynamics of posaconazole for invasive pulmonary aspergillosis: clinical implications for antifungal therapy. J Infect Dis 203(9):1324–1332
13. Lepak AJ, Marchillo K, Vanhecker J, Andes DR (2013) Posaconazole pharmacodynamic target determination against wild-type and Cyp51 mutant isolates of Aspergillus fumigatus in an in vivo model of invasive pulmonary aspergillosis. Antimicrob Agents Chemother 57(1):579–585
14. Andes D, Diekema DJ, Pfaller MA et al (2008) In vivo pharmacodynamic characterization of anidulafungin in a neutropenic murine candidiasis model. Antimicrob Agents Chemother 52(2):539–550
15. Mavridou E, Bruggemann RJ, Melchers WJ, Mouton JW, Verweij PE (2010) Efficacy of posaconazole against three clinical Aspergillus fumigatus isolates with mutations in the cyp51A gene. Antimicrob Agents Chemother 54(2):860–865
16. Petraitiene R, Petraitis V, Groll AH et al (2001) Antifungal activity and pharmacokinetics of posaconazole (SCH 56592) in treatment and prevention of experimental invasive pulmonary aspergillosis: correlation with galactomannan antigenemia. Antimicrob Agents Chemother 45(3):857–869
17. Petraitis V, Petraitiene R, Hope WW et al (2009) Combination therapy in treatment of experimental pulmonary aspergillosis: in vitro and in vivo correlations of the concentration- and dose- dependent interactions between anidulafungin and voriconazole by Bliss independence drug interaction analysis. Antimicrob Agents Chemother 53(6):2382–2391
18. Petraitis V, Petraitiene R, Lin P et al (2005) Efficacy and safety of generic amphotericin B in experimental pulmonary aspergillosis. Antimicrob Agents Chemother 49(4):1642–1645
19. Petraitis V, Petraitiene R, Sarafandi AA et al (2003) Combination therapy in treatment of experimental pulmonary aspergillosis: synergistic interaction between an antifungal triazole and an echinocandin. J Infect Dis 187(12):1834–1843
20. Berenguer J, Allende MC, Lee JW et al (1995) Pathogenesis of pulmonary aspergillosis. Granulocytopenia versus cyclosporine and methylprednisolone-induced immunosuppression. Am J Respir Crit Care Med 152(3):1079–1086
21. Sudan A, Livermore J, Howard SJ et al (2013) Pharmacokinetics and pharmacodynamics of fluconazole for cryptococcal meningoencephalitis: implications for antifungal therapy and in vitro susceptibility breakpoints. Antimicrob Agents Chemother 57(6):2793–2800

22. O'Connor L, Livermore J, Sharp AD et al (2013) Pharmacodynamics of liposomal amphotericin B and flucytosine for cryptococcal meningoencephalitis: safe and effective regimens for immunocompromised patients. J Infect Dis 208(2):351–361
23. Livermore J, Howard SJ, Sharp AD et al (2013) Efficacy of an abbreviated induction regimen of amphotericin B deoxycholate for cryptococcal meningoencephalitis: 3 days of therapy is equivalent to 14 days. mBio 5(1):e00725–e00713
24. Arendrup MC, Cuenca-Estrella M, Lass-Florl C, Hope WW (2013) Breakpoints for antifungal agents: an update from EUCAST focussing on echinocandins against Candida spp. and triazoles against Aspergillus spp. Drug Resist Updat 16(6):81–95
25. Warn PA, Livermore J, Howard S et al (2011) Anidulafungin for neonatal hematogenous Candida meningoencephalitis: identification of candidate regimens for humans using a translational pharmacological approach. Antimicrob Agents Chemother 56(2):708–714
26. Hope WW, Mickiene D, Petraitis V et al (2008) The pharmacokinetics and pharmacodynamics of micafungin in experimental hematogenous Candida meningoencephalitis: implications for echinocandin therapy in neonates. J Infect Dis 197(1):163–171
27. Denning DW, Hope WW (2010) Therapy for fungal diseases: opportunities and priorities. Trends Microbiol 18(5):195–204
28. Groll AH, Giri N, Petraitis V et al (2000) Comparative efficacy and distribution of lipid formulations of amphotericin B in experimental Candida albicans infection of the central nervous system. J Infect Dis 182(1):274–282
29. Andes D, Safdar N, Marchillo K, Conklin R (2006) Pharmacokinetic-pharmacodynamic comparison of amphotericin B (AMB) and two lipid-associated AMB preparations, liposomal AMB and AMB lipid complex, in murine candidiasis models. Antimicrob Agents Chemother 50(2):674–684
30. Groll AH, Lyman CA, Petraitis V et al (2006) Compartmentalized intrapulmonary pharmacokinetics of amphotericin B and its lipid formulations. Antimicrob Agents Chemother 50(10):3418–3423
31. Cornely OA, Maertens J, Bresnik M et al (2007) Liposomal amphotericin B as initial therapy for invasive mold infection: a randomized trial comparing a high-loading dose regimen with standard dosing (AmBiLoad trial). Clin Infect Dis 44(10):1289–1297
32. Andes D, van Ogtrop M (2000) In vivo characterization of the pharmacodynamics of flucytosine in a neutropenic murine disseminated candidiasis model. Antimicrob Agents Chemother 44(4):938–942
33. Hope WW, Warn PA, Sharp A et al (2006) Derivation of an in vivo drug exposure breakpoint for flucytosine against Candida albicans and Impact of the MIC, growth rate, and resistance genotype on the antifungal effect. Antimicrob Agents Chemother 50(11):3680–3688
34. Hope WW, Warn PA, Sharp A et al (2007) Optimization of the dosage of flucytosine in combination with amphotericin B for disseminated candidiasis: a pharmacodynamic rationale for reduced dosing. Antimicrob Agents Chemother 51(10):3760–3762
35. Stamm AM, Diasio RB, Dismukes WE et al (1987) Toxicity of amphotericin B plus flucytosine in 194 patients with cryptococcal meningitis. Am J Med 83(2):236–242
36. Andes D, van Ogtrop M (1999) Characterization and quantitation of the pharmacodynamics of fluconazole in a neutropenic murine disseminated candidiasis infection model. Antimicrob Agents Chemother 43(9):2116–2120
37. Troke PF, Hockey HP, Hope WW (2011) Observational study of the clinical efficacy of voriconazole and its relationship to plasma concentrations in patients. Antimicrob Agents Chemother 55(10):4782–4788
38. Lepak AJ, Marchillo K, Vanhecker J, Andes DR (2013) Isavuconazole (BAL4815) pharmacodynamic target determination in an in vivo murine model of invasive pulmonary aspergillosis against wild-type and cyp51 mutant isolates of Aspergillus fumigatus. Antimicrob Agents Chemother 57(12):6284–6289
39. Rex JH, Pfaller MA, Galgiani JN et al (1997) Development of interpretive breakpoints for antifungal susceptibility testing: conceptual framework and analysis of in vitro-in vivo correlation data for fluconazole, itraconazole, and candida infections. Subcommittee on Antifungal Susceptibility Testing of the National Committee for Clinical Laboratory Standards. Clin Infect Dis 24(2):235–247
40. Rodriguez-Tudela JL, Almirante B, Rodriguez-Pardo D et al (2007) Correlation of the MIC and dose/MIC ratio of fluconazole to the therapeutic response of patients with mucosal candidiasis and candidemia. Antimicrob Agents Chemother 51(10):3599–3604
41. Ashbee HR, Barnes RA, Johnson EM, Richardson MD, Gorton R, Hope WW (2013) Therapeutic drug monitoring (TDM) of antifungal agents: guidelines from the British Society for Medical Mycology. J Antimicrob Chemother 69(5):1162–1176
42. Andes D, Marchillo K, Lowther J, Bryskier A, Stamstad T, Conklin R (2003) In vivo pharmacodynamics of HMR 3270, a glucan synthase inhibitor, in a murine candidiasis model. Antimicrob Agents Chemother 47(4):1187–1192
43. Andes DR, Diekema DJ, Pfaller MA, Marchillo K, Bohrmueller J (2008) In vivo pharmacodynamic target investigation for micafungin against Candida albicans and C. glabrata in a neutropenic

murine candidiasis model. Antimicrob Agents Chemother 52(10):3497–3503
44. Louie A, Deziel M, Liu W, Drusano MF, Gumbo T, Drusano GL (2005) Pharmacodynamics of caspofungin in a murine model of systemic candidiasis: importance of persistence of caspofungin in tissues to understanding drug activity. Antimicrob Agents Chemother 49(12):5058–5068
45. Stevens DA, Ichinomiya M, Koshi Y, Horiuchi H (2006) Escape of Candida from caspofungin inhibition at concentrations above the MIC (paradoxical effect) accomplished by increased cell wall chitin; evidence for beta-1,6-glucan synthesis inhibition by caspofungin. Antimicrob Agents Chemother 50(9):3160–3161
46. Andes D, Diekema DJ, Pfaller MA, Bohrmuller J, Marchillo K, Lepak A (2010) In vivo comparison of the pharmacodynamic targets for echinocandin drugs against Candida species. Antimicrob Agents Chemother 54(6):2497–2506
47. Hope WW, Shoham S, Walsh TJ (2007) The pharmacology and clinical use of caspofungin. Expert Opin Drug Metab Toxicol 3(2):263–274
48. Petraitis V, Petraitiene R, Groll AH et al (2002) Comparative antifungal activities and plasma pharmacokinetics of micafungin (FK463) against disseminated candidiasis and invasive pulmonary aspergillosis in persistently neutropenic rabbits. Antimicrob Agents Chemother 46(6):1857–1869
49. Slater JL, Howard SJ, Sharp A et al (2011) Disseminated Candidiasis caused by Candida albicans with amino acid substitutions in Fks1 at position Ser645 cannot be successfully treated with micafungin. Antimicrob Agents Chemother 55(7):3075–3083
50. Arendrup MC, Perlin DS, Jensen RH, Howard SJ, Goodwin J, Hope W (2012) Differential in vivo activities of anidulafungin, caspofungin, and micafungin against Candida glabrata isolates with and without FKS resistance mutations. Antimicrob Agents Chemother 56(5):2435–2442
51. Andes D, Ambrose PG, Hammel JP et al (2011) Use of pharmacokinetic-pharmacodynamic analyses to optimize therapy with the systemic antifungal micafungin for invasive candidiasis or candidemia. Antimicrob Agents Chemother 55(5):2113–2121
52. Meletiadis J, Petraitis V, Petraitiene R et al (2006) Triazole-polyene antagonism in experimental invasive pulmonary aspergillosis: in vitro and in vivo correlation. J Infect Dis 194(7):1008–1018

Chapter 16

Pharmacokinetics and Pharmacodynamics of the Tuberculosis Drugs

Aline B. Barth, Eric F. Egelund, and Charles A. Peloquin

Abstract

In the last 40 years, only rifapentine and bedaquiline have been approved in the USA for the treatment of active tuberculosis. Therefore, one focus of research involves optimizing the current antituberculosis drugs' pharmacokinetic and pharmacodynamic properties. The aim of this chapter is to review both the pharmacokinetics and pharmacodynamics of the antituberculosis drugs. Specifically, the pharmacokinetic properties of absorption, distribution, metabolism, and elimination are reviewed for each drug. Regarding pharmacodynamics, we discuss pharmacodynamic modeling, mechanisms of resistance, and current methodologies used to evaluate a drug's susceptibility to *Mycobacterium tuberculosis*. As a whole, we highlight the importance of pharmacokinetic/pharmacodynamic (PK/PD) modeling and the challenges faced in applying PK/PD to tuberculosis. Finally, therapeutic drug monitoring (TDM) is discussed as a tool that provides clinicians a means to optimize a drug's PK/PD relationship for an individual patient.

Key words Pharmacokinetics, Pharmacodynamics, Tuberculosis, Therapeutic drug monitoring

1 Introduction

There is evidence of tuberculosis (TB) since prehistoric times, and it is hypothesized that *Mycobacterium tuberculosis* (*Mtb*) might have been responsible for more deaths than any other infection in history [1]. In 2012, an estimated 8.6 million people became ill with TB, and the disease caused an estimated 1.3 million deaths [2]. TB is considered to be the second leading killer as sole infectious agent, with the leading killer considered to be the human immunodeficiency virus (HIV). That said, TB is the leading cause of death among patients with HIV [3], and one of the major causes of death among women of reproductive age [2].

The initial drug used for TB treatment was streptomycin (SM) [4, 5]. However, the use of a single agent rapidly promoted the emergence of resistance [5]. In an effort to prevent drug resistance, combined therapy was evaluated. Initially p-aminosalicylic acid (PAS) was evaluated with SM, and in 1952, isoniazid (INH)

John C. Rotschafer et al. (eds.), *Antibiotic Pharmacodynamics*, Methods in Pharmacology and Toxicology, DOI 10.1007/978-1-4939-3323-5_16, © Springer Science+Business Media New York 2016

was introduced [4, 5]. INH has strong early bactericidal activity (EBA), rapidly reducing the number of bacilli in sputum. INH is continued throughout therapy in an effort to prevent resistance. A three-drug regimen, with an initial 6-month intensive phase of SM, PAS, and INH, followed by PAS and INH for 12 more months, proved to be more effective than the two drug regimen. This regimen helped introduce the concept of an initial intensive phase, followed by a continuation phase [5]. Murine studies with pyrazinamide (PZA) demonstrated its sterilizing activity when combined with INH against *Mtb* [6]. Studies with rifampin (RIF) demonstrate similar sterilizing behavior [7, 8]. Sterilizing activity is the ability to kill off persisting organisms, and to prevent post-treatment relapses. Sterilizing activity thus is the most sought-after characteristic in a TB drug. Regimens containing INH and RIF could be completed in only 9 months, half of the prior duration without RIF. Further, studies proved that RIF and PZA had synergistic activities [4]. The addition of PZA to INH and RIF reduced the duration of therapy from 9 to 6 months. PZA appeared to produce most of its sterilizing activity during the first 2 months of therapy, while RIF has this effect throughout treatment [4]. A randomized clinical trial demonstrated that an intensive phase regimen of INH, RIF, PZA, and SM, followed by a 4-month continuation phase of INH and RIF promoted very low relapse rates. The current "first-line" regimen, according to the World Health Organization (WHO) follows the same pattern, substituting ethambutol (EMB) for SM [9]. EMB is recommended as the fourth drug, along with INH, RIF, and PZA, to further prevent the emergence of resistance, since susceptibility data often are delayed, or absent altogether. Further studies aimed at shortening the duration of therapy to less than 6 months were unsuccessful, primarily in terms of preventing post-treatment relapses [10]. The structures of the TB drugs are shown in Fig. 1.

Resistance to at least INH and RIF characterizes multidrug-resistant tuberculosis (MDR-TB) [11]. The current treatment recommendation for MDR-TB is to use any remaining first-line drugs, plus a fluoroquinolone [levofloxacin (LEVO) or moxifloxacin (MOXI)], and an injectable agent [amikacin (AK), kanamycin (KM), SM or capreomycin (CM)]. Other "second-line" drugs that might be used, depending on susceptibility data, include cycloserine (CS), ethionamide (ETA), and PAS. "Third-line" drugs also used for TB include clofazimine, linezolid, amoxicillin/clavulanate, imipenem, macrolides, and high-dose isoniazid. These drugs are especially important for the treatment of extensively drug-resistant tuberculosis (XDR-TB), characterized by MDR-TB plus resistance to a fluoroquinolone and at least one injectable agent. In 2012, bedaquiline (TMC-207) was approved by the US Food and Drug Administration (FDA) for the treatment of multidrug resistance as a part of the combination therapy [12]. In 2013,

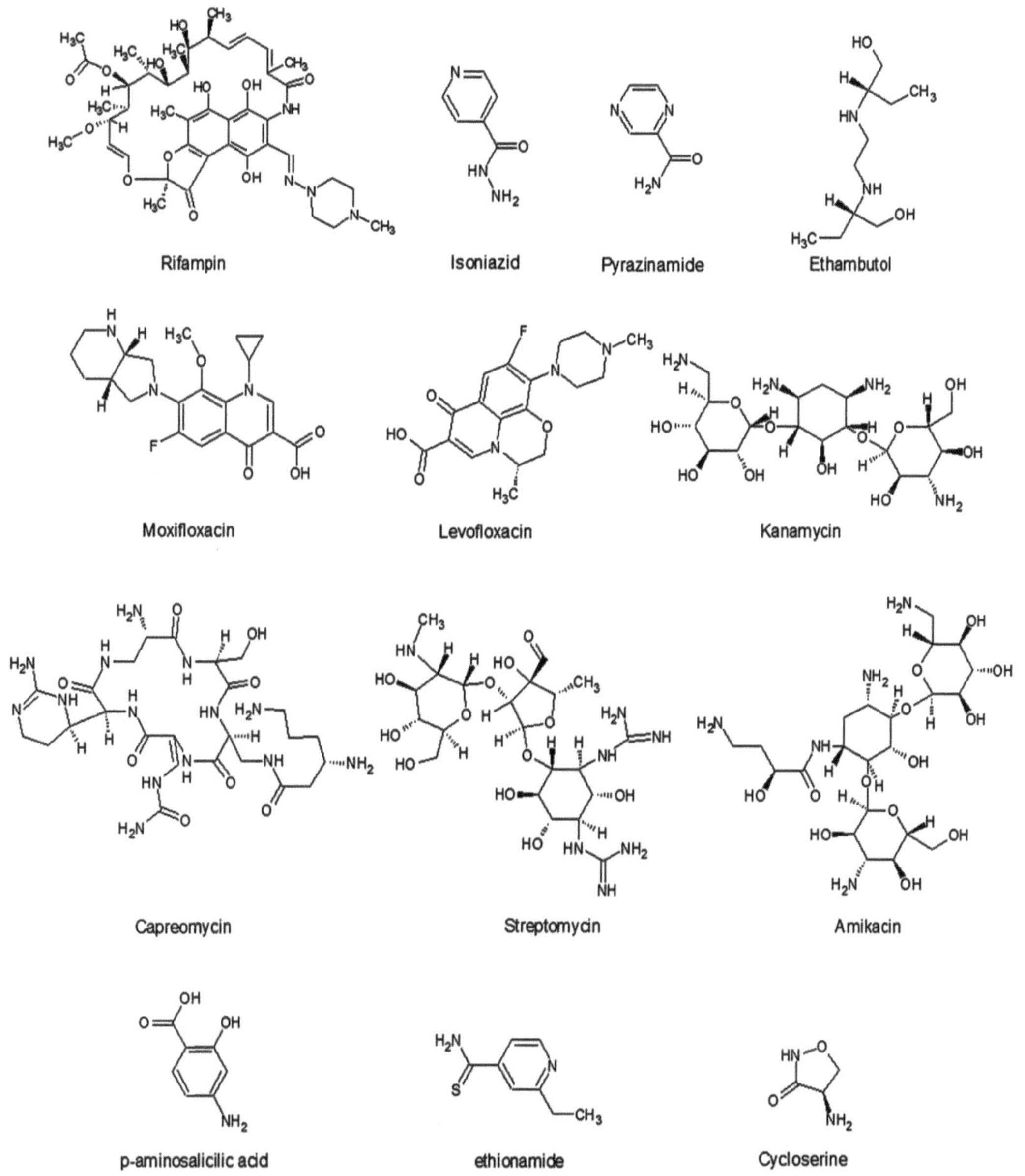

Fig. 1 Chemical structure of the main drugs used on the treatment of tuberculosis. The figures were drawn with the software Chemsketch version 14.01, 2012

delamanid (OPC-67683) was similarly approved by the European Medications Agency (EMA) [13].

The aim of this chapter is to review different aspects of the pharmacokinetics (PK) and pharmacodynamics (PD) of TB drugs. We begin with a review of the mechanisms of action and mechanisms of resistance for the TB drugs, followed by current methodologies to evaluate TB drug susceptibility. Next, we review PD models and their application to TB drugs. Finally, we highlight the use of therapeutic drug monitoring (TDM) as a means of optimizing treatment for individual patients. We note why the current drugs are used, and point out important gaps in our knowledge. As a whole, we highlight the importance of PK/PD and the challenges faced in applying it to TB treatment.

2 Mechanism of Action

A general overview of the mechanisms of action for the TB drugs is shown in Fig. 2.

2.1 First Line Drugs

RIF inhibits the DNA-dependent RNA-polymerase, thus preventing the transcription of DNA to RNA [14]. The RNA polymerase enzyme has the following subunits: $\alpha 2$, β, β', and σ. The inhibition occurs through the binding of the drug to the β subunit, encoded by the *rpoB* gene (same gene where mutations can cause drug resistance) [15]. RIF has potent, concentration-dependent bactericidal activity, and starts to kill microorganisms within minutes [8]. RIF displays sterilizing activity throughout the entire treatment period [4].

INH is a pro-drug, activated by the mycobacterial enzyme KatG [16]. The drug inhibits enzymes responsible for the synthesis of cell wall lipids. Specifically, INH inhibits the *inh*A protein activity for the synthesis of mycolic acids for the cell wall [17]. INH has strong bactericidal activity, and is particularly effective at the beginning of treatment against actively replicating microorganisms [18]. INH is not particularly effective against persisting bacilli [5]. INH use is maintained throughout treatment in an effort to prevent resistance. The absence of sterilizing activity is a characteristic seen among current TB drugs whose mechanism of action is based on cell wall inhibition.

PZA also is a pro-drug, and it is only active at an acidic pH. *Mtb* enzyme nicotinamidase/pyrazinamidase converts it to pyrazinoic acid (POA), which becomes trapped within the bacilli [19, 20]. Debate continues regarding its precise mode of action. It is hypothesized that POA, as an uncharged acidic conjugate (HPOA), causes acidification of the cytoplasm. This leads to the inhibition of important enzymes, and the disruption of the membrane potential. PZA only appears to kill microorganisms with low rates of metabolism, because they are unable to prevent HPOA accumulation and acidification [5]. The drug kills extracellular microorganisms, and in combination with RIF, it is responsible for the elimination of "persister" organisms. PZA's sterilizing activity is evident primarily during the first 2 months of therapy.

EMB inhibits mycobacterial cell wall synthesis [21, 22]. The drug inhibits the synthesis of arabinogalactan by preventing the polymerization of arabinose by an arabinosyl-transferase. The drug has moderate bactericidal activity in the initial phase of the

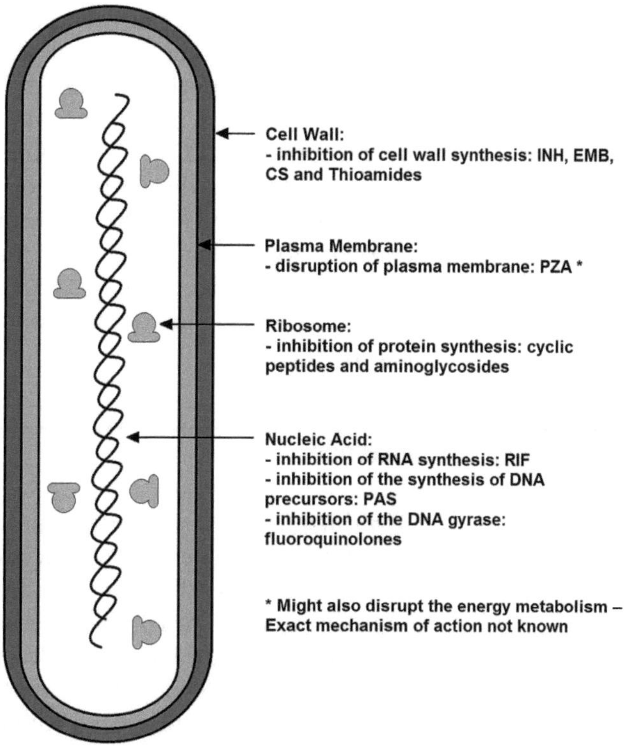

Fig. 2 Known or proposed targets for the TB drugs

treatment but it lacks sterilizing activity [4, 23, 24]. EMB's main use is to prevent further drug resistance while susceptibility data are pending. Once the susceptibility results are available, and if the microorganism is susceptible to the other three drugs, EMB can be stopped. EMB also is used as part of MDR-TB treatment regimens.

2.2 Second Line Drugs

Fluoroquinolones inhibit topoisomenrase II, also known as DNA gyrase, in *Mtb*. In other microorganisms these drugs also inhibit topoisomerase IV, absent in *Mtb* [25]. DNA gyrase is a bacterial enzyme responsible for preserving the superhelical twists in the DNA [26]. This enzyme consists of two subunits A and two subunits B, encoded by the genes *gyrA* and *gyrB*, respectively [25]. These drugs possess EBA and sterilizing activity [27].

Aminoglycosides inhibit protein synthesis by binding to the 16S ribosomal RNA sequence [28]. This inhibition does not affect human protein synthesis, since the ribosomal RNA structures are different [29]. Although CM is a polypeptide and not an aminoglycoside, it is often placed in the same category as the aminoglycosides, "the injectable agents," because of similarities in terms of dose, route of administration, pharmacokinetics, and toxicity [30]. All injectable agents are highly bactericidal against *Mtb* [31]. However, they lack potent sterilizing activity.

CS inhibits two enzymes, preventing peptidoglycan synthesis and d-alanine metabolism: d-alanine-d-alanine ligase, and alanine racemase, respectively [32]. ETA is a pro-drug, activated within the microorganism by a mono-oxygenase enzyme that is encoded by the ethA gene [17]. ETA inhibits the *inh*A protein activity that is responsible for the synthesis of cell wall mycolic acid (similar mechanism as INH). The mechanism of action of PAShas been debated for many years but may involve the inhibition of dihydrofolate reductase [33]. PAS displays tuberculostatic activity against *Mtb* [34]. In combination, it enhances the activity of SM and INH [33].

3 Development of Resistance

Mycobacterium tuberculosis acquires spontaneous chromosomal mutations that generate resistance to antimicrobials, with different frequencies depending on the drug [35]. The frequencies are approximately 1 in 10^6 microorganisms for INH and 1 in 10^8 microorganisms for RIF. Considering that a TB lesion may contain 10^8 microorganisms or more, mutant organisms are likely to be present. These will be spared when administering a single antimicrobial agent. When administering drugs with different mechanisms of resistance, the probability of resistance to both being present in a single bacterium is the sum of the probability for each drug. For INH and RIF, the probability of selecting a dual-resistant mutant would be 1 in 10^{14} microorganisms. INH and RIF have among the strongest early bactericidal effects, and therefore are effective in reducing the bacillary burden and preventing resistance in combined therapy. EMB has intermediate EBA, and PZA has the lowest EBA of the first line drugs.

Spontaneous mutations that confer resistance to fluoroquinolones happen in the frequency range of 2 in 10^6 microorganisms to 1 in 10^8 microorganisms [25]. Therefore 1–100 resistant *Mtb* are expected within the TB lesion. Cross-resistance also has been described for the fluoroquinolones. If there is diminished susceptibility to one of the drugs within the class, it is likely that the susceptibility is reduced for all fluoroquinolones [25].

The genes associated with resistance mutations, and the corresponding gene products, are shown for each TB drug in Table 1. The relationship with the mechanism of action with the resistance gene is described in Sect. 2 for the majority of the drugs.

Patient adherence to treatment is thought to play an important role in the prevention of drug resistance. This topic presents an important challenge, considering the long treatment duration, and the need for multiple drugs, each with adverse effects. After a study demonstrated the possibility of domiciliary treatment as opposed to long stays in a sanatorium, treatment costs were drastically

Table 1
Gene and product correlated with resistance for the tuberculosis drugs [130–132]

Drug	Gene correlated with resistance	Gene product
Rifampin	*rpoB*	β-Subunit of RNA polymerase
Isoniazid	*katG*	Catalase/peroxidase
	inhA	Enoyl reductase
	ahpC	Alkyl hydroperoxide reductase
Pyrazinamide	*pncA*	Pyrazinamidase/nicotinamidase
Ethambutol	*embB*	Arabinosyl transferase
Levofloxacin/moxifloxacin	*gyrA/gyrB*	DNA gyrase
Capreomycin	*tlyA*	rRNA methyltransferase
Amikacin/kanamycin	*rrs*	16S rRNA
Streptomycin	*rpsL*	S12 ribosomal protein
	rrs	16S rRNA
	gidB	7-Methylguanosine methyltransferase
Cycloserine	*alrA*[a]	d-alanine racemase
p-Aminosalicylic acid	*thyA*	Thymidylate synthase A
Ethionamide	*inhA*	Enoyl reductase

[a]Study with *Mycobacterium smegmatis*

reduced [5]. At the same time, the means for assuring regular drug administration, directly observed therapy (DOT), was initiated only gradually. Large numbers of patients failing to take drugs regularly often is blamed for much of the current drug resistance. In the US, DOT consists of the direct supervision of drug intake by a member of the healthcare team, and now is offered to a majority of TB patients throughout their treatment.

Considering the difficulty of seeing a patient 7 days a week, most TB programs provide a drug holiday over the weekend [36]. A study conducted by Drusano and colleagues evaluated the effect of drug holidays on the emergence of resistance to rifampin and moxifloxacin, using an in vitro system. They concluded that the 5/7 days regimen generated resistance to moxifloxacin, while the 7/7 days regimen did not. Another study by Srivastava et al., based on clinical trial simulations, concluded that around 1 % of TB patients develop drug resistance solely due to PK variability [37]. Dartois, however, points out the influence of PK variability on noncompliance [38]. She states that a patient with high drug exposure might not develop resistance because of missing doses while a patient with low drug exposure may. The impact of PK variability on resistance reinforces the importance of therapeutic drug monitoring (TDM) discussed in Sect. 17.

In addition to the factors discussed above, other limitations exist in the current treatment of TB. The flexibility of doses with regard to differences in body weight is low and this factor can provide variability in drug exposure among patients. The current doses were optimized many years ago when the mean population weight was significantly lower than today. In addition, due to evolution *Mtb* strains present MIC distributions that might differ from place to place [39, 40]. Therefore, there is a need for revising the current TB drug doses in order to avoid resistance.

4 Susceptibility Testing

The ultimate aim of the drug susceptibility test (DST) is to verify if the isolate differs from the wild-type *Mtb* in terms of susceptibility to specific antimicrobials [41]. DSTs can be classified as qualitative or quantitative. Qualitative tests suggest susceptibility or resistance, but do not provide a specific value. Quantitative tests determine the MIC, the smallest concentration that produces 99 % or more of inhibition on the microorganism population. The interpretation of the qualitative test is restricted to "susceptible," "intermediate," and "resistant" without a final MIC value. To interpret MIC results it is important to take into consideration the relationship with the drug concentrations achieved at the infection site, the correlation between the isolate MIC, and the MIC from other strains of the same species, as well as previous use of antimicrobial agents. The results of DST are solely suggestive. It is the clinician's responsibility to consider the drug's metabolism and pharmacology, patient specific characteristics, and the use of concomitant drugs, among other factors [42].

Drug susceptibility testing on TB patients' samples is performed with the objective of evaluating the adequacy of the drugs for treatment, to confirm if a treatment failure is due to drug resistance, and to estimate the prevalence of drug resistance [43]. Some of the limitations of drug susceptibility testing include the fact that the environment conditions are different than the ones in the host [42]. This includes the fact that a unique microorganism is grown in an environment with plenty of nutrients. However, one result that can always be used in the clinic is the evaluation of resistance. If the microorganism is resistant to a certain antibiotic in vitro, there is a good chance that it will be resistant in the patient as well.

Direct and indirect methods have been used for DST on TB isolates [44]. The direct method refers to the direct inoculation of the sample. The advantage of this approach is a shorter time for obtaining results. The indirect method requires the isolation of the microorganism prior to susceptibility testing. Advantages of the indirect approach include a more precise inoculum size, and reduced contamination by other organisms.

The most common solid media used for *Mtb* are the egg-based Löwenstein–Jensen (L–J) and the agar based 7H11 [45]. L–J media presents some disadvantages, such as a high batch-to-batch variation (depending on the egg quality), difficulties on distinguishing colonies from debris, and obtaining consistent drug concentrations. In contrast, the 7H11 media is transparent, promoting an easy differentiation of colonies from debris and therefore small colonies can be detected earlier. However, plates are expensive, with a short half-life (1 month) and they have to be protected from light that can cause degradation and formation of formaldehyde, toxic to the mycobacteria.

Both direct and indirect methods can be used in agar plates by the proportion method [44]. "Critical" drug concentrations are incorporated in the agar. Those concentrations are empirical without relationship to concentrations obtained in the human body. It is presumed that the patient will not respond to the treatment if the result of the test is "resistant." The sample is inoculated in quadrants with and without drug and the percentage of resistance is calculated based on this relationship. The isolate is considered susceptible if the drug completely inhibits growth and at least 100 colonies are found on the control (agar without drug), and resistant if there is at least 1 % of growth on the agar containing drug in relation to the control.

Different systems have been used for liquid media [45]. The Bactec 460 TB system is based on the use of radioisotopes. The microorganisms metabolize [^{14}C] palmitic acid to $^{14}CO_2$, detected by the equipment [45]. The production and quantity of $^{14}CO_2$ is directly proportional to the growth of the microorganism. Some limitations of this system include the impossibility of evaluating colony morphology, the overgrowth of contaminants, cost, the disposal of the radioisotopes and safety, considering the necessity of using syringes with needles. This system was discontinued due to the use of radioisotopes.

The BACTEC 960 MGIT system is a continuous monitoring system based on the use of mycobacterial growth indicator tubes (MGIT) [45]. These tubes contain a fluorescence sensor that is bound to oxygen. The sensor consists of silicon rubber that contains ruthenium pentahydrate. Initially, there is no fluorescence. However, as the mycobacteria (or other microorganisms) metabolize the bound oxygen, the indicator starts to fluoresce. The instrument then is able to detect the change in fluorescence, and it calculates a number (growth index) that is used in an algorithm to determine growth.

Both indirect qualitative and quantitative analysis can be performed for the BACTEC systems [44]. Regarding the qualitative analysis, resistance is indicated if the daily growth index in the drug containing-vial is higher than the observed growth of the control diluted 1:100. For the quantitative analysis (MIC definition), three drug concentrations are necessary. The lowest concentrations correspond to the highest MIC found for wild strains [41] and the sample is considered susceptible if the MIC is lower or equal to this concentration. The MIC is the sample with the lowest drug concentration where minimal or no growth index increase is detected.

It has been demonstrated that both sensitivity and time to growth are similar for Bactec 460 TB and BACTEC 960 MGIT system and superior to solid media [45]. The advantage of the BACTEC 960 MGIT system over the BACTEC 460 TB system is the lack of need for radioisotopes, the reduced potential for cross-contamination, reduced labor, the possibility of continuous monitoring and electronic data management [45].

To perform DST with PZA, the pH of the broth has to be reduced to 6 (usually 6.8–7), due to the fact that the drug is more active at lower pH values [44]. For more details about DST and critical drug concentrations we recommend the following books by Leonid Heifets [41, 44].

Molecular tools can be used to reduce diagnostic time through the evaluation of mutations associated with resistance [46]. Campbell and colleagues used molecular methods to detect TB drug resistance and compared the results with the phenotypic data, as well as calculated accuracy values. The results of the study support the use of molecular methods to detect resistance to TB drugs. However, it is important to emphasize that molecular tests do not replace the use of culture and the DST [47]. Phenotypic and genotypic results need to be evaluated together to provide more accurate clinical information.

The adequacy of the current recommended susceptibility breakpoints and their clinical relevance has been a topic of much discussion. *Mtb*'s evolution was pointed out as a reason for the inadequacy of the previously established breakpoints, as well as the variability in the MIC values according to different regions, in addition to PK variability [39, 48]. Gumbo evaluated the currently used critical concentrations in terms of the probability of achieving an area under the curve/MIC that correlates with 90 % or more of maximal *Mtb* kill in 90 % or more of patients [40]. This study embraced the use of Monte Carlo simulations using 10,000 virtual patients. The author proposed that the susceptibility breakpoints of isoniazid, rifampin, and pyrazinamide should be lowered, while the concentrations of moxifloxacin and ethambutol were adequate. A change in the current ofloxacin breakpoint from 2 to 0.5 μg/mL was suggested by a study that also used Monte Carlo simulations to evaluate the probability of target attainment [49].

5 PK/PD Indices

When evaluating the PK/PD indices it is important to take into account the role of protein binding. The binding of drugs to proteins is an important factor that influences the amount of drug that can penetrate into the tissues (at the site of infection) and exert its effect [50, 51]. The serum protein binding is especially important when it is higher than 70–80 %, considering that any small change in the binding can have a significant effect on the free fraction [51].

Anti-infective drugs have been classified into two major groups according to the killing profile: time-dependent killing and concentration-dependent killing [52, 53]. The parameters associated with the concentration-dependent killing drugs are given by the ratio of the area under the curve of the free drug concentration over the MIC (*f*AUC/MIC) or the ratio of the maximum drug concentration over the MIC (fC_{max}/MIC) [35]. The effect of the concentration-dependent drugs increases with an increase in dose. Fluoroquinolones, aminoglycosides and rifamycins are examples of concentration-dependent drugs. Once above the MIC by twofold to fourfold, the effects of the time-dependent drugs do not increase with an increase in dose. For these compounds the effect depends on the time that the drug concentration remains above the MIC (T > MIC). Beta-lactams are examples of time-dependent killing compounds. Considering that the effect within the PK/PD parameter is given by the ratio of an exposure variable to a potency variable (MIC), the higher the MIC value, the lower the microbiological effect of a drug [54].

5.1 Limitations of the Use of PK/PD Indices

The PK/PD indices use the drug concentrations in the plasma or serum [53]. This approach has the drawback of not taking into consideration the tissue distribution, and historically, protein binding was not considered. Additionally, the MIC provides important information regarding the potency of the interaction between the microorganism and the drug, but does not offer information about the effect of the drug over time [55]. The MIC does not generate specific information regarding the rate of antibactericidal effect and how different doses can affect this rate [53]. The MIC is a static parameter that relies on the bacterial count at a certain time point. It does not take into consideration that different microorganism growth and death rates can generate the same final MIC value. The MIC also does not supply information about a possible postantibiotic effect of the compound [55].

6 Pharmacodynamic Models

An alternative approach in relation to the PK/PD parameters is to evaluate the efficacy of antimicrobials with time-kill curves [53]. This methodology considers the microbial growth and kill as a function of time and drug concentration. In some systems, it is possible to mimic the human PK drug profile and therefore expose the microorganism to this change in concentration over the time. Mathematical models can be used to analyze the data and through the use of simulations, the optimal dosage regimen can be identified. This approach presents several advantages over the use of the MIC: direct comparison of the effect of different drug concentrations, more detailed information regarding the PK–PD relationship, and information about the effect of the antimicrobial over time. Time-kill curves can be obtained from in vitro systems as well as animal models. In this section we will provide information about some commonly used in vitro systems for mycobacteria, as well as animal models for TB.

6.1 *In Vitro Models*

Regarding in vitro models, the hollow fiber system (HFS) frequently has been used to perform time-kill curves with different drugs and *Mtb* [36, 56, 57]. The HFS contains hollow fiber cartridges and the microorganisms are placed in a peripheral compartment, as shown in Fig. 3a. Semipermeable hollow fibers separate the central compartment from the peripheral and allow the transference of nutrients and drug, but not microorganisms, according to the membrane pore cutoff [56]. The drug is added in a dosing port located in the central compartment. Peristaltic pumps continuously infuse broth into the central compartment and at the same rate remove broth containing drug from the central compartment to waste. The pump rates are set in such a manner that the human plasma drug profile can be mimicked within the system. Media samples are serially collected and plated. Time-kill curves are obtained by plotting the change in the colony-forming unit per mL (CFU/mL) over time.

An alternative model was developed by Budha and collaborators based on previously developed in vitro systems and is shown in Fig. 3b [58]. A peristaltic pump continuously infuses broth into the main double-armed flask while a second pump is set at the same rate and removes broth from the main flask through a filter that prevents microorganism elimination. Drug doses are added on a lateral arm. The rates at which the pumps work allow the bacteria to be exposed to the human PK profile of the drug within the main flask. The double-armed flask is kept at 37 °C by water recirculation through a water jacket and the culture is maintained homogeneous through the use of a magnetic stirrer. The samples are collected and further plated in the same manner as described for the HFS.

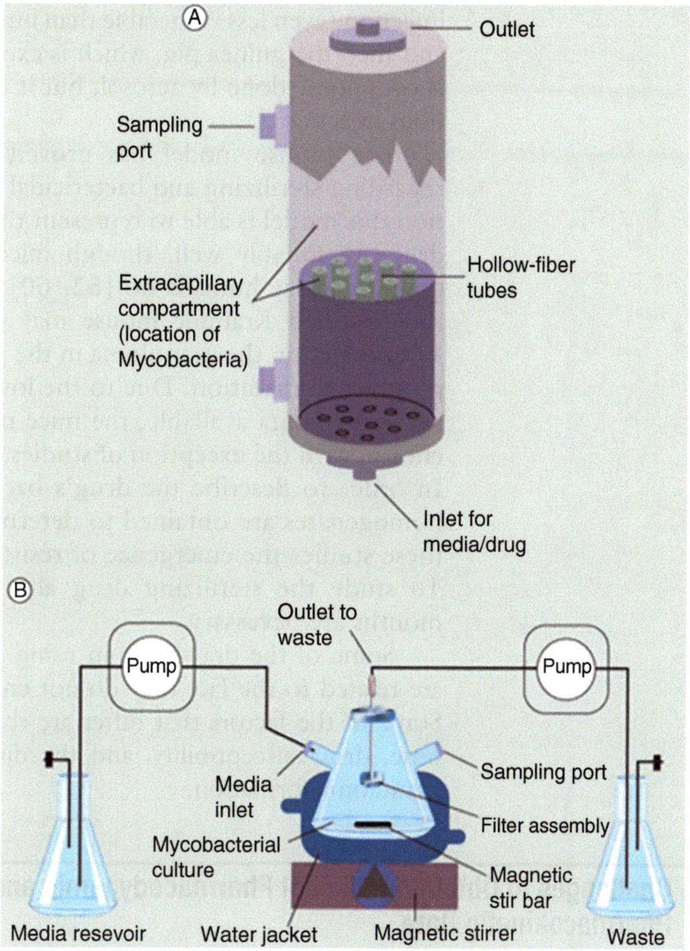

Fig. 3 The hollow fiber system cartridge (**a**) and the dilution system (**b**). Adapted from Vaddady PK et al. 2010 [59]

The in vitro models represent a simplification of what occurs in vivo [59]. The differences are related to pathogen, host and PK factors. Regarding the pathogen factors, the majority of the microorganisms present different growth rates in vitro in relation to in vivo. Additionally, host factors, such as the immune response, are not fully captured, and plasma protein binding may not be taken into account.

6.2 Animal Models

Animal models take into account the interaction between the microorganism, the host and the drug, which is not possible with in vitro systems [60]. The vast majority of preclinical TB studies were performed with mice, rabbits, and guinea pigs [61]. In addition, nonhuman primates and cattle models have been used. Considering the three species, mice are the least vulnerable to infection (even less vulnerable than humans) followed by the rabbit and then the guinea pig, which is extremely vulnerable. Infection is commonly done by aerosol, but it can also be done by intravenous injection.

The mouse model has proved to generate reliable data regarding sterilizing and bactericidal drug activity [60]. In addition this model is able to represent the activity of the current TB drugs reasonably well, though mice do not develop necrotic granulomas as humans do [52, 60]. More recent models with the so-called Kramnic mouse may be more human-like [62]. After infection the granuloma in the guinea pig and in the rabbit progress to caseation. Due to the low cost, small size, and large amount of data available, the mice model is still the method of choice, with the exception of studies that require caseation [63]. In order to describe the drug's bactericidal effect, lung tissue homogenates are obtained to determine the CFU/mL. During these studies the emergence of resistance also can be evaluated. To study the sterilizing drug activity, studies longer than 2 months are necessary.

Some of the drawbacks in using animal TB infection models are related to the fact they do not entirely reflect human disease. Some of the factors that differ are the course of the disease over time, drug susceptibility, and the disease characteristics such as granuloma formation.

7 Challenges to Obtaining Clinical Pharmacodynamic and Tissue Pharmacokinetic Data

Tuberculosis affects different organs in the human body. The main targets are the lungs, and for a drug to reach the site of action it needs to be transported from the blood to the lesions—which may not be vascularized—and penetrate into caseous granulomas to reach *Mtb* [64]. Doses for the first line TB treatment were established many years ago at a time when pharmacokinetics and pharmacodynamics were used sparingly as dose optimization tools. Therefore, drug penetration was not taken into account and this represents a major factor why today we have suboptimal doses. The unique structure of the lungs make the acquisition of human data difficult regarding drug penetration, information about the temporal kill profile of the microorganisms during treatment, as well as data about resistance patterns.

Data from drug concentrations in the epithelial lining fluid (ELF) is often equated to the extracellular drug concentrations in the pulmonary tissue [65]. Although these drug concentrations are considered to be in equilibrium with the extracellular fluid, it does not represent the drug concentration inside the TB lesion. The TB granuloma is protected by a fibrous wall and may contain caseous material with different pH values in relation to healthy tissue. These factors could promote different patterns of drug penetration into the lesions as compared to healthy tissue. Although this approach offers an alternative considering the protected location of the infection, its clinical significance has not been proven yet.

Sputum samples are used to evaluate the resistance of clinical isolates. However, it has been demonstrated that the lung cavity presents an environment that favors the development of resistance [66, 67]. Additional drug resistance has been demonstrated in the cavity in relation to sputum [66, 67]. The lack of vascularization in the caseous lesions results in diminished delivery of oxygen and nutrients, generating metabolic quiescence that leads to a reduction of *Mtb* cellular proliferation [64]. In addition, the lack of vascularization leads to a reduced penetration of drugs as well as T lymphocytes. These factors lead to an increase in drug tolerance within the lesion.

7.1 Rifamycins

The rifamycins consist of three drugs used in the treatment of TB: rifampin, rifabutin, and rifapentine. First introduced in the late 1960s, rifampin is the most important of TB drugs. The rifamycins work by inhibiting RNA polymerase. Consequently, mutations in the *rpoB* gene encoding RNA polymerase can result in the formation of resistant organisms.

The rifamycins are concentration-dependent killers of TB. Both C_{max}/MIC or AUC/MIC are associated with mycobacterial killing. Studies reveal that the rifamycins concentrate within macrophages, although higher intracellular concentrations may not equal higher intracellular activity [68]. Burman et al. point out that there is large variability in study results [69].

Clinically evaluating the PD properties of the rifamycins can be difficult. Rifamycin monotherapy leads to resistance by most pathogens, necessitating the use of combination therapy. However, separating the extent of the rifamycins' effectiveness from companion drugs is problematic. Additionally, unless measured in vitro, the immune system "interferes" with evaluating the killing of *Mtb* by rifampin (or any antimicrobial), thus, HFS are often used to assess the clinical utility of anti-TB drugs, including the rifamycins.

7.2 Rifampin

The current recommended rifampin dose for active TB disease is 600 mg. Arrival at this dose is somewhat cloudy, but Van Ingen et al. give three reasons initial investigators chose this particular dose: (1) cost of the drug at the time was prohibitive due to its semisynthetic nature (2), concern over possible toxicity at higher doses, and (3) a 600 mg dose provided a C_{max} between 8.8 and 12 μg/mL, which is 40–60 times the MIC of *Mtb*, not taking into account protein binding [70]. This C_{max}/MIC suggests that

600 mg would be more than sufficient to eradicate *Mtb*. However, even a modest reduction in dose to 450 mg resulted in a significant decline in rifampin's activity [71]. EBA also decreases with a 300 mg dose, but increases with higher doses [72].

For rifampin, many early studies pointed to C_{max}/MIC as the parameter most associated with efficacy. However, recent studies by Jayaram and Gumbo suggest a greater correlation with the AUC/MIC [57, 73]. Gumbo et al. used a HFS to show increased killing of *Mtb* with increasing AUC [57]. In agreement, Jayaram et al. identified the AUC/MIC as the PK/PD parameter most associated with microbial killing using an aerosol infection model [73]. However, C_{max}/MIC was the parameter most associated with prevention of resistance. Gumbo et al. noted that a $fC_{max}/MIC > 175$ is required for the prevention of rifampin monoresistance [57].

Caution is necessary when attempting to translate model results to humans. Human pulmonary TB primarily consists of extracellular bacilli while murine TB models are primarily intracellular. Additionally, as many researchers point out, animal models may have many features that limit their usefulness. We discuss this further in the rifapentine section.

7.3 Rifabutin

Rifabutin shares some structural features with rifampin, but differences exist in their PK properties due to rifabutin's increased lipid solubility [74]. This increased lipophilicity leads to a larger volume of distribution, a decreased clearance and, thus, a much longer half-life. Despite a much lower C_{max}/MIC (approximately 7.5 μg/mL) compared to rifampin, rifabutin seems to be as active as rifampin [69, 75]. Additionally; rifabutin's inductive capabilities are much less than rifampin's (~40 %) [76]. Unfortunately, rifabutin is a CYP3A4 substrate, resulting in many bidirectional interactions with CYP inhibitors (e.g., protease inhibitors). Rifabutin, unlike rifampin, is limited by concentration-related toxicities. The risk of patients experiencing anterior uveitis, neutropenia and thrombocytopenia increases with increasing concentrations.

7.4 Rifapentine

A cyclo-pentyl derivative of rifampin, rifapentine has a much longer half-life (~12 h) than rifampin. The longer half-life was thought to lend itself to intermittent dosing, but in humans, that has not proven to be the case. Additionally, early in vitro and murine studies indicated rifapentine was more potent than rifampin [77–79]. However, clinical trials show rifapentine to be no more active than rifampin [80–82]. Study 29 compared 10 mg/kg rifampin plus standard therapy (INH, PZA, EMB) to 10 mg/kg rifapentine plus standard therapy during the first 2 months of treatment. The study showed no difference in outcomes (time to culture conversion) between the two groups [81]. Three possible reasons were offered by the authors: (1) rifapentine's high protein binding might have detracted from its effect, (2) the dichotomous endpoint used in the study reduced statistical power, and (3) the medications generally were taken without food, which increases rifampin absorption but decreases rifapentine absorption.

One reason for this discrepancy between preclinical and clinical studies may be the animal model used. In the murine model, rifapentine looked superior to rifampin, but in the guinea pig model, the two rifamycins were similar, just as in Study 29 [83]. Guinea pigs, when infected with TB, develop necrotic granulomas similar to humans with *Mtb* concentrated extracellularly rather than intracellularly. Mice, on the other hand, do not develop necrotic granulomas and *Mtb* are primarily intracellular. Rifapentine is believed to penetrate macrophages better than rifampin, which would account for the greater efficacy in in vitro and murine studies [68]. Extracellular activity is comparable between the two [68].

Increasing the dose of rifapentine could result in greater efficacy. However, unlike rifampin, rifapentine's dose–response curve appears to flatten just short of a 1200 mg dose. Doubling the dose from 600 to 1200 mg does not result in a proportional increase in exposure. In a recent POP PK analysis by Savic et al., modeling and simulation showed that, while rifapentine exposure increased less than proportionally, there was no plateau in exposures from 450 to 1800 mg [84].

As with isoniazid, Dr. Mitchison makes a case for rifapentine's C_{max} as the parameter most associated with efficacy rather than AUC, citing Study 29 as an example [85]. He advises that future murine studies are conducted with a "chronic" disease model whereby mice are infected for months rather than a couple of weeks [86]. This model would allow for the presence of persister populations of *Mtb*. Further, he suggests using liquid media rather than solid media [85]. However, Neuremberger et al. argue that the duration infection in the murine studies is long enough to produce persisters [87].

8 Isoniazid

Along with rifampin, isoniazid is a main drug in TB treatment. The complex interplay between isoniazid pharmacokinetics and pharmacodynamics is often difficult to unravel. Mutations in the *N*-acetyl transferase (NAT-2) gene lead to two distinct rates of clearance. Whether or not this difference in clearance affects outcomes is often debated.

Isoniazid is a prodrug, converted to its active form by the catalase peroxidase enzyme (KatG). The activated intermediate is believed to be an isonicotinoyl radical which couples to NAD+/NADPH and forms an adduct [88]. This INH-NAD adduct is responsible for antitubercular activity by blocking mycolic acid synthesis [16]. Mutations disrupt catalase peroxidase's activity, resulting in an INH resistant organism [89, 90]. The most common mutation, accounting for 30–60 % of KatG mutations, is a point mutation, S315T [90, 91]. This alteration in the KatG enzyme confers complete resistance to INH at 1–2 μg/mL. A mutation in the *inhA* gene also confers resistance to isoniazid but to a lesser extent. InhA, an enoyl reductase enzyme, looks to be the main target for the INH-NAD adduct. Resistance to this target occurs in approximately 1 in 10^7 bacteria. Mutations in *inhA* confer resistance to not only isoniazid, but the structurally similar antitubercular drug ethionamide [92, 93]. Some evidence exists that higher doses of isoniazid (16–18 mg/kg/day) can overcome low-level resistance [94].

Isoniazid is considered bactericidal and produces a post-antibiotic effect which can last up to 5 days [95]. The clinical relevance of this effect is not known. Isoniazid eliminates *Mtb* in the log-phase stage of growth, causing a rapid decline in bacilli within the first few days of administration. This decline in bacillary rate is referred to as early bactericidal activity (EBA). Isoniazid's decline in bactericidal activity is attributed to the reduction of bacteria in log phase; however, Gumbo et al. believe it is due to the emergence of isoniazid resistance within the bacterial population [96]. Mitchison et al. disagree, stating there are no clinical data to support this and growth rates are slower in actual patients [97]. Regardless of the mechanism, the PD parameter primarily associated with efficacy is either C_{max} or AUC. Gumbo et al. identified the AUC/MIC as the PK/PD parameter primarily associated with both microbial kill and prevention of resistance [98]. However, Mitchison et al. maintain C_{max} as the PK parameter primarily associated with efficacy [85]. Knowing the appropriate PK parameter associated with efficacy may determine what TB drugs are used together. For instance, Weiner et al. state that the reason once weekly isoniazid/rifapentine was less effective than a twice weekly regimen was due to low isoniazid concentrations, in other words, a "pharmacokinetic mismatch." [99] The authors suggest a companion drug with a higher AUC may prove more effective. However, Srivastava et al. contend that a pharmacokinetic mismatch does not lead to emergence of resistance to either isoniazid or rifampin [100].

9 Pyrazinamide

A prodrug, PZA is converted to its active form, pyrazinoic acid, by the bacterial pyrazinamidase enzyme. Most mycobacterial species are resistant to PZA. PZA's activity is limited to *Mtb*, and *M. africanum*. Resistance is conferred through mutations in the *pncA* gene that encodes pyrazinamidase [101]. The exact mechanism of action has yet to be fully elucidated [102–104]. Pyrazinoic acid seems to be the active constituent. PZA is most effective in an acidic environment but *Mtb* appears not to consume any significant amount of acid, thus, it is believed that only pyrazinoic acid created within *Mtb* is active [19, 104]. PZA's preference for an acidic environment makes it difficult to assess resistance through culture methods. Alternative methods for assessing resistance include genetic sequencing of *pncA*, the Wayne Assay, a color metric assay, which assesses pyrazinamidase activity, or molecular based assays [105].

PZA's efficacy appears to be dose-dependent. Currently, the recommended US dose is 25 mg/kg daily or 50 mg/kg twice weekly. Some studies suggest higher doses should be used to maximize efficacy (>30 mg/kg/day). A murine and guinea pig study by Ahmad et al. showed dose-dependent activity at human-equivalent doses. Utilizing an in vitro PK/PD model examining PZA's sterilizing activity against *Mtb* (pH of 5.8) Gumbo et al. state that the current PZA dosing recommendation of 20–25 mg/kg/day is suboptimal. The authors' modeling suggests doses of 3000–4000 mg per day (40–60 mg/kg/day) are necessary.

The PK/PD parameter primarily associated with PZA activity is believed to be AUC/MIC [106]. Gumbo et al., utilizing a HFS, showed that PZA's sterilizing effect correlated best with AUC/MIC while the time above the MIC correlated with suppression of resistance [106]. However, as stated previously, the MIC depends on the pH of the media used. For example, the highest PZA MIC against 21 susceptible *Mtb* strains was shown to be eightfold lower at a pH of 5.5 (less than 50 μg/mL) than at a pH of 5.95 (400 μg/mL) [107]. The variability seen in vitro may be less than the variability seen within the lysosomes of macrophages, which is believed to range between a pH of 4.8–7 [108].

The primary concern with using higher doses is the fear of hepatotoxicity. INH and RIF are potential hepatotoxins, so the rate of hepatotoxicity due solely to PZA is difficult to determine. Early PZA studies using higher doses showed an association between PZA and an increased incidence of hepatotoxicity. However, a meta-analysis by Pasipanodya and Gumbo suggests that a majority of cases may be idiosyncratic [109]. Additional adverse reactions include GI upset, arthralgia and an increase in uric acid concentrations [110]. The 1959 USPHS study of PZA and INH showed PZA dose-related increases in hepatotoxicity. In the study, 4 of 160 (2 %) patients given PZA 25 mg/kg daily, developed hepatotoxicity while 11 of 167 (7 %) given PZA 40 mg/kg daily developed hepatotoxicity [111]. Hepatotoxicity in the high dose group was associated with elevated bilirubin and symptoms of liver dysfunction. A meta-analysis of 29 studies by Pasipanodya and Gumbo suggest hepatotoxicity is not dose related but idiosyncratic [109]. They did note a trend toward increasing frequency of hepatotoxicity at doses greater than 40 mg/kg but that doses of up to 60 mg/kg were not predicted to have a significant increase in hepatotoxicity. The mechanism through which toxicity occurs is unclear. In the same study, the most frequent adverse event was arthralgia which was associated with higher doses, however, the clinical importance of this side effect was considered "nonsevere" [109].

10 Ethambutol

EMB is a synthetic agent that was specifically designed to be used against *Mtb*. It is believed EMB targets arabinosyltransferases that are necessary for the synthesis of arabinan (in arabinogalactan), a cell wall component. Inhibiting this synthesis leads to mycolic acid accumulation and eventually cell death [21, 112]. EMB is bacteriostatic at lower doses with MICs in the 0.5–2 μg/mL range, depending upon the media used. Higher doses of EMB can be bactericidal in vitro. Resistance occurs from mutations primarily in one of the genes encoding arabinosyltransferases, designated *embC*, *embA*, and *embB* (*embCAB* operon).

The most important adverse event seen with EMB is optic neuritis. The incidence of optic neuritis is low with standard doses in patients with normal renal function. It may add to visual problems in patients with preexisting ocular conditions, such as cataracts or diabetic retinopathy. Ezer et al. report a cumulative incidence of visual impairment of 22.5 per 1000 persons with permanent impairment at 4.3 persons per 1000 [113]. Snellen charts are used to test for visual acuity while Ishihara color plates are used for green–red color discrimination. Tests should be conducted at baseline and throughout treatment. Adverse vision changes are dose related with an increased incidence seen with 30 mg/kg/day compared with 15–25 mg/kg/day. Visual changes in patients on EMB generally are reversible once EMB is discontinued, though not always. Additional adverse events include GI disturbance, arthralgia, and neutropenia and thrombocytopenia.

11 Fluoroquinolones

11.1 Levofloxacin and Moxifloxacin

Oral LEVO bioavailability is close to 100 % and absorption is fast, with a T_{max} range of 0.8–2.4 h [114]. The drug penetrates well into most tissues with a volume of distribution of 1.1 L/Kg. LEVO binds mainly to albumin with protein binding ranging from 24 to 38 %. The protein binding does not depend on serum drug concentrations. MOXI bioavailability is higher than 85 %. The T_{MAX} is about 2 h, while the volume of distribution is around 2.7 L/kg [115]. MOXI protein binding is around 50 %. Fluoroquinolones can cross the placenta and can be detected in breast milk. The kidneys primarily clear LEVO, while MOXI is eliminated by the liver (52 %) and by the kidney (20 %). The elimination half-life is 7.4 h for LEVO and 6.5 h for MOXI when measured in TB patients [116]. Considering that the kidneys eliminate the majority of LEVO, caution has to be taken with patients that present renal dysfunction and MOXI might be a better option [30]. The fluoroquinolones present GI side effects such as nausea, diarrhea and vomiting. They also can cause tendinitis, tendon rupture and phototoxicity. MOXI seems to be more toxic then LEVO in terms of QT interval prolongation. Currently, the recommended doses for LEVO are 750 and 1000 mg once a day (orally or intravenously), while the MOXI dose is 400 mg once a day.

In vitro and in vivo studies demonstrated absence of induction or inhibition of the cytochrome CYP P450 and as a consequence no drug interactions associated with this metabolizing enzyme are expected, however, RIF reduces MOXI concentrations 25–30%, probably through induced sulphation or glucuronidation [117]. An increase on the effect of warfarin and its derivatives was noticed in patients taking the drug concomitantly with LEVO [117]. In addition, altered blood glucose concentrations have been described for patients taking diabetic drugs. LEVO interactions with other drugs used for TB is not common [25]. The drug absorption might be reduced by the concomitant ingestion of antacids with multivalent cations [25].

12 Aminoglycosides and Polypeptides

12.1 Amikacin, Kanamycin, Streptomycin, and Capreomycin

These drugs are commonly prescribed once resistance to SM has been demonstrated [30]. The drugs are intravenously administered at a dose of 12–15 mg/kg 5–7 days a week, and 20–27 mg/kg 2 or 3 days per week [115]. When administered intramuscularly, the drugs take between 30 and 90 min to be absorbed. The intravenous infusions typically last 30 min. The drugs present low plasma protein binding, with a volume of distribution in the range of 0.25–0.30 L/kg. No metabolites have been described so far. The drugs are eliminated by the kidneys with elimination half-lives in the range of 2–4 h and with the clearance in parallel to the creatinine clearance. The main side effects for these drugs are related to auditory, vestibular and renal toxicities. Reversible non-oliguric acute tubular necrosis might increase the serum creatinine. Renal cation loss also has been demonstrated. Periodic monitoring of blood urea nitrogen, serum creatinine, calcium, potassium, magnesium is recommended. Physical examinations for vestibular changes also are recommended. Injectable TB drugs may enhance the nephrotoxicity of other drugs, such as amphotericin B, and they may enhance the effects of neuromuscular blocking agents in selected patients [115].

13 Ethionamide

A structural analog of INH, ETA also inhibits mycolic acid synthesis. Cross-resistance between INH and ETA is possible. Mutations in the *inhA* structural gene or in the promotor region typically cause resistance to both INH and ETA. Mutations in the *katg* gene affect only INH, allowing the use of ETA [118, 119].

ETA is usually administered twice a day at the doses of 250–500 mg [115]. The drug is adequately absorbed, and the T_{max} is in the range of 1.5–2.5 h (500 mg dose). The plasma protein binding ranges from 10 to 30 %. Some ETA reaches the CSF, but CSF concentrations may be below the MIC. It also promptly crosses the placenta. The PK/PD of ETA have not been adequately studied. Based on some similarity to INH, one might posit that AUC/MIC is the most important parameter. In light of that, it is easy to see why ETA is a weak TB drug, because both C_{max}/MIC and AUC/MIC are low. Further, Time > MIC is brief, so ETA has very little going for it. The drug is mostly metabolized in the liver and the sulphoxide metabolite can be converted back to the parent drug [30]. ETA has significant GI side effects manifested in the majority of patients as nausea and in many patients as vomiting. ETA suppositories can be taken together (or singularly) with a reduced oral dose in order to prevent the GI side effects [115]. Another important side effect is hypothyroidism that is more common in patients also treated with PAS.

14 Para-Amino Salicylic Acid

PAS, structurally similar to aspirin, is available as a granule dosage form. Its exact mechanism of action is unknown. It is believed PAS inhibits dihydropteroate synthase (DHPS) in *Mtb* by competing with its structural analog, para-aminobenzoate (PABA), a necessary precursor in folate synthase, though research continues [33, 120].

As with aspirin, PAS may cause GI upset. GI complaints are the most common side effects experienced with PAS and increases with increasing dose. PASER®, a sustained-release, enteric-coated, granule dosage form was created to lessen these side effects. The granules typically are administered as a packet of small beads, which can be sprinkled onto soft food (provided that they are not chewed), or poured into the mouth and washed down with liquid.

PAS is given two to three times daily. It is metabolized by N-acetyl transferase 1 (NAT-1). The parent drug is predominately cleared by the liver, with metabolites renally cleared. As noted, PAS has the potential to cause hypothyroidism and patients should be monitored for this side effect.

15 Cycloserine

Cycloserine, sometimes called "psycho-serine" because of its untoward CNS side effects, is one of the less pleasant drugs taken by TB patients. A small molecule (molecular weight = 102 g/mol), cycloserine easily penetrates the CNS. The drug works by disrupting the incorporation of d-alanine into peptidoglycan, an integral component of the bacterial cell wall. The appropriate PK/PD parameter associated with efficacy is unknown, while toxicity appears to be concentration-dependent. CNS side effects are the primary concern with administering cycloserine. Vega et al. estimate the incidence of anxiety, depression, and psychosis each occurs in 12–13 % of patients [121]. The exact mechanism for causing CNS effects is unknown, but may be through its actions as a partial agonist of the *N*-methyl-d-aspartate (NMDA) receptor [122, 123].

16 Bedaquiline

At the time of this writing, bedaquiline (Sirturo®) is the latest drug to be approved for use in TB treatment in the US. A diarylquinoline, bedaquiline represents the first novel class of anti-TB drugs in over four decades. Bedaquiline inhibits the proton pump of adenosine triphosphate (ATP) synthase, a necessary enzyme in the synthesis of *Mtb* [124]. No cross-resistance with first- and second-line TB drugs occurs, due to its unique mechanism of action. Some cross-resistance may be seen with the reserve TB drug clofazimine [125]. Currently only approved for use in MDR TB, bedaquiline shows bactericidal activity against other mycobacterial species. Bedaquiline is active against both sensitive and drug resistant strains with an MIC of 0.03 μg/mL [126]. An early murine study indicates AUC as the PD parameter most associated with efficacy [127]. Rouan et al. administered bedaquiline to mice at doses of 15, 30, or 60 mg/kg divided daily (5 days per week), twice weekly, or once weekly. Bactericidal activity correlated with total weekly dosing (and exposure) rather than frequency of administration [127].

The primary concern with bedaquiline is the potential for QT prolongation. An additive, or even synergistic, prolongation in the QT interval may be seen when administered with other QT-prolonging agents such as the FQs and the macrolides [128]. Thus, close monitoring of ECGs are necessary.

17 TDM

As with many other conditions, TDM can benefit TB patients by individualizing drug therapy. TDM can reduce the risk of toxicity, or increase the likelihood of efficacy. Drug therapy can be modified to achieve specific, targeted concentrations. Patients with TB often experience reduced serum drug concentrations because of (1) a low initial dose, (2) malabsorption, or (3) drug–drug interactions. All of these problems can be alleviated through TDM [129].

Multiple factors may influence drug absorption, including: disease states (e.g., diabetes, HIV), food, antacids, or gut transporters altered by concurrent medications. Drugs may be malabsorbed, undergo delayed absorption. Measuring serum concentrations at two time points (typically 2 and 6 h post dose) can distinguish between the two problems. TDM allows for a prompt change in dose, and contributes to a more rapid and complete response to treatment [129].

18 Conclusions

The clinical pharmacodynamics of the TB drugs were insufficiently studied in the past, but significant efforts have been made in recent years to better understand and control therapy. Many treatment centers in developing nations still rely on clinical diagnosis, perhaps supplemented with sputum microscopy. Under such conditions, treatment remains empiric. Other centers use cultures and susceptibility testing. Most often, "critical" concentrations are used, but more focus has been placed on using MICs, similar to what is done in most other infections. Combining MIC values with PK parameters, such as C_{max}, the AUC, or Time > MIC, gives clinicians the ability to target desired PK/PD values.

Determining the appropriate targets can be difficult with TB, because multiple drugs are used simultaneously. Lacking clear data regarding synergist combinations, it seems reasonable to optimize each drug within these combination regimens. New drugs are being developed to treat *Mtb* and MDR-TB, but these new drugs will be combined with older, weaker second- and third-line TB drugs. Further research is needed to optimize these new combination regimens.

Several studies suggest that higher doses of TB drugs should be used, especially RIF and PZA, in order to increase efficacy. Certain diseases, including diabetes and HIV, may reduce TB drug concentrations. Further, high interindividual and intraindividual PK variability can be seen with TB drugs. The current standard doses might not be adequate for certain patients. TDM is a useful tool for determining the appropriate doses of the TB drugs on a case-by-case basis.

Acknowledgements

Many thanks to Justin May for his technical expertise, and Natan Andres for graphical assistance.

References

1. Daniel TM (2006) The history of tuberculosis. Respir Med 100:1862–1870
2. World Health Organization (2013) WHO Global tuberculosis report 2013
3. World Health Organization (2012) HIV and TB (TB/HIV).
4. Fox W, Ellard GA, Mitchison DA (1999) Studies on the treatment of tuberculosis undertaken by the British Medical Research Council tuberculosis units, 1946-1986, with relevant subsequent publications. Int J Tuberc Lung Dis 3:S231–S279
5. Mitchison DA (2004) Antimicrobial therapy of tuberculosis: Justification for currently recommended treatment regimens. Semin Respir Crit Care Med 25:307–315
6. McCune RM Jr, Tompsett R (1956) Fate of Mycobacterium tuberculosis in mouse tissues as determined by the microbial enumeration technique. I. The persistence of drug-susceptible tubercle bacilli in the tissues despite prolonged antimicrobial therapy. J Exp Med 104:737–762
7. Grosset J (1978) The sterilizing value of rifampicin and pyrazinamide in experimental short-course chemotherapy. Bull Int Union Tuberc 53:5–12
8. Dickinson JM, Mitchison DA (1981) Experimental models to explain the high sterilizing activity of rifampin in the chemotherapy of tuberculosis. Am Rev Respir Dis 123:367–371
9. Organization WH (2010) Treatment of tuberculosis: guidelines, 4th edn. WHO Press, Geneva, Switzerland
10. Fox W (1981) Whither short-course chemotherapy? Br J Dis Chest 75:331–357
11. Francis J Curry National Tuberculosis Center and California Department of Public Health (2008) Drug resistant tuberculosis: a survival guide for clinicians, 2nd edn. Francis J Curry National Tuberculosis Center and California Department of Public Health
12. FDA news release (2012) http://www.fda.gov/NewsEvents/Newsroom/PressAnnouncements/ucm333695.htm. Accessed 2 Dec 2014.
13. EM Agency (2013) (CHMP) CfMPfHU, London
14. Wehrli W (1983) Rifampin: mechanisms of action and resistance. Rev Infect Dis 5(Suppl 3):S407–S411
15. Floss HG, Yu T-W (2005) Rifamycins-mode of action, resistance, and biosynthesis. Chem Rev 105(2):621–632
16. Timmins GS, Deretic V (2006) Mechanisms of action of isoniazid. Mol Microbiol 62:1220–1227
17. Vadwai V, Ajbani K, Jose M et al (2013) Can inhA mutation predict ethionamide resistance? Int J Tuberc Lung Dis 17:129–130
18. Jindani A, Dore CJ, Mitchison DA (2003) Bactericidal and sterilizing activities of antituberculosis drugs during the first 14 days. Am J Respir Crit Care Med 167:1348–1354
19. Zhang Y, Mitchison D (2003) The curious characteristics of pyrazinamide: a review. Int J Tuberc Lung Dis 7:6–21
20. Zhang Y, Wade MM, Scorpio A, Zhang H, Sun Z (2003) Mode of action of pyrazinamide: disruption of Mycobacterium tuberculosis membrane transport and energetics by pyrazinoic acid. J Antimicrob Chemother 52:790–795
21. Mikusova K, Slayden RA, Besra GS, Brennan PJ (1995) Biogenesis of the mycobacterial cell wall and the site of action of ethambutol. Antimicrob Agents Chemother 39:2484–2489
22. Sreevatsan S, Stockbauer KE, Pan X et al (1997) Ethambutol resistance in Mycobacterium tuberculosis: critical role of embB mutations. Antimicrob Agents Chemother 41:1677–1681
23. Botha FJ, Sirgel FA, Parkin DP, van de Wal BW, Donald PR, Mitchison DA (1996) Early bactericidal activity of ethambutol, pyrazinamide and the fixed combination of isoniazid, rifampicin and pyrazinamide (Rifater) in patients with pulmonary tuberculosis. S Afr Med J 86:155–158
24. Mitchison DA (2000) Role of individual drugs in the chemotherapy of tuberculosis. Int J Tuberc Lung Dis 4:796–806
25. Ginsburg AS, Grosset JH, Bishai WR (2003) Fluoroquinolones, tuberculosis, and resistance. Lancet Infect Dis 3:432–442
26. Wolfson JS, Hooper DC (1985) The fluoroquinolones: structures, mechanisms of action and resistance, and spectra of activity in vitro. Antimicrob Agents Chemother 28:581–586
27. Mitnick CD, McGee B, Peloquin CA (2009) Tuberculosis pharmacotherapy: strategies to optimize patient care. Expert Opin Pharmacother 10:381–401
28. Blanchard SC, Fourmy D, Eason RG, Puglisi JD (1998) rRNA chemical groups required for aminoglycoside binding. Biochemistry 37:7716–7724
29. Forge A, Schacht J (2000) Aminoglycoside antibiotics. Audiol Neurootol 5:3–22

30. Peloquin C. Pharmacometrics and tuberculosis. In: Derendorf HSS (ed), Applied pharmacometrics: (in press)
31. Heifets L, Lindholm-Levy P (1989) Comparison of bactericidal activities of streptomycin, amikacin, kanamycin, and capreomycin against Mycobacterium avium and M. tuberculosis. Antimicrob Agents Chemother 33:1298–1301
32. Prosser GA, de Carvalho LP (2013) Reinterpreting the mechanism of inhibition of Mycobacterium tuberculosis D-alanine:D-alanine ligase by D-cycloserine. Biochemistry 52:7145–7149
33. Rengarajan J, Sassetti CM, Naroditskaya V, Sloutsky A, Bloom BR, Rubin EJ (2004) The folate pathway is a target for resistance to the drug para-aminosalicylic acid (PAS) in mycobacteria. Mol Microbiol 53:275–282
34. Youmans GP, Raleigh GW, Youmans AS (1947) The tuberculostatic action of para-aminosalicylic acid. J Bacteriol 54:409–416
35. Nuermberger E, Grosset J (2004) Pharmacokinetic and pharmacodynamic issues in the treatment of mycobacterial infections. Eur J Clin Microbiol Infect Dis 23:243–255
36. Drusano GL, Sgambati N, Eichas A, Brown D, Kulawy R, Louie A (2011) Effect of administration of moxifloxacin plus rifampin against Mycobacterium tuberculosis for 7 of 7 days versus 5 of 7 days in an in vitro pharmacodynamic system. MBio 2:e00108–e00111
37. Srivastava S, Pasipanodya JG, Meek C, Leff R, Gumbo T (2011) Multidrug-resistant tuberculosis not due to noncompliance but to between-patient pharmacokinetic variability. J Infect Dis 204:1951–1959
38. Dartois V (2011) Drug forgiveness and interpatient pharmacokinetic variability in tuberculosis. J Infect Dis 204:1827–1829
39. Pasipanodya J, Srivastava S, Gumbo T (2012) New susceptibility breakpoints and the regional variability of MIC distribution in Mycobacterium tuberculosis isolates. Antimicrob Agents Chemother 56:5428
40. Gumbo T (2010) New susceptibility breakpoints for first-line antituberculosis drugs based on antimicrobial pharmacokinetic/pharmacodynamic science and population pharmacokinetic variability. Antimicrob Agents Chemother 54:1484–1491
41. Heifets L (1991) Drug susceptibility in the chemotheraphy of mycobacterial infections. CRC, Boca Raton
42. Isenberg HD (1988) Antimicrobial susceptibility testing: a critical evaluation. J Antimicrob Chemother 22(Suppl A):73–86
43. Canetti G, Froman S, Grosset J et al (1963) Mycobacteria: laboratory methods for testing drug sensitivity and resistance. Bull World Health Organ 29:565–578
44. Heifets L (1996) Clinics in laboratory medicine, Clinical mycobacteriology. WB Saunders, Philadelphia, PA
45. Murray PR (ed) (2003) Manual of clinical microbiology, 8th edn. American Society of Microbiology, Washington DC
46. Campbell PJ, Morlock GP, Sikes RD et al (2011) Molecular detection of mutations associated with first- and second-line drug resistance compared with conventional drug susceptibility testing of Mycobacterium tuberculosis. Antimicrob Agents Chemother 55:2032–2041
47. Metchock B (2013) National Consultancy on proposed CDC guidance for the use of bedaquiline in the treatment of multidrug-resistant tuberculosis: laboratory perspective and review of CDC laboratory services. National Center for HIV/AIDS, Viral Hepatitis, STD & TB Prevention. Division of Tuberculosis Elimination (Power Point presentation)
48. Pasipanodya J, Gumbo T (2011) An oracle: antituberculosis pharmacokinetics-pharmacodynamics, clinical correlation, and clinical trial simulations to predict the future. Antimicrob Agents Chemother 55:24–34
49. Chigutsa E, Meredith S, Wiesner L et al (2012) Population pharmacokinetics and pharmacodynamics of ofloxacin in South African patients with multidrug-resistant tuberculosis. Antimicrob Agents Chemother 56:3857–3863
50. Zeitlinger MA, Derendorf H, Mouton JW et al (2011) Protein binding: do we ever learn? Antimicrob Agents Chemother 55:3067–3074
51. Craig WA, Kunin CM (1976) Significance of serum protein and tissue binding of antimicrobial agents. Annu Rev Med 27:287–300
52. Budha NR, Lee RE, Meibohm B (2008) Biopharmaceutics, pharmacokinetics and pharmacodynamics of antituberculosis drugs. Curr Med Chem 15:809–825
53. Mueller M, de la Pena A, Derendorf H (2004) Issues in pharmacokinetics and pharmacodynamics of anti-infective agents: kill curves versus MIC. Antimicrob Agents Chemother 48:369–377
54. Drusano GL (2004) Antimicrobial pharmacodynamics: critical interactions of 'bug and drug'. Nat Rev Microbiol 2:289–300
55. Craig WA (1998) Pharmacokinetic/pharmacodynamic parameters: rationale for antibacterial dosing of mice and men. Clin Infect Dis 26:1–10, quiz 1-2

56. Gumbo T, Louie A, Deziel MR, Parsons LM, Salfinger M, Drusano GL (2004) Selection of a moxifloxacin dose that suppresses drug resistance in Mycobacterium tuberculosis, by use of an in vitro pharmacodynamic infection model and mathematical modeling. J Infect Dis 190:1642–1651
57. Gumbo T, Louie A, Deziel MR et al (2007) Concentration-dependent Mycobacterium tuberculosis killing and prevention of resistance by rifampin. Antimicrob Agents Chemother 51:3781–3788
58. Budha NR, Lee RB, Hurdle JG, Lee RE, Meibohm B (2009) A simple in vitro PK/PD model system to determine time-kill curves of drugs against Mycobacteria. Tuberculosis (Edinb) 89:378–385
59. Vaddady PK, Lee RE, Meibohm B (2010) In vitro pharmacokinetic/pharmacodynamic models in anti-infective drug development: focus on TB. Future Med Chem 2:1355–1369
60. Nuermberger E (2008) Using animal models to develop new treatments for tuberculosis. Semin Respir Crit Care Med 29:542–551
61. Dharmadhikari AS, Nardell EA (2008) What animal models teach humans about tuberculosis. Am J Respir Cell Mol Biol 39:503–508
62. Harper J, Skerry C, Davis SL et al (2012) Mouse model of necrotic tuberculosis granulomas develops hypoxic lesions. J Infect Dis 205:595–602
63. Davies GR, Nuermberger EL (2008) Pharmacokinetics and pharmacodynamics in the development of anti-tuberculosis drugs. Tuberculosis (Edinb) 88(Suppl 1):S65–S74
64. Dartois V (2014) The path of anti-tuberculosis drugs: from blood to lesions to mycobacterial cells. Nat Rev Microbiol 12:159–167
65. Rodvold KA, Yoo L, George JM (2011) Penetration of anti-infective agents into pulmonary epithelial lining fluid: focus on antifungal, antitubercular and miscellaneous anti-infective agents. Clin Pharmacokinet 50:689–704
66. Kempker RR, Rabin AS, Nikolaishvili K et al (2012) Additional drug resistance in Mycobacterium tuberculosis isolates from resected cavities among patients with multidrug-resistant or extensively drug-resistant pulmonary tuberculosis. Clin Infect Dis 54:e51–e54
67. Kaplan G, Post FA, Moreira AL et al (2003) Mycobacterium tuberculosis growth at the cavity surface: a microenvironment with failed immunity. Infect Immun 71:7099–7108
68. Mor N, Simon B, Mezo N, Heifets L (1995) Comparison of activities of rifapentine and rifampin against Mycobacterium tuberculosis residing in human macrophages. Antimicrob Agents Chemother 39:2073–2077
69. Burman WJ, Gallicano K, Peloquin C (2001) Comparative pharmacokinetics and pharmacodynamics of the rifamycin antibacterials. Clin Pharmacokinet 40:327–341
70. van Ingen J, Aarnoutse RE, Donald PR et al (2011) Why do we use 600 mg of rifampicin in tuberculosis treatment? Clin Infect Dis 52:E194–E199
71. Long MW, Snider DE Jr, Farer LS (1979) U.S. Public Health Service Cooperative trial of three rifampin-isoniazid regimens in treatment of pulmonary tuberculosis. Am Rev Respir Dis 119:879–894
72. Jindani A, Aber VR, Edwards EA, Mitchison DA (1980) The early bactericidal activity of drugs in patients with pulmonary tuberculosis. Am Rev Respir Dis 121:939–949
73. Jayaram R, Gaonkar S, Kaur P et al (2003) Pharmacokinetics-pharmacodynamics of rifampin in an aerosol infection model of tuberculosis. Antimicrob Agents Chemother 47:2118–2124
74. Blaschke TF, Skinner MH (1996) The clinical pharmacokinetics of rifabutin. Clin Infect Dis 22(Suppl 1):S15–S21, discussion S-2
75. McGregor MM, Olliaro P, Wolmarans L et al (1996) Efficacy and safety of rifabutin in the treatment of patients with newly diagnosed pulmonary tuberculosis. Am J Respir Crit Care Med 154:1462–1467
76. Li AP, Reith MK, Rasmussen A et al (1997) Primary human hepatocytes as a tool for the evaluation of structure-activity relationship in cytochrome P450 induction potential of xenobiotics: evaluation of rifampin, rifapentine and rifabutin. Chem Biol Interact 107:17–30
77. Rosenthal IM, Zhang M, Williams KN et al (2007) Daily dosing of rifapentine cures tuberculosis in three months or less in the murine model. PLoS Med 4:e344
78. Bemer-Melchior P, Bryskier A, Drugeon HB (2000) Comparison of the in vitro activities of rifapentine and rifampicin against Mycobacterium tuberculosis complex. J Antimicrob Chemother 46:571–576
79. Sirgel FA, Fourie PB, Donald PR et al (2005) The early bactericidal activities of rifampin and rifapentine in pulmonary tuberculosis. Am J Respir Crit Care Med 172:128–135
80. Tam CM, Chan SL, Kam KM, Goodall RL, Mitchison DA (2002) Rifapentine and isoniazid in the continuation phase of a 6-month regimen. Final report at 5 years: prognostic

value of various measures. Int J Tuberc Lung Dis 6:3–10

81. Dorman SE, Goldberg S, Stout JE et al (2012) Substitution of rifapentine for rifampin during intensive phase treatment of pulmonary tuberculosis: study 29 of the tuberculosis trials consortium. J Infect Dis 206:1030–1040
82. Benator D, Bhattacharya M, Bozeman L et al (2002) Rifapentine and isoniazid once a week versus rifampicin and isoniazid twice a week for treatment of drug-susceptible pulmonary tuberculosis in HIV-negative patients: a randomised clinical trial. Lancet 360:528–534
83. Dutta NK, Illei PB, Peloquin CA et al (2012) Rifapentine is not more active than rifampin against chronic tuberculosis in guinea pigs. Antimicrob Agents Chemother 56:3726–3731
84. Savic RM, Lu Y, Bliven-Sizemore E et al (2014) Population pharmacokinetics of rifapentine and desacetyl rifapentine in healthy volunteers: nonlinearities in clearance and bioavailability. Antimicrob Agents Chemother 58(6):3035–3042
85. Mitchison DA (2012) Pharmacokinetic/pharmacodynamic parameters and the choice of high-dosage rifamycins. Int J Tuberc Lung Dis 16:1186–1189
86. Coates AR, Hu Y, Jindani A, Mitchison DA (2013) Contradictory results with high-dosage rifamycin in mice and humans. Antimicrob Agents Chemother 57:1103
87. Nuermberger EL, Rosenthal IM, Tasneen R et al (2013) Reply to "Contradictory results with high-dosage rifamycin in mice and humans". Antimicrob Agents Chemother 57:1104–1105
88. Cade CE, Dlouhy AC, Medzihradszky KF, Salas-Castillo SP, Ghiladi RA (2010) Isoniazid-resistance conferring mutations in Mycobacterium tuberculosis KatG: catalase, peroxidase, and INH-NADH adduct formation activities. Protein Sci 19:458–474
89. Parsons LM, Salfinger M, Clobridge A et al (2005) Phenotypic and molecular characterization of Mycobacterium tuberculosis isolates resistant to both isoniazid and ethambutol. Antimicrob Agents Chemother 49:2218–2225
90. Barry CE 3rd, Slayden RA, Mdluli K (1998) Mechanisms of isoniazid resistance in Mycobacterium tuberculosis. Drug Resist Updat 1:128–134
91. Slayden RA, Barry CE 3rd (2000) The genetics and biochemistry of isoniazid resistance in mycobacterium tuberculosis. Microbes Infect 2:659–669
92. Banerjee A, Dubnau E, Quemard A et al (1994) inhA, a gene encoding a target for isoniazid and ethionamide in Mycobacterium tuberculosis. Science 263:227–230
93. Guo H, Seet Q, Denkin S, Parsons L, Zhang Y (2006) Molecular characterization of isoniazid-resistant clinical isolates of Mycobacterium tuberculosis from the USA. J Med Microbiol 55:1527–1531
94. Katiyar SK, Bihari S, Prakash S, Mamtani M, Kulkarni H (2008) A randomised controlled trial of high-dose isoniazid adjuvant therapy for multidrug-resistant tuberculosis. Int J Tuberc Lung Dis 12:139–145
95. Awaness AM, Mitchison DA (1973) Cumulative effects of pulsed exposures of mycobacterium tuberculosis to isoniazid. Tubercle 54(2):153–158
96. Gumbo T, Louie A, Liu W et al (2007) Isoniazid's bactericidal activity ceases because of the emergence of resistance, not depletion of Mycobacterium tuberculosis in the log phase of growth. J Infect Dis 195:194–201
97. Mitchison DA, Jindani A, Davies GR, Sirgel F (2007) Isoniazid activity is terminated by bacterial persistence. J Infect Dis 195:1871–1872, author reply 2-3
98. Gumbo T, Louie A, Liu W et al (2007) Isoniazid bactericidal activity and resistance emergence: integrating pharmacodynamics and pharmacogenomics to predict efficacy in different ethnic populations. Antimicrob Agents Chemother 51:2329–2336
99. Weiner M, Burman W, Vernon A et al (2003) Low isoniazid concentrations and outcome of tuberculosis treatment with once-weekly isoniazid and rifapentine. Am J Respir Crit Care Med 167:1341–1347
100. Srivastava S, Sherman C, Meek C, Leff R, Gumbo T (2011) Pharmacokinetic mismatch does not lead to emergence of isoniazid- or rifampin-resistant Mycobacterium tuberculosis but to better antimicrobial effect: a new paradigm for antituberculosis drug scheduling. Antimicrob Agents Chemother 55:5085–5089
101. Somoskovi A, Dormandy J, Parsons LM et al (2007) Sequencing of the pncA gene in members of the Mycobacterium tuberculosis complex has important diagnostic applications: Identification of a species-specific pncA mutation in "Mycobacterium canettii" and the reliable and rapid predictor of pyrazinamide resistance. J Clin Microbiol 45:595–599
102. Shi W, Zhang X, Jiang X et al (2011) Pyrazinamide inhibits trans-translation in Mycobacterium tuberculosis. Science 333:1630–1632

103. Zimhony O, Vilcheze C, Arai M, Welch JT, Jacobs WR Jr (2007) Pyrazinoic acid and its n-propyl ester inhibit fatty acid synthase type I in replicating tubercle bacilli. Antimicrob Agents Chemother 51:752–754
104. Boshoff HI, Mizrahi V, Barry CE 3rd (2002) Effects of pyrazinamide on fatty acid synthesis by whole mycobacterial cells and purified fatty acid synthase I. J Bacteriol 184:2167–2172
105. Martin A, Takiff H, Vandamme P, Swings J, Palomino JC, Portaels F (2006) A new rapid and simple colorimetric method to detect pyrazinamide resistance in Mycobacterium tuberculosis using nicotinamide. J Antimicrob Chemother 58:327–331
106. Gumbo T, Dona CS, Meek C, Leff R (2009) Pharmacokinetics-pharmacodynamics of pyrazinamide in a novel in vitro model of tuberculosis for sterilizing effect: a paradigm for faster assessment of new antituberculosis drugs. Antimicrob Agents Chemother 53:3197–3204
107. Salfinger M, Heifets LB (1988) Determination of pyrazinamide MICs for mycobacterium-tuberculosis at different pHs by the radiometric method. Antimicrob Agents Chemother 32:1002–1004
108. Chicurel M, Garcia E, Goodsaid F (1988) Modulation of macrophage lysosomal PH by mycobacterium-tuberculosis-derived proteins. Infect Immun 56:479–83
109. Pasipanodya JG, Gumbo T (2010) Clinical and toxicodynamic evidence that high-dose pyrazinamide is not more hepatotoxic than the low doses currently used. Antimicrob Agents Chemother 54:2847–2854
110. Girling DJ (1982) Adverse effects of antituberculosis drugs. Drugs 23:56–74
111. Girling DJ (1978) The hepatic toxicity of antituberculosis regimens containing isoniazid, rifampicin and pyrazinamide. Tubercle 59:13–32
112. Srivastava S, Ayyagari A, Dhole TN, Nyati KK, Dwivedi SK (2009) emb nucleotide polymorphisms and the role of embB306 mutations in Mycobacterium tuberculosis resistance to ethambutol. Int J Med Microbiol 299:269–280
113. Ezer N, Benedetti A, Darvish-Zargar M, Menzies D (2013) Incidence of ethambutol-related visual impairment during treatment of active tuberculosis. Int J Tuberc Lung Dis 17:447–455
114. Fish DN, Chow AT (1997) The clinical pharmacokinetics of levofloxacin. Clin Pharmacokinet 32:101–119
115. Peloquin C, Alsultan A. Clinical pharmacology of the anti-tuberculosis drugs. In: Davies PDO BP, Gordon SB (eds) Clinical tuberculosis. 5th edn. (in press)
116. Peloquin CA, Hadad DJ, Molino LP et al (2008) Population pharmacokinetics of levofloxacin, gatifloxacin, and moxifloxacin in adults with pulmonary tuberculosis. Antimicrob Agents Chemother 52:852–857
117. (2008) Levofloxacin. Tuberculosis (Edinb) 88: 119-121
118. Canetti G (1965) Present aspects of bacterial resistance in tuberculosis. Am Rev Respir Dis 92:687–703
119. Morlock GP, Metchock B, Sikes D, Crawford JT, Cooksey RC (2003) ethA, inhA, and katG loci of ethionamide-resistant clinical Mycobacterium tuberculosis isolates. Antimicrob Agents Chemother 47:3799–3805
120. Chakraborty S, Gruber T, Barry CE 3rd, Boshoff HI, Rhee KY (2013) Para-aminosalicylic acid acts as an alternative substrate of folate metabolism in Mycobacterium tuberculosis. Science 339:88–91
121. Vega P, Sweetland A, Acha J et al (2004) Psychiatric issues in the management of patients with multidrug-resistant tuberculosis. Int J Tuberc Lung Dis 8:749–759
122. Bakhla AK, Gore PS, Srivastava SL (2013) Cycloserine induced mania. Ind Psychiatry J 22:69–70
123. Emmett MR, Mick SJ, Cler JA, Rao TS, Iyengar S, Wood PL (1991) Actions of D-cycloserine at the N-methyl-D-aspartate-associated glycine receptor site in vivo. Neuropharmacology 30:1167–1171
124. Matteelli A, Carvalho AC, Dooley KE, Kritski A (2010) TMC207: the first compound of a new class of potent anti-tuberculosis drugs. Future Microbiol 5:849–858
125. Hartkoorn RC, Uplekar S, Cole ST (2014) Cross-resistance between clofazimine and bedaquiline through upregulation of MmpL5 in Mycobacterium tuberculosis. Antimicrob Agents Chemother 58:2979–2981
126. Andries K, Verhasselt P, Guillemont J et al (2005) A diarylquinoline drug active on the ATP synthase of Mycobacterium tuberculosis. Science 307:223–227
127. Rouan MC, Lounis N, Gevers T et al (2012) Pharmacokinetics and pharmacodynamics of TMC207 and its N-desmethyl metabolite in a murine model of tuberculosis. Antimicrob Agents Chemother 56:1444–1451

128. (2013) Sirturo [package insert]. Janssen, Titusville, NJ
129. Peloquin CA (2002) Therapeutic drug monitoring in the treatment of tuberculosis. Drugs 62:2169–2183
130. Almeida Da Silva PE, Palomino JC (2011) Molecular basis and mechanisms of drug resistance in Mycobacterium tuberculosis: classical and new drugs. J Antimicrob Chemother 66:1417–1430
131. Blanchard JS (1996) Molecular mechanisms of drug resistance in Mycobacterium tuberculosis. Annu Rev Biochem 65: 215–239
132. Caceres NE, Harris NB, Wellehan JF, Feng Z, Kapur V, Barletta RG (1997) Overexpression of the D-alanine racemase gene confers resistance to D-cycloserine in Mycobacterium smegmatis. J Bacteriol 179:5046–5055

Chapter 17

Pharmacodynamics of Antimalarial Agents

Rahul P. Bakshi and Theresa A. Shapiro

Abstract

Antimalarials were among the first, and today are among the most widely used, anti-infective agents. The fundamental pharmacodynamic endpoint for antimalarials is quite simple: elimination of this eukaryotic protozoal pathogen from its host; numerous surrogates for this have been developed. Antimalarial therapy is confounded by several key factors including the coexistence of multiple pharmacologically distinct *Plasmodium* life cycle forms in the human host; limited resources for discovery, development, and deployment of new drugs; and a high requirement for safety due to the enormous patient population and use for chemoprophylaxis of healthy travelers. Further, for any particular drug, myriad influences impact the pharmacological endpoint, including rapidity of the onset of action, potency, 'static vs. 'cidal activity, susceptibility to parasite resistance, immune status of the host, and the suitability of prevailing pharmacokinetics. Classic and recently described pharmacodynamic endpoints in preclinical models are presented, as are new insights into the pharmacokinetic drivers of antimalarial pharmacodynamics. The efficacy and safety of existing drugs are surveyed, and some novel experimental agents are discussed.

Key words Malaria, *Plasmodium*, Antimalarial, Pharmacokinetics, Pharmacodynamics, PK/PD, Parasite reduction ratio, Resistance, Combination therapy

1 Malaria

Malaria is a mosquito-borne infectious disease that afflicts hundreds of millions and kills nearly a million children every year in Africa. Recent efforts have brought encouraging progress toward eliminating this major public health challenge, via a combination of vector control, use of insecticide-impregnated bednets, improved diagnostics, and chemotherapy campaigns. Nevertheless, the lack of a vaccine and widespread drug resistance make the need for effective and safe new antimalarial agents compelling. Of the *Plasmodium* species pathogenic to humans, *falciparum* is most aggressive, causing life-threatening infection and having the greatest propensity for drug resistance [1, 2].

Malaria parasites have a complex life cycle (Fig. 1). From a therapeutic perspective, by far the most important forms are asexually dividing parasites that dwell within erythrocytes. They alone

John C. Rotschafer et al. (eds.), *Antibiotic Pharmacodynamics*, Methods in Pharmacology and Toxicology, DOI 10.1007/978-1-4939-3323-5_17, © Springer Science+Business Media New York 2016

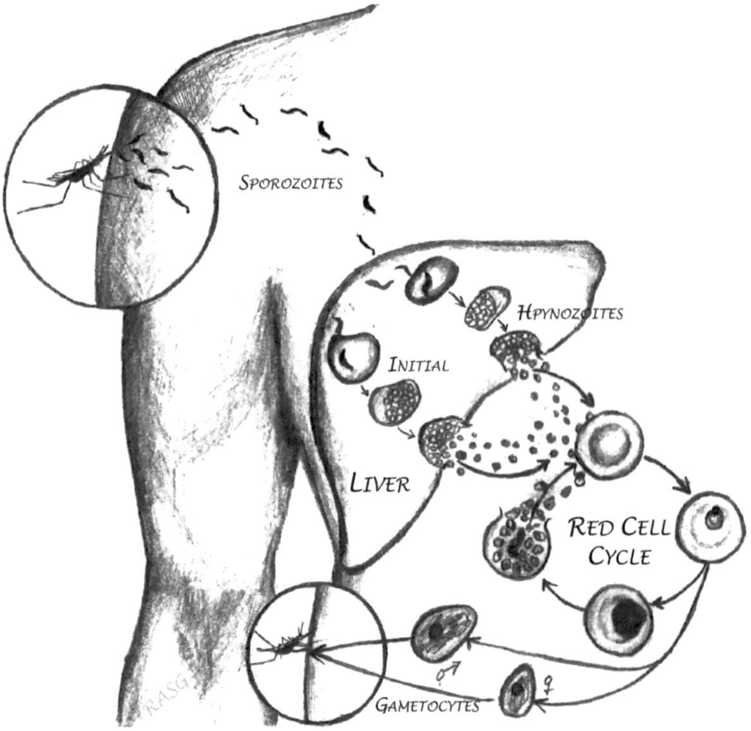

Fig. 1 Life cycle of malaria parasites. Sporozoites inoculated by a mosquito rapidly make their way to the liver and infect hepatocytes. Parasites replicate within the hepatocyte, rupture the cell, and enter the blood stream as merozoites. These merozoites invade erythrocytes, initiating the blood stage of the infection. Erythrocytic parasites amplify 8–32-fold over 48–72 h, rupture the red blood cell, invade new erythrocytes, and restart the cycle. All parasite proliferation within the human is asexual. Some erythrocytic forms differentiate into gametocytes that will infect a biting mosquito, reproduce sexually, and eventually generate sporozoites that complete the life cycle. Some liver stage parasites of *Plasmodium vivax* and *Plasmodium ovale* form latent hypnozoites that may remain quiescent for years, before activating and establishing symptomatic disease

are responsible for the morbidity and mortality of malaria, and in severe infection may number hundreds of millions per milliliter of blood. It is the cyclical release of naked parasites into the bloodstream that gives rise to the classic periodic agues of malaria. *P. falciparum*'s unique lethality stems from adherence of infected erythrocytes to blood vessel walls, which causes a cytokine response and functional vascular obstruction. In severe cases this results in cerebral malaria, extensive hemolysis, and multiple end-organ failures. The remaining life cycle stages (all of which may coexist simultaneously within the same patient) are responsible for transmission of infection to the mosquito and may cause late reactivation of symptomatic disease. Unfortunately, each life cycle form has a different profile of drug susceptibilities (Fig. 2) [3]; hence multiple drugs may be required for complete eradication of the infection from a patient. In addition to their obvious necessity for the treatment of established infection, antimalarial drugs will also remain essential for the chemoprophylaxis of travelers to malarious regions until a suitable vaccine becomes available.

The discovery and development of antimalarial drugs has proven challenging. *Plasmodium* parasites are host-specific, such that species pathogenic for humans rarely propagate in other animals, and they have proven equally difficult to study in vitro. Obligate intracellular pathogens with an ~80 % AT genome [4], long term in vitro cultivation was not accomplished until 1976, when the preference of *P. falciparum* for microaerophilic conditions was realized [5]. *P. vivax* still cannot be maintained in continuous culture. Over time, however, animal models and in vitro assay systems have matured to the point that important parameters such as potency, pharmacokinetic–pharmacodynamic linkage, and proof-of-principle in vivo efficacy can be measured. Though eukaryotic like its human host, *Plasmodium* has numerous unique

		Liver stages		Blood stages	
		Latent	Primary	Asexual	Gametocytes
Group I					
	Chloroquine	–	–	+	±
	Quinine	–	–	+	±
	Mefloquine	–	–	+	–
	Artemisinin	–	–	+	±
	FANSIDAR { Pyrimethamine, Sulfadoxine }	–	±	+	–
	Tetracyclines	–	–	±	–
Group II					
	MALARONE { Atovaquone, Proguanil }	–	+	+	–
Group III					
	Primaquine	+	+	–	±

Fig. 2 Simplified pharmacodynamic specificities of antimalarial drugs. Depicted are the classes of antimalarial drugs, in the context of their major activities against distinct forms of *Plasmodium* in a human host. Disease-initiating sporozoites are not listed since no drug has meaningful activity against this stage. Group I drugs primarily target the disease-causing asexual blood stages, and form the bulwark of antimalarial therapy. The Group II synergistic combination of atovaquone plus proguanil has reliable action against pathogenic red cell stages as well as the initial liver stage of *P. falciparum*; it is useful for prophylaxis as well as treatment. Group III primaquine targets regular and latent liver stages and gametocytes, but has no useful activity against asexual blood stages. Interspecies differences and unknown or unreliable activities are not shown

and distinguishing features exploitable for drug targeting. These include, for example, a chloroplast-like organelle whose self-contained genome and proteins have clinically useful susceptibility to several conventional antibacterials (e.g., tetracyclines, clindamycin) [6]; efficient hemoglobin digestion and corollary brisk detoxification of byproduct heme by chloroquine-sensitive crystallization [7]; and absolute dependence on pyrimidine biosynthesis disrupted by atovaquone-mediated blockade of mitochondrial electron transport [8]. In recent years availability of the complete genome sequence [4] and use of high throughput screens against libraries of millions of compounds [9–11] have provided much-needed promising new therapeutic leads (Sect. 4.7).

2 Pharmacodynamic Endpoints for Antimalarial Drugs

2.1 In Vivo

For most animal models of malaria neither the host nor the parasite is directly pertinent to human infection, and the time course and characteristics of human disease are not faithfully recapitulated. However, different animal model systems mimic some aspects of the host–parasite interaction and allow for biological and pharmacological investigations. In addition to humans, three major animal models have been utilized for studying antimalarial agents.

2.1.1 Avian

Avian malaria was the initial model of choice for chemotherapeutic development [12]. *P. gallinaceum* was particularly practical since both the mosquito vector and avian host (ducks, chickens) are easily infected. Although avian red cells are nucleated and the life cycle of *P. gallinaceum* differs significantly from that of human parasites, the erythrocytic stage is usefully mimicked. Mid-twentieth century development of major drugs chloroquine, primaquine, proguanil, and some antifolates was accomplished using *P. gallinaceum*-avian malaria. Subsequent discovery of rodent malaria, a system relatively easy to manipulate and with greater similarity to human physiology, resulted in a shift away from avian models.

2.1.2 Rodent

Rodent malaria parasites *P. berghei*, *P. yoelii*, and *P. chabaudi* have proven invaluable for pharmacodynamic screening of candidate compounds [13] and rodent models are now standard in antimalarial drug development [14]. However, no rodent model fully recapitulates the disease profile seen in human malaria, rodent parasite behavior in vivo can differ significantly from that of human-tropic *Plasmodium* species, and rodents may differ substantially in their handling of antimalarials. Controversy surrounds the use of the *P. berghei* ANKA-mouse model of cerebral malaria that reproduces some, but not all, pathophysiological aspects of human cerebral malaria [15]. Recent development of a mouse model in which human erythrocytes are maintained by immunosuppression enables pharmacodynamic evaluations against the parasites of greatest interest (asexual blood stages of *P. falciparum*), but in a mouse background [16].

2.1.3 Nonhuman Primate

Multiple *Plasmodium* species naturally infect nonhuman primates and mimic important features of human infection, arguably making them the best surrogates for human disease. However, the expense, limited availability, and ethical concerns surrounding use of primates severely limit their practical utility. Notable models include the *P. cynomolgi*-macaque that mimics human *P. vivax* infection, and the *P. coatneyi*- and *P. fragile*-macaque models that in many aspects resemble human *P. falciparum* infections [17]. In fact, the *P. cynomolgi*-macaque model proved critical in the development of primaquine, the only agent known to target latent liver forms (hypnozoites), thus preventing *P. vivax* and *P. ovale* relapses. The demonstration that *P. knowlesi*, normally infective to Old World Monkeys, can cause significant, sometimes lethal, zoonotic disease in humans has made this pathogen a subject of considerable study [18]. While monkey-to-human transmission is more frequent than previously estimated, human-to-human transmission has not been demonstrated. There have been efforts to infect nonhuman primates with human parasites. Some success has been obtained using the *Aotus* monkey host for *P. falciparum*, *P. vivax*, or *P. malariae*; however, results from these artificial self-curing infections need to be interpreted with caution.

2.1.4 Humans

Experimental malaria in humans has a long and checkered history [19], but thoughtful and safe studies conducted during the World War II era provided invaluable new knowledge on the complex biology (Fig. 1) and pathophysiology of *falciparum* and *vivax* malaria, and made possible the rapid development and deployment of amodiaquine, chloroquine, and proguanil to troops fighting in malarious areas of Africa, Europe, and the Pacific. Even today, studying some aspects of antimalarial pharmacodynamics depends heavily on experimental human infections. Prior to large and difficult to control field trials of prophylactic efficacy, small, tightly controlled studies in which well-informed and consenting healthy volunteers are challenged by the bite of malaria-infected mosquitoes or by the inoculation of malaria-infected blood, are standard in assessing drug [20] or vaccine candidates [21] for malaria prophylaxis.

Classical pharmacodynamic endpoints for antimalarial development and use have been clinical—both symptomatic (e.g., time to fever reduction) and microbiological (e.g., time to parasite clearance, 28 day cure rate). In recent years, new metrics have been devised for use in clinical trials. They take cognizance of the fact that unlike most other infections, the pathogenic forms of malaria are confined to erythrocytes in the bloodstream. In severe illness infected cells can number up to 10^{12}, and clinical success of a drug depends on reducing this burden rapidly and completely. From this realization have come clinical measures of rate of killing, rate of recrudescence and parasite reduction ratio (Sect. 2.2.3). In some cases these endpoints are now also being applied to animal and in vitro studies. Demonstrating and counting parasites in a blood smear by simple light microscopy remains the gold standard for measuring antimalarial pharmacodynamic activity. PCR- and antibody-based assays are now also available but logistical and resource limitations restrict their widespread field-deployment.

2.2 In Vitro

For much of the twentieth century, malaria research was restricted to in vivo models since human parasites could not be cultured in vitro. Trager and Jensen's breakthrough report of the continuous culture of *P. falciparum* erythrocytic stages in vitro enabled a veritable explosion in malaria research [5]. Unfortunately, this success has not translated to *P. vivax*, which preferentially infects immature red cells, or to liver stages of the *Plasmodium* life cycle. Nonetheless, *P. falciparum* blood stages maintained in vitro form the basis for numerous and diverse pharmacodynamic assays. The following pharmacodynamic endpoints all focus on the asexual erythrocytic parasites, which are responsible for symptomatic disease.

2.2.1 Growth Inhibition

As developed in a micro-titer format, this assay allows high throughput screens and facile measurement of dose–response relationships. Maximum sensitivity is provided by measuring the incorporation of [^{3}H]hypoxanthine into parasite nucleic acid polymers [22]; however, the use of dyes [23] and flow cytometry [24], though less sensitive, avoids the logistical restraints of radioisotopes. Growth inhibition assays do not discriminate between the 'static or 'cidal nature of growth inhibition (that is, whether or not the parasite proliferates once drug pressure is lifted). In addition, they provide limited information about the speed of effect—an important parameter for in vivo consideration. Nevertheless, this is a rapid, simple and important first step in screening for antimalarial activity.

2.2.2 Parasiticidal vs. Parasitistatic Activity

A logical follow-up to growth inhibition assay is to determine whether the effect is 'static, or 'cidal. In this method parasites are treated with drug, the drug is removed, and individual parasites are cloned out by limiting dilution. Survivors are detectable after a period of 3–6 weeks [25, 26]. The 48 h erythrocytic life cycle and frequent requirement for fresh medium and red cells make these assays cumbersome, time-consuming, costly, and subject to microbial contamination. Less rigorous approaches have been reported [27, 28] but not extensively validated by comparison with the classic method.

2.2.3 Speed of Action and Parasite Reduction Ratio (PRR)

The rapidity of drug action is important in clinical care, and may determine the utilization profile of a drug, particularly in the setting of patients with high parasitemia. Speed of action is measured via the Parasite Reduction Ratio (PRR), the number of parasites present before drug treatment divided by those remaining after treatment. PRR assays are constrained to one life cycle of the parasite; 48 h for *P. falciparum*. Thus, the higher the PRR, the more rapid is a drug's effect. PRR studies are usually performed in vivo (in humans or in nonhuman models) wherein high parasitemia before dosing makes measurement of the decline both straightforward and sensitive. Measurement of PRR in vitro has been accomplished, with log PRR values ranging from >8 for artemisinin to <3 for atovaquone [25]. However, in vitro assays rely on limiting dilution cloning and outgrowth, thus taking weeks to yield a result. The standard growth inhibition assay has recently been modified to yield information about speed-of-action of antimalarial drugs [29]. Output of this assay is binary, with compounds being classified as fast-acting or non-fast-acting.

2.2.4 Pharmacokinetic/Pharmacodynamic Linkage

Modifications of an existing hollow fiber cartridge apparatus have very recently made possible studies in which *P. falciparum* can be exposed in vitro to dynamically changing drug concentrations, akin to those that occur in vivo and distinctly different from the constant drug concentrations usually studied in vitro [30]. This system allows studies of the pharmacokinetics that drive many different antimalarial pharmacodynamics. For example, using known human pharmacokinetics, different dosing regimens can be tested to identify those that provide maximal parasite reduction and/or minimal emergence of resistance. Alternatively, the fundamental governance of drug action by either peak concentration or time of exposure can be discerned by applying a given dose of drug by two artificial (and extremely different) kinetic regimens (Sect. 3.4).

In summary, from a century ago when ducks and chickens were the major vehicle for antimalarial drug development, pharmacodynamic analysis has progressed to the stage where most microbiological endpoints can be assayed in vitro. Complexities of the parasite and the host give rise to a significant number of issues that must be addressed for successful antimalarial development and use, and no single model system or assay is sufficient to address all of them. Multiple approaches remain necessary.

3 Pharmacodynamic Issues

3.1 Life Cycle Stage Specificity

Antimalarial drugs can only be understood, and properly used, in the context of their activity against different forms of the parasite. *Plasmodium* has a multistage, complex, and dynamic life cycle, even just within the confines of the human host (Fig. 1). Human disease is initiated by the bite of an infected female Anopheline mosquito (the vector), which inoculates sporozoites in the course of taking a blood meal. This form circulates for just a few minutes before infecting hepatocytes, undergoing multiple rounds of asexual reproduction over several weeks, amplifying 10–30,000-fold, rupturing the cell and spilling progeny into the bloodstream. The released merozoites invade erythrocytes, differentiate and replicate asexually 8–32-fold over 48–72 h, before lysing the cell and infecting new erythrocytes. Severely ill patients may harbor up to 10^{12} erythrocytic parasites. Some erythrocytic forms differentiate into gametocytes, responsible for infecting and undergoing sexual reproduction within the mosquito, eventually to generate salivary gland-resident sporozoites that complete the life cycle. The above biology is common to all pathogenic species of *Plasmodium*, but *vivax* and *ovale* have the additional feature that some liver stage parasites, termed hypnozoites, are latent and may remain quiescent for decades after the mosquito bite, before activating and establishing an erythrocytic cycle [1].

The various life cycle forms within a patient are morphologically, biochemically, and pharmacologically distinct (Fig. 2). The activity of drugs against the various life cycle stages can be used to classify antimalarials into pharmacologically convenient groups [3]. No drug works against sporozoites, and, unfortunately, no drug is active against all forms other than sporozoites. Group I drugs primarily target asexual blood stages. They alone cause morbidity and mortality, hence are the major target of drug therapy. The Group II synergistic combination of atovaquone and proguanil has additional activity against the initial liver stage of *P. falciparum*. Group III primaquine targets liver stages and gametocytes, but has no useful activity against asexual blood stages. Primaquine's activity against latent hypnozoites of *P. vivax* or *ovale* prevents the late reactivation of symptomatic erythrocytic parasites that characterizes these species. Killing gametocytes prevents transmission of infection to the mosquito and is hence of public health importance.

Choice of appropriate drug is driven, in large part, by the desired outcome. Treatment of, or prophylaxis against, symptomatic malaria is provided by Group I and II agents. Public health campaigns, or regimens striving for complete cure, may include primaquine for its reliable activity against hypnozoites and gametocytes. Prophylaxis can also be obtained by drugs that target liver stage parasites (Groups II and III). Life cycle stage specificity is also important in new drug discovery, the ideal agent being one that has reliable activity against all parasite forms.

3.2 Drug Resistance

The World Health Organization (WHO) defines malaria drug resistance as "the ability of a parasite strain to survive or multiply despite the administration and absorption of a drug given in doses equal to or higher than those usually recommended but within the tolerance of the subject" [31]. Acquisition of resistance, which may be rapid and at a high level, negates the clinical utility of a drug and may jeopardize its entire chemical class. Recognized resistance mechanisms include amplification of, or most commonly point mutation(s) in, a target protein sequence. In recent years experimentally induced resistance to "lead" compounds in drug development has been exploited to obtain invaluable insight into molecular mechanism of action as well as long-term vulnerability to resistance. Interestingly, for leads that generate resistance in the lab, pharmacodynamic utility of the class may be preserved by screening for class members that retain activity against the primary resistance [32]. Additionally, emergence of resistance may be delayed if the molecular mechanism involves multiple molecular targets. As for other anti-infective classes, the most reliable route for precluding resistance in the field is to avoid monotherapy by use of drug combinations.

3.3 Drug Combinations

The pharmacological battle against malaria has laid bare the inadvisability of monotherapy, the end result of which has been emergence and dissemination of resistance to nearly every class of antimalarial drug that has been deployed. Laboratory, and in some cases field, data indicate that antimalarial drug resistance can be delayed, and perhaps avoided, by drug combinations. The earliest and best-studied antimalarial drug combinations stem from Nobel prize-winning studies by Hitchings and Elion on the antibacterial pairing of a sulfonamide inhibitor of dihydropteroate synthase plus a folate reductase inhibitor, both of which interfere with production of essential nutrient tetrahydrofolate [33]. Profound synergism is obtained against malaria parasites by this dual inhibition: when sulfadiazine and pyrimethamine are given in combination (as opposed to singly) the same efficacy is obtained by a 20-fold (or more) reduction in the dose of each drug [34]. (Interestingly, the first-ever inkling of sulfonamide/antifolate synergy against any organism came from Joseph Greenberg's studies of *P. gallinaceum* in chicks [35].) The ability to use lesser doses for maximal efficacy reduces cost and the likelihood of host toxicity. Synergism and the well-matched pharmacokinetics of this pair were designed to minimize the emergence of resistance. Two other antimalarial fixed dose combinations have since been marketed. Atovaquone plus proguanil (Sects. 4.4 and 4.5.1) relies on synergistic collapse of the parasite's transmitochondrial membrane potential [36]. The more empirical pairing of artemether and lumefantrine targets different processes and their pharmacokinetic mismatch (2–3 h vs. 3–6 days) results in long-term persistence of lumefantrine alone, a concern for resistance.

The now-accepted requirement for combination therapy and emergence of several promising new antimalarial leads (Sect. 4.7) have given rise to spirited discussions of the most rational basis for choosing drug pairs [37, 38]. The relative importance of (1) similarities/differences in molecular mechanism of action and in mechanisms of resistance; (2) synergistic, additive or antagonistic interaction; (3) matching half-life; (4) 'static/'cidal activity; are all under consideration. While thoughtful consideration and various in silico models can usefully examine these various factors, only experimental work will identify the key determinants of success.

3.4 Pharmacokinetic/Pharmacodynamic Linkage

Ironically, though malaria featured prominently in Paul Ehrlich's seminal studies toward rational drug discovery [39], and antimalarial drug concentrations were amongst the earliest to be measured in order to understand and guide therapy [40], today the status of pharmacokinetic/pharmacodynamic linkage is notably incomplete. Particularly lacking is an understanding of the fundamental PK governance of antimalarial activity. Extensive study of antibacterials has revealed that pharmacodynamic efficacy is usually driven by a specific pharmacokinetic parameter—C_{MAX} or T_{MIC} (Fig. 3) [41, 42]. Indeed, antibacterials are classified and clinically

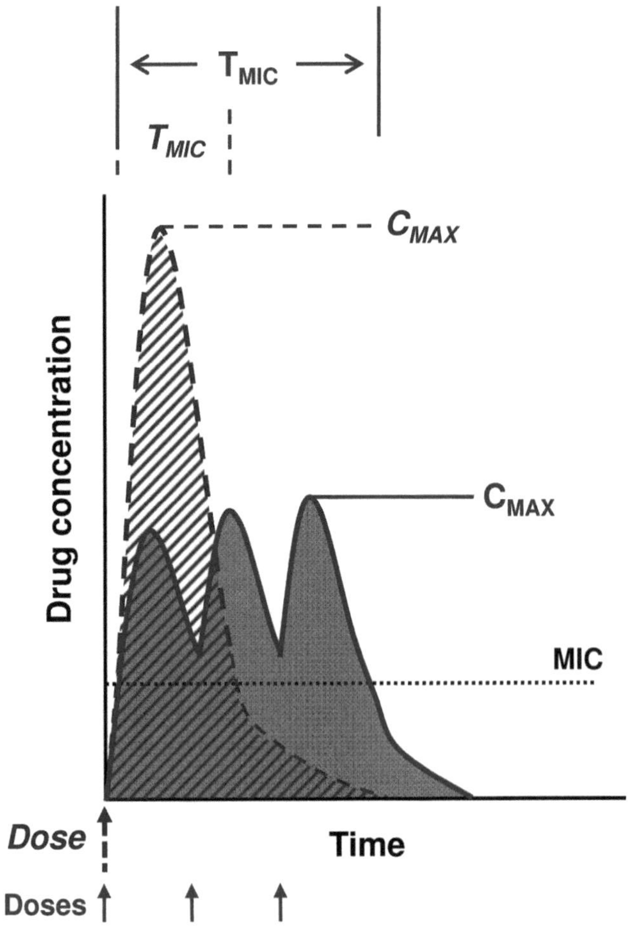

Fig. 3 Pharmacokinetic parameters of a drug in vivo. Following dosing, drug concentration in blood rises (*dashed line*) until reaching a peak (C_{MAX}), and then decays at a rate characteristic of the drug and the dosed organism, until all drug is cleared from the system. During this time, drug concentrations spend a certain interval (T_{MIC}) above a predetermined Minimal Inhibitory Concentration (MIC). The Area Under the concentration–time Curve (AUC, *diagonal black lines*) is an indicator of total drug exposure. The same amount of drug can be dosed via a different regimen using multiple smaller doses (*solid line*). This regimen yields lower C_{MAX}s but a longer T_{MIC} while maintaining the same AUC (*shaded area*)

dosed based this PK/PD link. Recent in vitro studies have demonstrated that such PK/PD governance also pertains for antimalarials. Initial proof of principle work indicates that antimalarials too can be classified as being driven by C_{MAX} or T_{MIC}, independent of their 'static or 'cidal action, and that this governance is class-wide [30]. This information may improve empirical dosing regimens [38], and, more importantly, provide new guidance in drug development. For example, an experimental compound that is C_{MAX}-driven may be fully efficacious in vivo, despite having a short-half life. However, short in vivo half-life for a compound that has been shown to be governed by time of exposure would suggest either a NOGO decision or efforts to modify its chemical structure so as to prolong plasma half-life.

3.5 Safety

Given the enormous number of people afflicted with malaria, the often limited health resources in malaria endemic areas, and the tens of millions of travelers to malarious countries every year who should take chemoprophylaxis (http://www.cdc.gov/malaria/travelers/index.html), it becomes immediately obvious that the requirement for safety is unusually high for antimalarial drugs. This imposing barrier of safety must be kept in mind when selecting candidates for development, and in designing studies to test potential drugs.

3.6 Considerations for New Drug Development

Rational drug development starts with the identification of a suitable molecular target. Screening small molecules in vitro for activity against the cell-free target is followed by testing and development of favored candidates in more complex whole cell assays and animal models. For *Plasmodium* this process presents several challenges. The eukaryotic nature of *Plasmodium*, and resultant similarity of basic biochemical mechanisms between the pathogen and its host, immediately narrows the list of unique molecular entities suitable for selective targeting. Intracellular residence of the parasite further complicates drug design. For a lead to be truly efficacious, its molecular target should be accessible and essential during all stages of the parasite life cycle, and preferably be present and required in all species of *Plasmodium* pathogenic to humans. Finally, there should be a high barrier to resistance, a facet influenced by both the function and redundancy of the target. Rational drug development schema can yield candidates that are tremendously effective in cell-free screens, but a great many of these prove ineffective against erythrocytic parasites in vitro or in vivo. An alternative strategy is to screen against whole cells or animal models; determination of molecular mechanism of action occurs later, if at all, in the process. Most successful antimalarials have been developed through this less-than-rational strategy, indeed chloroquine was discovered and developed using avian and rodent models [43] and its molecular mechanism of action was not described until 50 years later [44]. Artemisinins were co-opted from ancient Chinese remedies [45] and details of their mechanism of efficacy are debated.

The malaria research community has coalesced around the SERCaP—Single Exposure Radical Cure and Prophylaxis—as the ideal for new antimalarial drug development [46]. This sets a very high bar. SERCaP dictates that the treatment regimen be single dose, rapidly efficacious, target all forms of the parasite including latent stages, and have a long-lasting pharmacodynamic effect so as to prevent reinfection. Prudent drug development also demands that the agent be inexpensive, orally bioavailable, and provide a high barrier to resistance. It is improbable that any single molecule will satisfy all of these requirements. Instead, future malaria therapies will likely be based on the combination of multiple agents, each providing a unique spectrum of action. In subsequent sections, we discuss clinically used antimalarial drugs and some experimental agents in development, in context of the aspects described above.

4 Pharmacodynamics of Antimalarial Drugs

4.1 4-Substituted Quinolines

Agents in this class share structural similarities (Fig. 4) and a common molecular mechanism of action; however, resistance is mediated by multiple different mechanisms, not all of which have been characterized.

4.1.1 Chloroquine

Synthesized by the Germans as Resochin in 1934, and rediscovered by the Allies as SN7618 in 1944, chloroquine (Fig. 4, **1**) was for decades the mainstay of antimalarial chemotherapy [43]. Christened chloroquine by E. K. Marshall in 1945, the drug inhibits the essential parasite process of heme detoxification [44]. *Plasmodium* satisfies most of its amino acid requirements by digesting host cell hemoglobin, releasing free heme in the process. Heme-induced oxidative damage is avoided by nonenzymatic crystallization into the inert polymer hemozoin [7]. Chloroquine concentrates in parasites and inhibits heme crystallization, leading to oxidative damage and death.

While chloroquine-resistant parasites are not readily generated in vitro, the eventual emergence and global dissemination of resistance has rendered chloroquine useless in all but a few locales. Elegant parasite cross-breeding studies pinpointed resistance in *P. falciparum* to point mutations in PfCRT (*P. falciparum* chloroquine resistance transporter) [47]. Presence of resistance mutations decreases the accumulation, hence the cytotoxicity, of chloroquine. Curiously, although other 4-substituted quinolines also inhibit heme polymerization [48], and *P. vivax* may be chloroquine-resistant [31], PfCRT appears not to mediate these resistances [49].

Chloroquine's tremendous clinical success prior to resistance can be explained by its ability to satisfy many of the pharmacodynamic requirements for an ideal antimalarial. It targets a pathway not present in the human host, is parasiticidal, fast acting, and has a relatively high PRR. Furthermore, the pharmacokinetics of chloroquine are favorable. It persists with a plasma half-life of weeks to months [50]. This long half-life permits the convenient weekly dosing of chloroquine for antimalarial prophylaxis.

Chloroquine toxicity is both dose- and age-related; doses must be substantially reduced for safe use in children. At doses and regimens required to treat malaria, toxicity in adults is negligible [51]. Rare adverse events include diplopia and dizziness. Cumulative high doses of chloroquine used in anticancer [52] and immunosuppressive therapy [53] may lead to neurotoxicity, cardiotoxicity, and irreversible retinopathy.

4.1.2 Quinine

Quinine (Fig. 4, **2**), an alkaloid extracted from the bark of the cinchona tree, was used as an antipyretic by the Quechua in South America. It was transported to Rome by the Jesuits in the early seventeenth century and, in a vivid indication of today's great need for new antimalarials, this antique natural product remains a drug of choice for treating patients with severe falciparum malaria [54].

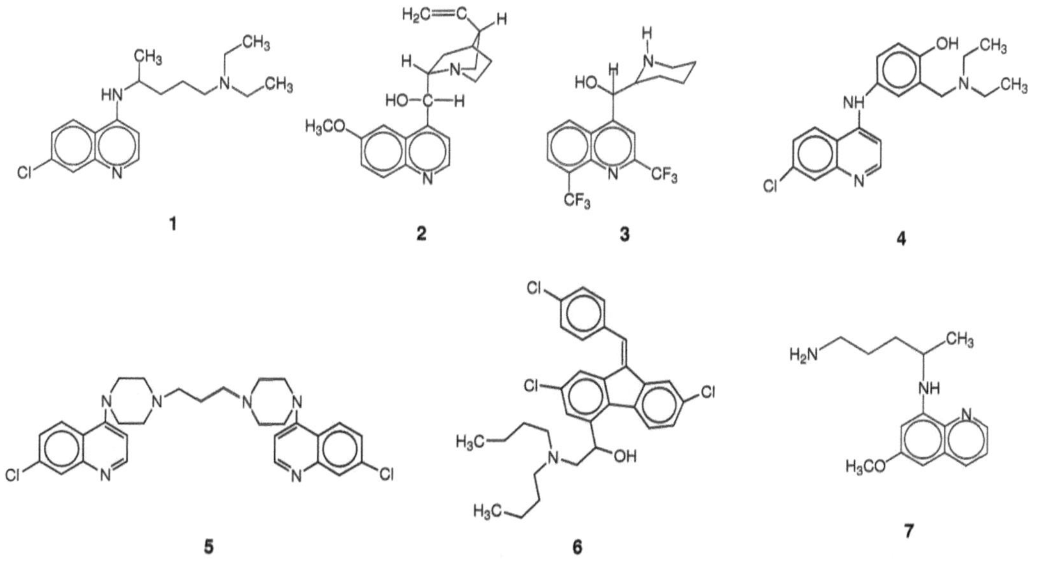

Fig. 4 The substituted quinolines and structurally related compounds. Drugs with substitutions at the 4-position include chloroquine (**1**), quinine (**2**), mefloquine (**3**), and amodiaquine (**4**). Piperaquine (**5**) is a bisquinoline while lumefantrine (**6**) is structurally similar to substituted quinolines. All have potent activity against asexual erythrocytic parasites. Primaquine (**7**), an 8-substituted quinoline, targets liver stages and gametocytes

Quinine differs from chloroquine in having an ~8 h plasma half-life [50]. This necessitates more frequent dosing, and in severely ill patients, a loading dose [55]. Quinine resistance has been observed in the field, with genetic studies indicating a multifactorial phenotype [56]. Quinine has significant toxicity [51]. Symptoms include the classic cinchonism (disturbances of vision and hearing, headache, nausea), as well as hypoglycemia and hypotension that may be life threatening. This toxicity profile and its relatively short half-life make quinine unsuitable as a prophylaxis agent. Quinidine, an efficacious antiarrhythmic, is a stereoisomer of quinine with potent antimalarial activity. In cases where quinine is unavailable, intravenous quinidine is an acceptable substitute for temporary management of severe malaria [55].

4.1.3 Mefloquine

Mefloquine (Fig. 4, **3**) was discovered in a whole-cell screen by the Walter Reed Institute of Medical Research [57], and became an immediate agent of choice for its high activity against drug-resistant *P. falciparum* [58]. PfCRT does not confer mefloquine-resistance [59]. This fact, combined with a weeks-long half-life [60], enables the use of mefloquine for prophylaxis against chloroquine-resistant malaria. Unfortunately, now-widespread resistance limits mefloquine's utility. Resistance appears to be multifactorial, and is usually associated with increased expression of multidrug-transporter proteins [59]. Mefloquine toxicity is dose-related, and usually mild at doses used for short-term prophylaxis [51]. The adverse event spectrum expands at higher doses, to include CNS toxicity and neuropsychiatric effects. For this reason, it is not utilized in long-term prophylaxis regimens.

4.1.4 Other 4-Substituted Quinolines and Structural Relatives

Amodiaquine (Fig. 4, **4**), an old antimalarial with structural and mechanistic features of chloroquine, has significant activity against chloroquine-resistant *Plasmodium* [61]. However, its use is disfavored due to an association with hepatotoxicity and agranulocytosis [51]. Piperaquine (Fig. 4, **5**) is also active against chloroquine-resistant malaria; its molecular mechanism of action is unclear [62]. It is clinically utilized in combination with dihydroartemisinin. Lumefantrine (Fig. 4, **6**), a molecule structurally similar to substituted quinolines, acts against asexual erythrocytic forms of *P. falciparum* by an unknown molecular mechanism of action [63]. Lumefantrine is FDA-approved and marketed as a fixed-dose combination with artemether (Sect. 4.3) for use against both drug-sensitive and drug-resistant malaria.

4.2 8-Aminoquinolines

8-aminoquinoline primaquine (Fig. 4, 7) is the only clinically used antimalarial with reliable activity against initial and latent liver stages and gametocytes (Fig. 2) [64]. Conversely, primaquine has no useful effect on blood stage asexual forms of *Plasmodium*, and hence it has no place in the acute treatment of symptomatic malaria.

Primaquine is the only agent known to eliminate hypnozoites of *P. vivax* and *P. ovale*, thus preventing late relapses of these infections. The molecular mechanism of action of primaquine is unclear, but appears to be mediated largely by its metabolites. Primaquine's vivid toxicities suggest that it acts by generating oxidative species and interfering with redox balance in the pathogen. Primaquine is associated with frequent gastrointestinal intolerance and at high doses causes methemoglobinemia in most people (primaquine use reviewed in [65]). Patients with glucose-6-phosphate dehydrogenase deficiency are particularly susceptible, even at therapeutic doses, to acute, sometimes life threatening, hemolysis and hemolytic anemia [66]. Indeed, primaquine-induced hemolysis led to the discovery of glucose-6-phosphate dehydrogenase deficiency, the first genetic abnormality associated with an enzyme [67].

4.3 The Artemisinins

Artemisinin (Fig. 5, **8**) or qinghaosu is the active moiety in *Artemesia annua*, a plant utilized by Chinese herbalists for over 2000 years [45]. A sesquiterpene lactone endoperoxide, the artemisinins currently form the last line of defense against multidrug-resistant *P. falciparum*. Their mechanism of action has been the subject of much study. It is generally accepted that the endoperoxide is the active pharmacophore. Iron- or heme-catalyzed cleavage of the oxygen-oxygen bond likely leads to subsequent formation of a carbon-centered radical [68] that in turn alkylates parasite macromolecules. Semisynthetic derivatives artemether (Fig. 5, **9**), arteether (Fig. 5, **10**), and artesunate (Fig. 5, **11**) are more soluble than parent artemisinin, but act in a similar fashion. While these compounds themselves have antimalarial activity, they also act as prodrugs in vivo. All derivatives (**8–11**) are rapidly converted in vivo to dihydroartemisinin (Fig. 5, **12**), itself an antimalarial [69]. The artemisinins have potent and rapid activity against asexual erythrocytic stages of *P. falciparum* and *P. vivax*, making them particularly useful in severely ill patients with high parasite burden.

A distinguishing characteristic of the artemisinins is their extremely short half-life [70]. Cleared from plasma within minutes, their great activity against a parasite with a complex 48 h life cycle has always been puzzling. However, in vitro PK/PD studies

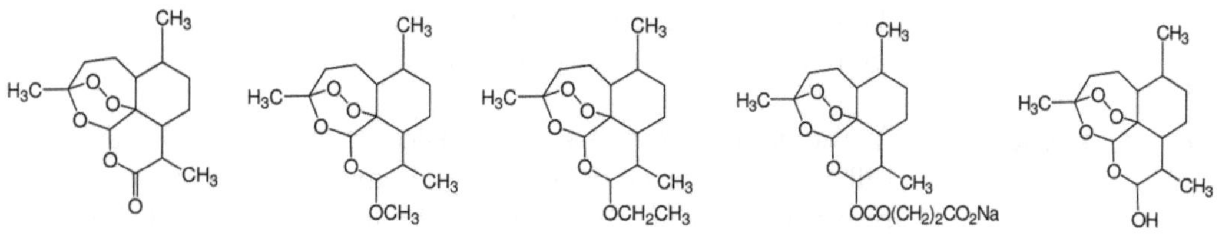

8 9 10 11 12

Fig. 5 The artemisinins. Members of this family include natural product artemisinin (**8**), and its semisynthetic derivatives artemether (**9**), arteether (**10**), artesunate (**11**), and dihydroartemisinin (**12**). These compounds are an obligate component of most clinically efficacious antimalarial drug regimens have demonstrated that artemisinin efficacy is C_{MAX}-driven, a mechanism that aligns ideally with its short half-life, providing a satisfactory explanation for the clinical success of such remarkably short-lived drugs [30]. Interestingly, daily dose artemisinin monotherapy, even for 7 days, invariably leads to recrudescence of parasitemia [71]. Explanations for this phenomenon include differential effects on life-cycle stages and/or induction of post-treatment "quiescence" in surviving parasites [72]. Long-lived endoperoxides (Sect. 4.7.4) have been developed in an effort to remedy this problem [73]. In any case, artemisinins are now almost always used in combination regimens.

Efficacy of the artemisinins has recently been threatened by the discovery of a resistance-like phenomenon. While not meeting WHO's definition of leading to treatment failure, the effect manifests pharmacodynamically as a slower rate of parasite clearance and longer persistence of parasites in vivo [74]. Genetic studies suggest that parasite genotype accounts only partially for the observed clinical phenotype, implying the existence of as-yet-undefined contributions from the human host [75]. Although geographically still restricted, this "resistance" phenotype has begun a slow march out of its initial focus in Southeast Asia. Recent genome-wide association studies on "resistant" parasites [76], as well as attempts to recapitulate resistance in vitro, have focused on polymorphisms in a region of chromosome 13 (encoding a protein containing a kelch 13 propeller domain) that appear to correlate with the phenotype [77]. Recent in vitro work has demonstrated that these kelch 13 polymorphisms are necessary and sufficient to enhance the survival of the parasite ring stage in the face of artemisinin pressure [78]. While the exact molecular mechanism is unclear, transcriptomic analysis suggests that this 'resistance' is mediated via an upregulation of the parasite's unfolded protein response [79]. Artemisinins currently form the last line of defense against drug-resistant malaria and the threat to their efficacy has, appropriately, spurred greater urgency in new antimalarial drug development.

Artemisinins are considered relatively safe, having been used for decades in millions of humans. Recognized toxicities include hemolysis and hypersensitivity reactions. Animal toxicology studies indicate that brain, liver, bone marrow, and fetus may be affected. This adverse event profile has not been unambiguously demonstrated in humans treated with therapeutic doses [51].

4.4 Atovaquone

Atovaquone (Fig. 6, **13**) is an analog of coenzyme Q that specifically targets the cytochrome bc_1 complex of the mitochondrial respiratory chain. It interferes with mitochondrial functions, including pyrimidine biosynthesis, by inhibiting electron transport and collapsing the mitochondrial transmembrane potential [80]. Potent activity against asexual erythrocytic forms of *P. falciparum* and *P. vivax*, and the ability to eliminate *P. falciparum* liver stage

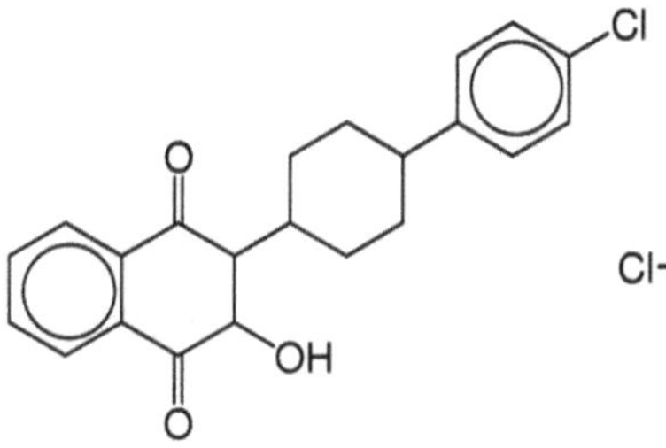

13

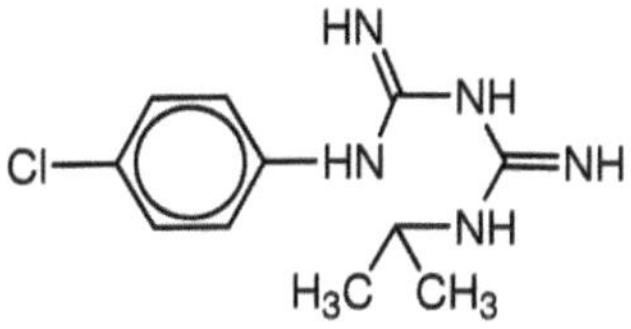

14

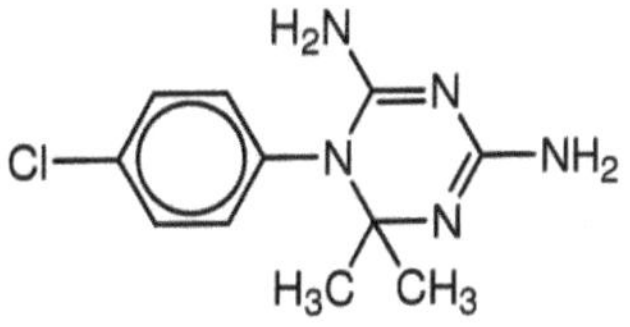

15

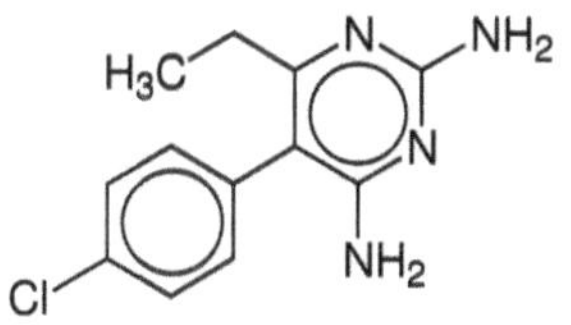

16

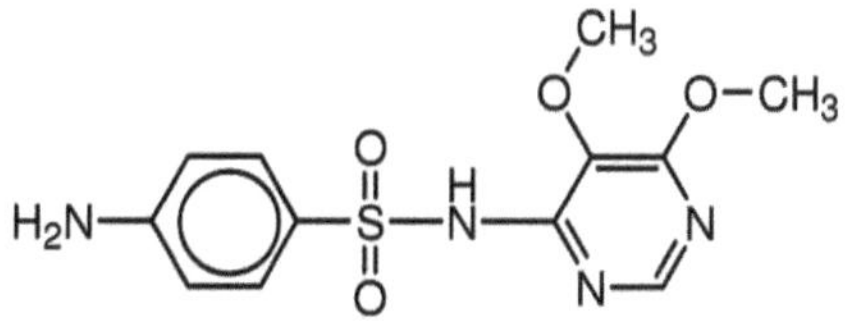

17

Fig. 6 Atovaquone, antifolates, and sulfonamides. Atovaquone (**13**) is a cytochrome bc_1 inhibitor that is effective on its own, synergizes with the biguanide proguanil (**14**), and is clinically always used in combination. Proguanil is a prodrug metabolized in vivo to cycloguanil (**15**), a dihydrofolate reductase inhibitor. Pyrimethamine (**16**) also targets dihydrofolate reductase and is used in synergistic combination with sulfadoxine (**17**), a dihydropteroate synthase-targeting sulfonamide

parasites makes this agent especially useful for prophylaxis. Atovaquone is relatively safe—common adverse events include headache, rash, abdominal pain, vomiting, and diarrhea.

In its very first clinical trials atovaquone failed spectacularly, and quite unexpectedly, thanks to the rapid emergence of drug-resistant *P. falciparum*, mediated by point mutations in target cytochrome b (atovaquone reviewed in [36]). Utility of this potent, safe, relatively long-lived candidate was saved by its synergistic combination, demonstrable both in lab and clinic, with veteran antimalarial proguanil (Sect. 4.5.1).

4.5 Antifolates and Sulfonamides

Sulfonamides and antifolates were among the earliest synthetic antimalarial agents, and were developed primarily using avian models of malaria.

4.5.1 Proguanil and Cycloguanil

The biguanide proguanil (Fig. 6, **14**) targets *Plasmodium* in multiple ways. Best known as a prodrug, in vivo it is metabolized by CYP2C19 to cycloguanil (Fig. 6, **15**) [81], which inhibits *P. falciparum* dihydrofolate reductase [82]. However, proguanil is also active in vitro (where it is not converted to cycloguanil) suggesting other direct (and unknown) targets [83]. Pharmacogenetic differences in CYP2C19 can affect the conversion to cycloguanil, and patients with CYP2C19*2–CYP2C19*8 alleles (poor metabolizers) may not fully convert proguanil to cycloguanil [81]. Clinical relevance of the poor metabolizer phenotype with respect to malaria is the subject of debate. Proguanil is remarkably safe at therapeutic doses. Resistance against cycloguanil is conferred by point mutations in *Plasmodium* dihydrofolate reductase [84], and these arose and spread rapidly in the era of proguanil monotherapy. Clinical use of proguanil is now largely confined to its synergistic combination with atovaquone (Sect. 4.4). While proguanil itself displays no effect on the mitochondrial membrane potential, it greatly enhances atovaquone's effect [85].

4.5.2 Pyrimethamine

Pyrimethamine (Fig. 6, **16**) is a diaminopyrimidine that targets *Plasmodium* dihydrofolate reductase [82]. The effects of inhibiting folate metabolism manifest late in the replication cycle of asexual erythrocytic forms, making pyrimethamine a slow-acting drug. Pharmacodynamic efficacy of pyrimethamine can be augmented by host immunity, and significantly inhibited by dietary *p*-aminobenzoic acid or folate. Point mutations in *Plasmodium* dihydrofolate reductase confer resistance to this drug [86]. Therapeutic doses of pyrimethamine are safe; excessive doses can recapitulate symptoms of folate deficiency [51]. Pyrimethamine is usually dosed in combination with a sulfonamide or sulfone to create a synergistic effect. However, the utility of this combination is limited by widespread drug resistance, as well as by intrinsic toxicity of the sulfonamides.

4.5.3 Sulfonamides and Sulfones

Sulfonamides and sulfones inhibit *Plasmodium* dihydropteroate synthase [87], an enzyme involved in folate biosynthesis that has no counterpart in humans. These agents are slow acting and readily generate mutations in target protein dihydropteroate synthase [88], which confers class-wide resistance. Clinical utility is confined to coadministration with an antifolate partner drug. The combination of sulfadoxine (Fig. 6, **17**) with pyrimethamine is particularly effective since multiple steps of the same biosynthetic pathway are affected. This particular combination was designed to include partners with matched in vivo pharmacokinetics (both drugs are long-lived), thus avoiding functional monotherapy with either agent towards the end of the dosing interval. The use of sulfonamides and sulfonamide-containing combinations is limited by toxicity, including Stevens–Johnson syndrome and exfoliative dermatitis [51]. Additionally, widespread resistance of *Plasmodium* to both partner drugs has compromised the utility of this drug class and its combinations.

4.6 Antibacterials

Tetracycline (Fig. 7, **18**) and doxycycline (Fig. 7, **19**) are slow acting agents [61] that target the apicoplast, a chloroplast-like organelle in malaria parasites. Interference with apicoplast function results in delayed death of the parasite: effects of the drug are not manifest until the next replication cycle [89]. This delayed effect makes

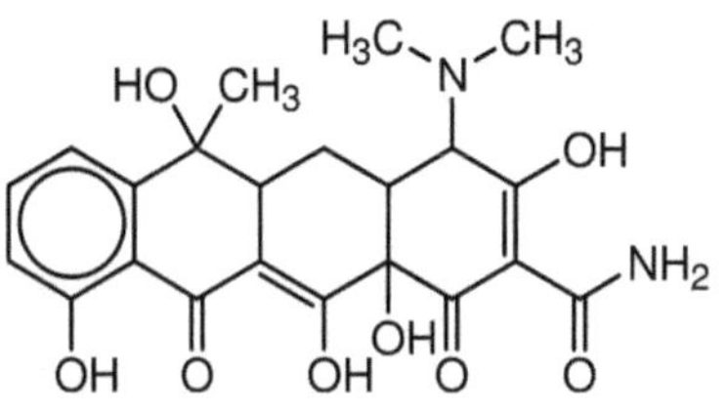

18

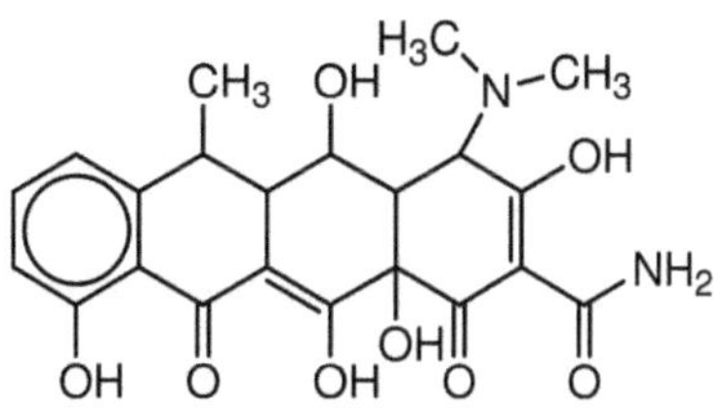

19

Fig. 7 Antibacterials. Tetracycline (**18**) and doxycycline (**19**) are slow-acting antimalarials useful for adjunctive therapy and short-term prophylaxis

the tetracyclines unsuitable for treatment of established severe infections; however, they are useful as adjunctive therapy and for short-term prophylaxis. Adverse effects that limit their use include discoloring depositions in bones and teeth, and a tendency to cause photosensitivity [90].

4.7 Experimental Agents

Today's global development of new antimalarial drugs is largely coordinated by the Medicines for Malaria Venture (MMV), a non-profit public–private foundation. MMV coordinates industrial and academic antimalarial efforts and facilitates progress of drug candidates through the long and complex development pathway [91]. A current snapshot of the global antimalarial development portfolio can be found on the foundation's website (www.mmv.org). There are multiple new drugs or drug combinations in various stages of development [92], ranging from the discovery phase to post-approval management. The following are agents currently in human trials, with a focus on novel pharmacophores, molecular targets, or pharmacokinetics.

4.7.1 DSM265

Developed by a multinational academic collaboration, DSM265 (Fig. 8, **20**) targets dihydroorotate dehydrogenase, a mitochondrial enzyme in *P. falciparum* essential for pyrimidine biosynthesis and parasite survival [93]. The compound achieves several important benchmarks in that it is potent, selective, active against chloroquine-resistant parasites, bioavailable and metabolically stable. It will likely be deployed in combination therapy with a suitable partner.

4.7.2 KAE609

KAE609 (Fig. 8, **21**) is a spiroindolone that targets a P-type ATPase Na(+) channel of *P. falciparum* [94]. Developed from a natural product screen in an industry–academia collaboration, KAE609 is a novel pharmacophore targeting a subsequently described and hitherto unexplored *Plasmodium* function, and has successfully completed Phase IIA clinical trials. The relative ease of generating resistance in vitro is somewhat worrisome; however, this efficacious compound will provide much-needed diversity to the antimalarial armamentarium.

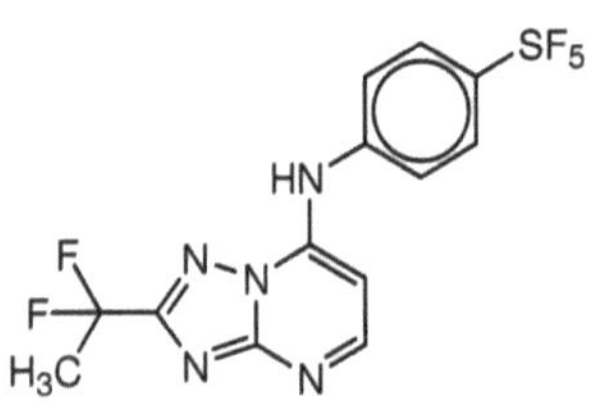

20

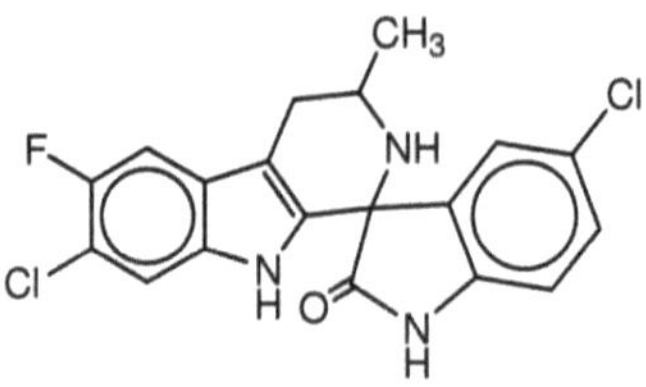

21

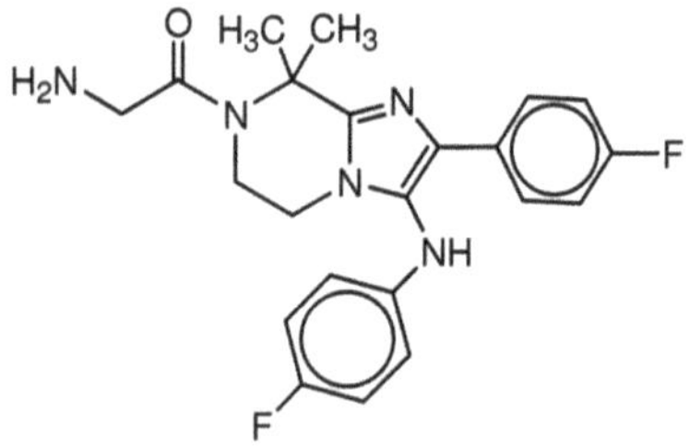

22

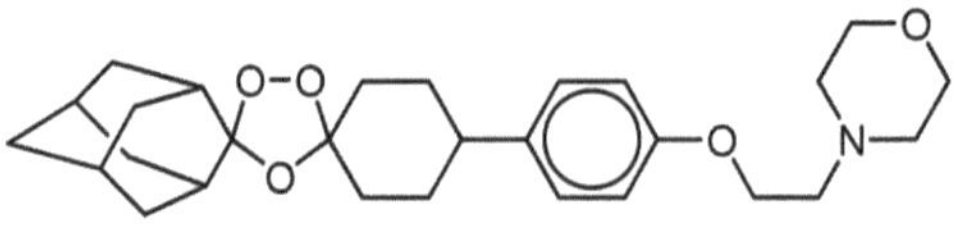

23

Fig. 8 Experimental antimalarials. Triazolopyrimidine DSM265 (**20**) inhibits dihydroorotate dehydrogenase, an essential malarial enzyme. KAE609 (**21**) targets the *Pf*ATP4 (Na+) channel and KAF156 (**22**) is an imidazolopiperazine active against both blood and liver stages of the parasite life cycle. OZ439 (**23**) contains the endoperoxide pharmacophore of the artemisinins, but is designed to persist in the blood

4.7.3 KAF 156

An imidazopyrazine derivative discovered and developed through a whole cell screening approach, KAF156 (Fig. 8, **22**) targets both liver and blood stages of *Plasmodium* [95]. This multistage activity, coupled with acceptable pharmacokinetics, suggests that KAF156 has potential to provide both the Radical Cure and the Protection demanded by the SERCaP model.

4.7.4 OZ439

OZ439 (Fig. 8, **23**) is member of the synthetic ozonides [96]. Its endoperoxide motif mimics that of the artemisinins, and their mechanism of action is likely in common. The unique feature of OZ439 is its metabolic stability: a terminal half-life of 25–30 h compared to half-lives of just minutes for the artemisinins [73]. Recent in vitro research on artemisinin resistance has yielded the intriguing suggestion that the resistance phenotype may be mediated by a quiescence or dormancy mechanism that simply allows the parasite to outlast the short-lived drug [72]. If so, long-$t_{1/2}$ endoperoxide OZ439 will be crucial for combating and perhaps reversing artemisinin resistance in the field.

5 Summary

Malaria is a public health problem of immense proportions. The complex biology of malaria makes drug development and use particularly challenging, a situation exacerbated by drug resistance. The parasite is a eukaryote, which limits the availability of targets unique to the pathogen. Plasmodium species pathogenic to humans will not infect other animals, rendering animal models deficient. Finally, human parasites are difficult, and in some cases impossible, to culture in vitro, limiting development of laboratory assays.

The asexual erythrocytic stages that cause symptomatic illness are the primary targets of treatment. However, prevention and public health strategies necessitate the targeting of liver stages and gametocytes, both of which are pharmacologically distinct from the asexual blood stages.

Initial pharmacodynamic endpoints for antimalarial development were clinical and required human studies. Surrogate animal models and in vitro assays have matured to the point where a rational combination of assays yields adequate information to aid drug development, and these in conjunction with contemporary screening methods have yielded a number of highly promising experimental drug candidates.

Successful antimalarial drugs must fulfil certain criteria. The drug must be potent; provide a single-dose cure; act rapidly; and target all stages of the parasite life cycle. Drug pharmacokinetics in vivo must align with the essential pharmacokinetic–pharmacodynamic linkage. The molecule must possess a high barrier to resistance. And ultimately, the drug must be extremely safe, given expected administration to millions of patients and to healthy uninfected travelers. No single drug currently fulfils all these criteria. Indeed, it is unlikely any agent ever will. Successful antimalarial regimens will require combinations of drugs, rationally selected to provide best activity.

Existing antimalarials have proven successful because they fulfill some of the requirements listed above. New drug development efforts have formalized these benchmarks and progress along the development pathway is now governed by these criteria. While there are several new pharmacophores targeting novel targets, and some old ones aiming for different processes, antimalarial drug development is likely to remain a challenging endeavor for the foreseeable future.

Acknowledgements

We thank Drs. David Sullivan and Kartiki Desai for their careful reading of the manuscript and thoughtful comments; Dr. Elizabeth Nenortas for proofing chemical structures; and Rachel Shapiro Grasmick for drawing the malaria life cycle. This project was supported by the Johns Hopkins Malaria Research Institute, the Bloomberg Family Foundation, and by NIH grants R01AI095453 and R01AI111962.

References

1. Fairhurst RM, Wellems TE (2010) Plasmodium species (Malaria). In: Mandell GL, Bennett JE, Donlin R (eds) Mandel, Douglas and Bennett's principles and practice of infectious diseases, vol 2, Churchill. Livingstone, Philadelphia, PA, pp 3437–3462
2. White NJ, Pukrittayakamee S, Hien TT et al (2014) Malaria. Lancet 383(9918):723–735. doi:10.1016/S0140-6736(13)60024-0
3. Shapiro TA, Goldberg DE (2006) Chemotherapy of protozoal infections: malaria. In: Brunton LL, Lazo JS, Parker KL (eds) Goodman and Gilman's the pharmacological basis of therapeutics, 11th edn. McGraw-Hill, New York, pp 1021–1047
4. Gardner MJ, Hall N, Fung E et al (2002) Genome sequence of the human malaria parasite Plasmodium falciparum. Nature 419(6906):498–511. doi:10.1038/nature01097
5. Trager W, Jensen JB (1976) Human malaria parasites in continuous culture. Science 193(4254):673–675
6. Dahl EL, Rosenthal PJ (2008) Apicoplast translation, transcription and genome replication: targets for antimalarial antibiotics. Trends Parasitol 24(6):279–284. doi:10.1016/j.pt.2008.03.007
7. Francis SE, Sullivan DJ Jr, Goldberg DE (1997) Hemoglobin metabolism in the malaria parasite Plasmodium falciparum. Annu Rev Microbiol 51:97–123. doi:10.1146/annurev.micro.51.1.97
8. Painter HJ, Morrisey JM, Mather MW et al (2007) Specific role of mitochondrial electron transport in blood-stage Plasmodium falciparum. Nature 446(7131):88–91. doi:10.1038/nature05572
9. Gamo FJ, Sanz LM, Vidal J et al (2010) Thousands of chemical starting points for antimalarial lead identification. Nature 465(7296):305–310. doi:10.1038/nature09107
10. Guiguemde WA, Shelat AA, Bouck D et al (2010) Chemical genetics of Plasmodium falciparum. Nature 465(7296):311–315. doi:10.1038/nature09099
11. Rottmann M, McNamara C, Yeung BK et al (2010) Spiroindolones, a potent compound class for the treatment of malaria. Science 329(5996):1175–1180. doi:10.1126/science.1193225
12. McGhee RB (1988) Major animal models in malaria research: avian. In: Wernsdorfer WH, McGregor I (eds) Malaria: principles and practice of malariology, vol 2. Churchill Livingstone, Edinburgh, pp 1545–1567
13. Cox FEG (1988) Major animal models in malaria research: rodent. In: Wernsdorfer WH, McGregor I (eds) Malaria: principles and practice of malariology, vol 2. Churchill Livingstone, Edinburgh, pp 1503–1543
14. Fidock DA, Rosenthal PJ, Croft SL et al (2004) Antimalarial drug discovery: efficacy models for compound screening. Nat Rev Drug Discov 3(6):509–520. doi:10.1038/nrd1416
15. Craig AG, Grau GE, Janse C et al (2012) The role of animal models for research on severe malaria. PLoS Pathog 8(2):e1002401. doi:10.1371/journal.ppat.1002401
16. Angulo-Barturen I, Jimenez-Diaz MB, Mulet T et al (2008) A murine model of falciparum-malaria by in vivo selection of competent strains in non-myelodepleted mice engrafted with human erythrocytes. PLoS One 3(5):e2252. doi:10.1371/journal.pone.0002252
17. Collins WE (1988) Major animal models in malaria research: simian. In: Wernsdorfer WH, McGregor I (eds) Malaria: principles and practice of malariology, vol 2. Churchill Livingstone, Edinburgh, pp 1473–1501
18. Cox-Singh J (2012) Zoonotic malaria: Plasmodium knowlesi, an emerging pathogen. Curr Opin Infect Dis 25(5):530–536. doi:10.1097/QCO.0b013e3283558780
19. Bruce-Chwatt LJ (1967) Clinical trials of antimalarial drugs. Trans R Soc Trop Med Hyg 61(3):412–426
20. Shapiro TA, Ranasinha CD, Kumar N et al (1999) Prophylactic activity of atovaquone against Plasmodium falciparum in humans. Am J Trop Med Hyg 60(5):831–836
21. Seder RA, Chang LJ, Enama ME et al (2013) Protection against malaria by intravenous immunization with a nonreplicating sporozoite vaccine. Science 341(6152):1359–1365. doi:10.1126/science.1241800
22. Desjardins RE, Canfield CJ, Haynes JD et al (1979) Quantitative assessment of antimalarial activity in vitro by a semiautomated microdilution technique. Antimicrob Agents Chemother 16(6):710–718
23. Bennett TN, Paguio M, Gligorijevic B et al (2004) Novel, rapid, and inexpensive cell-based quantification of antimalarial drug efficacy. Antimicrob Agents Chemother 48(5):1807–1810
24. Karl S, Wong RP, St Pierre TG et al (2009) A comparative study of a flow-cytometry-based assessment of in vitro Plasmodium falciparum drug sensitivity. Malar J 8:294. doi:10.1186/1475-2875-8-294

25. Sanz LM, Crespo B, De-Cozar C et al (2012) P. falciparum in vitro killing rates allow to discriminate between different antimalarial mode-of-action. PLoS One 7(2):e30949. doi:10.1371/journal.pone.0030949
26. Young RD, Rathod PK (1993) Clonal viability measurements on Plasmodium falciparum to assess in vitro schizonticidal activity of leupeptin, chloroquine, and 5-fluoroorotate. Antimicrob Agents Chemother 37(5): 1102–1107
27. Paguio MF, Bogle KL, Roepe PD (2011) Plasmodium falciparum resistance to cytocidal versus cytostatic effects of chloroquine. Mol Biochem Parasitol 178(1–2):1–6. doi:10.1016/j.molbiopara.2011.03.003
28. Painter HJ, Morrisey JM, Vaidya AB (2010) Mitochondrial electron transport inhibition and viability of intraerythrocytic Plasmodium falciparum. Antimicrob Agents Chemother 54(12):5281–5287. doi:10.1128/AAC.00937-10
29. Le Manach C, Scheurer C, Sax S et al (2013) Fast in vitro methods to determine the speed of action and the stage-specificity of anti-malarials in Plasmodium falciparum. Malar J 12:424. doi:10.1186/1475-2875-12-424
30. Bakshi RP, Nenortas E, Tripathi AK et al (2013) Model system to define pharmacokinetic requirements for antimalarial drug efficacy. Sci Transl Med 5(205):205ra135. doi:10.1126/scitranslmed.3006684
31. Barrette A, Ringwald P (2010) Global report on antimalarial drug efficacy and drug resistance: 2000–2010. World Health Organization, Switzerland
32. Zhao X, Xu C, Domagala J et al (1997) DNA topoisomerase targets of the fluoroquinolones: a strategy for avoiding bacterial resistance. Proc Natl Acad Sci U S A 94(25):13991–13996
33. Hitchings GH (1969) A quarter century of chemotherapy. JAMA 209(9):1339–1340
34. Richards WHG (1966) Antimalarial activity of sulphonamides and a sulphone, singly and in combination with pyrimethamine, against drug resistant and normal strains of laboratory plasmodia. Nature 212(5069):1494–1495
35. Greenberg J, Boyd BL, Josephson ES (1948) Synergistic effect of chlorguanide and sulfadiazine against Plasmodium gallinaceum in the chick. J Pharmacol Exp Ther 94(1):60–64
36. Vaidya A (2001) Atovaquone-proguanil combination. In: Rosenthal PJ (ed) Antimalarial chemotherapy. Humana Press Inc., Totowa, NJ, pp 203–218
37. Hastings IM, Hodel EM (2014) Pharmacological considerations in the design of anti-malarial drug combination therapies—is matching half-lives enough? Malar J 13(1):62. doi:10.1186/1475-2875-13-62
38. White NJ (2013) Pharmacokinetic and pharmacodynamic considerations in antimalarial dose optimization. Antimicrob Agents Chemother 57(12):5792–5807. doi:10.1128/AAC.00287-13
39. Lazarus A (1922) Paul Ehrlich, vol 2. Rikola, Wien
40. Lipkin IJ, Ramsden W (1918) Nephelometric estimation of quinine in blood and urine. Br Med J 1(2994):560–561
41. Craig WA (1998) Pharmacokinetic/pharmacodynamic parameters: rationale for antibacterial dosing of mice and men. Clin Infect Dis 26(1):1–10, quiz 11–12
42. Drusano GL (2004) Antimicrobial pharmacodynamics: critical interactions of 'bug and drug'. Nat Rev Microbiol 2(4):289–300. doi:10.1038/nrmicro862
43. Coatney GR (1963) Pitfalls in a discovery: the chronicle of chloroquine. Am J Trop Med Hyg 12:121–128
44. Sullivan DJ Jr, Gluzman IY, Russell DG et al (1996) On the molecular mechanism of chloroquine's antimalarial action. Proc Natl Acad Sci U S A 93(21):11865–11870
45. Klayman DL (1985) Qinghaosu (artemisinin): an antimalarial drug from China. Science 228(4703):1049–1055
46. Alonso PA, Djimde A, Magill A et al (2011) A research agenda for malaria eradication: drugs. PLoS Med 8(1):e1000402. doi:10.1371/journal.pmed.1000402
47. Fidock DA, Nomura T, Talley AK et al (2000) Mutations in the P. falciparum digestive vacuole transmembrane protein PfCRT and evidence for their role in chloroquine resistance. Mol Cell 6(4):861–871
48. Sullivan DJ Jr, Matile H, Ridley RG et al (1998) A common mechanism for blockade of heme polymerization by antimalarial quinolines. J Biol Chem 273(47):31103–31107
49. Nomura T, Carlton JM, Baird JK et al (2001) Evidence for different mechanisms of chloroquine resistance in 2 Plasmodium species that cause human malaria. J Infect Dis 183(11):1653–1661. doi:10.1086/320707
50. Krishna S, White NJ (1996) Pharmacokinetics of quinine, chloroquine and amodiaquine. Clinical implications. Clin Pharmacokinet 30(4):263–299
51. Taylor WR, White NJ (2004) Antimalarial drug toxicity: a review. Drug Saf 27(1):25–61
52. Amaravadi RK, Lippincott-Schwartz J, Yin XM et al (2011) Principles and current strategies for targeting autophagy for cancer treatment.

Clin Cancer Res 17(4):654–666. doi:10.1158/1078-0432.CCR-10-2634
53. Meyer KC, Decker C, Baughman R (2010) Toxicity and monitoring of immunosuppressive therapy used in systemic autoimmune diseases. Clin Chest Med 31(3):565–588. doi:10.1016/j.ccm.2010.05.006
54. Achan J, Talisuna AO, Erhart A et al (2011) Quinine, an old anti-malarial drug in a modern world: role in the treatment of malaria. Malar J 10:144. doi:10.1186/1475-2875-10-144
55. Warrell DA (1989) Treatment of severe malaria. J R Soc Med 82(Suppl 17):44–50, discussion 50–51
56. Foley M, Tilley L (1998) Quinoline antimalarials: mechanisms of action and resistance and prospects for new agents. Pharmacol Ther 79(1):55–87
57. Osdene TS, Russell PB, Rane L (1967) 2,4,7-Triamino-6-ortho-substituted Arylpteridines. A new series of potent antimalarial agents. J Med Chem 10(3):431–434. doi:10.1021/jm00315a031
58. Trenholme CM, Williams RL, Desjardins RE et al (1975) Mefloquine (WR 142,490) in the treatment of human malaria. Science 190(4216):792–794
59. Price RN, Uhlemann AC, Brockman A et al (2004) Mefloquine resistance in Plasmodium falciparum and increased pfmdr1 gene copy number. Lancet 364(9432):438–447. doi:10.1016/S0140-6736(04)16767-6
60. Karbwang J, White NJ (1990) Clinical pharmacokinetics of mefloquine. Clin Pharmacokinet 19(4):264–279. doi:10.2165/00003088-199019040-00002
61. Rieckmann KH (1971) Determination of the drug sensitivity of Plasmodium falciparum. JAMA 217(5):573–578
62. Davis TM, Hung TY, Sim IK et al (2005) Piperaquine: a resurgent antimalarial drug. Drugs 65(1):75–87
63. White NJ, van Vugt M, Ezzet F (1999) Clinical pharmacokinetics and pharmacodynamics and pharmacodynamics of artemether-lumefantrine. Clin Pharmacokinet 37(2):105–125
64. Arnold J, Alving AS, Hockwald RS et al (1955) The antimalarial action of primaquine against the blood and tissue stages of falciparum malaria (Panama, P-F-6 strain). J Lab Clin Med 46(3):391–397
65. Hill DR, Baird JK, Parise ME et al (2006) Primaquine: report from CDC expert meeting on malaria chemoprophylaxis I. Am J Trop Med Hyg 75(3):402–415
66. Beutler E (1959) The hemolytic effect of primaquine and related compounds: a review. Blood 14(2):103–139
67. Alving AS, Carson PE, Flanagan CL et al (1956) Enzymatic deficiency in primaquine-sensitive erythrocytes. Science 124(3220): 484–485
68. Posner GH, Park SB, Gonzalez L et al (1996) Evidence for the importance of high-valent Fe=O and of a diketone in the molecular mechanism of action of antimalarial trioxane analogs of artemisinin. J Am Chem Soc 118:3537–3538
69. Newton PN, Barnes KI, Smith PJ et al (2006) The pharmacokinetics of intravenous artesunate in adults with severe falciparum malaria. Eur J Clin Pharmacol 62(12):1003–1009. doi:10.1007/s00228-006-0203-2
70. Benakis A, Paris M, Loutan L et al (1997) Pharmacokinetics of artemisinin and artesunate after oral administration in healthy volunteers. Am J Trop Med Hyg 56(1):17–23
71. Hassan Alin M, Ashton M, Kihamia CM et al (1996) Multiple dose pharmacokinetics of oral artemisinin and comparison of its efficacy with that of oral artesunate in falciparum malaria patients. Trans R Soc Trop Med Hyg 90(1):61–65
72. Klonis N, Xie SC, McCaw JM et al (2013) Altered temporal response of malaria parasites determines differential sensitivity to artemisinin. Proc Natl Acad Sci U S A 110(13):5157–5162. doi:10.1073/pnas.1217452110
73. Moehrle JJ, Duparc S, Siethoff C et al (2013) First-in-man safety and pharmacokinetics of synthetic ozonide OZ439 demonstrates an improved exposure profile relative to other peroxide antimalarials. Br J Clin Pharmacol 75(2):524–537. doi:10.1111/j.1365-2125.2012.04368.x
74. Dondorp AM, Yeung S, White L et al (2010) Artemisinin resistance: current status and scenarios for containment. Nat Rev Microbiol 8(4):272–280. doi:10.1038/nrmicro2331
75. Anderson TJ, Nair S, Nkhoma S et al (2010) High heritability of malaria parasite clearance rate indicates a genetic basis for artemisinin resistance in western Cambodia. J Infect Dis 201(9):1326–1330. doi:10.1086/651562
76. Takala-Harrison S, Clark TG, Jacob CG et al (2013) Genetic loci associated with delayed clearance of Plasmodium falciparum following artemisinin treatment in Southeast Asia. Proc Natl Acad Sci U S A 110(1):240–245. doi:10.1073/pnas.1211205110
77. Ariey F, Witkowski B, Amaratunga C et al (2014) A molecular marker of artemisinin-resistant Plasmodium falciparum malaria.

Nature 505(7481):50–55. doi:10.1038/nature12876

78. Hudson AT (1993) Atovaquone—a novel broad-spectrum anti-infective drug. Parasitol Today 9(2):66–68
79. Desta Z, Zhao X, Shin JG et al (2002) Clinical significance of the cytochrome P450 2C19 genetic polymorphism. Clin Pharmacokinet 41(12):913–958. doi:10.2165/00003088-200241120-00002
80. Ferone R, Burchall JJ, Hitchings GH (1969) Plasmodium berghei dihydrofolate reductase. Isolation, properties, and inhibition by antifolates. Mol Pharmacol 5(1):49–59
81. Watkins WM, Sixsmith DG, Chulay JD (1984) The activity of proguanil and its metabolites, cycloguanil and p-chlorophenylbiguanide, against Plasmodium falciparum in vitro. Ann Trop Med Parasitol 78(3):273–278
82. Foote SJ, Galatis D, Cowman AF (1990) Amino acids in the dihydrofolate reductase-thymidylate synthase gene of Plasmodium falciparum involved in cycloguanil resistance differ from those involved in pyrimethamine resistance. Proc Natl Acad Sci U S A 87(8):3014–3017
83. Srivastava IK, Vaidya AB (1999) A mechanism for the synergistic antimalarial action of atovaquone and proguanil. Antimicrob Agents Chemother 43(6):1334–1339
84. Peterson DS, Walliker D, Wellems TE (1988) Evidence that a point mutation in dihydrofolate reductase-thymidylate synthase confers resistance to pyrimethamine in falciparum malaria. Proc Natl Acad Sci U S A 85(23):9114–9118
85. Triglia T, Menting JG, Wilson C et al (1997) Mutations in dihydropteroate synthase are responsible for sulfone and sulfonamide resistance in Plasmodium falciparum. Proc Natl Acad Sci U S A 94(25):13944–13949
86. Wang P, Read M, Sims PF et al (1997) Sulfadoxine resistance in the human malaria parasite Plasmodium falciparum is determined by mutations in dihydropteroate synthetase and an additional factor associated with folate utilization. Mol Microbiol 23(5):979–986
87. Dahl EL, Shock JL, Shenai BR et al (2006) Tetracyclines specifically target the apicoplast of the malaria parasite Plasmodium falciparum. Antimicrob Agents Chemother 50(9):3124–3131. doi:10.1128/AAC.00394-06
88. Clendenning WE (1965) Complications of tetracycline therapy. Arch Dermatol 91:628–632
89. Burrows JN, Burlot E, Campo B et al (2014) Antimalarial drug discovery—the path towards eradication. Parasitology 141(1):128–139. doi:10.1017/S0031182013000826
90. Flannery EL, Chatterjee AK, Winzeler EA (2013) Antimalarial drug discovery—approaches and progress towards new medicines. Nat Rev Microbiol 11(12):849–862. doi:10.1038/nrmicro3138
91. Coteron JM, Marco M, Esquivias J et al (2011) Structure-guided lead optimization of triazolopyrimidine-ring substituents identifies potent Plasmodium falciparum dihydroorotate dehydrogenase inhibitors with clinical candidate potential. J Med Chem 54(15):5540–5561. doi:10.1021/jm200592f
92. Spillman NJ, Allen RJ, McNamara CW et al (2013) Na(+) regulation in the malaria parasite Plasmodium falciparum involves the cation ATPase PfATP4 and is a target of the spiroindolone antimalarials. Cell Host Microbe 13(2):227–237. doi:10.1016/j.chom.2012.12.006
93. McNamara CW, Lee MC, Lim CS et al (2013) Targeting Plasmodium PI(4)K to eliminate malaria. Nature 504(7479):248–253. doi:10.1038/nature12782
94. Vennerstrom JL, Arbe-Barnes S, Brun R et al (2004) Identification of an antimalarial synthetic trioxolane drug development candidate. Nature 430(7002):900–904. doi:10.1038/nature02779

Chapter 18

Pharmacodynamics of Antiviral Agents

Renee-Claude Mercier, Bernadette Jakeman, and Larry Pineda

Abstract

The first antiviral drugs developed in the 1960s targeted herpes viruses. Discovery and research surrounding antiviral drugs lagged behind antibacterial agents due to the difficulties associated with isolating viruses and defining experimental treatment outcomes. Antiviral drug discovery was accelerated in the 1980s due to a better understanding of viral replication drug targeting sites and the advent of new technologies like viral genome sequencing. Most antiviral research has focused on the Human Immunodeficiency Virus (HIV) and most recently on the Hepatitis viruses, leaving very little new drug discovery against either the Herpesviridae family of viruses or influenza viruses. Unfortunately, herpesviruses have the ability to establish lifelong infections requiring patients to take multiple courses of the same antiviral agents during their lifetime. Chronic exposure has been linked to the development of viral resistance. Influenza viruses have the ability to spread easily from person to person and lead to severe disease in susceptible populations. Unfortunately, in vitro susceptibility has yet to be linked to clinical outcomes and pharmacodynamic studies have rarely been conducted with antiviral drugs. The chapter focuses on the pharmacodynamic parameters known with commonly used antiviral agents. Hopefully, by the end of the chapter it would become evident that there is much need to dedicate future research efforts towards clarifying how antiviral pharmacodynamics can help optimize dosing strategies. Especially, given the limited number of compounds currently available coupled with the development of resistance that is threatening to further eliminate treatment options for patients afflicted by such viral diseases.

Key words Antivirals, Herpesviridae family, Acyclovir, Valacyclovir, Famciclovir, IC_{50}, Thymidine kinase, Plaque reduction assay, Influenza, Zanamivir, Oseltamivir

1 Introduction

Herpesviridae viruses are DNA viruses that are able to establish latent infections. This family of viruses includes the herpes simplex viruses (HSV) type 1 and type 2, varicella-zoster virus (VZV), Epstein-Barr virus (EBV), and cytomegalovirus (CMV). Infections with herpesviruses are common and usually self-limiting, with the majority of adults infected with HSV-1, VZV, and EBV. Life-threatening conditions can occur, with increased risk in immunosuppressed patients. Antivirals used in the treatment of these infections typically inhibit viral DNA synthesis, but do not cure the

John C. Rotschafer et al. (eds.), *Antibiotic Pharmacodynamics*, Methods in Pharmacology and Toxicology,
DOI 10.1007/978-1-4939-3323-5_18, © Springer Science+Business Media New York 2016

viral infection. When the treatment is complete and the medication is stopped reactivation may occur in some patients.

HSV most commonly results in mucocutaneous infections. Transmission occurs through skin-to-skin contact or exposure to infected oral or genital secretions. HSV-1 is the most common strain of HSV and typically causes oral herpes. Seroprevalence of HSV-1 amongst persons aged 14–49 is 57.7 % [1]. HSV-2 is the most common cause of genital lesions [2, 3]. Seroprevalence of HSV-2 in persons aged 20–49 was 18.9 % [4]. HSV infections can also enhance the transmission of other sexually transmitted diseases [5].

VZV primary infection, referred to as chickenpox, typically results in a self-limiting vesicular rash. It is transmitted person to person via respiratory droplets or direct exposure to the rash. More than 90 % of cases occur in childhood [3]. Reactivation, referred to as herpes zoster or shingles, results in a painful dermatomal vesicular rash. Risk of reactivation increases with age and immunosuppression [3].

CMV is a common infection that is usually self-limited. The majority of healthy children and adults infected with CMV have no symptoms and are unaware that they have been infected. By the age of 40 approximately 50–80 % of US adults have been infected with CMV [6]. When symptoms are present they most commonly resemble flu-like illness and include fever, sore throat, fatigue, and swollen glands. CMV is of great concern in immunocompromised patients, notably transplant recipients, and patients with HIV and acquired-immunodeficiency syndrome (AIDS). CMV disease in immunocompromised patients most commonly presents as retinitis in AIDS patients, pneumonitis in bone marrow transplant patients and hepatitis in liver transplant patients. Other diseases associated with CMV include gastrointestinal invasion, encephalopathy, polyradiculopathy, and myelosuppression to name only those. The incidence of most CMV-related disease has been declining with more aggressive prophylaxis in high-risk populations and the use of potent antiretroviral agents in HIV patients [6, 7]. Congenital CMV is still of great concern today, and accounts for approximately 1 % of all live births in the USA (~40,000 infants/year). Congenital CMV is a frequent viral cause of mental retardation and hearing loss. Up to 90 % of infants with symptomatic CMV diseases at birth will develop neurologic deficits, including hearing loss in 30–65 % of the patients [8, 9].

Influenza, also commonly called the flu, is an acute, febrile, and highly contagious respiratory tract infection caused by influenza virus. The influenza virus is an encapsulated, single-stranded RNA orthomyxovirus that is transmitted from person to person via respiratory droplets. There are three distinct types of influenza; however, the two most clinically relevant types are influenza A and influenza B. The host range for influenza A includes a variety of species including humans, swine, equine, avian, and marine mammals. Type B however only infects humans [10, 11].

Awareness of the viral morphologic characteristics is essential for understanding influenza virus pathogenesis and pharmacologic agents. The influenza viral envelope contains several membrane proteins including two sialic acid-recognizing glycoproteins (hemagglutinin and neuraminidase), as well as a proton-selective matrix (M)-2 ion channel. All are key targets for antiviral agents. Hemagglutinin binds to sialic acid-containing receptors found on the surface of host respiratory tract cells [12]. Attachment leads to endocytosis by the host cell and subsequent viral uncoating. The M2 ion channel, via passage of hydrogen ions, is instrumental in acidifying the interior of the endosome [13]. This allows for release of the viral RNA into the cytoplasm. Intracellular viral replication follows with ultimate exocytosis of viral progeny bound to the host cell wall [11]. The final release of virions from infected host cells is mediated by the enzymatic action of neuraminidase upon sialic acid moieties [14]. Neuraminidase also facilitates viral spread throughout the upper respiratory tract by cleaving off sialic acid on respiratory mucin [15]. Viral replication in the respiratory tract reaches a peak between 24 and 72 h after the onset of illness [16].

Vaccination remains the primary means of preventing and controlling influenza virus infections [17], but its effectiveness is limited mainly due to seasonal antigenic changes [11, 13]. Therefore, augmentation with antiviral agents is necessary to achieve optimal management of influenza infections.

2 Acyclovir/Valacyclovir and Penciclovir/Famciclovir

Acyclovir and penciclovir are nucleoside analogues that inhibit viral DNA polymerase. Acyclovir was one of the first orally available drugs used in the treatment of HSV and is still one of the most commonly used antivirals today. However, due to limited oral bioavailability of acyclovir and penciclovir, their prodrugs (valacyclovir and famciclovir, respectively) were developed to provide alternative oral formulations. Valacyclovir and famciclovir are rapidly converted to their respective parent drugs after first-pass metabolism and block viral DNA synthesis through the same mechanism [18]. Today these compounds are mainly used for the treatment and suppression of HSV and VZV infections.

Clinical use of acyclovir and penciclovir is limited due to poor oral bioavailability (15–30 % and 5 %, respectively) [19–21]. Penciclovir is currently only available in a topical preparation. Acyclovir is available in topical, oral, and intravenous formulations. Topical formulations of penciclovir and acyclovir are used for herpes labialis and genital HSV. The oral formulations of acyclovir, valacyclovir, and famciclovir are used for the treatment and suppression of genital HSV and VZV infections. Oral acyclovir has been shown to decrease VZV-associated post-herpetic neuralgia

[22–24], and data show a protective benefit when these agents are used for VZV prophylaxis in high-risk patients [25, 26]. Oral therapies can also be used for treatment of mucocutaneous HSV in immunocompromised patients, who tend to have more severe infections. Acyclovir is the only compound that is available as an intravenous formulation. It is reserved for severe HSV or VZV infections, including encephalitis.

2.1 Pharmacodynamics

Acyclovir/valacyclovir and penciclovir/famciclovir have in vitro and in vivo inhibitory activity against HSV type 1 and type 2, and VZV. HSV and VSV encode a viral thymidine kinase (TK) required for viral DNA synthesis. Both acyclovir and penciclovir have a high affinity for the HSV- and VZV-encoded TK and low affinity for human TK, preferentially targeting infected cells. Early in vitro studies using human cell lines determined that drug activity varies between herpes viruses, with HSV-1 being the most susceptible virus to these agents [27]. These compounds have limited activity against EBV and CMV [19].

After cellular uptake, both compounds are converted to the monophosphate form by the viral-encoded TK. Acyclovir monophosphate and penciclovir monophosphate are then converted to the active triphosphate form by host cellular kinases. After activation the compounds bind viral DNA polymerase and are incorporated into the viral DNA chain. Acyclovir triphosphate does not contain the 3′-hydroxyl group required for DNA elongation, causing termination of the chain. Penciclovir triphosphate contains the 3′-hydroxyl group, making it a short-chain terminator. Host DNA polymerases do not effectively use the activated forms of these compounds as substrates. This specificity for viral enzymes explains the low toxicity associated with these drugs [19, 28–30].

Serum half-lives of acyclovir and penciclovir are short [31, 32]. However, in vitro studies comparing intracellular drug activity have found that penciclovir has a higher affinity for viral TK as compared to acyclovir, which results in higher intracellular concentrations of penciclovir triphosphate. An in vitro cell culture analysis using human MRC-5 cell lines determined that the intracellular half-life of activated penciclovir triphosphate is 10 h in HSV-1-infected cells, 20 h in HSV-2-infected cells and 7 h in VZV-infected cells; compared with the intracellular half-life of acyclovir triphosphate, which is ≤1 h [33]. Acyclovir triphosphate, however, has a higher affinity for viral DNA polymerase compared to penciclovir triphosphate. As a result, clinical efficacy appears to be similar with these compounds [20, 34–36].

Steady-state C_{max} concentrations following oral administration of acyclovir 200 mg, 400 mg, and 800 mg every 4 h were 0.8, 1.2, and 1.6 μg/mL, respectively. Corresponding steady-state C_{min} concentrations were 0.4, 0.6, and 0.8 μg/mL [37]. Higher concentrations are achieved with intravenous administration of acyclovir. Steady-state C_{max} concentrations for 2.5, 5.0, 10.0, and 15.0 mg/kg administered intravenously every 8 h were 6.7, 9.7, 20.0, and 20.6 μg/mL respectively. Corresponding mean steady-state C_{min} concentrations were 0.5, 0.7, 2.3, and 2.0 μg/mL [38–40]. High serum concentrations are achieved with oral valacyclovir. Administration of the lowest dose of valacyclovir 250 mg four times daily resulted in slightly higher concentrations, with less variability in AUC, than acyclovir 800 mg five times daily. Peak acyclovir concentrations seen after valacyclovir 2000 mg four times daily, are similar to what is attained with intravenous acyclovir 5 mg/kg administered every 8 h (~9 μg/mL), with an AUC similar to intravenous 10 mg/kg administered every 8 h [41]. Acyclovir concentrations are not routinely measured in practice. Because median IC_{50} concentrations are seen with VZV isolates, higher doses of acyclovir are used clinically for VZV infections (acyclovir 800 mg PO five times daily or 10 mg/kg/dose every 8 h).

Data to support a correlation between serum drug concentrations and antiviral effects is lacking [37]. The gold standard phenotypic method for evaluating the susceptibility of viral isolates to these antiviral drugs is the plaque reduction assay (PRA) [42, 43]. PRA results are determined by the IC_{50}, or concentration of drug at which viral replication is inhibited by 50 % in cell culture. In vitro cell culture analyses have shown acyclovir inhibitory concentrations for HSV-1, HSV-2, and VZV to range from 0.02 to 1.9 μg/mL, 0.3 to 2.9 μg/mL, and 0.8 to 5.2 μg/mL, respectively [3]. In vitro cell culture analyses have shown penciclovir inhibitory concentrations for HSV-1, HSV-2, and VZV to range from 0.02 to 1.8 μg/mL, 0.3 to 2.4 μg/mL, and 0.9 to 5.1 μg/mL, respectively [3]. Susceptibility results can vary greatly between different cell lines used for viral isolation in vitro, and assay sensitivities may vary between laboratories even when identical viruses are used in the same cell line [44].

Limited data is available to help establish a correlation between in vitro susceptibility and clinical outcomes. The correlation between clinical response to acyclovir and in vitro susceptibility results was evaluated using PRAs in Vero cells for 243 clinical isolates of HSV (80 % HSV-2) collected from 115 patients with orofacial, genital, and perirectal lesions. Effective concentration (EC_{50}) values ≥2 μg/mL were associated with poor clinical response (P<0.001). However, the positive predictive value of PRA results of <2 μg/mL was only 62 % [45]. In addition to lab variability, host immune status and heterogenous viral populations could have affected the ability to predict clinical response. Regardless, for acyclovir and penciclovir, a breakpoint of 2 μg/mL is typically used when interpreting PRAs [30, 44, 45]. For the vast majority of isolates, this is an acceptable breakpoint. However, to identify unusual isolates with borderline susceptibility, it has been suggested that an additional breakpoint be used internally, based on ten-times the IC_{50} of a sensitive control strain [46]. The PK-PD parameter most predictive of efficacy has not been determined.

2.2 Clinical Application

Findings from a number of clinical studies suggest that time above the IC_{50} is an important criterion for efficacy [47–51]. For episodic treatment of HSV, high-dose therapy does not appear to have additional benefit. A valacyclovir 500 mg twice-daily regimen was compared to a valacyclovir 1000 mg twice-daily regimen in the treatment of recurrent genital HSV episodes in 987 immunocompetent patients [47]. No difference was found between the two dosing regimens. Both dosing regimens were effective at reducing the duration of episode when compared to placebo. In another study by Saiag and colleagues [48], valacyclovir was self-administered as 1000 mg daily or 500 mg twice-daily by 922 immunocompetent patients during an episode of recurrent genital HSV. The two regimens were found to be equivalent at reducing episodic duration and pain. Correlations between clinical results and serum drug concentrations were not evaluated.

For prophylaxis, a large placebo-controlled trial [49] evaluated different dosing regimens in 1479 immunocompetent patients with genital HSV. A dose–response relationship was found when comparing once-daily valacyclovir regimens. Recurrence-free rates after 1 year of treatment with valacyclovir 250 mg, 500 mg, and 1000 mg daily were 22 %, 40 %, and 48 %, respectively; with acyclovir AUCs of 22.0 mg h/L, 45.8 mg h/L, and 80.4 mg h/L, respectively. However, a regimen of valacyclovir 250 mg given twice daily had a higher recurrence-free rate (50 %) compared with both valacyclovir 500 mg daily and 1000 mg daily, even though the acyclovir AUC was only 55.1 mg h/L for the valacyclovir 250 mg twice-daily regimen. Again, this suggests that longer exposure above inhibitory concentrations is important for efficacy, but more data is needed.

Because of acyclovir's limited oral bioavailability and short half-life, multiple daily dosing schedules are required. It has been suggested that short serum drug half-lives lead to sub-inhibitory serum concentrations for a significant portion of the dosing period, which may contribute to viral breakthrough [50]. Viral breakthrough occurs frequently and is often subclinical. Suppressive therapy reduces the risk of transmission, but does not eliminate it completely [51–53]. Breakthroughs can occur while patients are on standard- or high-dose regimens [51].

Acyclovir is mainly eliminated unchanged by the kidneys, by both glomerular filtration and tubular secretion [54]. AUC will be directly affected by changes in clearance. In patients with impaired renal function receiving valacyclovir and acyclovir dosage adjustments should be made [29, 37]. Because acyclovir is small and has low protein-binding capacity, it is removed during hemodialysis, dropping serum drug concentrations by 60 % [37].

As mentioned above, acyclovir's high specificity for infected cells makes it a fairly well-tolerated medication. Side effects described with intravenous formulations include phlebitis (14 %), skin rash (4.7 %), neurologic side effects (<1 %; headache, hallucinations, dizziness, confusion, somnolence, convulsions), and transient elevations in serum creatinine (4.7 %) or acute kidney injury (AKI) caused by crystallization of drug in the renal tubules [37, 41, 55, 56]. Risk of AKI appears to be greatest with high-dose IV formulations and lower with oral formulations. In a large retrospective cohort of 160,915, patients receiving oral acyclovir and valacyclovir (N=76,269) had a relative risk of AKI of 1.00 (95 % CI, 0.83–1.21) when compared with famciclovir, which has not been associated with AKI [57]. Because acyclovir is hydrophilic, weight-based dosing of IV acyclovir should be based on ideal body weight. There have been a number of case reports describing acyclovir-induced renal failure in obese patients when actual body weight was used [58, 59]. Because the mechanism is thought to be due to crystallization of the drug, it is recommended that IV formulations be slowly infused and given with adequate hydration.

2.3 Resistance

Acyclovir resistance is low in immunocompetent patients, with rates reported to be <1 % [60–63]. Risk factors for resistance include chronic antiviral prophylaxis or treatment and immunosuppression [64–66]. Resistance rates in immunosuppressed patients range from 4 to 7 % [60, 61, 67], with the highest frequency (7–14.3 %) seen in bone marrow transplant patient [60, 68].

Mechanisms of resistance seen in HSV-1, HSV-2, and VZV include TK gene mutations, resulting in enzyme deficiency or decreased drug affinity, and/or alterations in viral DNA polymerase, decreasing drug affinity [65, 69–71]. TK gene mutation that results in enzyme deficiency is the most common mechanism of resistance identified in both immunocompetent and immunocompromised patients [67, 69, 72]. It appears that TK deficient viruses may be less virulent causing less severe disease [73]. However, a number of cases reports have recently described encephalitis caused by acyclovir-resistant viruses [74–76]. Due to similar drug mechanisms of action, viral isolates resistant to acyclovir are also resistant to valacyclovir, famciclovir, and penciclovir. TK deficiency appears to be the main mechanism of resistance to penciclovir as well [30, 46]. Overall, the prevalence of penciclovir resistance was found to be similar to that of acyclovir in immunocompetent patients [46].

Drug susceptibility testing is generally not recommended, especially in immunocompetent patients. However, it may be considered in immunocompromised patients with severe or persistent infections. PRA resistance testing requires isolation of the virus in cell culture, delaying results for 7–14 days. The lag time may also delay initiation of appropriate treatment. Another disadvantage of phenotypic testing is a lack of standardization with varying results within and between laboratories [44]. Gene sequencing can also be used when timely results are required or when viral yield for culture is low, such as in CSF fluid. Gene sequencing reveals mutations in viral TK or viral DNA polymerase that confer resistance. A drawback to gene sequencing is that mutations of unknown significance are frequently detected [69, 77–80]. In such cases, phenotypical susceptibility testing is still required. Ganciclovir/valganciclovir, foscarnet, and cidofovir are potential alternative therapies in these cases (*see* Sect. 3).

3 Ganciclovir/Valganciclovir, Foscarnet, and Cidofovir

Ganciclovir is a deoxyguanosine analogue similar in structure to acyclovir however it contains an additional hydroxymethyl group on the acyclic side chain [81, 82]. Valganciclovir is the l-valyl ester prodrug of ganciclovir [83]. Ganciclovir has potent antiviral activity against Herpesviruses including CMV, HSV, and VZV. Its primary therapeutic role is in the treatment of CMV infections [81–83]. Foscarnet, a pyrophosphate analogue, has activity against Herpesviruses and HIV. Clinical uses most commonly include treatment of ganciclovir-resistant CMV and acyclovir-resistant HSV infections as most remain susceptible to foscarnet. Its utility as a clinical agent, however, is limited by its toxicity profile [84, 85]. Cidofovir is an acyclic phosphonate nucleotide analogue of deoxycytidine monophosphate with antiviral properties against human herpesviruses (HHV), including CMV, EBV, HHV-6, HHV-8, and other DNA viruses such as papillomaviruses, polyomaviruses, poxviruses and adenoviruses. Similar to foscarnet, cidofovir's side effect profile limits its use to ganciclovir-resistant CMV and acyclovir-resistant HSV infections [85–88]. Ganciclovir, foscarnet and cidofovir have been commonly use since their approval many decades ago yet little is known about their pharmacodynamic properties.

3.1 Pharmacodynamics

Antiviral agents with activity against cytomegalovirus have been approved at doses that would likely lead to concentrations above the IC_{50} while trying to minimize toxicity. Unfortunately, very little is known about how to optimize dosing in order to provide desired clinical outcomes, minimize toxicity and limit the development of resistance. Few studies have been conducted to determine the most appropriate pharmacodynamic parameters that predict positive outcomes with ganciclovir and valganciclovir. Conversely, the data is very limited with foscarnet and non-existent for cidofovir.

Ganciclovir inhibits viral DNA polymerase by competing with dGTP as a substrate. Ganciclovir first enters CMV infected cells where it is monophosphorylated by viral protein kinase (UL97 gene). Cellular kinases further phosphorylate ganciclovir into its active triphosphate form which then competitively competes with dGTP. The triphosphate form of ganciclovir achieves 10 to 100-fold higher intracellular concentrations in CMV infected cells than uninfected cells. Ganciclovir also has much higher affinity for viral DNA polymerase than host cell DNA polymerase. The average IC_{50} for CMV susceptible strains ranges from 0.1 to 2.0 mg/L. No correlation exists as of yet between in vitro sensitivity and clinical response for ganciclovir. Valganciclovir is a pro-drug of ganciclovir with enhanced bioavailability due to its active transport across the gastrointestinal wall via the intestinal peptide transporter PEPT1. Once across the membrane barrier, valganciclovir is hydrolyzed into ganciclovir and possesses the same pharmacodynamic properties as the parent drug ganciclovir [89, 90].

A recent in vitro study utilizing a pharmacodynamic model demonstrated that a new dosing strategy for ganciclovir against CMV would optimize the antiviral effect while minimizing toxicity [91]. This study supported the findings that ganciclovir exhibits concentration-dependent antiviral activity and toxicity. The study was carried out in vitro in lymphoblastoid cell cultures, with subsequent data analysis using a mathematical model to characterize ganciclovir pharmacodynamics. Briefly, high doses of ganciclovir for short exposure time maximized antiviral efficacy while limiting toxicity. Complete viral suppression was achieved at 20 mg/L. This concentration was associated with cellular toxicity, although, the toxicity was predicted to become significant only after long-term exposure of ≥7 days. The model predicted that an optimal dosing regimen for ganciclovir in patients with stem cell transplant with normal renal function would translate to 10 mg/kg every 12 h for 2 days, followed by doses 180, 192, 204, and 216 h after first dose for a total of eight doses.

3.2 Clinical Applications

Pharmacokinetic parameters differ among patients with solid organ transplant, HIV/AIDS or healthy volunteers. Primarily the time to achieve C_{max} was longer in transplant patients (3.0 ± 1 h) as compared to healthy volunteers or patients with HIV/AIDS (1.6 ± 0.6 h). The AUCs achieved with doses of valganciclovir of 450–900 mg were also 1.7–2.5 times higher in transplant patients compared to healthy volunteers and patients with HIV/AIDS. Consequently, the ganciclovir $t_{1/2}$ is longer in transplant patients than in healthy volunteers and HIV/AIDS persons (4.7 ± 1.4 h vs. 3.7 ± 1.1 h, respectively). The differences are most likely due to an increase in ganciclovir clearance of 13.6 ± 4.2 L/h in healthy volunteers and HIV/AIDS patients compared to 8.0 ± 2.9 L/h in transplant patients. The terminal Vd was 50 ± 16 L in transplant patients and 71 ± 37 L in the healthy volunteer and HIV/AIDS cohort. Therefore, transplant patients who require ganciclovir or valganciclovir may benefit from a reduced dose in order to achieve optimal concentrations as compared to patients with HIV/AIDS. In addition, valganciclovir bioavailability is on average 66 ± 10 %. Food intake may increase the AUC by 24–30 % which could account for the pharmacokinetic alterations [92].

It is important to understand the characteristics that influence the pharmacokinetic properties of ganciclovir and valganciclovir in different patient populations such as HIV/AIDS patients. For example, a study demonstrated that HIV patients with CMV retinitis had a 40 % increase in ganciclovir clearance compared to patients who were only shedding virus in the urine. It is unclear whether the difference could be attributed to the inflammatory state of the patients or perhaps interactions with concomitantly administered medications [93, 94].

Ganciclovir is primarily eliminated via glomerular and tubular secretion, making the presence of renal impairment a significant pharmacokinetic determinant. Approximately 85 % [73–99 %] of ganciclovir is recovered unchanged in the urine. With decreased renal function a parallel increase in AUC and $t_{1/2}$ is expected. Weight may also influence ganciclovir's pharmacokinetics as obese patients have been shown to have an increased absolute clearance and larger Vd than thinner patients. Heavier patients may require higher dosage or conversely smaller patients may need reduced dose of ganciclovir to achieve appropriate therapeutic concentrations. While this may be important to prevent toxicity in patients with lower BMIs, most of the studies evaluating dosing in obese patients did not account for other confounding factors such as sex, age or race. This makes clear dosing recommendations based on weight impossible at this time [94–97].

3.2.1 Prophylactic Use

The use of ganciclovir in the prevention and treatment of CMV in solid organ transplant recipients was investigated in two prospective clinical trials [98, 99]. Steady-state peak and trough concentrations were measured and correlated with treatment outcomes. Among both the patients receiving prophylaxis ($n = 43$) and the treatment ($n = 25$) groups, no correlation was found between ganciclovir serum concentrations, total dose or duration and CMV disease or relapse. Interestingly, two liver transplant recipients D+R– (donor positive, recipient negative) developed CMV disease and both had ganciclovir trough concentrations less than 0.31 mg/L [98].

Later in 2005, Wiltshire and colleagues published the results of their study investigating the pharmacodynamics of oral ganciclovir and valganciclovir in solid organ transplant recipients. The authors aimed to establish the relationship between ganciclovir concentrations and prevention of CMV viremia, CMV disease, and the incidence of hematologic toxicity. The mean daily AUC was 46.3 ± 15.2 μg•h/mL with valganciclovir compared to 28.0 ± 10.9 μg•h/mL with oral ganciclovir, an average 1.65-fold greater increase with valganciclovir (95 % CI 1.58–1.81) than oral ganciclovir. The difference in ganciclovir exposure between the two groups resulted in a significant lower incidence of viremia during the prophylactic period (2.9 % valganciclovir vs. 19.4 % oral ganciclovir; $P = 0.001$). Ganciclovir exposure resulting in an AUC

>45 μg•h/mL was associated with low incidence of viremia (3 %). This was characteristically achievable with valganciclovir although less than 10 % of patients on oral ganciclovir achieved such an AUC. After 100 days of prophylactic treatment, a logistic regression demonstrated that an AUC of 50 μg•h/mL predicted an average incidence of viremia of 1.3 %. An AUC of 25 μg•h/mL had an eightfold higher risk of viremia. The ganciclovir exposure did not predict the incidence of viremia in the post-prophylactic period at 4 and 12 months post-transplant. Additionally, most of the CMV disease reported in this study occurred between 3 and 6 months post-transplant [99].

A ganciclovir AUC greater than 50 mg•h/L appears to prevent CMV viremia while trough concentrations below 0.31 mg/L are insufficient to prevent CMV disease in high risk liver transplant patients. However, further RCT are needed to confirm these findings [98, 99].

Foscarnet pharmacodynamics relationships were explored in a prospective study of asymptomatic patients with CMV viremia over a 10-day period. Subjects were randomized to receive one of four foscarnet dosing schemes: 15 mg/kg q8h, 30 mg/kg q8h, 45 mg/kg q12h, or 90 mg/kg q12h. A significant relationship was demonstrated between both foscarnet peak concentrations and AUC with a decrease in the level of CMV antigenemia. Reduced CMV viremia was also correlated with foscarnet exposure. A foscarnet dose of 45 mg/kg q12h corresponded to a 50 % decrease in CMV antigenemia. Toxicity was limited due to short courses of foscarnet, and CMV susceptibility to foscarnet was not altered after the 10-day course. This study was instrumental in promoting the use of higher doses of foscarnet during induction therapy for CMV disease [100].

3.2.2 Induction Therapy

Pharmacokinetic studies of ganciclovir conducted in newborns [101, 102] have shown that newborns have an increased clearance of ganciclovir in the first 6 weeks of life, with a parallel decrease in AUC. Contrarily, oral valganciclovir's AUC was only marginally decreased probably due to an increase in bioavailability by 32 % over the same period [101, 102]. Twenty-four newborns of whom 18 had positive CMV viral load upon enrollment were studied by Kimberlin and colleagues. The authors targeted a ganciclovir AUC_{0-12} of 27 mg•h/L in this population. The ganciclovir pharmacokinetic parameters (C_{max}, T_{last}, C_{last}, AUC_{12}, and clearance) over the course of the 56 days of blood sampling were not correlated with changes in the viral load. Ultimately the study showed that valganciclovir doses of 16 mg/kg provided ganciclovir concentration similar to IV ganciclovir 6 mg/kg in newborns [101].

Trough values have also been investigated as a potential marker of efficacy with ganciclovir. Twelve of 15 HIV patients with CMV retinitis treated with IV ganciclovir had trough concentrations below 0.6 mg/L. Of these six experienced treatment failure. Once the dose was increased to achieve trough concentrations above 0.6 mg/L, four of the patients who had previously failed responded to therapy [103]. In a cohort of 11 pediatric renal transplant patients receiving preemptive ganciclovir treatment, the mean trough concentration of 1.3 ± 0.8 mg/L was linked to good virologic response. Only one patient out of 11 developed CMV disease and the patient was mistakenly administered too low of a dose (trough of 0.35 mg/L). The patient failed ganciclovir and the CMV strain when tested was ganciclovir-resistant [104]. Hence, with the limited data available supporting the use of ganciclovir trough concentrations to guide therapy, one can only conclude that concentrations below 0.6 mg/L are insufficient to treat CMV retinitis and concentrations above 1.3 mg/L appear to prevent CMV disease in pediatric renal transplant patients [103, 104].

Foscarnet pharmacodynamic parameters were also studied in a subset of HIV patients with CMV retinitis. The study demonstrated that foscarnet exposure was correlated with increased time to disease progression. AUC and C_{max} were both associated with delayed time to progression. Most important was the finding that patients with baseline positive CMV blood culture were more likely to benefit from higher dosage as they were more likely to have rapid disease progression. Foscarnet nephrotoxicity has also been associated with increased drug exposure, which limits clinicians' ability to significantly adjust the dose upwardly [105].

3.2.3 Maintenance Therapy

AIDS patients with a history of CMV disease will continue on ganciclovir (usually administered as valganciclovir) maintenance therapy until a significant rebound is seen with CD4 cell count to prevent disease relapse. Fourteen patients with AIDS on maintenance therapy for CMV retinitis had ganciclovir trough concentrations measured and correlated with disease progression. Lower trough concentrations <0.6 mg/L appeared associated with an increased risk of disease progression although the findings were not significant [106]. Moreover, in a study looking at ganciclovir dose intensification to prevent CMV relapse, average ganciclovir AUC_{0-24} was highly predictive of time to CMV retinitis progression. C_{max} was also found to be a predictor of time to progression, however, in the multivariate model, only AUC_{0-24} maintained a significant predictive value. C_{min} had no correlation with treatment outcome [107]. This data strengthens the evidence for ganciclovir total exposure over time as the best predictor of treatment outcomes.

A small study of nine patients receiving foscarnet as maintenance therapy for CMV retinitis demonstrated an association between increased foscarnet AUC and a decreased risk of disease progression, although this was not statistically significant [108].

3.2.4 Toxicity

Ganciclovir has been used for prophylaxis, and preemptive treatment of CMV disease. Its use has often been limited by its adverse effects including hematologic, neurologic, and possibly hepatic toxicity [89, 96]. A dose-dependent hematologic toxicity profile has been demonstrated in vitro. Ganciclovir IC_{50} ranged from 0.7 to 4.8 mg/L in granulocyte-macrophage progenitors and 0.4 to 7.4 mg/L for erythroid progenitors [109]. Despite these in vitro findings, no clear correlation between ganciclovir serum concentrations and bone marrow suppression has been reported in clinical trials. In one study done in bone marrow transplant recipients, 3 of 5 patients who received IV ganciclovir developed bone marrow suppression with mean peak and trough plasma concentrations exceeding 12.8 mg/L and 2.6 mg/L, respectively [110]. In contrast, neutropenia was reported with ganciclovir peak and trough concentrations of 3.9 mg/L and 0.7 mg/L in one bone marrow transplant recipient. However when all 11 patients' ganciclovir concentrations were taken into consideration, the authors found no correlation between ganciclovir concentrations and bone marrow suppression [111].Other studies suggest similar lack of correlation between ganciclovir concentrations and bone marrow suppression [98, 112, 113]. In solid organ transplant patients, an increased ganciclovir AUC did not correlate with increased anemia and was only weakly associated with increased neutropenia and leucopenia [99]. Because of the inconsistencies among studies investigating the relationship between hematologic toxicity and ganciclovir serum concentrations, a toxic range cannot be established. Close monitoring however is warranted as these adverse events are commonly reported and treatment limiting.

Reports of ganciclovir associated neurotoxicity and hepatotoxicity have been published [114–117]. Although neurotoxicity appears to be related to high ganciclovir plasma and CSF concentrations, the limited amount of data precludes an accurate description of toxic range [114–116].

3.3 Resistance

Ganciclovir resistance in CMV is defined as an IC_{50} >1.5–3 mg/L in vitro. Resistance has been attributed to two different mechanisms: (1) alteration via point mutation or deletions in the phosphotransferase encoded by the UL97 gene preventing phosphorylation of ganciclovir into ganciclovir monophosphate; and (2) alteration in the DNA polymerase UL54 gene. Alterations in the UL97 gene will confer resistance to ganciclovir alone while mutation in the UL54 gene will confer resistance to cidofovir as well as ganciclovir. Valganciclovir achieves higher serum concentrations and therefore would be expected to lead to a reduced rate of resistance when compared to oral ganciclovir. CMV strains resistant to both ganciclovir and cidofovir usually remain sensitive to foscarnet, although cross-resistance to all three agents has been seen. Foscarnet resistance is attributed to mutations in the DNA polymerase and is define as IC_{50} >400 μmol/L in plaque reduction or >600 μmol/L in DNA hybridization assays. Resistance is rarely seen in naïve patients and tends to develop over the course of long term therapy. For example, 7 % of patients with CMV retinitis developed ganciclovir resistance by 3 months (28 % by 9 months), 37 % by 12 months with foscarnet, and 29 % by 3 months with cidofovir [89, 90, 118].

In a study of solid organ transplant recipients who received 100 days of valganciclovir or oral ganciclovir, the incidence of CMV UL97 mutation leading to ganciclovir resistance was 0 % in the valganciclovir group compared to 1.9 % in the oral ganciclovir group at the end of prophylaxis. The incidence of the UL97 mutation 1 year after transplantation remained at 0 % for valganciclovir but was 6 % for oral ganciclovir [99].

4 Influenza Antiviral Agents

Currently, there are four antiviral agents approved in the USA for the treatment and prevention of influenza: the adamantanes or M-2 inhibitors amantadine (Symmetrel) and rimantadine (Flumadine), and the neuraminidase inhibitors zanamivir (Relenza) and oseltamivir (Tamiflu) [10]. Other neuraminidase inhibitors like peramivir and laninamivir are not approved for use in the USA at this time. The utility of the adamantanes is limited mainly due to the development of resistance among influenza A strains. The CDC/ACIP and WHO no longer recommend the use of adamantanes for treatment and chemoprophylaxis of influenza virus. Therefore, this pharmacodynamic overview will focus primarily on the neuraminidase inhibitors.

4.1 Pharmacodynamics

4.1.1 Adamantanes (M-2 Inhibitors)

The adamantanes are tricyclic amines which hamper influenza A replication by inhibiting the action of M2 ion channel proteins. This hinders the pH changes necessary for viral uncoating and subsequent ribonucleoprotein transport to the nucleus [90]. Adamantanes do not exhibit antiviral activity against influenza B isolates.

Amantadine is well-absorbed orally and is available in tablet, capsule, and syrup preparations. Likewise, rimantadine is available as a tablet for oral administration. To date, no data is available to support a correlation between serum drug concentrations and antiviral effects. In vitro cell culture analyses have shown inhibitory levels for influenza A virus to range from 0.1 to 25.0 μg/mL for amantadine [90, 119] and from 0.1 to 0.4 μg/mL for rimantadine [90]. However, both agents are marketed with notations that quantitative relationships between susceptibility in cell culture and clinical response to therapy have not been established [119, 120]. Given the limited clinical utility of the adamantanes for treatment and chemoprophylaxis of influenza, it is unlikely that such data will be further pursued.

4.1.2 Neuraminidase Inhibitors

Neuraminidase inhibitors are structural analogues of sialic acid. As a class, they competitively inhibit the activity of influenza neuraminidases. Without cleavage of sialic acid residues, new virions remain bound to the infected host cell wall and viral spread is inhibited [121]. The neuraminidase inhibitors have antiviral activity against both influenza A and B.

Oseltamivir and zanamivir are the primary pharmaceutical options in this class of antivirals. Oseltamivir is available for oral administration as the ethyl ester prodrug oseltamivir phosphate. It is rapidly and extensively converted to the active form, oseltamivir carboxylate, via hepatic esterase hydrolysis [122]. Oseltamivir carboxylate in the bloodstream then distributes to both the upper and lower respiratory tract [123]. Due to poor oral bioavailability and rapid renal elimination, zanamivir is marketed as a dry powder for oral inhalation [124]. In healthy volunteers, 10 mg of zanamivir via inhalation achieved 13.2 % whole lung deposition with 77.6 % oropharynx deposition [125]. Laninamivir octanoate is a novel long-acting neuraminidase inhibitor which only requires one intranasal administration. Within 24 h, the prodrug is converted in the lungs to the active metabolite laninamivir [126]. An unmet medical need for a parenteral formulation has prompted ongoing investigations into oseltamivir and zanamivir [127] intravenous pharmacokinetics and efficacy. In addition, peramivir, an investigational intravenous neuraminidase inhibitor, was made available for emergency use authorization during the 2009 H1N1 influenza pandemic [10].

The susceptibility of various influenza A and B strains to neuraminidase inhibitors has been investigated in several in vitro analyses [121, 123, 128]. Neuraminidase enzymatic assays utilize fluorescence or chemiluminescence to quantify the activity of viral neuraminidase on a detectable substrate. Varying concentrations of the study compound are compared to a control in order to derive an inhibitory concentration. In comparison, cell culture assays measure inhibition of viral plaque formation, a cytopathic effect or viral proteins to determine antiviral activity [129]. In vivo susceptibilities have been shown to better correlate with enzymatic assays, and more variability is generally observed with culture assays [128, 130–132]. In fact, both zanamivir and oseltamivir are marketed with the notation that a relationship between cell culture inhibition and inhibition of replication in humans has not been established [124, 133]. The observed oseltamivir carboxylate concentration which reduces activity by 50 % (IC_{50}) range from 0.17 to 44 μg/L in cell culture, with a narrower range of 0.08 to 0.57 μg/L in neuraminidase enzymatic assays [121]. These values are similar to those of zanamivir against most strains, but oseltamivir carboxylate displayed more potent activity against influenza A (H3N2) in both enzymatic and culture assays [128]. These agents are highly specific for influenza virus neuraminidase with little to no activity against neuraminidases from other viruses, bacteria or human liver microsomes observed in vitro [128].

The efficacy of neuraminidase inhibitors has been tested in in vivo animal studies which confirmed observations noted in the in vitro studies [128, 134]. Both ferret and mouse models have been used to demonstrate the efficacy against influenza [129]. Oral administration of oseltamivir has produced sustained plasma concentrations in mice and ferrets. Mendel et al. evaluated the efficacy of oseltamivir in influenza infected mice. Efficacy was based on survival at 21 days post-infection as compared to untreated controls. Oseltamivir administered for 5 days increased survival rates for mice infected with influenza A (H1N1, H3N2) and influenza B isolates. In addition, a decrease in virus titers was detected in the lungs of mice infected with influenza A H1N1 as compared to controls [128].

The PK-PD parameters most predictive of efficacy and resistance have yet to be determined. Experimental infections trials were unable to demonstrate a dose–response effect in humans, most likely due to small sample sizes and variability in virus sensitivity [123]. In field trials, both the 75 mg and the 150 mg twice daily dosages elicited similar clinical efficacy for treatment of common influenza [123]. It is assumed that adequate oseltamivir carboxylate exposure is achieved with 75 mg twice daily dosing, but the pharmacodynamics of oseltamivir carboxylate are not completely defined in in vivo studies. The PD variable linked to efficacy of neuraminidase inhibitors against influenza was investigated in in vitro hollow-fiber infection models [135–137]. The 24-h area under the concentration–time curve ($AUC_{0\text{–}24}$) to IC_{50} or IC_{90} was identified as the PD index associated with oseltamivir carboxylate efficacy [135]. Likewise, in a murine model of influenza infection, AUC was found to be the linked PD variable for peramivir [138]. Interestingly, the index predictive of intravenous zanamivir efficacy was not AUC, but time above the 50 % effective concentration (EC_{50}) [137]. It was hypothesized that this finding was due to the short half-life of zanamivir (2.5 h). Therefore, a dose fractionation study was performed including a simulated half-life similar to oseltamivir (8 h). In contrast to the 2.5 h half-life, viral inhibition was similar for all dosage regimens simulated with the 8 h half-life suggesting that $AUC_{0\text{–}24}$:EC_{50} was the best PK-PD linked predictor at this half-life [137]. These results provide great insight into pharmacodynamic indexes, but clinical confirmation is still needed.

Currently available clinical trials contain sufficient efficacy data but lack concurrent plasma PK data. This is a major barrier in determining exposure–response relationships. Recently, a study group developed a population PK model from pooled clinical trial data in order to help determine the time course of oseltamivir carboxylate in adult and pediatric subjects [139]. With this model, patient demographics can be used to estimate the missing plasma concentration PK data in clinical trials. The study group used clinical data from two phase two inoculation studies and applied the predicted oseltamivir carboxylate exposure data to explore the exposure–response relationships for oseltamivir carboxylate efficacy [140]. Their findings suggested that a relationship between oseltamivir carboxylate AUC_{0-24} and efficacy did indeed exist. The researchers were, however, unable to determine if AUC alone was the exposure most associated with efficacy (C_{min} or C_{max} could not be excluded). They also observed that a higher AUC_{0-24} (>14,000 ng•h/mL) than that achieved by approved oseltamivir dosing (~6000 ng•h/mL) was associated with greater efficacy. Further studies are, however, still needed to determine the clinical applicability of such findings.

4.2 Clinical Application

The adamantanes are only active against influenza A and are associated with several toxic side effects. With the potential for rapid emergence of drug resistance, the value of this class for the treatment of influenza is limited. Their role in therapy against influenza is therefore limited for use in combination therapy or prophylaxis in certain instances when a neuraminidase inhibitor cannot be used. Amantadine is also licensed for use in the treatment of Parkinson's disease [119]. Conversely, the low rate of resistance and tolerability of the neuraminidase inhibitors makes them ideal first line agents. The effectiveness of oseltamivir for prophylaxis and treatment of influenza has been shown in several clinical studies. Randomized, control trials in outpatient settings conducted primarily among subjects with mild infection demonstrate that both zanamivir and oseltamivir can reduce the duration of influenza A and B by approximately 1 day when administered within 48 h of illness onset when compared against placebo [141]. Minimal to no benefit was observed when treatment was initiated after this treatment window [10, 121, 122]. It is worth noting that recent observational studies in hospitalized patients have indicated a benefit of antiviral treatment even if treatment is initiated more than 48 h and up to 96 h after onset of illness [142–144].

Zanamivir is FDA approved for treatment and prophylaxis of adults with influenza A or B, but not for children under the age of 5 [124]. The recommended dosage for treatment is 10 mg (two inhalations) twice daily. The chemoprophylaxis dosing is 10 mg once daily. For both oseltamivir and zanamivir, treatment duration is 5 days and chemoprophylaxis duration is 10 days. Some studies have shown persistent viral shedding in critically ill and immunocompromised patients. In such cases, extending treatment duration is warranted. Oseltamivir is FDA approved for treatment and chemoprophylaxis of influenza in adults and children ≥1 year of age [133]. In 2012, the FDA expanded oseltamivir's use to include treatment in children as young as 2 weeks old. The labeled dosing for oseltamivir in adults is 75 mg by mouth twice daily. However, some experts suggest that this may not be the most optimal dosing strategy in all populations. Studies of the 2009 H1N1 influenza pandemic observed that obese and critically ill patients had worse clinical outcomes. This led to the proposal that an increased dose of oseltamivir (150 mg twice daily) should be considered in patients who are morbidly obese or critically ill [145–147]. While the safety of oseltamivir 150 mg twice daily dosing has been established [148], there is no data available to evaluate if higher oseltamivir doses are superior in reducing the severity or duration of influenza. Pharmacokinetic studies have concluded that oseltamivir carboxylate exposure (AUC) from 75 mg dosing is largely unchanged in obesity when compared to nonobese patients [149, 150]. Some experts suggest that there may be some benefit to using higher doses in certain populations (H5N1 infection, critically ill, immunocompromised). A recent review article of patients infected with avian influenza strain (H5N1) suggest that higher doses, along with an increased duration of 10 days, may be beneficial due to the high levels of replication and the observation of progressive disease despite adequate treatment with standard dosing [151]. The absorption and distribution of oseltamivir carboxylate is still quite uncertain in critically ill patients. Additionally, prolonged shedding of influenza virus has been described in immunocompromised patients [10, 152, 153]. Considering the overall safety profile of oseltamivir, the acuity of illness in such patients, the lack of PD clinical data to guide optimal dosing and the uncertainty of systemic exposure; it is reasonable to use higher doses of oseltamivir in these patient populations.

Since zanamivir is almost completely eliminated renally, persons with renal impairment have higher serum AUCs [125]. It is likely that patients with renal disease would have a PK/PD index of AUC:EC and healthy individuals would have index of time above EC [137]. Oseltamivir phosphate (the oral pro-drug that is in the capsule) is metabolized to oseltamivir carboxylate that has a volume of distribution roughly equivalent to total body water. The active carboxylate metabolite has low protein binding and is excreted unchanged by glomerular filtration and tubular secretion so serum concentration might be predicted to decrease moderately. Therefore, it is recommended to adjust the dose of oseltamivir in patients with creatinine clearance less than 30 mL/min.

In early clinical trials investigating oseltamivir, approximately 10–20 % of patients were reported to experience self-limiting adverse effects. The most often reported toxicity of oseltamivir was gastrointestinal disturbance [121]. These include nausea, vomiting and abdominal pain. Initially, no differences in rate of side effects were noted when increasing doses up to 1000 mg were administered [123]. However, a recent surveillance study showed that adverse events could be correlated with increasing plasma concentrations (AUC) [154]. The intensity of the effects are typically mild to moderate, and are minimized when administered with food. Some neuropsychiatric side effects have been reported, however, postmarketing surveillance has since concluded that no important safety concerns need be mentioned for oseltamivir [155].

4.3 Resistance

Influenza A resistance to adamantanes has steadily increased worldwide since 2003. Resistance develops when single amino acid mutations occur at residues 27, 30 or 31 [130]. Adamantine resistant isolates increased from 0.4 %, during the 1994–1995 season, to 12.3 % during 2003–2004 season [156]. Ninety-two percent of influenza A (H3N2) viruses during the 2005–2006 season possessed a change in the M2 gene at position 31 which confers resistance [157]. Currently, all H3N2 and 2009 H1N1 viruses demonstrate resistance to adamantanes [141]. Resistance develops rapidly against adamantanes, and resistant isolates maintain virulence and transmissibility [130, 158, 159]. For this reason, adamantanes are not recommended for treatment or chemoprophylaxis of influenza A virus [10, 160].

Development of resistance to the neuraminidase inhibitors is not as common [161], and transmission of resistance mutations is rare [162, 163]. However, neuraminidase inhibitor resistance has been reported to occur during treatment/prophylaxis and in the absence of drug pressure [15]. Oseltamivir has become the most widely used neuraminidase inhibitor, making it vital to monitor resistance through ongoing surveillance. From 1999 to 2004, the incidence of oseltamivir resistance was reported as 0.33 % in adults and 4.0 % in children [164, 165]. Other studies have reported rates as high as 18 % in certain populations including children and immunocompromised patients [166, 167]. The most infamous account of oseltamivir resistance to date is the seasonal A (H1N1) with H274Y (H275Y in N1 numbering) neuraminidase mutation during the 2007–2008 and 2008–2009 influenza seasons where the majority of these strains were noted to be resistant [15]. Since then, the level of the resistant 2009 H1N1 pandemic strain has remained low in the USA (~1 %) [168]. Furthermore, greater than 99 % of all influenza strains circulating since 2009 have been oseltamivir susceptible [10].

Mutations in influenza neuraminidase enzyme elicit resistance to neuraminidase inhibitors by either direct or indirect alteration of the catalytic site. This conformational change reduces the binding affinity of neuraminidase inhibitors [169]. Neuraminidase mutations generally lead to a less functional enzyme and therefore less fit virus [169]. In vitro studies have also described hemagglutinin receptor mutations which can lead to resistance, but the clinical relevance is unknown [170]. The H274Y is the predominant neuraminidase mutation which confers resistance to oseltamivir [171]. Using a fluorimetry-based neuraminidase inhibition assay, Pizzorno et al. determined that the H247Y mutation increases the oseltamivir IC_{50} by almost 1000-fold. The mutations R292K and N294S have also been associated with reduced oseltamivir sensitivity while S246N, I117V, and I222R in the 2009 H1N1 pandemic strain have been shown to have a synergistic resistance effect with H274Y [15]. The I222R substitution may even aid with the restoration of fitness in H274Y mutants [172].

Structurally, zanamivir does not contain a bulky side chain like oseltamivir so binding with the active site occurs in a different manner [169]. Therefore, neuraminidase mutations which cause resistance to oseltamivir do not confer resistance to zanamivir. Incidentally, all influenza A and B types remain susceptible to zanamivir [173], but infrequent utilization may also factor into this observation. Even so, zanamivir resistant influenza strains with Q136K, I222R/K, E119G/V, and D198G substitutions have been described in the literature so surveillance will continue to be important as the antiviral use increases [15]. Peramivir is structurally similar to both oseltamivir and zanamivir, and hence mutations which affect their activity can also affect peramivir activity [15]. For example, Pizzorno et al. found H274Y to increase peramivir IC_{50} by 661-fold as compared to wild-type virus. Of note, no laninamivir resistant mutations have been reported to date [172].

Due to the ease of administration, oseltamivir remains the most utilized neuraminidase inhibitor today. Oseltamivir resistance is however a growing concern. The 2009 H1N1 pandemic highlighted the need for alternative therapies in these instances. Laninamivir as a single, long-acting inhalation has been shown to be as effective as oseltamivir for the treatment of influenza in adult patients (including oseltamivir-resistant influenza virus) [174], but it is not available for use in the USA. Zanamivir remains the most viable option for treatment of oseltamivir-resistant influenza. In cases where administration via inhalation is not feasible, parenteral administration is essential. Intravenous formulations of oseltamivir, peramivir, and zanamivir have been developed, but only zanamivir is currently available on a compassionate use basis for suspected/confirmed oseltamivir-resistant influenza.

5 Conclusions

Until recently, most of the research related to viral resistance in relationship to drug exposure has been done with HIV and antiretroviral drugs. With the increased incidence of HSV and CMV resistant infections and a lack of treatment options more emphasis should be placed on optimizing the pharmacodynamics of antiviral drugs, such as acyclovir and ganciclovir/valganciclovir. A better understanding of the relationship between drug exposure and therapeutic outcomes including efficacy and toxicity for all antiviral drugs would favor complete viral suppression which in return should lead to a decrease in resistance and minimize toxicity.

Similarly with influenza, new strategies will need to be developed to help combat the growing threat of NAI-resistant influenza. One such strategy currently being investigated is using the combination of amantadine, oseltamivir, and ribavirin [175]. Zanamivir intravenously is likely to be approved in the future and an enhanced understanding of dose–response relationship in critically ill patients would be essential prior to marketing.

References

1. Xu F, Sternberg MR, Kottiri BJ et al (2006) Trends in herpes simplex virus type 1 and type 2 seroprevalence in the United States. JAMA 296:964–973
2. Reeves WC, Corey L, Adams HG et al (1981) Risk of recurrence after first episodes of genital herpes. Relation to HSV type and antibody response. N Engl J Med 305:315–319
3. Mandell GL, Bennett JE, Dolin R (eds) (2010) Principles and practice of infectious diseases, 7th edn. Elsevier, Philadelphia, PA
4. Centers for Disease Control and Prevention (2010) Seroprevalence of herpes simplex virus type 2 among persons aged 14–19 years – United states 2005–2008. MMWR Morb Mortal Wkly Rep 59:456–459
5. Hook EW, Cannon RO, Nahmias AJ et al (1992) Herpes simplex virus infection as a risk factor for human immunodeficiency virus infection in heterosexuals. J Infect Dis 165:251–255
6. Crumpacker CS, Zhang JL (2010) Cytomegaloviruses. In: Mandell GL, Bennett JC, Dolin R (eds) Mandell, Douglas, and Bennett's: principles and practice of infectious disease, vol 2, 7th edn. Elsevier, Philadelphia, PA, pp 1971–1988
7. Emery VC (2001) Investigation of CMV disease in immunocompromised patients. J Clin Pathol 54:84–88
8. Kenneson A, Cannon MJ (2007) Review and meta-analysis of the epidemiology of congenital cytomegalovirus (CMV) infection. Rev Med Virol 17:253–276
9. Demmler GJ (1991) Infectious Diseases Society of America and Centers for Disease Control. Summary of a workshop on surveillance for congenital cytomegalovirus disease. Rev Infect Dis 13:315–329
10. Centers for Disease Control and Prevention (2011) Antiviral agents for the treatment and chemoprophylaxis of influenza. MMWR Morb Mortal Wkly Rep 60(1):1–25
11. Treanor JJ (2010) Influenza viruses, including avian influenza and swine influenza. In: Mandell GL, Bennett JE, Dolin R (eds) Principles and practice of infectious diseases, 7th edn. Elsevier Inc, Philadelphia, PA, pp 2265–2288
12. Luo M (2012) Influenza virus entry. In: Rossmann MG, Rao VB (eds) Advances in experimental medicine and biology, vol 726. Springer, Berlin
13. Astrahan P, Arkin IT (2010) Resistance characteristics of influenza to amino-adamantyls. Biochim Biophys Acta 1808:547–553
14. Gamblin SJ, Skehel JJ (2010) Influenza hemagglutinin and neuraminidase membrane glycoproteins. J Biol Chem 285(37):28403–28409. doi:10.1074/jbc.R110.129809
15. Samson M, Pizzorno A, Abed Y et al (2013) Influenza virus resistance to neuraminidase inhibitors. Antiviral Res 98:174–185
16. Moscona A (2005) Neuraminidase inhibitors for influenza. N Engl J Med 353(13):1363–1373
17. Centers for Disease Control and Prevention. Summary* recommendations: Prevention and control of influenza with vaccines: recommendations of the Advisory Committee on Immunization Practices (ACIP) (2013–14)
18. Soul-Lawton J, Seaber E, On N et al (1995) Absolute bioavailability and metabolic disposition of valacyclovir, the L-valyl ester of acyclovir, following oral administration to humans. Antimicrob Agents Chemother 39:2759–2764
19. Fletcher C, Bean B (1985) Evaluation of oral acyclovir therapy. Drug Intell Clin Pharm 19:518–524
20. Beutner KR (1995) Valacyclovir: a review of its antiviral activity, pharmacokinetic properties, and clinical efficacy. Antiviral Res 28:281–290
21. de Miranda P, Blum MR (1983) Pharmakokinetics of acyclovir after intravenous and oral administration. J Antimicrob Chemother 12(Suppl B):29–37
22. Rasi A, Behzadi AH, Rabet M et al (2010) The efficacy of time-based short-course acyclovir therapy in treatment of post-herpetic pain. J Infect Dev Ctries 4:754–760

23. Huff JC, Drucker JL, Clemmer A et al (1993) Effect of oral acyclovir on pain resolution in herpes zoster: a re-analysis. J Med Virol Suppl 1:93–96
24. Jackson JL, Gibbons R, Meyer G et al (1997) The effect of treating herpes zoster with oral acyclovir in preventing post-herpetic neuralgia: a meta-analysis. Arch Intern Med 157:909–912
25. Kim DH, Kumar D, Messner HA et al (2008) Clinical efficacy of prophylactic strategy for long-term low-dose acyclovir for Varicella-Zoster virus infection after allogeneic peripheral blood stem cell transplantation. Clin Transplant 22:770–779
26. Erard V, Guthrie KA, Varley C et al (2007) One-year acyclovir prophylaxis for preventing varicella-zoster virus disease after hematopoietic cell transplantation: no evidence of rebound varicella-zoster virus disease after drug continuation. Blood 110:3071–3077
27. Biron KK, Elion GB (1980) In vitro susceptibility of varicella-zoster virus to acyclovir. Antimicrob Agents Chemother 18:443–447
28. Whitley RJ, Gnann JW Jr (1992) Acyclovir: a decade later. N Engl J Med 327:782–789
29. Brantley JS, Hicks L, Sra K et al (2006) Valacyclovir for the treatment of genital herpes. Expert Rev Anti Infect Ther 4:367–376
30. Bacon TH, Levin MJ, Leary JJ et al (2003) Herpes simplex virus resistance to acyclovir and penciclovir after two decades of antiviral therapy. Clin Microbiol Rev 16:114–128
31. de Miranda P, Whitley RJ, Blum MR et al (1979) Acyclovir kinetics after intravenous infusion. Clin Pharmacol Ther 26:718–728
32. Richards DM, Carmine AA, Brogden RN et al (1983) Acyclovir: a review of its pharmacodynamic properties and therapeutic efficacy. Drugs 26:378–438
33. Earnshaw DL, Bacon TH, Darlison SJ et al (1992) Mode of antiviral action of penciclovir in MRC-5 cells infected with herpes simplex virus type 1 (HSV-1), HSV-2, and varicella zoster virus. Antimicrob Agents Chemother 36:2747–2757
34. Shafran SD, Tyring SK, Ashton R et al (2004) Once, twice, or three times daily famciclovir compared with aciclovir for the oral treatment of herpes zoster in immunocompetent adults: a randomized, multicenter, double-blind clinical trial. J Clin Virol 29:248–253
35. Shen MC, Lin HH, Lee SS et al (2004) Double-blind, randomized, acyclovir-controlled, parallel group trial comparing the safety and efficacy of famciclovir and acyclovir in patients with uncomplicated herpes zoster. J Microbiol Immunol Infect 37:75–81
36. Ormrod D, Goa K (2000) Valacyclovir: a review of its use in the management of herpes zoster. Drugs 59:1317–1340
37. Acyclovir tablets: prescribing information 20. Apotex Corp., Weston, FL. http://www.apotex.com/us/en/products/downloads/pil/acya_imtb_ins.pdf. Accessed 3 Feb 2014
38. Whitley RJ, Blum MR, Barton N et al (1982) Pharmacokinetics of acyclovir in humans following intravenous administration. Am J Med 73:165–170
39. Blum RM, Liao SHT, de Miranda P (1982) Overview of acyclovir pharmacokinetic disposition in adults and children. Am J Med 73:186–192
40. Brigden D, Bye A, Fowle AS et al (1981) Human pharmacokinetics of acyclovir (an antiviral agent) following rapid intravenous injection. J Antimicrob Chemother 7:399–404
41. Weller S, Blum MR, Doucette M et al (1993) Pharmacokinetics of the acyclovir pro-drug after escalating single- and multiple-dose administration to normal volunteers. Clin Pharmacol Ther 54:595–605
42. Piret J, Boivin G (2011) Resistance of herpes simplex viruses to nucleoside analogues: mechanisms, prevalence, and management. Antimicrob Agents Chemother 55:459–472
43. Frobert E, Cortay JC, Ooka T et al (2008) Genotypic detection of acyclovir-resistant HSV-1: characterization of 67 ACV-sensitive and 14 ACV-resistant viruses. Antiviral Res 79:28–36
44. Leary JJ, Wittrock R, Sarisky RT et al (2002) Susceptibilities of herpes simplex viruses to penciclovir and acyclovir in eight cell lines. Antimicrob Agents Chemother 46:762–768
45. Safrin S, Elbeik T, Phan L et al (1994) Correlation between response to acyclovir and foscarnet therapy *in vitro* susceptibility result for isolates of herpes simplex virus from HIV-infected patients. Antimicrob Agents Chemother 38:1246–1250
46. Sarisky RT, Crosson P, Cano R et al (2002) Comparison of methods for identifying resistant herpes simplex virus and measuring antiviral susceptibility. J Clin Virol 23:191–200
47. Spruance SL, Tyring SK, DeGregorio B et al (1996) A large-scale, placebo-controlled, dose-ranging trial for peroral valaciclovir for episodic treatment of recurrent herpes genitalis. Arch Intern Med 156:1729–1735
48. Saiag P, Praindhui D, Chastang C (1999) A double-blind randomized study for assessing the equivalence of valaciclovir 1000 mg once daily versus 500 mg twice daily in the early treatment of recurrent genital herpes. J Antimicrob Chemother 44:525–531

49. Reitano M, Tyring S, Lang W et al (1998) Valaciclovir for the suppression of recurrent genital HSV infection: a large-scale dose range-finding study. J Infect Dis 1998(178): 603–610
50. Schiffer JT, Swan DA, Lawrence C et al (2013) Rapid viral expansion and short drug half-life explain the incomplete effectiveness of current herpes simplex virus 2-directed antiviral agents. Antimicrob Agents Chemother 57:5820–5829
51. Johnston C, Saracino M, Kuntz S et al (2010) Standard-dose and high-dose daily antiviral therapy for short episodes of genital HSV-2 reactivation: three randomized, open-label, cross-over trials. Lancet 379:641–647
52. Corey L, Wald A, Patel R et al (2004) Once-daily valacyclovir to reduce the risk of transmission of genital herpes. N Engl J Med 350:11–20
53. Sperling RS, Fife KH, Warren TJ et al (2008) Effect of daily valacyclovir suppression on Herpes Simplex Type 2 viral shedding in HSV-2 seropositive subjects without a history of genital herpes. Sex Transm Dis 35: 286–290
54. Laskin OL, Longstreth JA, Saral R et al (1982) Pharmacokinetics and tolerance of acyclovir, a new anti-herpesvirus agent, in humans. Antimicrob Agents Chemother 21: 393–398
55. Mason WJ, Nickols HH (2008) Images in clinical medicine. Crystalluria from acyclovir use. N Engl J Med 358:e14
56. Fleischer R, Johnson M (2010) Acyclovir nephrotoxicity: a case report highlighting the importance of prevention, detection, and treatment of acyclovir-induced nephropathy. Case Rep Med. doi:10.1155/2010/602783
57. Lam NN, Weir MA, Yao Z et al (2013) Risk of acute kidney injury from oral acyclovir: a population-based study. Am J Kidney Dis 61:723–729
58. Hernandez JO, Norstrom J, Wysock G (2009) Acyclovir-induced renal failure in an obese patient. Am J Health Syst Pharm 66:1288–1291
59. Seedat A, Winnett G (2012) Acyclovir-induced acute renal failure and the importance of an expanding waist line. BMJ Case Rep. doi:10.1136/bcr-2012-006264
60. Stranska R, Schuurman R, Nienhuis E et al (2005) Survey of acyclovir-resistant herpes simplex virus in the Netherlands: prevalence and characterization. J Clin Virol 32:7–18
61. Christophers J, Clayton J, Craske J et al (1998) Survey of resistance of herpes simplex virus to acyclovir in northwest England. Antimicrob Agents Chemother 42:868–872
62. Boon RJ, Bacon TH, Robey HL et al (2000) Antiviral susceptibilities of herpes simplex virus from immunocompetent subjects with recurrent herpes labialie: a UK-based survey. J Antimicrob Chemother 2000(46):32–325
63. Bacon TH, Boon RJ, Schultz M et al (2002) Surveillance for antiviral-agent-resistant herpes simplex virus in the general population with recurrent herpes labialis. Antimicrob Agents Chemother 46:3042–3044
64. van Velzen M, van de Vijver DAMC, van Loenen FB et al (2013) Acyclovir prophylaxis predisposes to antiviral-resistant recurrent herpetic keratitis. J Infect Dis 208: 1359–1365
65. Levin MJ, Bacon TH, Leary JJ (2004) Resistance of herpes simplex virus infections to nucleoside analogues in HIV-infected patients. Clin Infect Dis 39(Suppl 5): S248–S257
66. Tenser RB (1991) Role of herpes simplex virus thymidine kinase expression in viral pathogenesis and latency. Intervirology 32: 76–92
67. Englund JA, Zimmerman ME, Swierkosz EM et al (1990) Herpes simplex virus resistant to acyclovir: a study in a tertiary care center. Ann Intern Med 112:416–422
68. Chen Y, Scieux C, Garrait V et al (2000) Resistant herpes simplex virus type 1 infection: an emerging concern after allogeneic stem cell transplantation. Clin Infect Dis 31:927–935
69. Burrel S, Aime C, Hermet L et al (2013) Surveillance of herpes simplex virus resistance to antivirals: a 4-year survey. Antiviral Res 100:365–372
70. Matthews JT, Carroll RD, Stevens JT et al (1989) In vitro mutagenesis of the herpes simplex virus type 1 DNA polymerase gene results in altered drug sensitivity of the enzyme. J Virol 63:4913–4918
71. Coen DM, Schaffer PA (1980) Two distinct loco confer resistance to acycloguanosine in herpes simplex virus type 1. Microbiology 77:2265–2269
72. Gaudreau A, Hill E, Balfour HH et al (1998) Phenotypic and genotypic characterization of acyclovir-resistant herpes simplex viruses from immunocompromised patients. J Infect Dis 178:297–303
73. Field HJ, Darby G (1980) Pathogenicity in mice of strains of herpes simplex virus which are resistant to acyclovir *in vitro* and *in vivo*. Antimicrob Agents Chemother 17:209–216

74. Schepers K, Hernandez A, Adrei G et al (2014) Acyclovir-resistant herpes simplex encephalitis in a patient treated with anti-tumor necrosis factor-alpha monoclonal antibodies. J Clin Virol 59:67–70
75. Kakiuchi S, Nonoyama S, Wakamatsu H et al (2013) Neonatal herpes encephalitis caused by a virologically confirmed acyclovir-resistant herpes simplex virus 1 strain. J Clin Microbiol 51:356–359
76. Schulte EC, Sauerbrei A, Hoffman D et al (2010) Acyclovir resistance in herpes simplex encephalitis. Ann Nuerol 67:830–833
77. van der Beek MT, Claas ECJ, van der Blij-de Brouwer CS et al (2013) Rapid susceptibility testing for herpes simplex virus type 1 using real-time PCR. J Clin Virol 56:19–24
78. Burrel S, Deback C, Agut H et al (2010) Genotypic characterization of UL23 thymidine kinase and UL30 DNA polymerase of clinical isolates of herpes simplex virus: natural polymorphism and mutations associated with resistance to antivirals. Antimicrob Agents Chemother 54:4833–4842
79. Sauerbrei A, Deinhardt S, Zell R et al (2010) Testing of herpes simplex virus for resistance to antiviral drugs. Virulence 1:555–557
80. Chibo D, Druce J, Sasadeusz J et al (2004) Molecular analysis of clinical isolates of acyclovir resistant herpes simplex virus. Antiviral Res 61:83–91
81. Crumpacker CS (1996) Ganciclovir. N Engl J Med 335:721–729
82. Faulds D, Heel RC (1990) Ganciclovir. A review of its antiviral activity, pharmacokinetic properties and therapeutic efficacy in cytomegalovirus infections. Drugs 39:597–638
83. Cvetković RS, Wellington K (2005) Valganciclovir: a review of its use in the management of CMV infection and disease in immunocompromised patients. Drugs 65:859–878
84. Wagstaff AJ, Bryson HM (1994) Foscarnet. A reappraisal of its antiviral activity, pharmacokinetic properties and therapeutic use in immunocompromised patients with viral infections. Drugs 48:199–226
85. Le Page AK, Jager MM, Iwasenko JM et al (2013) Clinical aspects of cytomegalovirus antiviral resistance in solid organ transplant recipients. Clin Infect Dis 56:1018–1029
86. De Clercq E (2003) Clinical potential of the acyclic nucleoside phosphates cidofovir, adefovir, and tenofovir in treatment of DNA virus and retrovirus infections. Clin Microbiol Rev 16:569–596
87. Hitchcock MJ, Jaffe HS, Martin JC et al (1996) Cidofovir, a new agent with potent anti-herpesvirus activity. Antivir Chem Chemother 7:115–127
88. Safrin S, Cherrington JM, Jaffe HS (1997) Clinical uses of cidofovir. Rev Med Virol 7:145–156
89. Ganciclovir (Cytovene-IV). Package insert. (2010). Genentech USA, Inc, San Francisco, CA.
90. Aoki FY, Hayden FG, Dolin R (2010) Antiviral drugs (other than antiretrovirals). In: Mandell GL, Bennett JC, Dolin R (eds) Mandell, Douglas, and Bennett's: principles and practice of infectious disease, vol 1, 7th edn. Elsevier, Philadelphia, PA, pp 565–610
91. Janoly-Dumenil A, Rouvet I, Bleyzac N, Morfin F, Zabot M, Tod M (2012) A pharmacodynamic model of ganciclovir antiviral effect and toxicity for lymphoblastoid cells suggests a new dosing regimen to treat cytomegalovirus infection. Antimicrob Agents Chemother 56:3732–3738
92. Brown F, Banken L, Saywell K et al (1999) Pharmacokinetics of valganciclovir and ganciclovir following multiple oral dosages of valganciclovir in HIV- and CMV-seropositive volunteers. Clin Pharmacokinet 37:167–176
93. Yuen GJ, Drusano GL, Fletcher C et al (1995) Population differences in ganciclovir clearance as determined by nonlinear mixed-effects modelling. J Antimicrob Chemother 39: 2350–2352
94. Preston SL, Drusano GL (1996) Nonparametric expectation maximization population modeling of ganciclovir. J Clin Pharmacol 36:301–310
95. Wiltshire H, Hirankarn S, Farrell C, the Valganciclovir Solid Organ Transplant Study Group et al (2005) Pharmacokinetic profile of ganciclovir after its oral administration and from its prodrug, valganciclovir, in solid organ transplant recipients. Clin Pharmacokinet 44:495–507
96. Perrottet N, Decosterd LA, Meylan P, Pascual M, Biollaz J, Buclin T (2009) Valganciclovir in adult solid organ transplant recipients: pharmacokinetic and pharmacodynamic characteristics and clinical interpretation of plasma concentration measurements. Clin Pharmacokinet 48(6):399–418
97. Zhao W, Baudouin V, Zhang D, Deschênes G, Le Guellec C, Jacqz-Aigrain E (2009) Population pharmacokinetics of ganciclovir following administration of valganciclovir in paediatric renal transplant patients. Clin Pharmacokinet 48(5):321–328
98. Fishman JA, Doran MT, Volpicelli SA et al (2000) Dosing of intravenous ganciclovir for

the prophylaxis and treatment of cytomegalovirus infection in solid organ transplant recipients. Transplantation 69:389–394
99. Wiltshire H, Paya CV, Pescovitz MD, Humar A, Dominguez E, Washburn K, Blumberg E, Alexander B, Freeman R, Heaton N, Zuideveld KP, the Valganciclovir Solid Organ Transplant Study Group (2005) Pharmacodynamics of oral ganciclovir and valganciclovir in solid organ transplant recipients. Transplantation 79:1477–1483
100. Balfour HH Jr, Fletcher CV, Erice A, Henry WK, Acosta EP, Smith SA, Holm MA, Boivin G, Shepp DH, Crumpacker CS, Eaton CA, Martin-Munley SS (1996) Effect of foscarnet on quantities of cytomegalovirus and human immunodeficiency virus in blood of persons with AIDS. Antimicrob Agents Chemother 40:2721–2726
101. Kimberlin DW, Acosta EP, Sánchez PJ, Sood S, Agrawal V, Homans J, Jacobs RF, Lang D, Romero JR, Griffin J, Cloud GA, Lakeman FD, Whitley RJ, National Institute of Allergy and Infectious Diseases Collaborative Antiviral Study Group (2008) Pharmacokinetic and pharmacodynamic assessment of oral valganciclovir in the treatment of symptomatic congenital cytomegalovirus disease. J Infect Dis 197:836–845
102. Acosta EP, Brundage RC, King JR, Sánchez PJ, Sood S, Agrawal V, Homans J, Jacobs RF, Lang D, Romero JR, Griffin J, Cloud G, Whitley R, Kimberlin DW, National Institute of Allergy and Infectious Diseases Collaborative Antiviral Study Group (2007) Ganciclovir population pharmacokinetics in neonates following intravenous administration of ganciclovir and oral administration of a liquid valganciclovir formulation. Clin Pharmacol Ther 81:867–872
103. Piketty C, Bardin C, Gilquin J et al (1996) Low plasma concentrations achieved with conventional schedules of administration of ganciclovir in patients with AIDS. J Infect Dis 174:188–190
104. Zhang D, Lapeyraque AL, Popon M et al (2003) Pharmacokinetics of ganciclovir in pediatric renal transplant recipients. Pediatr Nephrol 18:943–948
105. Drusano GL, Aweeka F, Gambertoglio J, Jacobson M, Polis M, Lane HC, Eaton C, Martin-Munley S (1996) Relationship between foscarnet exposure, baseline cytomegalovirus (CMV) blood culture and the time to progression of CMV retinitis in HIV-positive patients. AIDS 10:1113–1119
106. Piketty C, Bardin C, Gilquin J et al (2000) Monitoring plasma levels of ganciclovir in AIDS patients receiving oral ganciclovir as maintenance therapy for CMV retinitis. Clin Microbiol Infect 6:117–120
107. Lalezari JP, Friedberg DN, Bissett J et al, Roche Cooperative Oral Ganciclovir Study Group (2002) High dose oral ganciclovir treatment for cytomegalovirus retinitis. J Clin Virol 24:67–77
108. Jacobson MA, Polsky B, Causey D, Davis R, Tong W, O'Donnell JJ, Kuppermann BD, Heinemann MH, Feinberg J, Lizak P et al (1994) Pharmacodynamic relationship of pharmacokinetic parameters of maintenance doses of foscarnet and clinical outcome of cytomegalovirus retinitis. Antimicrob Agents Chemother 38:1190–1193
109. Sommadossi JP, Carlisle R (1987) Toxicity of 30-azido-30-deoxythymidine and 9-(1,3-dihydroxy-2-propoxymethyl) guanine for normal human hematopoietic progenitor cells in vitro. Antimicrob Agents Chemother 31:452–454
110. Shepp DH, Dandliker PS, de Miranda P et al (1985) Activity of 9-[2-hydroxy-1-(hydroxymethyl) ethoxymethyl]guanine in the treatment of cytomegalovirus pneumonia. Ann Intern Med 10:368–373
111. Erice A, Jordan MC, Chace BA et al (1987) Ganciclovir treatment of cytomegalovirus disease in transplant recipients and others immunocompromised hosts. JAMA 22:3082–3087
112. Fletcher C, Sawchuk R, Chinnock B et al (1986) Human pharmacokinetics of the antiviral drug DHPG. Clin Pharmacol Ther 40:281–286
113. Buhles W Jr, Mastre BJ, Tinker AJ et al (1988) Ganciclovir treatment of life- or sight-threatening cytomegalovirus infections: experience in 314 immunocompromised patients. Rev Infect Dis 10(Suppl 3):495–503
114. Manuel O, Venetz JP, Fellay J et al (2007) Efficacy and safety of universal valganciclovir prophylaxis combined with a tacrolimus/mycophenolate-based regimen in kidney transplantation. Swiss Med Wkly 137:669–676
115. Combarnous F, Fouque D, Chossegros P et al (1994) Neurologic side-effects of ganciclovir. Clin Nephrol 42:279–280
116. Peyrière H, Jeziorrsky E, Jalabert A et al (2006) Neurotoxicity related to valganciclovir in a child with impaired renal function: usefulness of therapeutic drug monitoring. Ann Pharmacother 40:143–146
117. Figge HL, Baille GR, Briceland LL et al (1992) Possible ganciclovir-induced hepatotoxicity in patients with AIDS. Clin Pharm 11:432–434

118. Limaye AP, Corey L, Koelle DM, Davis CL, Boeckh M (2000) Emergence of ganciclovir-resistant cytomegalovirus disease among recipients of solid-organ transplants. Lancet 356:645–649
119. Endo Pharmaceuticals Inc. (2007) Symmetrel® (amantadine) full prescribing information. Endo Pharmaceuticals Inc., Chadds Ford, PA
120. Forest Pharmaceuticals, Inc. (2007) Flumadine® (rimantadine). Full prescribing information. Forest Pharmaceuticals, Inc., St. Louis, MO
121. Widmer N, Meylan P, Ivanyuk A et al (2010) Oseltamivir in seasonal, avian H5N1 and pandemic 2009 A/H1N1 influenza. Clin Pharmacokinet 49(11):741–765
122. McNicholl IR, McNicholl JJ (2001) Neuraminidase inhibitors: zanamivir and oseltamivir. Ann Pharmacother 35:57–70
123. He G, Massarella J, Ward P (1999) Clinical pharmacokinetics of the prodrug oseltamivir and its active metabolite Ro 64-0802. Clin Pharmacokinet 37(6):471–484
124. GlaxoSmithKline (2013) Relenza® (zanamivir). Full prescribing information. GlaxoSmithKline, Research Triangle Park, NC
125. Cass LM, Efthymiopoulos C, Marsh J et al (1999) Pharmacokinetics of zanamivir after intravenous, oral, inhaled or intranasal administration to healthy volunteers. Clin Pharmacokinet 36(S1):1–11
126. Kubo S, Tomozawa T, Kakuta M et al (2010) Laninamivir prodrug CS-8958, a long-acting neuraminidase inhibitor, shows superior anti-influenza virus activity after a single administration. Antimicrob Agents Chemother 54: 1256–1264
127. Weller S, Jones LS, Lou Y et al (2013) Pharmacokinetics of zanamivir following intravenous administration to subjects with and without renal impairment. Antimicrob Agents Chemother 57(7):2967–2971
128. Mendel DB, Tai CY, Escarpe PA et al (1998) Oral administration of a prodrug of the influenza virus neuraminidase inhibitor GS 4071 protects mice and ferrets against influenza infection. Antimicrob Agents Chemother 42(3):640–646
129. Sidwell RW, Smee DF (2000) In vitro and in vivo assay systems for study of influenza virus inhibitors. Antiviral Res 48:1–16
130. Tisdale M (2000) Monitoring of viral susceptibility: new challenges with the development of influenza NA inhibitors. Rev Med Virol 10:45–55
131. Woods JM, Bethell RC, Coates JAV et al (1993)4-Guanidino-2,4-dideoxy-2,3-dehydro-n-acetylneuraminic acid is a highly effective inhibitor both of the sialidase (neuraminidase) and of growth of a wide range of influenza A and B viruses in vitro. Antimicrob Agents Chemother 37:1473–1479
132. Hayden FG, Rollins BS, Madren LK (1994) Anti-influenza virus activity of the neraminidase inhibitor 4-guanidino-Neu5Ac2en in cell culture and in human respiratory epithelium. Antiviral Res 25:123–131
133. Gilead Sciences, Inc. (2011) Tamiflu® (oseltamivir). Full prescribing information. Gilead Sciences, Inc., Foster City, CA
134. Li W, Escarpe EJ, Eisenburg K et al (1998) Identification of GS 4104 as an orally bioavailable prodrug of the influenza virus neuraminidase inhibitor GS 4071. Antimicrob Agents Chemother 42:647–653
135. McSharry JJ, Weng Q, Brown A et al (2009) Prediction of the pharmacodynamically linked variable of oseltamivir carboxylate for influenza A virus using an in vitro hollow-fiber infection model system. Antimicrob Agents Chemother 53(6):2375–2381
136. Brown AN, Bulitta JB, McSharry JJ et al (2011) Effect of half-life on the pharmacodynamic index of zanamavir against influenza virus delineated by a mathematical model. Antimicrob Agents Chemother 55(4): 1747–1753
137. Brown AN, McSharry JJ, Weng Q et al (2011) Zanamivir, at 600 milligrams twice daily, inhibits oseltamivir-resistant 2009 pandemic H1N1 influenza virus in an in vitro hollow-fiber infection model system. Antimicrob Agents Chemother 55(4):1740–1746
138. Drusano GL, Preston SL, Smee D et al (2001) Pharmacodynamic evaluation of RWJ-270201, a novel neuraminidase inhibitor, in a lethal murine model of influenza predicts efficacy for once-daily dosing. Antimicrob Agents Chemother 45(7):2115–2118
139. Kamal MA, Van Wart SA, Rayner CR et al (2013) Population pharmacokinetics of oseltamivir: pediatrics through geriatrics. Antimicrob Agents Chemother 57(8): 3470–3477
140. Rayner CR, Bulik CC, Kamal MA et al (2013) Pharmacokinetic-pharmacodynamic determinants of oseltamivir efficacy using data from phase 2 inoculation studies. Antimicrob Agents Chemother 57(8):3478–3487
141. Centers for Disease Control and Prevention (2010) Update: influenza activity-United States, 2009–10 season. MMWR Morb Mortal Wkly Rep 59:901–908
142. McGeer A, Green KA, Plevneshi A et al (2007) Antiviral therapy and outcomes of

influenza requiring hospitalization in Ontario, Canada. Clin Infect Dis 45:1568–1575

143. Lee N, Cockram CS, Chan PK et al (2008) Antiviral treatment for patients hospitalized with severe influenza infection may affect clinical outcomes. Clin Infect Dis 46:1323–1324
144. Lee N, Chan PK, Hui DS et al (2009) Viral loads and duration of viral shedding in adult patients hospitalized with influenza. J Infect Dis 200(4):492–500
145. Napolitano LM, Park PK, Sihler KC et al (2009) Intensive-care patients with severe novel influenza A (H1N1) virus infection – Michigan, June 2009. MMWR Morb Mortal Wkly Rep 58(27):749–752
146. Jain S, Kamimoto L, Bramley AM et al (2009) Hospitalized patients with 2009 H1N1 influenza in the United States, April–June 2009. N Engl J Med 361:1935–1944
147. Louie JK, Acosta M, Winter K (2009) Factors associated with death or hospitalization due to pandemic 2009 influenza A (H1N1) infection in California. JAMA 302:1896–1902
148. Nicholson KG, Aoki FY, Osterhaus ADME et al (2000) Efficacy and safety of oseltamivir in treatment of acute influenza: a randomized controlled trial. Lancet 355:1845–1850
149. Thorne-Humphrey LM, Goralski KB, Slayter KL et al (2011) Oseltamivir pharmacokinetics in morbid obesity (OPTIMO trial). J Antimicrob Chemother 66:2083–2091
150. Manjunath PP, Thomas PL (2011) Oseltamivir and oseltamivir carboxylate pharmacokinetics in obese adults: dose modification for weight is not necessary. Antimicrob Agents Chemother 55(12):5640–5645
151. Writing Committee of the Second World Health Organization Consult Aspects of Human Infection with Avian Influenza A (H5N1) Virus (2008) Update on avian influenza A (H5N1) virus infection in humans. N Engl J Med 358:261–273
152. Weinstock DM, Gubareva LV, Zuccotti G (2003) Prolonged shedding of multidrug-resistant influenza A virus in an immunocompromised patient. N Engl J Med 348(9):867
153. Baz M, Abed Y, McDonald J et al (2006) Characterization of multidrug-resistant influenza A/H3N2 viruses shed during 1 year by an immunocompromised child. Clin Infect Dis 43:1555–1561
154. Wattanagoon Y, Stepniewska K, Lindegardh N (2009) Pharmacokinetics of high-dose oseltamivir in healthy volunteers. Antimicrob Agents Chemother 53(3):945–952
155. Dutkowski R, Thakrar B, Froehlich E et al (2003) Safety and pharmacology of oseltamivir in clinical use. Drug Saf 26(11):787–801
156. Bright RA, Medina MJ, Xu X et al (2005) Incidence of adamantane resistance among influenza A (H3N2) viruses isolated worldwide from 1994 to 2005: a cause for concern. Lancet 366:1175–1181
157. Bright RA, Shay DK, Shu B et al (2006) Adamantane resistance among influenza A viruses isolated early during the 2005–2006 influenza season in the United States. JAMA 295:891–894
158. Englund JA, Champlin RE, Wyde PR et al (1998) Common emergence of amantadine and rimantadine-resistant influenza A viruses in symptomatic immunocompromised adults. Clin Infect Dis 26:1418–1424
159. Hayden FG, Belshe RB, Clover RD et al (1989) Emergence and apparent transmission of rimantadine-resistant influenza A virus in families. N Engl J Med 321:1696–1702
160. World Health Organization (2010) WHO guidelines for pharmacological management of pandemic influenza A(H1N1) 2009 and other influenza viruses. http://www.who.int/csr/resources/publications/swineflu/h1n1_use_antivirals_20090820/en/
161. McKimm-Breschkin J, Trivedi T, Hampson A et al (2003) Neuraminidase sequence analysis and susceptibilities of influenza virus clinical isolates to zanamivir and oseltamivir. Antimicrob Agents Chemother 47:2264–2272
162. Le QM, Wertheim HF, Tran ND et al (2010) A community cluster of oseltamivir-resistant cases of 2009 H1N1 influenza. N Engl J Med 362:86–87
163. Hatakeyama S, Sugaya N, Ito M et al (2007) Emergence of influenza B viruses with reduced sensitivity to neuraminidase inhibitors. JAMA 297:1435–1442
164. Aoki FY, Boivin G, Roberts N (2007) Influenza virus susceptibility and resistance to oseltamivir. Antivir Ther 12(4 Pt B): 603–616
165. Ward P, Small I, Smith J et al (2005) Oseltamivir (Tamiflu®) and its potential for use in the event of an influenza pandemic. J Antimicrob Chemother 55(S1):i5–i21
166. Kiso M, Mitamura K, Sakai-Tagawa Y et al (2004) Resistant influenza A viruses in children treated with oseltamivir: descriptive study. Lancet 364:759–765
167. Ison MG, Gubareva LV, Atmar RL (2006) Recovery of drug-resistant influenza virus from immunocompromised patients: a case series. J Infect Dis 193:760–764
168. Storms AD, Gubareva LV, Su S et al (2012) Oseltamivir-resistant pandemic (H1N1) 2009 virus infections, United States, 2010–11. Emerg Infect Dis 18:308–311

169. Moscona A (2005) Oseltamivir resistance – disabling our influenza defenses. N Engl J Med 353(25):2633–2636
170. Ginting TE, Shinya K, Kyan Y et al (2012) Amino acid changes in hemagglutinin contribute to the replication of oseltamivir-resistant H1N1 influenza viruses. J Virol 86:121–127
171. Govorkova EA, Baranovich T, Seiler P et al (2013) Antiviral resistance among highly pathogenic influenza A (H1N1) viruses isolated worldwide in 2002–2012 shows need for continued monitoring. Antiviral Res 98: 297–304
172. Pizzorno A, Abed Y, Bouhy X et al (2012) Impact of mutations at residue I223 of the neuraminidase protein on the resistance profile, replication level, and virulence of the 2009 pandemic influenza virus. Antimicrob Agents Chemother 56(3):1208–1214
173. Thorlund K, Awad T, Boivin G et al (2011) Systematic review of influenza resistance to the neuraminidase inhibitors. BMC Infect Dis 11(134)
174. Watanabe A, Change SC, Kim MJ et al (2010) Long-acting neuraminidase inhibitor laninamivir octanoate versus oseltamivir for treatment of influenza: a double-blind, randomized, noninferiority clinical trial. Clin Infect Dis 51(10):1167–1175
175. Seo S, Englund JA, Nguyen JT et al (2013) Combination therapy with amantadine, oseltamivir and ribavirin for influenza A infection: safety and pharmacokinetics. Antivir Ther 18(3):377–386

Chapter 19

Pharmacodynamics of Antiretroviral Agents

Kajal B. Larson and Edward P. Acosta

Abstract

The identification of drug targets against the human immunodeficiency virus has led to the development and approval of several antiretroviral agents. Drug monotherapy and non-adherence to prescribed regimen have led to the emergence of drug resistance and current drug regimens consisting of at least three drugs are recommended. The relationship between drug exposure or concentrations and response has been described for most agents, both as single agents and in combination with other drugs. The introduction of fixed-dose formulation and the fact that new drugs are only tested in combination with other antiretrovirals introduces issues in determining the exact pharmacodynamics of single agents. However, favorable responses such as viral suppression, now defined as HIV-1 RNA level <20–50 copies/mL, and restoration of immune function as evidenced by increased CD4+ cell counts, remain the benchmark in efficacy comparison. Further, HIV-RNA levels, CD4+ cell counts, and resistance-associated mutations at baseline often predict virological failure or success of HIV drugs. Although therapeutic drug monitoring may have advantages in specific populations, it is not indicated for routine use and has limited utility for some drug classes such as nucleoside reverse transcriptase inhibitors and protease inhibitors.

Key words Pharmacokinetics, Pharmacodynamics, Antiretrovirals, Concentration–response, Protease inhibitors, Non-nucleoside reverse transcriptase inhibitors

1 Overview of HIV Infection

In the early 1980s, several cases of a cellular-immune dysfunction were reported in the USA [1] and soon after, the term Acquired Immune Deficiency Syndrome (AIDS) was coined. The patients presented with fever, rash, and lymphadenopathy and were more susceptible to opportunistic infections such as pneumocystis pneumonia and cytomegalovirus infections. In May 1983, the human immunodeficiency virus (HIV) was isolated and later confirmed to be the causative pathogen of AIDS. Two strains, HIV-1 and HIV-2, are known to exist, with HIV-1 infections being more prevalent worldwide and while HIV-2 is more common in some countries, this strain is less readily transmitted and pathogenic than HIV-1 [2, 3]. Dual infections with both strains have also been reported [4].

John C. Rotschafer et al. (eds.), *Antibiotic Pharmacodynamics*, Methods in Pharmacology and Toxicology,
DOI 10.1007/978-1-4939-3323-5_19, © Springer Science+Business Media New York 2016

HIV is an RNA retrovirus (*Lentivirus* genus) that contains two single strands of RNA, enclosed by a nucleocapsid and an outer lipid envelop. Of the nine HIV genes, three genes, namely *gag*, *pol*, and *env* are mainly responsible for the synthesis of structural proteins needed for virus replication, including reverse transcriptase, protease, and integrase, which are known HIV drug targets. HIV targets T cells such as CD4+ lymphocytes, macrophages, and dendritic cells, by first binding to the CD4 receptor through the viral glycoprotein gp120. This interaction is then followed by binding to a co-receptor, either chemokine receptor 5 (CCR5) or chemokine receptor 4 (CXCR4), which causes a conformational change in the viral envelope, activating gp41, a fusion peptide that allows viral entry into host cells. The *env* gene encodes the two glycoproteins, gp120 and gp41. Another receptor, integrin α-4 β-7, appears to be important for the attachment, of HIV-1 to dendritic cells in the gut, enabling the transport of HIV to lymphoid organs and infection of T-cells. Major HIV genes and proteins and their functions are summarized in Table 1.

Table 1
Major HIV genes, proteins, and functions

Gene	Protein(s)	Major function(s)	Notes
Gag	p24, p7, p6 p17	Capsid protein Matrix protein	p24 antigen assay can be used to detect HIV infection
Pol	Reverse transcriptase	Transcribes viral RNA to DNA	Drug target
	Integrase	Integrates viral DNA into host genome	Drug target
	Protease	Cleaves viral polyproteins into functional units	Drug target
Vif	Vif	Degrades host cell defense protein APOBEC3G	
Vpr	Vpr	Regulates nuclear import of pre-integration complex	
Tat	Tat	Promotes transcription of viral DNA	
Rev	Rev	Allows export of unspliced viral RNA from nucleus	
Vpu	Vpu	Intracellular degradation of CD4	
Env	gp120	Binds CD4, CCR5, CXCR4	Drug target
	gp41	Promotes fusion of virus to host cell	Drug target
Nef	Nef	Downregulates CD4 and other receptors	

Untreated HIV infection starts with primary infection followed by dissemination of virus to lymphoid organs, clinical latency, elevated HIV expression, clinical disease, and death. After primary infection, there is a sharp decrease in the number of CD4 T-cells in peripheral blood. An immune response to HIV ensues within 1 week to 3 months after infection, which results in a decrease in plasma viremia and an increase in CD4 cells. This is a phase of prolonged clinical latency, which can last for as long as 10 years. During this time, viral replication is still active, with an estimated turnover of ten billion HIV particles. However, the immune system cannot completely clear the HIV infection and the virus-infected cells persist in the lymph nodes. Eventually, the patient starts to show symptoms as the CD4 T-cell count continues to decrease until it reaches a critical level below which there is a substantial risk of opportunistic diseases. In untreated cases, death usually occurs within 2 years after the onset of clinical symptoms.

Sensitive assays have been developed to detect HIV RNA in plasma and a single measurement of plasma viral load about 6 months after infection can predict the subsequent risk of developing AIDS in untreated male patients, making RNA viral load a useful prognostic tool. High viral loads tend to correlate with rapid disease progression and poorer responses to treatment. In women, viral load has been suggested to be less predictive of progression to AIDS. Nonetheless, the plasma viral load appears to be the best predictor of long-term clinical outcome, whereas the CD4 lymphocyte counts are the best predictor of short-term risk of developing an opportunistic disease. Further, it has been shown that suppression of HIV-1 RNA to <20–50 copies/mL is a better predictor of durable virologic success than suppression to <400–500 copies/mL [5]. Virologic efficacy is related to initial CD4 counts, which depends on unpredictable presentation of patients for care. In an attempt to reduce the variation in drug efficacy which decreases the risk of disease progression, guidelines that strongly recommend ART initiation when CD4 count are less than 350 cells/mm^3 or between 350 and 500 cell/mm^3 have been implemented [6].

2 HIV Therapy

In 2012, there were 2.3 million new HIV infections worldwide [7]. Significant advances in ARV therapy in the past three decades have reduced the mortality and morbidity due to AIDS, and there were about 35 million people living with HIV at the end of 2012 [7]. There are currently 26 antiretroviral (ARV) drugs spanning six drug classes that are approved for the treatment of HIV with standard treatment consisting of a combination of at least three drugs from two different classes (HAART, highly active antiretroviral therapy). Table 2 summarizes the recommended guidelines for the use of ARV drugs for the treatment of HIV infections (Current HIV treatment guidelines can be found at https://aidsinfo.nih.gov/contentfiles/lvguidelines/AdultandAdolescentGL.pdf).

3 General Pharmacodynamic Principles

Pharmacodynamics (PD) is the study of the biochemical, molecular and/or physiological effects of a drug on the body, and defines the relationship between drug exposure and therapeutic effect. In HIV research, the most commonly used parameters to define ARV success or drug efficacy are CD4 return, decrease in HIV RNA, and suppression of the viral antigen, p24. The development of sensitive drug assays has enabled the measurement of plasma drug concentrations, which are also used to determine PD relationships. However, ARV drug concentration at the site of action may be different from plasma drug concentrations. For example, nucleoside reverse transcriptase inhibitors (NRTIs) are activated intracellularly and therefore the concentration of the phosphorylated active entities could better describe the PD of NRTIs. PD relationships are intricately connected to drug concentrations, which can vary because of changes in pharmacokinetics (drug absorption, distribution, metabolism, and elimination) as shown in Figs. 1 and 2. For example, raltegravir, an integrase inhibitor, has been shown to have high inter- and intra-patient variability [8] and protease inhibitors (PIs) are highly variable, presumably because of fluctuations in plasma proteins, to which these drugs are highly bound. Drug concentration can also vary because of non-adherence to therapy, which leads to exposure of replicating virus to suboptimal drug concentration that will eventually lead to the selection of drug-resistant isolates. In ARV therapy, cross-resistance, whereby the virus does not respond to some drugs from the same category can occur. In these situations, higher drug doses can be used to try to achieve an effect but in most cases, drug class switching is prescribed.

In this chapter, we review the pharmacodynamics of antiretrovirals in humans, including safety, efficacy, and tolerability data and therapeutic drug monitoring.

4 Nucleoside Reverse Transcriptase Inhibitors

Nucleoside reverse transcriptase inhibitors (NRTIs) are the oldest drug class in ARV therapy, with zidovudine being the first drug approved by the US Food and Drug Administration (FDA) for the treatment of HIV. Agents in this class are activated by an intracellular phosphorylation cascade and are incorporated into viral DNA. The viral enzyme reverse transcriptase cannot recognize the NRTI-bound DNA and chain elongation is stopped.

Table 2
US guidelines for antiretroviral regimens in treatment-naïve patients [6]

Antiretroviral drugs	Dosing
Preferred regimens	
Non-nucleoside reverse transcriptase regimen	
Efavirenz/tenofovir/emtricitabine[a]	600/300/200 mg once a day
Protease inhibitor regimens	
Atazanavir Ritonavir Tenofovir/emtricitabine[a]	300 mg once a day 100 mg once a day 300/200 mg once a day
Darunavir Ritonavir Abacavir/lamivudine[a]	800 mg once a day 100 mg once a day 300/200 mg once a day
Integrase inhibitor regimen	
Raltegravir Tenofovir/emtricitabine[a]	400 mg twice a day 300/200 mg once a day
Alternative regimens	
Non-nucleoside reverse transcriptase regimen	
Efavirenz Abacavir/lamivudine[a]	600 mg once a day 600/300 mg once a day
Rilpivirine/tenofovir/emtricitabine[a]	25/300/200 mg once a day
Rilpivirine Abacavir/lamivudine[a]	25 mg once a day 600/300 mg once a day
Protease inhibitor regimens	
Atazanavir Ritonavir Abacavir/lamivudine[a]	300 mg once a day 100 mg once a day 600/300 mg once a day
Darunavir Ritonavir Abacavir/lamivudine[a]	800/100 mg once a day 100 mg once a day 600/300 mg once a day
Fosamprenavir/ritonavir Abacavir/lamivudine[a] or Tenofovir/emtricitabine[a]	1400/200 mg once a day[b] or 700/100 mg twice a day 600/300 mg once a day 300/200 mg once a day
Lopinavir/ritonavir[a] Abacavir/lamivudine[a] or Tenofovir/emtricitabine[a]	400/100 mg twice daily or 800/200 mg once a day 600/300 mg once a day 300/200 mg once a day
Integrase inhibitor regimen	
Elvitegravir/cobicistat/ tenofovir/emtricitabine[a]	150/150/300/200 mg once a day
Raltegravir Abacavir/lamivudine[a]	400 mg twice a day 600/300 mg once a day

[a]Fixed dose combination
[b]Ritonavir can also be given at 100 mg once a day

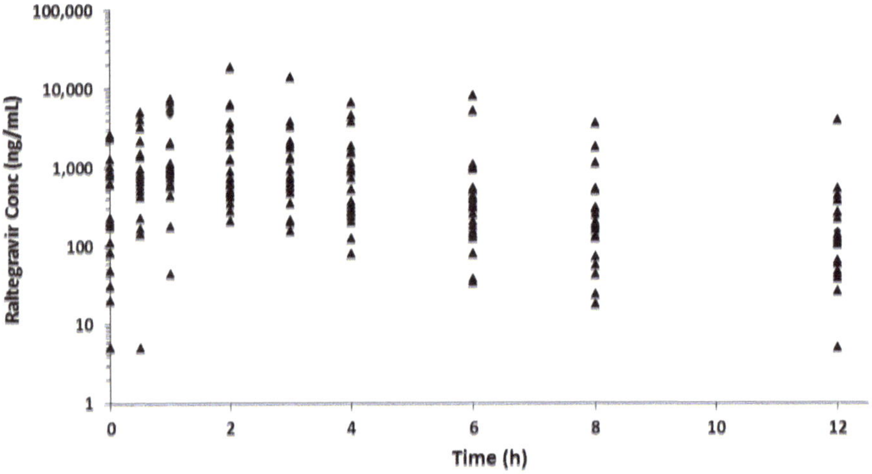

Fig. 1 Variability in raltegravir concentrations following 400 mg twice daily dosing in HIV-positive patients from ≥6 to <19 years of age (n=22). *Triangles* are individual raltegravir concentrations. Data are from Nachman S et al. Pharmacokinetics, safety, and 48-week efficacy of oral raltegravir in HIV-1-infected children aged 2 through 18 years. *Clinical Infectious Diseases*, 2014;58:413–22

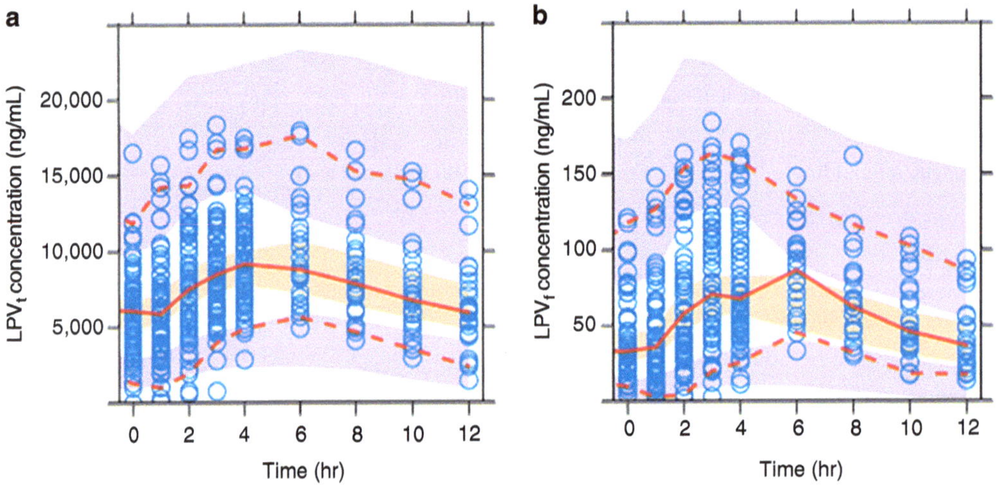

Fig. 2 Variability in lopinavir concentrations in HIV-positive treatment-naïve patients. Individual total (**a**) and free (**b**) lopinavir concentrations are displayed in *circles. Solid line* is the population pharmacokinetic prediction of median concentration. The *dashed lines* are the 5th and 95th percentiles of the observed data and the *shaded areas* are the corresponding 95 % confidence interval of the simulated data. Reproduced from K. Wang et al. *Clin Pharmacokinet* 2014; 53: 361–71

4.1 Zidovudine

Zidovudine was the first ARV approved by the FDA for the treatment of HIV infection in 1987. In one of the initial trials with zidovudine, 145 patients received zidovudine and 137 received placebo. Patients who received zidovudine had a statistically significant increase in CD4 cell counts compared to patients on placebo [9]. A high number of deaths were noted in the placebo group and the trial was stopped. Soon after the discovery of zidovudine resistance, combination therapy was investigated in clinical trials. In a double-blind, randomized trial, during with treatment-naïve, HIV-infected patients received either lamivudine 300 mg twice a day plus zidovudine 200 mg every 8 h or zidovudine monotherapy, revealed that combination therapy led to a significant increase in CD4 cell counts and decrease in HIV-1 viral load without any significant differences in incidence or severity in safety events [10]. These results were similar to other studies, including one that compared combination zidovudine therapy to zidovudine monotherapy in zidovudine-experienced patients [11–13]. The efficacy of zidovudine plus lamivudine was also shown to be superior compared to stavudine in the ACTG 302 study, during which zidovudine-experienced patients had been switched to either stavudine or lamivudine plus zidovudine [14]. Nowadays, zidovudine (300 mg) is available as a fixed-dose combination (FDC) with lamivudine (150 mg).

The major side effects of zidovudine include dose-related mitochondrial toxicity and severe anemia and neutropenia. Although a zidovudine plus lamivudine combination is not a preferred agent in the USA [6], it is a preferred regimen in pregnant women in the USA [6] and has been recommended by the World Health Organization in cases where tenofovir, lamivudine (or emtricitabine), and efavirenz are contraindicated or not available [15].

4.2 Didanosine

Approved by the FDA in 1991, didanosine is an NRTI whose dosing is based on body weight. Fatal and nonfatal adverse reactions have been observed with the use of didanosine and include pancreatitis, lactic acidosis, severe hepatomegaly with steatosis, hepatic toxicity, non-cirrhotic portal hypertension, peripheral neuropathy, retinal changes and optic neuritis, immune reconstitution syndrome, and fat redistribution.

In an early comparison of zidovudine with didanosine, patients who were switched to receive didanosine (either 750 or 500 mg per day) had better response than those who received zidovudine, with respect to CD4 cell counts and p24 antigen levels, suggesting that a change from zidovudine to didanosine may be favorable [16]. The long-term efficacy of didanosine, stavudine, and nelfinavir was compared to zidovudine, lamivudine, and nelfinavir in HIV-infected, treatment-naïve patients. The two arms had similar proportion of patients who achieved HIV RNA <400 copies/mL or experienced virologic failure. Further, a similar median increase in CD4 cell counts was observed in both groups, indicating that didanosine-containing therapy was noninferior to zidovudine plus lamivudine and nelfinavir [17, 18].

4.3 Stavudine

Stavudine was approved for the treatment of HIV in 1994 but its use has become rare in developed countries and is being phased out in resource-limited settings because of concerns about long-term cumulative toxicity. Further, tenofovir, zidovudine, or stavudine were compared as part of first-line ARV therapy in resource-limited setting and while virologic suppression was similar for all agents, zidovudine had the lowest CD4 cell count rise and tenofovir had the least mortality [19]. In the USA, stavudine can be administered at 40 mg twice daily while the international dose is 30 mg twice daily, highlighting the lack of optimal dosing information.

The clinical efficacy of monotherapy stavudine was investigated in a study in 822 HIV infected adults who were zidovudine-experienced [20]. While the authors found that stavudine was well tolerated, there were no significant differences between stavudine or zidovudine monotherapy in the study population. In treatment-naïve and -experienced HIV-infected individuals, combination therapy (stavudine plus lamivudine) led to a decrease in HIV-1 RNA and an increase in CD4 cell counts with 17 % of subjects experiencing grade 3 or 4 toxicity [21].

Intermittent exposure to NRTIs was explored using high doses of stavudine in NRTI-experienced patients [22]. Patients received 280 mg per day of stavudine for 4 weeks, a dosage predicted to achieve a steady-state concentration of 336 ng/mL. Stavudine treatment was discontinued for 4 weeks and started again for an additional 4 weeks. The authors found that this approach was well tolerated, with a decrease in viral load and increase in CD4 cell count. A significant relationship was observed between stavudine exposure and change in viral load. Although an increase in viral load and a decrease in CD4 cell counts were seen when patients were not receiving stavudine ("off" cycles), resistance to study drugs was not likely as evidenced by detection of only one new NRTI resistance mutation in the study population. This work suggested that intermittent treatment with ARVs could be a viable option for patients with treatment failure.

4.4 Lamivudine

Lamivudine is a cytidine analog that has activity against both HIV-1 and HIV-2 and can also inhibit the reverse transcriptase of the Hepatitis B virus. Approved by the FDA in 1995, lamivudine can be administered at 300 mg once daily or 150 mg twice daily. Weight-based dosing of lamivudine in children 3 months and older is also approved. In 2004, lamivudine was approved as a combination pill with abacavir. As with other NRTIs, lamivudine resistance is of concern. Clinical trials have showed that in patients receiving lamivudine monotherapy or combination therapy with lamivudine plus zidovudine, most subjects became resistant to lamivudine within 12 weeks of treatment initiation. However, the combination treatment delayed the emergence of zidovudine resistance [23].

Further, most lamivudine-resistant strains of HIV are cross-resistant to didanosine, and zalcitabine (an NRTI that is no longer manufactured).

Lamivudine has been studied extensively as part of combination regimens. In treatment-naïve adults, a lamivudine plus zidovudine regimen had greater increases in CD4 cell counts and decreases in viral load compared to monotherapy with these agents at week 24, with sustained virologic effects at week 48 [10]. While the combination treatment delayed the emergence of zidovudine resistance, lamivudine resistance developed rapidly. At week 48 of treatment with twice-daily lamivudine and zidovudine as a combination tablet plus abacavir, 56 % of patients had achieved HIV-1 RNA <50 copies/mL [24]. Further, the authors found that prior use of lamivudine or zidovudine and the presence of the reverse transcriptase mutation M184V did not have an effect on virologic outcome. In the ACTG trial A5202, where treatment-naïve patients were randomized to receive tenofovir-emtricitabine or abacavir-lamivudine, combined with efavirenz or atazanavir/ritonavir, similar viral load declines at week 4 were observed in patients receiving tenofovir or lamivudine [25]. However, patients who had a high baseline viral load (≥100,000 copies/mL), increased virologic failure rates were observed in the lamivudine treatment group. In virologically suppressed patients who received lopinavir/ritonavir as part of their ARV regimen and had raised cholesterol levels, switching from lamivudine/abacavir to tenofovir/emtricitabine led to improvements in fasting lipid profiles without a deterioration in virological control, suggesting that tenofovir/emtricitabine may have a superior safety profile compared to lamivudine/abacavir [26]. While lamivudine/abacavir is not one of the preferred ARV regimens in treatment naïve patients in the USA, emtricitabine and lamivudine can be switched as these two agents were found to be clinically equivalent [6, 27]. Lamivudine/abacavir remains an important, albeit alternative regimen.

4.5 Abacavir

In 1998, abacavir became the 15th ARV drug approved by the FDA. Abacavir exists as co-formulated pills, either with lamivudine or with zidovudine plus lamivudine. The major adverse effects associated with abacavir are hypersensitivity reaction, lactic acidosis, and severe hepatomegaly. Patients with the HLA-B*5701 allele have a significantly increased risk for the hypersensitivity reaction, which is a multi-organ clinical syndrome and can be fatal. Screening for this specific allele is recommended prior to taking abacavir. Underlying heart conditions should be considered before starting treatment with abacavir as patients may be at an increased risk for myocardial infarction.

In a dose-ranging study in antiretroviral-naïve patients, the pharmacokinetics of abacavir were dose proportional over the doses studied [28]. While the incidence of adverse effects was not correlated to abacavir exposure, a relationship was observed between nausea and maximum plasma concentration (C_{max}). Further, C_{max} and area under the concentration–time curve from 0 to infinity ($AUC_{0-\infty}$) were significantly associated with virologic and immunologic function. Only a small difference in the change in HIV-1 RNA levels when the dose was increased from 300 to 600 mg was observed, suggesting that the appropriate dose of abacavir is 300 mg twice a day.

The data from A5202 showed that patients with high viral loads had an increased risk for virologic failure when taking lamivudine/abacavir compared to tenofovir/emtricitabine. Therefore, similar to lamivudine, treatment with abacavir is not preferred over tenofovir/emtricitabine as an initial treatment regimen [6].

4.6 Emtricitabine

Similar to lamivudine, emtricitabine is a cytidine analog that has activity against HIV and hepatitis B infections. It was approved by the FDA for the treatment of HIV infections in 2003. Emtricitabine exists as a component of three fixed-dose combinations, namely Truvada (tenofovir and emtricitabine), Atripla (tenofovir, emtricitabine, and efavirenz), and Stribild (elvitegravir, cobicistat, tenofovir, and emtricitabine). These combinations are advantageous because they lower pill burden and simplify dosing regimens. Emtricitabine in its co-formulated form is part of most of the preferred regimens in treatment-naïve, HIV-infected patients [6].

Similar to most NRTIs, emtricitabine is phosphorylated intracellularly to emtricitabine triphosphate, which is present at high concentration and has a long half-life in peripheral blood mononuclear cells (PBMC) following 200 mg, once-daily dosing [29]. Further, HIV-1 RNA suppression was associated with emtricitabine triphosphate levels in these cells. In a 96-week safety and efficacy comparison of efavirenz with either emtricitabine/tenofovir or lamivudine/abacavir, there were no significant differences in virological failure and adverse events between the two regimens [30]. While patients on lamivudine/abacavir had greater increases in lipid profiles, patients on emtricitabine/tenofovir had greater decreases in bone density and increases in tubular dysfunction and bone turnover. In a different study, emtricitabine/tenofovir and lamivudine/abacavir both given with atazanavir/ritonavir had comparable efficacy and safety profiles in the Japanese population [31]. In general, emtricitabine is a well-tolerated and efficacious drug, recommended in combination with other ARVs.

4.7 Tenofovir

Tenofovir is a nucleotide reverse transcriptase inhibitor available for the treatment of HIV-1. Tenofovir disoproxil fumarate is cleaved by esterases to tenofovir, which is then phosphorylated intracellularly to tenofovir diphosphate. It was also approved for the treatment of hepatitis B. Used with emtricitabine, tenofovir is an essential component of all initial ARV regimens, irrespective of backbone.

In an interaction study between abacavir and tenofovir, treatment-naïve patients received 7 days of abacavir or tenofovir monotherapy, followed by a 35-day washout period and 7 days of abacavir plus tenofovir dual therapy [32]. The authors found that the slopes of viral decay were similar during dual therapy and abacavir monotherapy, leading the authors to conclude that the coadministration of these drugs has a non-additive antiviral effect.

The major safety concerns with tenofovir are lactic acidosis, severe hepatomegaly, and post-treatment exacerbation of hepatitis B infections [33]. The use of tenofovir has been associated with greater decreases in bone mineral density and increases in biochemical markers of bone metabolism, which suggest increased bone turnover. Serum parathyroid hormone and vitamin D concentrations were also elevated. Because tenofovir is renally eliminated, its use is accompanied with renal toxicity concerns. Cases of renal impairment such as renal failure and Fanconi syndrome have been observed in patients using tenofovir. Estimated creatinine clearance assessments are recommended prior to initiation of and during therapy with tenofovir. A similar compound, tenofovir alafenamide fumarate, has also been recently approved.

5 Non-nucleoside Reverse Transcriptase Inhibitors

Non-nucleoside reverse transcriptase inhibitors (NNRTIs) are important components of HAART with five NNRTIs currently approved for HIV treatment in the USA. Similar to NRTIs, these drugs inhibit the HIV reverse transcriptase, but unlike the NRTIs, they bind to a site distinct from the active site of the enzyme. NNRTIs have no activity against HIV-2 strains, or HIV-1 strains in group O, which are usually only found in West and Central Africa [34]. NNRTIs are also metabolized by the cytochrome P450 (CYP) system of enzymes, which they can inhibit or induce and therefore can affect other drugs that also use CYP enzymes. Glucuronidation of NNRTIs has also been reported. In general, NNRTIs are safe and well-tolerated. Notable adverse events include hepatotoxicity and severe rash with nevirapine, central nervous system effects with efavirenz. Most have a long plasma half-life, except for delavirdine, and are administered once daily. Because only a single mutation in the HIV reverse transcriptase enzyme is needed to create a resistant strain of the virus, NNRTIs are considered to have a low genetic barrier to resistance and cross-resistance. While resistance to second generation NNRTIs such as etravirine and rilpivirine can develop, they are rare and thus these agents have a higher genetic barrier to resistance and remain an important treatment option for patients with virologic failure.

5.1 Nevirapine

Nevirapine was the first NNRTI to be approved in the USA in 1996 for HIV-infected patients, 15 days and older [35]. With an oral bioavailability >90 %, nevirapine is widely distributed in tissues, including central nervous system and breast milk and can cross the placenta. It is administered at 200 mg once a day for the first 14 days of treatment, followed by 200 mg twice daily. This lead-in period has been shown to reduce the frequency of rash, which can be severe and life-threatening. Sex-related differences, such as elevated plasma concentration and lower clearance in women, and ethnicity-related differences, with higher drug concentrations in blacks compared to white patients, have been reported [35, 36]. Treatment with nevirapine is not recommended in adult women with CD4 cell counts >250 cell/mm^3 or adult men with CD4 cell counts >400 cells/mm^3 [35].

In an initial Phase I/II evaluation of nevirapine alone and in combination with zidovudine in 62 HIV-infected patients with CD4 counts <400 mm^3, suppression of p24 antigen and increase in CD4 cell counts were observed but by week 8, all patients developed resistance. The INCAS trial compared the virologic effects of various combinations of nevirapine, didanosine, and zidovudine in 151 HIV-infected, ARV-naïve patients who had a CD4 cell count of 200–600 cells/mm^3 at baseline [37]. At week 8, plasma HIV-1 RNA levels were decreased by log 2.18, 1.55, and 0.90 in the triple drug therapy, zidovudine plus didanosine, and zidovudine plus nevirapine groups, respectively. Further, the rates of disease progression or death were 12 % (6/51), 25 % (13/53), and 23 % (11/47) in the triple drug therapy, zidovudine plus didanosine, and zidovudine plus nevirapine groups, respectively. The authors concluded that the triple drug therapy containing nevirapine led to greater and sustained decrease in viral plasma load than the other drug combinations. In a subset of INCAS study patients ($n = 15$) who received at least 1 year of double or triple therapy, there was a statistically significant negative correlation between magnitude of treatment effect and plasma and lymph node viral load, suggesting that combinations of ARV drugs that decreased plasma viremia can also reduce viral load in lymphoid tissues [38].

BI 1090 was a large placebo-controlled, double-blind, randomized trial comparing nevirapine plus lamivudine to lamivudine only in 2249 HIV-infected, NNRTI-naïve patients. Patients had initial CD4 counts <200 cells/mm^3 (median count of 96 cells/mm^3) and also received background therapy. At 48 weeks, 18 % of patients receiving nevirapine had an HIV-1 RNA <50 copies/mL compared to 2 % in the placebo group [35, 39]. The group also compared nevirapine/zidovudine/lamivudine to zidovudine/lamivudine/placebo regimens and found that after 1 year, 45 % of patients on the nevirapine arm had plasma viral load <50 copies/mL compared to 3 % in the placebo group [39]. Other clinical trials such as the Spanish efavirenz versus nevirapine comparison

(SENC) and Atlantic also found that nevirapine-containing regimens had good virological and immunological responses. The 2NN study compared various doses of nevirapine alone, efavirenz alone, or nevirapine plus efavirenz in 1216 ARV-naïve, HIV-infected patients who also received stavudine and lamivudine. The authors found that there were no significant differences between study groups, with regard to the proportions achieving plasma viral load of <50 copies/mL or increases in CD4 cell count [40]. Two of the 25 deaths during the trial were attributed to nevirapine. Overall, the authors found that ARV regimens that contained nevirapine or efavirenz had similar efficacy and that combining nevirapine with efavirenz led to more adverse events [40].

5.2 Delavirdine

Delavirdine was approved in the USA in 1998 but is now rarely used. Unlike nevirapine and efavirenz, delavirdine does not induce CYP but has been shown to inhibit CYP3A4, and can therefore enhance the pharmacokinetics of protease inhibitors, which are all metabolized by CYP3A4.

Delavirdine has been shown to have a mean half maximal inhibitory concentration (IC_{50}) of 0.038 μmol/L, and in vitro had an additive or synergistic ARV activity when combined with zidovudine, didanosine, lamivudine, or zalcitabine. Several trials evaluated the efficacy and safety of delavirdine. Similar to the nevirapine studies, delavirdine had superior virological responses when used in a triple-drug regimen compared to a dual-drug regimen. Protocol 0021 showed that at week 24, 61 % of patients who received the triple-drug combination had plasma viral load <40 copies/mL compared with only 3 and 9 % of patients who received zidovudine plus delavirdine and zidovudine plus lamivudine, respectively [41]. Similar results were seen at week 52. The ACTG 370 trial compared the virologic activity of continued lamivudine versus delavirdine switching when initiating protease inhibitor therapy in lamivudine experienced, HIV infected patients [42]. At week 48, 77 % of patients had achieved plasma viral load <50 copies/mL when on the delavirdine/zidovudine/indinavir regimen. This was significantly higher than the lamivudine/zidovudine/indinavir group (39 %, $p=0.005$). While both groups had considerable increases in CD4 cell counts, there were no statistically differences in this outcome between the two groups. The better virologic suppression in the delavirdine arm can be attributed to the enhanced pharmacokinetics of indinavir in the presence of delavirdine [42]. A prospective, randomized 2×3 factorial study by ACTG 359 compared saquinavir with ritonavir or nelfinavir together with delavirdine, adefovir (a drug originally developed as an ARV but now only approved for hepatitis infections) or both in HIV infected adults, who experienced virologic failure on indinavir [43]. At week 16, 40 % (34/85) of patients in the pooled delavirdine groups had plasma viral load ≤500 copies/mL compared to

18 % (16/88) of patients in the pooled adefovir groups and 33 % (27/81) of patients in the pooled delavirdine plus adefovir groups. The authors concluded that adefovir decreased the systemic concentrations of saquinavir and delavirdine, leading to inferior virological effect in patients receiving adefovir (with and without delavirdine) [43]. On the other hand, the superior virological effect seen in patients receiving delavirdine without adefovir could be attributed to the use of a new class of ARV drug and pharmacokinetic enhancement of PIs by delavirdine [43].

5.3 Efavirenz

Efavirenz was approved in the USA in 1998 and is the preferred NNRTI-based regimen, with tenofovir and emtricitabine in an FDC [6]. In HIV-infected patients at steady-state, pharmacokinetic parameters are dose proportional for 200, 400, and 600 mg efavirenz doses. However, C_{max} and AUC were less than proportional at the 1600 mg efavirenz dose, suggesting reduced absorption at higher doses. The median plasma efavirenz concentration has been reported to be higher in women that in men; however, these changes were not clinically relevant and dose adjustments based on gender are not needed. More recently, pharmacogenetic variations were suggested to be partly responsible for differences in efavirenz pharmacokinetics between HIV infected patients in Tanzania and Ethiopia [44].

The antiviral activity of efavirenz, in combination with indinavir or NRTIs has been investigated in 450 HIV-infected individuals [45]. Patients received efavirenz (600 mg once daily) plus zidovudine (300 mg twice daily) and lamivudine (150 mg twice daily), indinavir (800 mg every 8 h) plus zidovudine and lamivudine, or efavirenz plus indinavir (1000 mg every 8 h). The authors found that at 48 weeks, 70 % of patients who received efavirenz/NRTIs achieved a plasma viral load of <400 copies/mL compared to 48 % in the indinavir/NRTIs group [45]. Similarly, at week 48, a significantly higher number of patients on the efavirenz/NRTIs regimen achieved HIV-1 RNA levels <50 copies/mL compared to patients who received the indinavir/NRTIs regimen (90 % versus 75 %, $p < 0.05$). CD4 cell counts were increased across all regimens without any significant difference among the groups. In a study of 1147 HIV-infected, treatment-naïve subjects, three regimens were compared: zidovudine/lamivudine/abacavir, zidovudine/lamivudine/efavirenz, and zidovudine/lamivudine/abacavir/efavirenz [46]. The group found that more patients in the NRTI group had protocol-defined virologic failure compared to patients in the combined efavirenz group (21 % versus 11 %). Further, the time to virologic failure was significantly shorter in the NRTI group and the authors concluded that in treatment-naïve patients, the abacavir/zidovudine/lamivudine regimen was virologically inferior to the efavirenz regimens [46].

5.4 Etravirine

Considered a second-generation NNRTI because it is structurally different from the other agents in this class, etravirine has limited cross-resistance as it retains activity against HIV-1 isolates with K103N and Y181C mutations, which confer resistance to efavirenz and nevirapine, respectively. Etravirine is indicated for the treatment of HIV-1 infection in treatment-experienced patients 6 years and older with viral strains resistant to an NNRTI and other ARV drugs. In adults, it is administered at 200 mg twice daily. Weight based dosing not exceeding the adult dose is recommended for pediatric patients.

The effect of etravirine exposure on virologic and immunologic responses were evaluated in HIV-infected, treatment-experienced patients enrolled in two Phase III clinical trials [47]. The pharmacodynamic model identified baseline CD4 count, fold change in viral susceptibility to darunavir and etravirine, baseline viral load, phenotypic sensitivity score, adherence, and use of enfuvirtide as predictors of virologic response. However, pharmacokinetic exposure parameters for etravirine and darunavir were not prognostic factors for virologic response, and since their trials did not identify a relationship between the pharmacokinetics of etravirine and either efficacy or safety, the use of therapeutic drug monitoring (TDM) is not warranted [47]. In the GRACE trial, the pharmacodynamics of darunavir and etravirine in HIV-infected, treatment-experienced adults was evaluated [48]. Gender or race did not affect etravirine or darunavir exposures [48]. The group reported that patients with etravirine AUC_{0-12} and trough concentration (C_{trough}) in the lowest quartiles had the smallest change in viral load and the lowest response rates compared with the other pharmacokinetic quartiles. Again, no relevant relationships were found between etravirine pharmacokinetic parameters and safety. Similar results were seen in the SENSE trial, which evaluated the pharmacodynamics of etravirine administered at 400 mg once daily to treatment-naïve, HIV-infected adults [49].

5.5 Rilpivirine

Rilpivirine is the latest NNRTI drug developed and was approved in the USA in 2011. It is also available as a co-formulated pill, with tenofovir and emtricitabine (Complera®). It is indicated for the treatment of HIV-infected treatment adults with HIV-1 RNA ≤100,000 copies/mL. Severe depressive disorders and hepatic adverse events have been reported, although most cases of hepatic events were in patients with underlying liver disease, such as hepatitis B or C coinfection [50].

Two Phase II trials, ECHO and THRIVE, compared efficacy of rilpivirine (25 mg once daily) to efavirenz (600 mg once daily) in treatment-naïve adults who also received two NRTIs [50, 51]. At 48 and 96 weeks, the rilpivirine arm was noninferior to the efavirenz arm. However, higher rates of virologic failure were observed in patients taking rilpivirine [51–53]. In patients with viral load

≤100,000 copies/mL, rilpivirine and efavirenz had similar antiviral efficacy [50, 54], with similar frequencies of virological failure and NRTI resistance-associated mutations in both arms [54]. These findings support the indication of rilpivirine in patients with HIV-1 RNA ≤100,000 copies/mL [50].

6 Protease Inhibitors

PIs inhibit the HIV protease enzyme by mimicking the natural substrate and binding to the active site of the enzyme. CYPs, in particular hepatic CYP3A4, are responsible for the metabolism of all PIs. Intestinal enterocytes express CYP3A4 and P-glycoprotein, which decrease the oral bioavailability of PIs [55–57]. Pharmacokinetic enhancement of PIs, where ritonavir or cobicistat is administered to increase PI drug concentration to improve the low oral bioavailability, decrease pill burden, alleviate strict dietary restrictions, and avoid low plasma trough concentrations, which are all limitations of PI therapy. Ritonavir was introduced to the market in 1996 as a protease inhibitor but was shown to be a potent CYP3A4 inhibitor, and quickly became the most common boosting agent used in ARV therapy. As a boosting agent, ritonavir is used at low doses, which reduce the risk of ritonavir-associated adverse side effects. Cobicistat is a potent and specific inhibitor of CYP3A [58] and has been shown to inhibit intestinal P-glycoprotein in vitro [59]. Unlike ritonavir, cobicistat does not have any ARV activity and acts solely as a pharmacokinetic enhancer. Cobicistat is approved in Europe and in the US as Stribild and Genvoya. Co-formulations of cobicistat-PIs are under investigation.

In a 20-month follow-up study, predictors of virological rebound in HIV-1 infected patients receiving PI regimens were found to include previous ARV treatment, CD4 cell count $<500 \times 10^6$/L, higher viral load baseline, low adherence, and discontinuation of therapy at 4 months [60]. While young age was also found to predict virological rebound [60, 61], more work is needed to fully understand the relationship between age and virological outcome.

6.1 Saquinavir

Saquinavir, as a hard-gel capsule (Invirase) was the first PI to be approved by the FDA in 1995. A soft-gel capsule (Fortovase) with improved bioavailability compared to the hard gel capsule was approved shortly after. However, the soft-gel capsule was discontinued and saquinavir is now only available as the hard-gel capsule to be coadministered with ritonavir.

In early clinical trials, the efficacy of high-dose saquinavir monotherapy was investigated in 40 HIV-infected adults, who received either 3600 or 7200 mg saquinavir per day for 24 weeks [62]. The authors found that patients receiving high-dose saquinavir had a greater decrease in plasma HIV RNA levels and a greater increase in CD4 cell counts than the low-dose group. Further, a correlation between higher saquinavir exposure and greater reduction in plasma HIV RNA was found. With only four patients (20 %) developing resistance to saquinavir in the high-dose group, the authors concluded that higher doses of saquinavir should be further investigated. However, with the advent of ritonavir-boosting, high-dose saquinavir can be avoided. In a heterogeneous population (42 treatment-naïve and 106 treatment-experienced), HIV-infected individuals received saquinavir/ritonavir 1000/100 mg twice daily and 61 % of patients had HIV RNA levels <400 copies/mL at week 48 [63]. The recommended dose of saquinavir is 1000 mg twice daily in combination with ritonavir, 100 mg twice daily.

The safety and efficacy of saquinavir as part of a five-drug regimen were studied in HIV infected adults who had failed on conventional triple ARV therapy [64]. When saquinavir, ritonavir, and efavirenz were added to the two NRTIs, a significant increase in CD4 cell counts and a sustained reduction in plasma HIV RNA were observed at week 24. Further, the authors suggested that outcome of salvage therapy might be better predicted by measuring phenotypic resistance instead of resistance mutations.

6.2 Nelfinavir

Approved in 1997 by the FDA, nelfinavir is indicated for patients as young as 2 years old. It is metabolized by CYP3A and CYP2C19, and can inhibit CYP3A. While the AUC of nelfinavir and its metabolite were increased in the presence of low-dose ritonavir [65, 66], the safety and efficacy of a ritonavir-boosted nelfinavir regimen have not been studied and therefore nelfinavir is the one PI not used with ritonavir enhancement. Nelfinavir's metabolite also has antiretroviral activity and therefore ritonavir boosting may not be needed.

In a monotherapy study in HIV-infected, PI-naïve men, nelfinavir was shown to be efficacious [67]. Patients received nelfinavir at either 300 mg three times a day ($n = 10$) or 600 mg twice a day ($n = 10$). Amongst patients who had a reduction in plasma HIV RNA of at least 1 log during the 28-day study time, a dose–response relationship was observed in four and six patients receiving the 300 mg and the 600 mg doses, respectively. This was sustained in five patients past the 28 days. Over longer periods of time (8–15 months), virologic responses were sustained in six patients.

In the dose-ranging Agouron 511 study, ARV-naïve, HIV-infected patients ($n = 297$) received nelfinavir at 750 mg, 500 mg, or placebo, three times daily in addition to zidovudine and lamivudine [68]. At week 24, plasma viral load <50 copies/mL was achieved in 55 % and 30 % of patients receiving 750 mg and 500 mg, respectively. This was further sustained for an additional 6 months, in 61 % and 37 % of patients receiving 750 mg and 500 mg, respectively, indicating that the higher dose was better.

Increases in CD4 cell counts were greater among patients receiving nelfinavir triple therapy than zidovudine plus lamivudine, indicating superiority of nelfinavir plus zidovudine and lamivudine to placebo plus zidovudine and lamivudine. This supports the recommended dose of nelfinavir, 750 mg three times a day [65]. Nelfinavir can also be administered at 1250 mg twice a day.

The efficacy of nelfinavir in combination regimens has also been shown with a comparison between fosamprenavir/ritonavir (once daily) and nelfinavir (twice daily), in a background of abacavir and lamivudine. At week 48, similar number of patients had HIV RNA <50 copies/mL (55 % fosamprenavir and 53 % nelfinavir). However, more patients in the nelfinavir group experienced virological failure (17 % versus 7 %) [69]. Another study showed that compared to patients who received lopinavir/ritonavir plus stavudine and lamivudine, ARV-naïve patients receiving nelfinavir plus stavudine and lamivudine had a higher risk of losing virologic response ($p < 0.001$), which was associated with higher baseline viral load and CD4 counts [70].

6.3 Indinavir

Indinavir (Crixivan) is administered at 800 mg every 8 h for the treatment of HIV. Since high-fat meals reduce and delay absorption [71], administration of indinavir is recommended with lighter meals [72]. In a comparative study of five initial PI-containing and nevirapine containing regimens, 63 % of patients ($n = 690$), achieved an undetectable viral load within 5 months of starting treatment with saquinavir, indinavir, nelfinavir, ritonavir, saquinavir plus ritonavir, or nevirapine [73]. Relative to saquinavir, viral load rebound and CD4 cell count responses were similar between all groups. Prior NRTI exposure was associated with viral load rebound and lower baseline viral load and CD4 cell count were associated with reduced CD4 response. Further, saquinavir was found to be inferior to the other regimens, while the use of nelfinavir and indinavir was associated with the highest rates of achieving an undetectable viral load.

In a prospective study of 59 HIV-infected, treatment-experienced adults who were started on a salvage regimen with two NRTIs plus indinavir/ritonavir, 61 % of patients had a decrease in viral load with 38 % of patients achieving HIV RNA <50 copies/mL after 24 weeks [74], indicating that ritonavir/indinavir 100/800 mg twice daily could elicit a significant virologic response in patients with ARV treatment failure. This was also shown by Campo et al., who suggested that indinavir/ritonavir regimens could overcome indinavir resistance [75]. Although patients receiving indinavir/ritonavir are at a higher risk for nephrolithiasis compared to unboosted indinavir [72], indinavir/ritonavir (400/100 mg twice daily) is an important component of ARV, especially in resource-limited settings [76].

6.4 Lopinavir

An understanding of the acquisition of ritonavir-resistance mutations led to the development lopinavir, which interacts differently with the HIV protease enzyme than ritonavir and is thus active against ritonavir-resistant strains of HIV-1. Today, lopinavir is available as a co-formulated pill with ritonavir, known as Kaletra. The efficacy of lopinavir/ritonavir monotherapy for maintenance of HIV suppression has been shown. After 4 years of treatment, 67 % of patients (14/21) maintained HIV RNA <50 copies/mL [77]. Five patients had virological rebound, which was resolved by the addition of two nucleosides. In a larger study ($n = 197$), 95 % and 82.3 % of patients maintained virological success at 48 and 96 weeks [78], respectively, further supporting the use of lopinavir/ritonavir monotherapy as a maintenance regimen.

Lopinavir is highly protein bound and since only unbound drug can exert a pharmacological action, the link between total and free lopinavir exposure and pharmacodynamics has been assessed. A pharmacokinetic–pharmacodynamic model was developed using data from 35 treatment-naïve patients who received lopinavir/ritonavir 400/100 mg twice daily [79]. This novel model-based approach enabled a more accurate determination of viral dynamic parameters such as C_{trough} values for the effective concentration at 90 % (EC_{90}) and effective concentration at 95 % (EC_{95}) and virion clearance rate.

6.5 Atazanavir

Atazanavir is a PI used in treatment-naïve and -experienced individuals with HIV-1 infection. Atazanavir is approved at 400 mg once daily, and the recommended dose of atazanavir/ritonavir is 300/100 mg once daily in both treatment-naïve and -experienced patients. Atazanavir/ritonavir plus tenofovir and emtricitabine is an alternative PI-based regimen in the USA (https://aidsinfo.nih.gov/contentfiles/lvguidelines/AdultandAdolescentGL.pdf). However, it is not recommended for patients who require >20 mg omeprazole per day.

The pharmacokinetics and pharmacodynamics of atazanavir with and without ritonavir were investigated in 200 HIV-infected, treatment-naïve patients [80]. Atazanavir C_{trough} was five times greater in the presence of ritonavir and the C_{trough} values of HIV EC_{90} were achieved in 98 % and 100 % of patients on atazanavir (400 mg) and atazanavir/ritonavir (300/100 mg), respectively. The authors also found that atazanavir C_{trough} was associated with low HIV RNA but not with changes in CD4 cell count at week 48. Moreover, higher atazanavir C_{trough} was associated with increases in total bilirubin or jaundice, and modest increases in lipids were observed in the ritonavir group. Using logistic regression, the relationship between unboosted atazanavir pharmacokinetics and clinical outcome was studied in HIV-infected, treatment-experienced adults [81]. Seven ($n = 58$) patients, who had been identified as low absorbers, experienced virologic failure. Further, absorption rate and atazanavir C_{trough} were significant predictors of virologic failure, suggesting that in this population twice daily administration of unboosted atazanavir may be warranted.

6.6 Fosamprenavir

Fosamprenavir is the calcium phosphate ester prodrug of amprenavir, a PI that was discontinued due to the large capsule size, high pill burden, and complicated excipient requirements. Fosamprenavir is converted to amprenavir following ingestion [82, 83] and can be administered with or without ritonavir [84]. The efficacy of fosamprenavir with and without ritonavir has been studied. In the TRIAD study, HIV-infected patients who had virologic failure with PI regimens, received fosamprenavir/ritonavir (700/100 mg twice daily, $n=24$), fosamprenavir/ritonavir (1400/100 mg twice daily, $n=25$), or fosamprenavir/lopinavir/ritonavir (1400/533/133 mg twice daily, $n=25$) [85]. At week 24, a similar number of patients from each regimen achieved HIV RNA <50 copies/mL and the high-dose fosamprenavir regimen was not superior to the standard dose (700/100 mg twice daily) in this population. However, the authors found that lower baseline background drug resistance and higher fosamprenavir genotypic inhibitory quotient was associated with better antiviral responses. Nonetheless, fosamprenavir/ritonavir can be used in salvage therapy as shown by the sustained rate of virologic and immunologic responses at week 96 in the study by Quercia et al. [86].

6.7 Tipranavir

Tipranavir is a potent, non-peptidic PI that was approved by the FDA in 2005. Tipranavir has been shown to be active against HIV mutants that were resistant to other PIs, indicating a lack of PI cross-resistance to tipranavir [87–89]. In a 14-day trial, treatment-naïve patients received tipranavir (1200 mg twice daily) or tipranavir/ritonavir (300/200 mg or 1200/200 mg twice daily) [90]. The group receiving tipranavir/ritonavir at 1200/200 mg had the largest drop in viral load with a 70-fold increase in tipranavir exposure (compared to unboosted tipranavir), indicating that boosted tipranavir was effective. Similar results were also observed in treatment-experienced patients who received one of three dose combinations of tipranavir/ritonavir in addition to ARV regimens containing nevirapine, efavirenz, lamivudine, stavudine, or didanosine [91]. Following the addition of tipranavir/ritonavir, more patients achieved an HIV RNA <50 copies/mL (67.6 % compared to 40.4 %). Further, the long-term efficacy of boosted tipranavir in patients failing multiple PI regimens has also been reported [92].

6.8 Darunavir

Darunavir, the latest addition to the PIs, is approved for the treatment of HIV in combination with low-dose ritonavir. It is indicated for treatment-naïve and -experienced adults with no darunavir resistance mutation at 800 mg with ritonavir 100 mg once daily with food. Patients with at least one darunavir resistance mutation receive 600 mg with ritonavir 100 mg twice daily with food. Once daily darunavir/ritonavir plus tenofovir and emtricitabine is a preferred PI-based regimen in the USA [6].

When darunavir/ritonavir (800/100 mg) was compared to lopinavir/ritonavir (800/200 mg) in the ARTEMIS trial, a similar number of patients achieved HIV-1 RNA <50 copies/mL in both arms, although fewer discontinuations were seen in the darunavir/ritonavir group [93, 94]. Moreover, earlier 96-week ARTEMIS results showed that virologic response rates to darunavir/ritonavir were similar across different genders, age groups, races, and coinfection status in treatment-naïve patients [95]. In treatment-experienced patients, 39 % of patients who received darunavir/ritonavir 600/100 mg twice daily achieved HIV-1 RNA <50 copies/mL compared to 9 % of patients who received investigator-selected control PI at week 96, indicating that twice daily darunavir/ritonavir was appropriate for this population [96]. Analysis of a subgroup of this trial at week 24 showed that virologic response to darunavir was decreased when the fold change in half maximal effective concentration (EC_{50}) to darunavir at baseline was >40, or when three or more darunavir resistance-associated mutations, in addition to other PI mutations, were present [97].

7 Integrase Strand Transfer Inhibitors

The HIV-1 integrase enzyme catalyzes the insertion of viral DNA into the genome of the host cell, which is an essential step in the viral life cycle. While many inhibitors of the integrase enzyme were discovered, few had antiviral activity in cells and today, only three inhibitors are on the market. S/GSK1265744 is currently under development as a long acting inhibitor that would be administered monthly or quarterly. Overall, integrase inhibitors have potent HIV-1 activity with less drug interactions compared to NNRTIs and PIs.

7.1 Raltegravir

Raltegravir was the first integrase inhibitor approved by the FDA in 2007 in combination with other ARV drugs for the treatment of HIV-infected adults. In 2011, raltegravir was also approved for use in children and adolescents, ages 2–18 years [98] and additional studies in the pediatric population, especially in children less than 2 years of age, are ongoing. Raltegravir, in combination with tenofovir and emtricitabine is one of the preferred regiments in treatment-naïve patients [6]. Raltegravir, available as a 400 mg film-coated tablet, is administered orally twice daily. Raltegravir has been shown to be potent, with an in vitro 95 % inhibitory concentration (IC_{95}) of 33 nM (0.014 mg/L) in 50 % human serum [99] and an apparent in vitro 50 % inhibitory concentration (IC_{50}) of 2–7 nM (0.0008–0.003 mg/L)[100]. This compound is effective against both wild-type and multidrug-resistant HIV-1 (isolates resistant to protease inhibitors, nucleoside reverse transcriptase inhibitors and non-nucleoside reverse transcriptase) and in both treatment-naïve and treatment-experienced HIV infected adults [99, 100]. Raltegravir is primarily metabolized by uridine diphosphate (UDP)-glucuronosyltransferase (UGT) 1A1 and does not induce or inhibit CYP enzymes. In patients who receive rifampin, an antituberculosis drug, and raltegravir, the recommended dose of raltegravir is 800 mg twice daily, due to the UGT1A1 inducing properties of rifampin that leads to decreased raltegravir exposures.

The pharmacokinetics and pharmacodynamics of once-daily raltegravir were compared to the twice-daily dose in treatment-naïve patients in a Phase III clinical trial, QDMRK. At 48 weeks, the authors found that daily exposures, measured as AUC_{0-24}, were similar in both arms [101]. However, patients on the 800 mg once daily regimen had higher C_{max} and lower C_{trough} values compared to patients on the 400 mg twice daily arm [101]. Virologic response (HIV-1 RNA <50 copies/mL) was seen in 83 % and 87 % of patients receiving the once daily and twice daily regimen, respectively [102]. The authors concluded that although both regimens had high response rates, once-daily dosing of raltegravir is not recommended over twice-daily dosing. While there was no significant pharmacokinetic/pharmacodynamics association over the range of tested pharmacokinetic parameters in the twice daily arm, the authors found that virologic failure was associated with high baseline viral load and lower C_{trough} values in the once daily arm [101]. Similar results were seen in a sub-study of ANRS 139 TRIO trial, which evaluated virological outcome in highly treatment-experienced patients receiving raltegravir (400 mg twice daily), etravirine (200 mg twice daily), and darunavir/ritonavir (600/100 twice daily) [103]. The authors found that patients with virologic success ($n = 61$) had a baseline median HIV-1 DNA of 2.34 $\log_{10}$ copies/10^6 PBMC compared to 2.68 in patients with virologic failure ($n = 11$), which suggested that baseline HIV-1 DNA might predict virological response [103].

The efficacy of raltegravir (400 mg twice daily) was compared to efavirenz (600 mg once daily) in treatment-naïve patients, who had HIV-1 RNA >5000 copies/mL and also received tenofovir and emtricitabine in the STARTMRK trial [104]. At week 156, 75.4 % of patients on raltegravir had viral loads <50 copies/mL compared to 68.1 % of patients in the efavirenz arm [104]. There was a greater increase in CD4 cell counts in patients in the raltegravir arm compared to the efavirenz arm (332 versus 295 cells/mm^3) and the authors conclude that through 156 weeks, raltegravir was at least equivalent to efavirenz, with respect to viral suppression and immune restoration [104]. Similarly, Protocol 004 showed that at week 240, 68.8 % of patients (raltegravir, 400 mg twice daily) had HIV-1 RNA <50 copies/mL compared to 63.2 % of patients receiving efavirenz [105].

Nucleoside-sparing regimens plus raltegravir have been evaluated. In the SPARTAN study, the efficacy, safety, and resistance profile of atazanavir (300 mg twice daily) plus raltegravir (400 mg twice daily) was compared to atazanavir/ritonavir (300/100 mg once daily) plus tenofovir/emtricitabine (300/200 mg once daily). Viral load <50 copies/mL was achieved in 74.6 % of patients in the raltegravir arm compared to 63.3 % in the non-raltegravir arm. The authors noted higher systemic exposure of atazanavir and higher incidence of grade 4 hyperbilirubinemia in the raltegravir-containing arm [106]. Six patients (out of 63) were considered to experience virologic failure on the raltegravir arm, and four of these had developed resistance to raltegravir. In contrast, only 1 patient (out of 30) in the non-raltegravir treatment had virologic failure. Based on the observed resistance and adverse events results, the authors concluded that an atazanavir plus raltegravir regimen was not optimal. ACTG A5262 evaluated darunavir/ritonavir (800/100 mg once daily) plus raltegravir (400 mg twice daily) in treatment-naïve patients [107]. By week 48, virologic failure was seen in 26 % of patients which was associated with baseline viral load >100,000 copies/mL and a lower baseline CD4 cell count [107]. The KITE study evaluated the efficacy and safety of switching patients from standard ARV care to a reverse transcriptase sparing combination of lopinavir/ritonavir plus raltegravir in HIV-infected patients with plasma viral load <50 copies/mL [108]. At week 48, 92 % and 88 % remained virologically suppressed while on the raltegravir and standard care regimens, respectively, and no differences in CD4 cell counts were observed between the two arms [108]. Similarly, switching from an enfuvirtide-based regimen to a raltegravir-based regimen was generally well tolerated and patients with multidrug resistance had sustained antiviral activity [109].

7.2 Elvitegravir

Elvitegravir was approved by the FDA in 2012 as a co-formulated product with cobicistat, tenofovir, and emtricitabine for treatment-naïve patients. This FDC is not recommended in patients with a creatinine clearance of <70 mL/min. Elvitegravir is metabolized by CYP3A4 and because ritonavir and cobicistat can inhibit CYP3A4, these agents can boost elvitegravir exposures.

A Phase III clinical trial compared the elvitegravir FDC to efavirenz plus emtricitabine and tenofovir (also as an FDC) in treatment-naïve patients and found at week 48, 87.6 % of patients on the elvitegravir FDC had HIV RNA concentrations <50 copies/mL compared to 84.1 % of patients on the efavirenz FDC, suggesting noninferiority [110]. Similar efficacy results were seen by Cohen et al., who also reported fewer central nervous system and psychiatric events in patients using the elvitegravir FDC compared to the efavirenz FDC [111]. A Phase III study compared the elvitegravir FDC to atazanavir/ritonavir plus tenofovir and emtricitabine and did not find a statistical difference in RNA suppression between the two arms and the authors concluded that the elvitegravir FDC was noninferior to the atazanavir regimen [112].

The efficacy and safety of elvitegravir (150 mg once daily; 85 mg if given with atazanavir or ritonavir/lopinavir) were compared to raltegravir (400 mg twice daily) in a ritonavir-boosted PI backbone in treatment-experienced patients [113]. Similar virologic response (HIV-1 RNA <50 copies/mL) were observed in both arms, suggesting noninferiority. Three elvitegravir patients had serious events (seven in the raltegravir arm), with two elvitegravir patient deaths (eight in the raltegravir arm). Because of the similar efficacy profiles, the authors suggested that elvitegravir use may improve patients' adherence since elvitegravir can be given once daily whereas raltegravir requires twice daily dosing.

7.3 Dolutegravir

Dolutegravir is the latest addition to this drug class and was approved by the FDA in 2013. A second generation integrase inhibitor, dolutegravir is primarily metabolized by UGT1A1 and is not considered an inhibitor or inducer of CYP3A [114]. While patients who are resistant to elvitegravir also have raltegravir resistance [115], dolutegravir has limited cross-resistance with raltegravir [116–118].

The SPRING-1 trial was a dose ranging study of dolutegravir (10, 25 or 50 mg once daily) compared to efavirenz (600 mg once daily) in combination with two NRTIs in treatment-naïve patients [119]. At 96 weeks, the 50 mg dose of dolutegravir led to the highest proportion of patients with virological success (HIV RNA <50 copies/mL). Further, more patients receiving dolutegravir (including the lowest dose) achieved virological success compared to patients receiving efavirenz [119]. The SPRING-2 trial compared dolutegravir (50 mg once daily) to raltegravir (400 mg twice daily) in an NRTI background, in treatment-naïve, HIV-infected adults [120]. Similar viral suppression (81 % on dolutegravir and 76 % on raltegravir) and restoration of CD4 cell counts between the two regimens indicated that dolutegravir was noninferior to raltegravir at week 96 [120]. At week 48 of the SINGLE trial, a significantly higher proportion of treatment-naïve patients who received dolutegravir, abacavir, and lamivudine achieved virologic success compared to patients who received efavirenz, tenofovir, and emtricitabine [121]. The dolutegravir arm had a shorter median time to viral suppression than the efavirenz arm (28 versus 84 days, $p<0.001$) and greater increases in CD4 cell counts ($p<0.001$). While rash and neuropsychiatric events were more common in the efavirenz group, insomnia was more common in the dolutegravir group. Taken together, these data indicated that the dolutegravir regimen was superior to the efavirenz regimen. Similar results supporting the superiority of dolutegravir regimens were described in the SAILING trial, where once daily dolutegravir with investigator selected background therapy had a greater virological effect compared twice daily raltegravir in treatment-experienced adults [122]. In a cohort of patients with documented raltegravir resistance, week 24 data showed that dolutegravir at 50 mg twice daily had a greater virologic effect than at 50 mg once daily, demonstrating the lack of cross-resistance between dolutegravir and raltegravir [117]. To further confirm the results, the VIKING-3 study was designed and enrolled patients with documented raltegravir and/or elvitegravir resistance. Multivariate analyses showed that response (day 8) was affected by baseline HIV-1 RNA, dolutegravir phenotype, integrase inhibitor genotype, and pre-dose dolutegravir concentration (day 8) [118]. For week 24 response, baseline genotypic or phenotypic integrase inhibitor resistance and viral load but not pre-dose dolutegravir concentrations were significant prognostic factors.

8 Fusion Inhibitor

Enfuvirtide (T20) is a synthetic peptide that mimics the second heptad repeat (HR)-2 sequence of gp41 [123]. Enfuvirtide binds to HR-1, thereby blocking the formation of a six-helix bundle, which is essential for viral fusion to the host cell [124]. Enfuvirtide is indicated for the treatment of HIV infection in treatment-experienced patients. It is administered as a subcutaneous injection in the upper arm, anterior thigh, or abdomen, twice daily at a recommended adult dose of 90 mg [123]. Enfuvirtide resistance has been shown to appear within the first 14 days of treatment in four patients who received an intermediate dose of 30 mg twice a day [125] and mutations were most common in the HR-1 domain of the gp41 gene, between codons 38 and 45 [126].

A four-way crossover study in 12 HIV-infected patients, who received four single doses of enfuvirtide showed that an inverse Gaussian density function-input model linked to a two-compartment open distribution model with first-order elimination from the central compartment was found to best describe the pharmacokinetics of this drug [127]. Enfuvirtide has been shown to have a dose-related antiviral response with a maximal antiviral effect using the 90 mg twice daily dose [128–132]. Using data from two Phase III clinical trials, the relationship between pharmacokinetic exposure and plasma HIV-1 RNA levels in treatment-experienced, HIV-infected patients was investigated [133]. At week 24, the AUC_{0-12} and C_{max} were comparable between responders and nonresponders, an effect that was independent on the phenotypic sensitivity score, which is a measure of the number of drugs to which the virus is sensitive. These results indicated that virologic failure was not related to low enfuvirtide exposure. Further, using an empiric 2-parameter maximum effect (E_{max}) model to describe the exposure–response relationship of enfuvirtide, the authors found that when the E_{max} model used AUC_{0-12} as exposure, the model predicted that at week 24, the 90 mg twice-daily dose achieved 73 % and 92 % of maximal effect in patients with functional monotherapy and combination therapy, respectively. These results were similar when the model used C_{trough} as a measure of exposure. No difference in treatment efficacy was seen between males and females and the AUC_{0-12} was not related to the frequency of adverse events [133]. In a pediatric study, a population viral pharmacodynamics model was built but no statistically significant relationship was seen between pharmacokinetic-based exposure measure and virologic response measure [134].

9 Entry Inhibitor

Maraviroc is the only member in the entry inhibitor class of drugs and was approved in the USA and Europe in 2007. Maraviroc selectively and reversibly binds to the host cell CCR5 receptor, which is also the binding partner of viral gp120 and thus HIV cannot bind to and enter T-cells. Because HIV can use another receptor, CXCR4, to enter the cell, a HIV tropism test is needed prior to initiating maraviroc therapy.

The MOTIVATE 1 and 2 studies evaluated the safety and efficacy of maraviroc or placebo in treatment-experienced adults who were also receiving an optimized background regimen. At week 96, 39 % of patients who received maraviroc 300 mg once daily had viral load <50 copies/mL compared 41 % of patients (maraviroc 150 mg twice daily) [135]. While increased CD4 counts were seen with both once daily and twice daily regimens, these increases were significant between patients who received maraviroc compared to those who receive placebo. The authors concluded that maraviroc-containing regimens maintained durable responses in the population studied through 96 weeks of treatment. In a subgroup multivariate analysis of the MOTIVATE trials, race (or ethnic group), clade, viral load at screening, baseline CD4 cell count, overall susceptibility score, and first use of enfuvirtide were associated with virologic response at week 48 [136]. In the subgroup analyses, changes in viral tropism were investigated. In patients with mixed tropism, the rate of virologic suppression was greater in the maraviroc arm than in the placebo arm. Further, the median time to failure of twice-daily maraviroc was 98 days in CXCR4 patients compared to 149 days in CCR5 patients. Data from the MOTIVATE studies were also used to assess exposure–response relationship using a generalized additive model. The authors found that treatment success was associated with maraviroc treatment, high-weighted overall susceptibility to background treatment, absence of an undetectable maraviroc concentration (measure of adherence), high CD4 count at baseline, low viral load, race, absence of non-R5 baseline tropism, and absence of fosamprenavir. The authors also concluded that the doses of maraviroc used in the MOTIVATE studies produced concentrations high on the concentration–response curve and thus no concentration–response relationships were found after prognostic factors were taken into account [137].

10 Therapeutic Drug Monitoring

Therapeutic drug monitoring (TDM) of ARV, which is the adjustment of a patient's dosage regimen based on in vivo drug concentration, is a practice that is increasingly being used, especially in the USA and Europe, even though its clinical utility is debatable. As such, TDM of ARV agents is not recommended for routine use [6], largely because of the lack of evidence showing that TDM improves clinical and virologic outcomes. The characteristics of drugs amenable to TDM are summarized in Table 3.

Understanding the relationship between drug exposure or concentration and viral and immunological outcomes is essential in guiding TDM use in HIV-infected individuals. For most ARVs, sensitive and specific assays are available for detection of plasma

Table 3
Characteristics of drugs applicable to therapeutic drug monitoring (taken from Acosta el al., CID 2000)

Pharmacological
Pharmacokinetic data concerning the drug are available
Plasma concentration of the drug reflects the concentration at the site of action
Narrow range between therapeutic and toxic concentrations
Pharmacological effect is related to the drug concentration
Clinical
Clinical studies have documented the therapeutic range of the drug
Significant between-patient variability in drug absorption and disposition
Lack of an effect may be detrimental to the patient
Analytical
A sensitive drug assay is available
The assay has acceptable accuracy and precision with high specificity
Analysis time is short, required sample volume is small, and cost is minimal

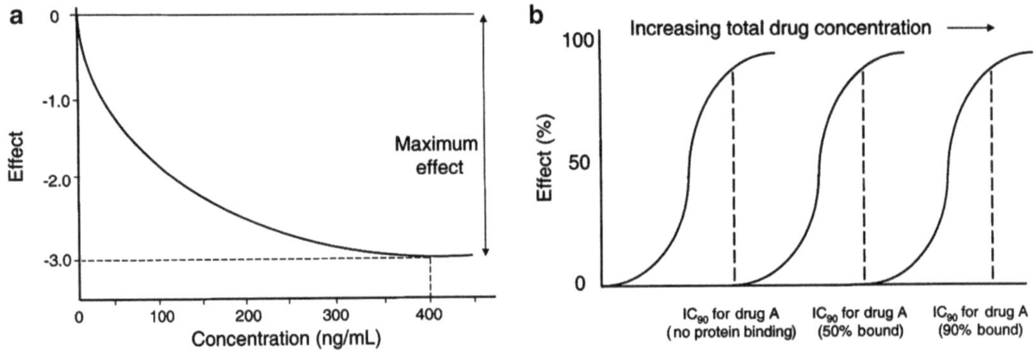

Fig. 3 Representative maximum effect (E_{max}) curve (**a**) illustrating an inhibitory E_{max} concentration–response relationship. Change in the concentration–effect curve (**b**) caused by protein binding that shifts the 90 % inhibitory concentration (IC_{90}) and a higher total drug concentration is required in the presence of increasing plasma protein concentrations to elicit the same pharmacological effect. Reproduced from E.P. Acosta et al. *Clin Infect Dis* 2000; 30(Suppl 2): S151–9

concentrations. However, because NRTIs are activated intracellularly, plasma concentration may not be a good surrogate for drug concentration at site of action and therefore TDM is of limited use for this drug class. Intra-patient and inter-patient can produce suboptimal plasma trough concentrations, which can lead to the selection of drug-resistant mutants. Pharmacokinetic boosting of PIs can reduce but not eliminate inter-patient variability. However, the effect of ritonavir varies depending on the coadministered PI. For example, when ritonavir affects the first pass effect, increases in AUC, C_{max}, and C_{min} but not half-life are observed. When ritonavir affects hepatic clearance of PIs, C_{max} increases are small, but AUC, C_{min} and half-life are considerably increased. Irrespective, the boosting properties of ritonavir and cobicistat are likely to reduce the risk of suboptimal PI concentration, which may render TDM for PI regimen pointless. Some ARVs are highly protein bound and therefore, changes in overall binding could affect total drug concentration and active (unbound) drug concentration (Fig. 3). Patients, who are not adherent to their ARV regimen with respect to pill count, dietary requirements, or dosing frequency, could have low plasma drug concentrations, which could be misinterpreted as a pharmacokinetic effect and lead to an unnecessary increased dosage. For some ARVs, there is a lack of established therapeutic ranges for ARV drug concentrations needed to achieve virologic success. This is especially true for PIs and NNRTIs, which have absorption, metabolic, and tolerability issues that limit the ability to determination of maximally tolerated doses. Moreover, the pharmacokinetic parameter that best defines therapeutic and toxic exposures of the ARVs has yet to be determined for many of the ARVs. Because of the ease on the patient and investigator, C_{trough} is mostly used for determination of efficacy, which can be tricky for drugs with multiple dosing schedules. On the other hand, AUC is most demanding in the clinical setting as multiple blood draws are required and can be costly. Nonetheless, TDM can be useful when dealing with special populations such as the hepatic impaired, children, women, ethnic groups, and pregnant women, which have age-related, metabolic, and physiological changes that can alter ARV exposure.

11 Summary and Conclusions

Use of ARV drugs for the treatment of HIV infection has considerably decreased mortality and morbidity. The pharmacodynamics of ARVs are mostly studied in the context of efficacy as demonstrated by viral suppression and immune function restoration. Because HIV infections cannot be cured, life-long treatment with ARVs are needed and will likely result in increased drug resistance, which justifies the use of triple or quadruple drug combinations and the need for appropriate concentration– and dose–response curves. While routine TDM of ARV drugs is not currently recommended, special population may benefit from TDM.

References

1. Centers for Disease Control (CDC) (1981) Pneumocystis pneumonia--Los Angeles. MMWR Morb Mortal Wkly Rep 30:250–252
2. Reeves JD, Doms RW (2002) Human immunodeficiency virus type 2. J Gen Virol 83: 1253–1265
3. Marlink R, Kanki P, Thior I, Travers K, Eisen G, Siby T et al (1994) Reduced rate of disease development after HIV-2 infection as compared to HIV-1. Science 265:1587–1590
4. Andersson S, Norrgren H, Dias F, Biberfeld G, Albert J (1999) Molecular characterization of human immunodeficiency virus (HIV)-1 and -2 in individuals from Guinea-Bissau with single or dual infections: predominance of a distinct HIV-1 subtype A/G recombinant in West Africa. Virology 262:312–320
5. Raboud JM, Montaner JS, Conway B, Rae S, Reiss P, Vella S et al (1998) Suppression of plasma viral load below 20 copies/ml is required to achieve a long-term response to therapy. AIDS 12:1619–1624
6. Guidelines for the Use of Antiretroviral Agents in HIV-1-Infected Adults and Adolescents [Internet]. AIDSinfo. [cited 2013 May 23]. Available from http://aidsinfo.nih.gov/guidelines/html/1/adult-and-adolescent-arv-guidelines/0
7. WHO|HIV/AIDS [Internet]. World Health Organization. [cited 2013 Mar 15]. Available from http://www.who.int/mediacentre/factsheets/fs360/en/index.html
8. Cattaneo D, Gervasoni C, Meraviglia P, Landonio S, Fucile S, Cozzi V et al (2012) Inter- and intra-patient variability of raltegravir pharmacokinetics in HIV-1-infected subjects. J Antimicrob Chemother 67:460–464
9. Fischl MA, Richman DD, Grieco MH, Gottlieb MS, Volberding PA, Laskin OL et al (1987) The efficacy of azidothymidine (AZT) in the treatment of patients with AIDS and AIDS-related complex. A double-blind, placebo-controlled trial. N Engl J Med 317:185–191
10. Katlama C, Ingrand D, Loveday C, Clumeck N, Mallolas J, Staszewski S et al (1996) Safety and efficacy of lamivudine-zidovudine combination therapy in antiretroviral-naive patients. A randomized controlled comparison with zidovudine monotherapy. Lamivudine European HIV Working Group. JAMA 276:118–125
11. Eron JJ, Benoit SL, Jemsek J, MacArthur RD, Santana J, Quinn JB et al (1995) Treatment with lamivudine, zidovudine, or both in HIV-positive patients with 200 to 500 CD4+ cells per cubic millimeter. North American HIV

Working Party. N Engl J Med 333: 1662–1669

12. Staszewski S, Loveday C, Picazo JJ, Dellarnonica P, Skinhøj P, Johnson MA et al (1996) Safety and efficacy of lamivudine-zidovudine combination therapy in zidovudine-experienced patients. A randomized controlled comparison with zidovudine monotherapy. Lamivudine European HIV Working Group. JAMA 276:111–117
13. Staszewski S, Hill AM, Bartlett J, Eron JJ, Katlama C, Johnson J et al (1997) Reductions in HIV-1 disease progression for zidovudine/lamivudine relative to control treatments: a meta-analysis of controlled trials. AIDS 11: 477–483
14. Katzenstein DA, Hughes M, Albrecht M, Hammer S, Para M, Murphy R et al (2000) Virologic and CD4+ cell responses to new nucleoside regimens: switching to stavudine or adding lamivudine after prolonged zidovudine treatment of human immunodeficiency virus infection. ACTG 302 Study Team. AIDS Clinical Trials Group. AIDS Res Hum Retroviruses 16:1031–1037
15. WHO|Summary: Consolidated guidelines on the use of ARV drugs for treating and preventing HIV infection [Internet]. WHO. [cited 2014 Jan 27]. Available from http://www.who.int/hiv/pub/guidelines/arv2013/short_summary/en/index.html
16. Kahn JO, Lagakos SW, Richman DD, Cross A, Pettinelli C, Liou SH et al (1992) A controlled trial comparing continued zidovudine with didanosine in human immunodeficiency virus infection. The NIAID AIDS Clinical Trials Group. N Engl J Med 327:581–587
17. Bristol-Myers Squibb Company (2000) A randomized study of the long term suppression of plasma HIV RNA levels by triple combination regimens in treatment naive subjects [Internet]. Available from http://ctr.bms.com/OneBmsCtd/ResultDetailAction.do?prodid=7&trialid=723
18. VIDEX EC (didanosine USP) Prescribing Information [Internet]. [cited 2014 Feb 4]. Available from packageinserts.bms.com/pi/pi_videx_ec.pdf
19. Velen K, Lewis JJ, Charalambous S, Grant AD, Churchyard GJ, Hoffmann CJ (2013) Comparison of tenofovir, zidovudine, or stavudine as part of first-line antiretroviral therapy in a resource-limited-setting: a cohort study. PLoS One 8:e64459
20. Spruance SL, Pavia AT, Mellors JW, Murphy R, Gathe J Jr, Stool E et al (1997) Clinical efficacy of monotherapy with stavudine compared with zidovudine in HIV-infected, zidovudine-experienced patients. A randomized, double-blind, controlled trial. Bristol-Myers Squibb Stavudine/019 Study Group. Ann Intern Med 126:355–363
21. Katlama C, Valantin MA, Matheron S, Coutellier A, Calvez V, Descamps D et al (1998) Efficacy and tolerability of stavudine plus lamivudine in treatment-naive and treatment-experienced patients with HIV-1 infection. Ann Intern Med 129:525–531
22. Acosta EP, Balfour HH Jr (2003) Intermittent administration of high-dose stavudine to nucleoside-experienced individuals infected with HIV-1. J Acquir Immune Defic Syndr 33:343–348
23. EPIVIR (lamivudine) Prescribing Information [Internet]. [cited 2014 Feb 4]. Available from www.viivhealthcare.com/media/32160/us_epivir.pdf
24. Henry K, Wallace RJ, Bellman PC, Norris D, Fisher RL, Ross LL et al (2001) Twice-daily triple nucleoside intensification treatment with lamivudine-zidovudine plus abacavir sustains suppression of human immunodeficiency virus type 1: results of the TARGET Study. J Infect Dis 183:571–578
25. Grant PM, Tierney C, Budhathoki C, Daar ES, Sax PE, Collier AC et al (2013) Early virologic response to abacavir/lamivudine and tenofovir/emtricitabine during ACTG A5202. HIV Clin Trials 14:284–291
26. Behrens G, Maserati R, Rieger A, Domingo P, Abel F, Wang H et al (2012) Switching to tenofovir/emtricitabine from abacavir/lamivudine in HIV-infected adults with raised cholesterol: effect on lipid profiles. Antivir Ther 17:1011–1020
27. Ford N, Shubber Z, Hill A, Vitoria M, Doherty M, Mills EJ et al (2013) Comparative efficacy of Lamivudine and emtricitabine: a systematic review and meta-analysis of randomized trials. PLoS One 8:e79981
28. Weller S, Radomski KM, Lou Y, Stein DS (2000) Population pharmacokinetics and pharmacodynamic modeling of abacavir (1592U89) from a dose-ranging, double-blind, randomized monotherapy trial with human immunodeficiency virus-infected subjects. Antimicrob Agents Chemother 44: 2052–2060
29. Wang LH, Begley J, St Claire RL III, Harris J, Wakeford C, Rousseau FS (2004) Pharmacokinetic and pharmacodynamic characteristics of emtricitabine support its once daily dosing for the treatment of HIV infection. AIDS Res Hum Retroviruses 20:1173–1182

30. Moyle GJ, Stellbrink H-J, Compston J, Orkin C, Arribas JR, Domingo P et al (2013) 96-Week results of abacavir/lamivudine versus tenofovir/emtricitabine, plus efavirenz, in antiretroviral-naive, HIV-1-infected adults: ASSERT study. Antivir Ther 18: 905–913
31. Nishijima T, Takano M, Ishisaka M, Komatsu H, Gatanaga H, Kikuchi Y et al (2013) Abacavir/lamivudine versus tenofovir/emtricitabine with atazanavir/ritonavir for treatment-naive Japanese patients with HIV-1 infection: a randomized multicenter trial. Intern Med 52:735–744
32. Goicoechea M, Jain S, Bi L, Kemper C, Daar ES, Diamond C et al (2010) Abacavir and tenofovir disoproxil fumarate co-administration results in a nonadditive antiviral effect in HIV-1-infected patients. AIDS 24:707–716
33. VIREAD® (tenofovir disoproxil fumarate) Prescribing Information [Internet]. [cited 2013 Nov 5]. Available from gilead.com/pdf/viread_pi.pdf
34. Peeters M, Gueye A, Mboup S, Bibollet-Ruche F, Ekaza E, Mulanga C et al (1997) Geographical distribution of HIV-1 group O viruses in Africa. AIDS 11:493–498
35. Viramune® (nevirapine) Prescribing Information [Internet]. Available from http://www.viramune.com/Landingpage.html
36. Von Hentig N, Carlebach A, Gute P, Knecht G, Klauke S, Rohrbacher M et al (2006) A comparison of the steady-state pharmacokinetics of nevirapine in men, nonpregnant women and women in late pregnancy. Br J Clin Pharmacol 62:552–559
37. Montaner JS, Reiss P, Cooper D, Vella S, Harris M, Conway B et al (1998) A randomized, double-blind trial comparing combinations of nevirapine, didanosine, and zidovudine for HIV-infected patients: the INCAS Trial. Italy, The Netherlands, Canada and Australia Study. JAMA 279:930–937
38. Harris M, Patenaude P, Cooperberg P, Filipenko D, Thorne A, Raboud J et al (1997) Correlation of virus load in plasma and lymph node tissue in human immunodeficiency virus infection. INCAS Study Group. Italy, Netherlands, Canada, Australia, and (United) States. J Infect Dis 176:1388–1392
39. Lange JMA (2003) Efficacy and durability of nevirapine in antiretroviral drug näive patients. J Acquir Immune Defic Syndr 34(Suppl 1):S40–S52
40. Van Leth F, Phanuphak P, Ruxrungtham K, Baraldi E, Miller S, Gazzard B et al (2004) Comparison of first-line antiretroviral therapy with regimens including nevirapine, efavirenz, or both drugs, plus stavudine and lamivudine: a randomised open-label trial, the 2NN Study. Lancet 363:1253–1263
41. Conway B (2000) Initial therapy with protease inhibitor-sparing regimens: evaluation of nevirapine and delavirdine. Clin Infect Dis 30(Suppl 2):S130–S134
42. Kuritzkes DR, Bassett RL, Johnson VA, Marschner IC, Eron JJ, Sommadossi JP et al (2000) Continued lamivudine versus delavirdine in combination with indinavir and zidovudine or stavudine in lamivudine-experienced patients: results of Adult AIDS Clinical Trials Group protocol 370. AIDS 14:1553–1561
43. Gulick RM, Hu XJ, Fiscus SA, Fletcher CV, Haubrich R, Cheng H et al (2000) Randomized study of saquinavir with ritonavir or nelfinavir together with delavirdine, adefovir, or both in human immunodeficiency virus-infected adults with virologic failure on indinavir: AIDS Clinical Trials Group Study 359. J Infect Dis 182:1375–1384
44. Ngaimisi E, Habtewold A, Minzi O, Makonnen E, Mugusi S, Amogne W et al (2013) Importance of ethnicity, CYP2B6 and ABCB1 genotype for efavirenz pharmacokinetics and treatment outcomes: a parallel-group prospective cohort study in two sub-Saharan Africa populations. PLoS One 8:e67946
45. Staszewski S, Morales-Ramirez J, Tashima KT, Rachlis A, Skiest D, Stanford J et al (1999) Efavirenz plus zidovudine and lamivudine, efavirenz plus indinavir, and indinavir plus zidovudine and lamivudine in the treatment of HIV-1 infection in adults. Study 006 Team. N Engl J Med 341:1865–1873
46. Gulick RM, Ribaudo HJ, Shikuma CM, Lustgarten S, Squires KE, Meyer WA III et al (2004) Triple-nucleoside regimens versus efavirenz-containing regimens for the initial treatment of HIV-1 infection. N Engl J Med 350:1850–1861
47. Kakuda TN, Wade JR, Snoeck E, Vis P, Schöller-Gyüre M, Peeters MP et al (2010) Pharmacokinetics and pharmacodynamics of the non-nucleoside reverse-transcriptase inhibitor etravirine in treatment-experienced HIV-1-infected patients. Clin Pharmacol Ther 88:695–703
48. Kakuda T, Sekar V, Vis P, Coate B, Ryan R, Anderson D et al (2012) pharmacokinetics and pharmacodynamics of darunavir and etravirine in HIV-1-infected, treatment-experienced patients in the gender, race, and clinical experience (GRACE) trial. AIDS Res Treat 2012:186987

49. Di Perri G, Green B, Morrish G, Hill A, Faetkenheuer G, Bickel M et al (2013) Pharmacokinetics and pharmacodynamics of etravirine 400 mg once daily in treatment-naïve patients. HIV Clin Trials 14:92–98
50. Edurant® (rilpivirine) Prescribing Information [Internet]. [cited 2013 Nov 5]. Available from http://www.edurant.com/patients/full-product-information
51. Nelson MR, Elion RA, Cohen CJ, Mills A, Hodder SL, Segal-Maurer S et al (2013) Rilpivirine versus efavirenz in HIV-1-infected subjects receiving emtricitabine/tenofovir DF: pooled 96-week data from ECHO and THRIVE Studies. HIV Clin Trials 14:81–91
52. Cohen CJ, Andrade-Villanueva J, Clotet B, Fourie J, Johnson MA, Ruxrungtham K et al (2011) Rilpivirine versus efavirenz with two background nucleoside or nucleotide reverse transcriptase inhibitors in treatment-naive adults infected with HIV-1 (THRIVE): a phase 3, randomised, non-inferiority trial. Lancet 378:229–237
53. Molina J-M, Cahn P, Grinsztejn B, Lazzarin A, Mills A, Saag M et al (2011) Rilpivirine versus efavirenz with tenofovir and emtricitabine in treatment-naive adults infected with HIV-1 (ECHO): a phase 3 randomised double-blind active-controlled trial. Lancet 378:238–246
54. Molina J-M, Clumeck N, Orkin C, Rimsky LT, Vanveggel S, Stevens M et al (2014) Week 96 analysis of rilpivirine or efavirenz in HIV-1-infected patients with baseline viral load ≤100,000 copies/mL in the pooled ECHO and THRIVE phase 3, randomized, double-blind trials. HIV Med 15:57–62
55. Chiba M, Hensleigh M, Lin JH (1997) Hepatic and intestinal metabolism of indinavir, an HIV protease inhibitor, in rat and human microsomes. Major role of CYP3A. Biochem Pharmacol 53:1187–1195
56. Fitzsimmons ME, Collins JM (1997) Selective biotransformation of the human immunodeficiency virus protease inhibitor saquinavir by human small-intestinal cytochrome P4503A4 potential contribution to high first-pass metabolism. Drug Metab Dispos 25:256–266
57. Koudriakova T, Iatsimirskaia E, Utkin I, Gangl E, Vouros P, Storozhuk E et al (1998) Metabolism of the human immunodeficiency virus protease inhibitors indinavir and ritonavir by human intestinal microsomes and expressed cytochrome P4503A4/3A5: mechanism-based inactivation of cytochrome P4503A by ritonavir. Drug Metab Dispos 26:552–561
58. Mathias AA, German P, Murray BP, Wei L, Jain A, West S et al (2010) Pharmacokinetics and pharmacodynamics of GS-9350: a novel pharmacokinetic enhancer without anti-HIV activity. Clin Pharmacol Ther 87:322–329
59. Lepist E-I, Phan TK, Roy A, Tong L, Maclennan K, Murray B et al (2012) Cobicistat boosts the intestinal absorption of transport substrates, including HIV protease inhibitors and GS-7340, in vitro. Antimicrob Agents Chemother 56:5409–5413
60. Le Moing V, Chêne G, Carrieri MP, Alioum A, Brun-Vézinet F, Piroth L et al (2002) Predictors of virological rebound in HIV-1-infected patients initiating a protease inhibitor-containing regimen. AIDS 16: |21–29
61. Paredes R, Mocroft A, Kirk O, Lazzarin A, Barton SE, Van Lunzen J et al (2000) Predictors of virological success and ensuing failure in HIV-positive patients starting highly active antiretroviral therapy in Europe: results from the EuroSIDA study. Arch Intern Med 160:1123–1132
62. Schapiro JM, Winters MA, Stewart F, Efron B, Norris J, Kozal MJ et al (1996) The effect of high-dose saquinavir on viral load and CD4+ T-cell counts in HIV-infected patients. Ann Intern Med 124:1039–1050
63. INVIRASE® (saquinavir mesylate) Prescribing Information [Internet]. Available from www.gene.com/gene/products/information/invirase/pdf/pi.pdf
64. Piketty C, Race E, Castiel P, Belec L, Peytavin G, Si-Mohamed A et al (1999) Efficacy of a five-drug combination including ritonavir, saquinavir and efavirenz in patients who failed on a conventional triple-drug regimen: phenotypic resistance to protease inhibitors predicts outcome of therapy. AIDS 13:F71–F77
65. Viracept® (nelfinavir mesylate) Prescribing Information [Internet]. Available from www.viivhealthcare.com/media/32259/us_viracept.pdf
66. Kurowski M, Kaeser B, Sawyer A, Popescu M, Mrozikiewicz A (2002) Low-dose ritonavir moderately enhances nelfinavir exposure. Clin Pharmacol Ther 72:123–132
67. Moyle GJ, Youle M, Higgs C, Monaghan J, Prince W, Chapman S et al (1998) Safety, pharmacokinetics, and antiretroviral activity of the potent, specific human immunodeficiency virus protease inhibitor nelfinavir: results of a phase I/II trial and extended follow-up in patients infected with human immunodeficiency virus. J Clin Pharmacol 38:736–743

68. Saag MS, Tebas P, Sension M, Conant M, Myers R, Chapman SK et al (2001) Randomized, double-blind comparison of two nelfinavir doses plus nucleosides in HIV-infected patients (Agouron study 511). AIDS 15:1971–1978
69. Gathe JC Jr, Ive P, Wood R, Schürmann D, Bellos NC, DeJesus E et al (2004) SOLO: 48-week efficacy and safety comparison of once-daily fosamprenavir/ritonavir versus twice-daily nelfinavir in naive HIV-1-infected patients. AIDS 18:1529–1537
70. King MS, Bernstein BM, Walmsley SL, Sherer R, Feinberg J, Sanne I et al (2004) Baseline HIV-1 RNA level and CD4 cell count predict time to loss of virologic response to nelfinavir, but not lopinavir/ritonavir, in antiretroviral therapy-naive patients. J Infect Dis 190: 280–284
71. Yeh KC, Deutsch PJ, Haddix H, Hesney M, Hoagland V, Ju WD et al (1998) Single-dose pharmacokinetics of indinavir and the effect of food. Antimicrob Agents Chemother 42:332–338
72. CRIXIVAN® (Indinavir sulfate) Prescribing Information [Internet]. Available from www.merck.com/product/usa/pi_circulars/c/crixivan/crixivan_pi.pdf
73. Easterbrook PJ, Newson R, Ives N, Pereira S, Moyle G, Gazzard BG (2001) Comparison of virologic, immunologic, and clinical response to five different initial protease inhibitor-containing and nevirapine-containing regimens. J Acquir Immune Defic Syndr 27: 350–364
74. Casado JL, Moreno A, Sabido R, Martí-Belda P, Antela A, Dronda F et al (2000) A clinical study of the combination of 100 mg ritonavir plus 800 mg indinavir as salvage therapy: influence of increased plasma drug levels in the rate of response. HIV Clin Trials 1: 13–19
75. Campo RE, Moreno JN, Suarez G, Miller N, Kolber MA, Holder DJ et al (2003) Efficacy of indinavir-ritonavir-based regimens in HIV-1-infected patients with prior protease inhibitor failures. AIDS 17:1933–1939
76. Cressey TR, Plipat N, Fregonese F, Chokephaibulkit K (2007) Indinavir/ritonavir remains an important component of HAART for the treatment of HIV/AIDS, particularly in resource-limited settings. Expert Opin Drug Metab Toxicol 3:347–361
77. Pulido F, Delgado R, Pérez-Valero I, González-García J, Miralles P, Arranz A et al (2008) Long-term (4 years) efficacy of lopinavir/ritonavir monotherapy for maintenance of HIV suppression. J Antimicrob Chemother 61:1359–1361
78. Lopez-Cortes LF, Ruiz-Valderas R, Sánchez-Rivas E, Lluch A, Gutierrez-Valencia A, Torres-Cornejo A et al (2013) Lopinavir plasma concentrations and virological outcome with lopinavir-ritonavir monotherapy in HIV-1-infected patients. Antimicrob Agents Chemother 57:3746–3751
79. Wang K, D'Argenio DZ, Acosta EP, Sheth AN, Delille C, Lennox JL et al (2014) Integrated population pharmacokinetic/viral dynamic modelling of lopinavir/ritonavir in HIV-1 treatment-naïve patients. Clin Pharmacokinet 53:361–371
80. Bertz RJ, Persson A, Chung E, Zhu L, Zhang J, McGrath D et al (2013) Pharmacokinetics and pharmacodynamics of atazanavir-containing antiretroviral regimens, with or without ritonavir, in patients who are HIV-positive and treatment-naïve. Pharmacotherapy 33:284–294
81. Goutelle S, Baudry T, Gagnieu M-C, Boibieux A, Livrozet J-M, Peyramond D et al (2013) Pharmacokinetic-pharmacodynamic modeling of unboosted Atazanavir in a cohort of stable HIV-infected patients. Antimicrob Agents Chemother 57:517–523
82. Falcoz C, Jenkins JM, Bye C, Hardman TC, Kenney KB, Studenberg S et al (2002) Pharmacokinetics of GW433908, a prodrug of amprenavir, in healthy male volunteers. J Clin Pharmacol 42:887–898
83. Furfine ES, Baker CT, Hale MR, Reynolds DJ, Salisbury JA, Searle AD et al (2004) Preclinical pharmacology and pharmacokinetics of GW433908, a water-soluble prodrug of the human immunodeficiency virus protease inhibitor amprenavir. Antimicrob Agents Chemother 48:791–798
84. LEXIVA (fosamprenavir calcium) Prescribing Information [Internet]. Available from http://www.accessdata.fda.gov/drugsatfda_docs/label/2013/021548s031,022116s015lbl.pdf
85. Molina J-M, Ait-Khaled M, Rinaldi R, Penco G, Baril J-G, Cauda R et al (2009) Fosamprenavir/ritonavir in advanced HIV disease (TRIAD): a randomized study of high-dose, dual-boosted or standard dose fosamprenavir/ritonavir in HIV-1-infected patients with antiretroviral resistance. J Antimicrob Chemother 64:398–410
86. Quercia R, Garnier E, Ferré V, Morineau P, Bonnet B, Soulard C et al (2005) Salvage therapy with ritonavir-boosted amprenavir/fosamprenavir: virological and immunological

response in two years follow-up. HIV Clin Trials 6:73–80

87. Thaisrivongs S, Strohbach JW (1999) Structure-based discovery of Tipranavir disodium (PNU-140690E): a potent, orally bioavailable, nonpeptidic HIV protease inhibitor. Biopolymers 51:51–58

88. Larder BA, Hertogs K, Bloor S, Van den Eynde CH, DeCian W, Wang Y et al (2000) Tipranavir inhibits broadly protease inhibitor-resistant HIV-1 clinical samples. AIDS 14: 1943–1948

89. Rusconi S, La Seta Catamancio S, Citterio P, Kurtagic S, Violin M, Balotta C et al (2000) Susceptibility to PNU-140690 (Tipranavir) of human immunodeficiency virus type 1 isolates derived from patients with multidrug resistance to other protease inhibitors. Antimicrob Agents Chemother 44:1328–1332

90. McCallister S, Valdez H, Curry K, MacGregor T, Borin M, Freimuth W et al (2004) A 14-day dose-response study of the efficacy, safety, and pharmacokinetics of the nonpeptidic protease inhibitor tipranavir in treatment-naive HIV-1-infected patients. J Acquir Immune Defic Syndr 35:376–382

91. Goebel FD, MacGregor TR, Sabo JP, Castles M, Johnson PA, Legg D et al (2010) Pharmacokinetic characterization of three doses of tipranavir boosted with ritonavir on highly active antiretroviral therapy in treatment-experienced HIV-1 patients. HIV Clin Trials 11:28–38

92. Markowitz M, Slater LN, Schwartz R, Kazanjian PH, Hathaway B, Wheeler D et al (2007) Long-term efficacy and safety of tipranavir boosted with ritonavir in HIV-1-infected patients failing multiple protease inhibitor regimens: 80-week data from a phase 2 study. J Acquir Immune Defic Syndr 45:401–410

93. Orkin C, DeJesus E, Khanlou H, Stoehr A, Supparatpinyo K, Lathouwers E et al (2013) Final 192-week efficacy and safety of once-daily darunavir/ritonavir compared with lopinavir/ritonavir in HIV-1-infected treatment-naïve patients in the ARTEMIS trial. HIV Med 14:49–59

94. Mills AM, Nelson M, Jayaweera D, Ruxrungtham K, Cassetti I, Girard P-M et al (2009) Once-daily darunavir/ritonavir vs. lopinavir/ritonavir in treatment-naive, HIV-1-infected patients: 96-week analysis. AIDS 23:1679–1688

95. Fourie J, Flamm J, Rodriguez-French A, Kilby D, Domingo P, Lazzarin A et al (2011) Effect of baseline characteristics on the efficacy and safety of once-daily darunavir/ritonavir in HIV-1-infected, treatment-naïve ARTEMIS patients at week 96. HIV Clin Trials 12:313–322

96. Arastéh K, Yeni P, Pozniak A, Grinsztejn B, Jayaweera D, Roberts A et al (2009) Efficacy and safety of darunavir/ritonavir in treatment-experienced HIV type-1 patients in the POWER 1, 2 and 3 trials at week 96. Antivir Ther 14:859–864

97. Pozniak A, Opravil M, Beatty G, Hill A, De Béthune M-P, Lefebvre E (2008) Effect of baseline viral susceptibility on response to darunavir/ritonavir versus control protease inhibitors in treatment-experienced HIV type 1-infected patients: POWER 1 and 2. AIDS Res Hum Retroviruses 24:1275–1280

98. Isentress Package Insert [Internet]. [cited 2013 Mar 15]. Available from http://www.accessdata.fda.gov/drugsatfda_docs/label/2009/022145s004lbl.pdf

99. Markowitz M, Morales-Ramirez JO, Nguyen B-Y, Kovacs CM, Steigbigel RT, Cooper DA et al (2006) Antiretroviral activity, pharmacokinetics, and tolerability of MK-0518, a novel inhibitor of HIV-1 integrase, dosed as monotherapy for 10 days in treatment-naive HIV-1-infected individuals. J Acquir Immune Defic Syndr 43:509–515

100. Miller M, Witmer M, Stillmock K, Felock P, Etco L, Flynn J et al (2006) Biochemical and antiviral activity of MK-0518, a potent HIV integrase inhibitor. [cited 2013 May 23]. Available from http://www.iasociety.org/Default.aspx?pageId=11&abstractId=2191670

101. Rizk ML, Hang Y, Luo W-L, Su J, Zhao J, Campbell H et al (2012) Pharmacokinetics and pharmacodynamics of once-daily versus twice-daily raltegravir in treatment-naive HIV-infected patients. Antimicrob Agents Chemother 56:3101–3106

102. Eron JJ Jr, Rockstroh JK, Reynes J, Andrade-Villanueva J, Ramalho-Madruga JV, Bekker L-G et al (2011) Raltegravir once daily or twice daily in previously untreated patients with HIV-1: a randomised, active-controlled, phase 3 non-inferiority trial. Lancet Infect Dis 11:907–915

103. Charpentier C, Fagard C, Colin C, Katlama C, Molina J-M, Jacomet C et al (2013) Role of baseline HIV-1 DNA level in highly-experienced patients receiving raltegravir, etravirine and darunavir/ritonavir regimen (ANRS139 TRIO trial). PLoS One 8:e53621

104. Rockstroh JK, Lennox JL, Dejesus E, Saag MS, Lazzarin A, Wan H et al (2011) Long-term treatment with raltegravir or efavirenz combined with tenofovir/emtricitabine for

treatment-naive human immunodeficiency virus-1-infected patients: 156-week results from STARTMRK. Clin Infect Dis 53: 807–816

105. Gotuzzo E, Markowitz M, Ratanasuwan W, Smith G, Prada G, Morales-Ramirez JO et al (2012) Sustained efficacy and safety of raltegravir after 5 years of combination antiretroviral therapy as initial treatment of HIV-1 infection: final results of a randomized, controlled, phase II study (Protocol 004). J Acquir Immune Defic Syndr 61:73–77

106. Kozal MJ, Lupo S, DeJesus E, Molina J-M, McDonald C, Raffi F et al (2012) A nucleoside- and ritonavir-sparing regimen containing atazanavir plus raltegravir in antiretroviral treatment-naïve HIV-infected patients: SPARTAN study results. HIV Clin Trials 13:119–130

107. Taiwo B, Zheng L, Gallien S, Matining RM, Kuritzkes DR, Wilson CC et al (2011) Efficacy of a nucleoside-sparing regimen of darunavir/ritonavir plus raltegravir in treatment-naive HIV-1-infected patients (ACTG A5262). AIDS 25:2113–2122

108. Ofotokun I, Sheth AN, Sanford SE, Easley KA, Shenvi N, White K et al (2012) A switch in therapy to a reverse transcriptase inhibitor sparing combination of lopinavir/ritonavir and raltegravir in virologically suppressed HIV-infected patients: a pilot randomized trial to assess efficacy and safety profile: the KITE study. AIDS Res Hum Retroviruses 28:1196–1206

109. Gallien S, Braun J, Delaugerre C, Charreau I, Reynes J, Jeanblanc F et al (2011) Efficacy and safety of raltegravir in treatment-experienced HIV-1-infected patients switching from enfuvirtide-based regimens: 48 week results of the randomized EASIER ANRS 138 trial. J Antimicrob Chemother 66: 2099–2106

110. Sax PE, DeJesus E, Mills A, Zolopa A, Cohen C, Wohl D et al (2012) Co-formulated elvitegravir, cobicistat, emtricitabine, and tenofovir versus co-formulated efavirenz, emtricitabine, and tenofovir for initial treatment of HIV-1 infection: a randomised, double-blind, phase 3 trial, analysis of results after 48 weeks. Lancet 379:2439–2448

111. Cohen C, Elion R, Ruane P, Shamblaw D, DeJesus E, Rashbaum B et al (2011) Randomized, phase 2 evaluation of two single-tablet regimens elvitegravir/cobicistat/emtricitabine/tenofovir disoproxil fumarate versus efavirenz/emtricitabine/tenofovir disoproxil fumarate for the initial treatment of HIV infection. AIDS 25:F7–F12

112. DeJesus E, Rockstroh JK, Henry K, Molina J-M, Gathe J, Ramanathan S et al (2012) Co-formulated elvitegravir, cobicistat, emtricitabine, and tenofovir disoproxil fumarate versus ritonavir-boosted atazanavir plus co-formulated emtricitabine and tenofovir disoproxil fumarate for initial treatment of HIV-1 infection: a randomised, double-blind, phase 3, non-inferiority trial. Lancet 379: 2429–2438

113. Molina J-M, Lamarca A, Andrade-Villanueva J, Clotet B, Clumeck N, Liu Y-P et al (2012) Efficacy and safety of once daily elvitegravir versus twice daily raltegravir in treatment-experienced patients with HIV-1 receiving a ritonavir-boosted protease inhibitor: randomised, double-blind, phase 3, non-inferiority study. Lancet Infect Dis 12:27–35

114. Min S, Song I, Borland J, Chen S, Lou Y, Fujiwara T et al (2010) Pharmacokinetics and safety of S/GSK1349572, a next-generation HIV integrase inhibitor, in healthy volunteers. Antimicrob Agents Chemother 54: 254–258

115. Garrido C, Villacian J, Zahonero N, Pattery T, Garcia F, Gutierrez F et al (2012) Broad phenotypic cross-resistance to elvitegravir in HIV-infected patients failing on raltegravir-containing regimens. Antimicrob Agents Chemother 56:2873–2878

116. Canducci F, Ceresola ER, Saita D, Castagna A, Gianotti N, Underwood M et al (2013) In vitro phenotypes to elvitegravir and dolutegravir in primary macrophages and lymphocytes of clonal recombinant viral variants selected in patients failing raltegravir. J Antimicrob Chemother 68:2525–2532

117. Eron JJ, Clotet B, Durant J, Katlama C, Kumar P, Lazzarin A et al (2013) Safety and efficacy of dolutegravir in treatment-experienced subjects with raltegravir-resistant HIV type 1 infection: 24-week results of the VIKING Study. J Infect Dis 207:740–748

118. Castagna A, Maggiolo F, Penco G, Wright D, Mills A, Grossberg R et al (2014) Dolutegravir in antiretroviral-experienced patients with raltegravir- and/or elvitegravir-resistant HIV-1: 24-week results of the phase III VIKING-3 study. J Infect Dis 210:354–362

119. Stellbrink H-J, Reynes J, Lazzarin A, Voronin E, Pulido F, Felizarta F et al (2013) Dolutegravir in antiretroviral-naive adults with HIV-1: 96-week results from a randomized dose-ranging study. AIDS 27: 1771–1778

120. Raffi F, Jaeger H, Quiros-Roldan E, Albrecht H, Belonosova E, Gatell JM et al (2013) Once-daily dolutegravir versus twice-daily

raltegravir in antiretroviral-naive adults with HIV-1 infection (SPRING-2 study): 96 week results from a randomised, double-blind, non-inferiority trial. Lancet Infect Dis 13: 927–935

121. Walmsley SL, Antela A, Clumeck N, Duiculescu D, Eberhard A, Gutiérrez F et al (2013) Dolutegravir plus abacavir-lamivudine for the treatment of HIV-1 infection. N Engl J Med 369:1807–1818

122. Cahn P, Pozniak AL, Mingrone H, Shuldyakov A, Brites C, Andrade-Villanueva JF et al (2013) Dolutegravir versus raltegravir in antiretroviral-experienced, integrase-inhibitor-naive adults with HIV: week 48 results from the randomised, double-blind, non-inferiority SAILING study. Lancet 382:700–708

123. FUZEON ®(enfuvirtide) for injection Prescribing Information [Internet]. [cited 2013 Nov 5]. Available from www.gene.com/gene/products/information/fuzeon/pdf/pi.pdf

124. Chan DC, Chutkowski CT, Kim PS (1998) Evidence that a prominent cavity in the coiled coil of HIV type 1 gp41 is an attractive drug target. Proc Natl Acad Sci U S A 95: 15613–15617

125. Wei X, Decker JM, Liu H, Zhang Z, Arani RB, Kilby JM et al (2002) Emergence of resistant human immunodeficiency virus type 1 in patients receiving fusion inhibitor (T-20) monotherapy. Antimicrob Agents Chemother 46:1896–1905

126. Descamps D, Assoumou L, Masquelier B, Marcelin A-G, Saidi S, Tamalet C et al (2008) HIV-1-infected patients from the French National Observatory experiencing virological failure while receiving enfuvirtide. J Antimicrob Chemother 62:451–455

127. Zhang X, Nieforth K, Lang J-M, Rouzier-Panis R, Reynes J, Dorr A et al (2002) Pharmacokinetics of plasma enfuvirtide after subcutaneous administration to patients with human immunodeficiency virus: inverse Gaussian density absorption and 2-compartment disposition. Clin Pharmacol Ther 72:10–19

128. Kilby JM, Hopkins S, Venetta TM, DiMassimo B, Cloud GA, Lee JY et al (1998) Potent suppression of HIV-1 replication in humans by T-20, a peptide inhibitor of gp41-mediated virus entry. Nat Med 4:1302–1307

129. Kilby JM, Lalezari JP, Eron JJ, Carlson M, Cohen C, Arduino RC et al (2002) The safety, plasma pharmacokinetics, and antiviral activity of subcutaneous enfuvirtide (T-20), a peptide inhibitor of gp41-mediated virus fusion, in HIV-infected adults. AIDS Res Hum Retroviruses 18:685–693

130. Wheeler DA, Lalezari JP, Kilby JM, Wheat J, Delehanty J, DeMasi R et al (2004) Safety, tolerability, and plasma pharmacokinetics of high-strength formulations of enfuvirtide (T-20) in treatment-experienced HIV-1-infected patients. J Clin Virol 30:183–190

131. Lalezari JP, DeJesus E, Northfelt DW, Richmond G, Wolfe P, Haubrich R et al (2003) A controlled Phase II trial assessing three doses of enfuvirtide (T-20) in combination with abacavir, amprenavir, ritonavir and efavirenz in non-nucleoside reverse transcriptase inhibitor-naive HIV-infected adults. Antivir Ther 8:279–287

132. Lalezari JP, Henry K, O'Hearn M, Montaner JSG, Piliero PJ, Trottier B et al (2003) Enfuvirtide, an HIV-1 fusion inhibitor, for drug-resistant HIV infection in North and South America. N Engl J Med 348: 2175–2185

133. Mould DR, Zhang X, Nieforth K, Salgo M, Buss N, Patel IH (2005) Population pharmacokinetics and exposure-response relationship of enfuvirtide in treatment-experienced human immunodeficiency virus type 1-infected patients. Clin Pharmacol Ther 77:515–528

134. Soy D, Aweeka FT, Church JA, Cunningham CK, Palumbo P, Kosel BW et al (2003) Population pharmacokinetics of enfuvirtide in pediatric patients with human immunodeficiency virus: searching for exposure-response relationships. Clin Pharmacol Ther 74: 569–580

135. Hardy WD, Gulick RM, Mayer H, Fätkenheuer G, Nelson M, Heera J et al (2010) Two-year safety and virologic efficacy of maraviroc in treatment-experienced patients with CCR5-tropic HIV-1 infection: 96-week combined analysis of MOTIVATE 1 and 2. J Acquir Immune Defic Syndr 55: 558–564

136. Fätkenheuer G, Nelson M, Lazzarin A, Konourina I, Hoepelman AIM, Lampiris H et al (2008) Subgroup analyses of maraviroc in previously treated R5 HIV-1 infection. N Engl J Med 359:1442–1455

137. Jacqmin P, Wade JR, Weatherley B, Snoeck E, Marshall S, McFadyen L (2013) Assessment of Maraviroc exposure-response relationship at 48 weeks in treatment-experienced HIV-1-infected patients in the MOTIVATE studies. CPT Pharmacometrics Syst Pharmacol 2:e64

Part IV

Pharmacodynamic Considerations and Special Populations

Chapter 20

Implementing a Continuous or Prolonged Infusion Beta-Lactam Program in the Hospital Setting

Shawn H. MacVane, Nathaniel J. Rhodes, Marc H. Scheetz, and Joseph L. Kuti

Abstract

The increasing prevalence of antimicrobial resistance coupled with the paucity of novel antimicrobial therapies calls for the optimization of currently available anti-infective agents. Continuous (CI) and prolonged infusions (PI) are infusion techniques used to optimize the percentage of the dosing interval that free drug concentrations remain above the minimum inhibitory concentration or fT% > MIC. fT% > MIC is the recognized pharmacodynamic driver of efficacy for time-dependent antibiotics such as beta-lactams. A growing body of evidence, including pharmacokinetic-pharmacodynamic modeling, pharmacoeconomic analyses, and clinical and microbiologic outcome studies, supports the utility of CI and PI dosing as an alternative administration technique compared to traditional intermittent infusion. Consequently, CI and PI dosing regimens are of utmost interest to antimicrobial stewardship programs at both large academic and small community hospitals. The aim of this chapter is to provide a comprehensive review of the theoretical advantages, available clinical studies, and process by which an institution can implement a successful CI and PI protocol of beta-lactam antibiotics.

Key words Antimicrobial stewardship, Beta-lactam, Continuous-infusion, Extended-infusion, Monte-Carlo simulation, Pharmacokinetic-pharmacodynamic model, Prolonged-infusion

1 Introduction

1.1 Needs Assessment

The prolonged or continuous infusion of beta-lactam antibiotics has become an increasingly utilized therapeutic modality to optimize the pharmacodynamics of this popular antibiotic class. Prospective and retrospective studies have demonstrated improvements in clinical success for these dosing modalities, with mortality benefits particularly observed in patients of higher acuity [1]. Continuous (CI) and prolonged infusions (PI) are also advocated for the treatment of multidrug-resistant (MDR) organisms by the Infectious Diseases Society of America (IDSA) and Society for Healthcare Epidemiology of America (SHEA) Guidelines for Antimicrobial Stewardship [2]. Although many hospitals and

John C. Rotschafer et al. (eds.), *Antibiotic Pharmacodynamics*, Methods in Pharmacology and Toxicology,
DOI 10.1007/978-1-4939-3323-5_20,

health systems have implemented continuous or prolonged infusion administration protocols for some beta-lactam antibiotics, there is variable uptake of these dosing strategies within the USA [3]. There are many institution-specific concerns to navigate and critical data to be considered when implementing a CI and PI protocol, but most organizations are able to implement these dosing strategies and realize their clinical benefit when effort is dedicated [1, 4, 5]. Importantly, implementation of a successful CI and PI protocol has been shown to be achievable at both large academic and small community hospitals [5–7]. Partnering with key stakeholders, selecting the best institution-specific agents, and measuring and delivering clinical and pharmacoeconomic outcomes are essential for success. This chapter discusses the justification and evidence for alternative administration techniques of beta-lactams and outlines the process by which an institution can implement a successful continuous infusion or prolonged infusion protocol.

2 Materials

2.1 Background/Evidence/Review Published Data

In regard to CI and PI administration, the primary objective of these alternate administration techniques is to optimize the PK-PD of beta-lactams. Specifically, the goal is to maximize the proportion of the dosing interval that target site concentrations of free drug remain above the minimum inhibitory concentration (MIC), or *f*T%>MIC. The goal *f*T%>MIC for each beta-lactam will vary according to known pharmacodynamic effects of the individual agent. Administration of beta-lactams by CI and PI will increase the likelihood of reaching those goals, which is also referred to as the probability of target attainment (PTA). To that end, this section reviews the evidence that CI and PI administration can achieve improved PTA for beta-lactam antibiotics.

2.1.1 Beta-Lactam PK-PD

Beta-lactams are among the oldest classes of antimicrobials used in modern clinical practice. Some of the first formal investigations into the PK-PD profile of beta-lactams were conducted by Harry Eagle in the early 1950s using animal models of infection and in vitro techniques, laying the foundation for future investigations. Eagle and colleagues described the relationship between the *f*T%>MIC ("the aggregate time penicillin remains at effectively bactericidal levels," as he called it) and bacterial killing as early as 1950 [8]. Despite this knowledge, much of the clinical practice has lagged behind: relying on intermittent infusion dosing of beta-lactams. Subsequently, additional investigations using animal studies and hollow fiber models have more accurately classified the PK-PD profiles of various beta-lactams. The interested reader is

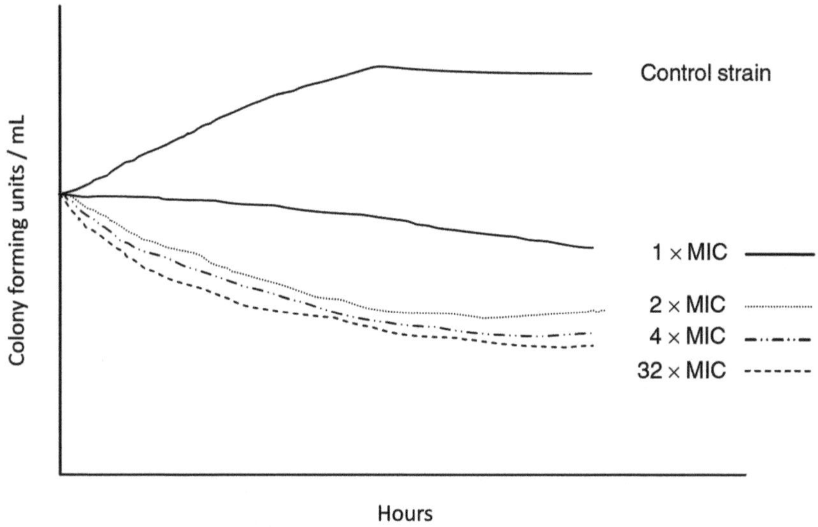

Fig. 1 Log-kill profile of beta-lactams at varying concentrations in multiples of the minimum inhibitory concentration (MIC). Originally published in Scheetz MH, Hurt KM, Noskin GA, Oliphant CM. Applying antimicrobial pharmacodynamics to resistant gram-negative pathogens. Am J Health Syst Pharm. © 2006, American Society of Health-System Pharmacists, Inc. All rights reserved. Reprinted with permission

referred to a more in-depth treatment of the history of animal infection model development and validation [9–14].

While beta-lactams are often classified as "concentration-independent" drugs, several studies have found that outcomes improve when drug concentrations are fourfold higher than the MIC for a prolonged period [15, 16]. As illustrated in Fig. 1, the impact of increasing drug concentrations of a typical beta-lactam on the log-kill profile becomes attenuated at approximately 4 × MIC. Once this threshold is achieved, minimal additional kill is observed with increasing multiples of the MIC, and antibacterial effects predominantly become time dependent. The three primary classes of beta-lactams have differing general requirements for *f* T% > MIC to achieve optimal arrest of bacterial growth. Penicillins have been observed to require 29–34 % *f* T% > MIC, cephalosporins have been observed to require approximately 35–53 % *f* T% > MIC, and carbapenems have been observed to require approximately 20–26 % *f* T% > MIC for bacteriostasis in a neutropenic murine thigh model of infection [17]. In the clinical setting, similar *f* T% > MIC requirements for efficacy have been observed in patients treated with beta-lactams for acute otitis media [18]. However, for more severe infections such as hospital-acquired pneumonia, clinical efficacy of beta-lactams in patients has better correlated with the bactericidal (1 to 2-log reduction) exposures from animal infection models (50–70 % *f* T% > MIC), particularly against Gram-negative bacteria [19–21]. While the above targets provide a general guide, the specific $fT\% > MIC$ necessary for optimal killing is dependent on the beta-lactam in question, the infectious organism, and host factors (i.e., the presence of neutropenia) [17, 22]. As the selection of a given beta-lactam for an institutional CI and PI protocol will depend on formulary status and contract pricing, discussion of specific beta-lactams will be limited to agents for which significant evidence exists.

Both the agent-specific pharmacokinetic parameters (i.e., protein binding, total body clearance) and the pathogen MIC influence the $fT\% > MIC$; yet only maximization of PTA can be controlled by the clinician through manipulation of the dosing regimen as the pathogen MIC cannot be altered. Therefore, the clinician wishing to optimize $fT\% > MIC$ for a known infection with a given MIC may choose to administer a beta-lactam by CI or PI, to administer a beta-lactam with similar activity to the patient's current regimen with a longer comparative half-life, or to administer the same beta-lactam initially chosen at a more dose dense (greater frequency) or dose intense (higher dose) [22]. The choice between these options will center on the patient's clinical status, the patient's disposition, and the local institution's capacity to administer beta-lactams in alternate fashions. In the following section, evidence to support the selection of a CI or PI dosing scheme over increasing dose intensity is described.

2.1.2 Administration Techniques to Optimize Beta-Lactam PK-PD

Of the available methods of maximizing $fT\% > MIC$, the focus of this chapter is on the use of CI and PI administration techniques. A PI regimen extends (or prolongs) the traditional infusion time in the approved product labeling (usually 30 min for most beta-lactams). The resulting single-dose concentration time profile produces a blunted peak (C_{max}) and a delayed time to trough (C_{min}). CI and PI regiments generally increase in $fT\% > MIC$, which is illustrated in Fig. 2. Similarly, CI regimens will produce even greater reductions in C_{max} and with significant increases in $fT\% > MIC$ (Fig. 2).

Prospective studies evaluating CI and PI demonstrate clinical outcomes that range from no benefit to mortality benefit conferred. Importantly, few studies have identified substantial risk to using a CI or PI approach. In spite of the theoretical benefit that CI and PI dosing regimens are expected to provide, the observed impact on clinical outcomes tends to be most profound in the critically ill patients. A potential explanation for why observed outcomes sometimes fail to correspond with the predicted benefit is the "Hawthorne effect," wherein compliance with a given CI and PI protocol appears high during the period surrounding the implementation and then later regresses to baseline levels of noncompliance. Several studies have described successful implementation of CI and PI protocols during the observation period [6, 7, 23], but long-term follow-up studies are less prevalent. It is prudent to

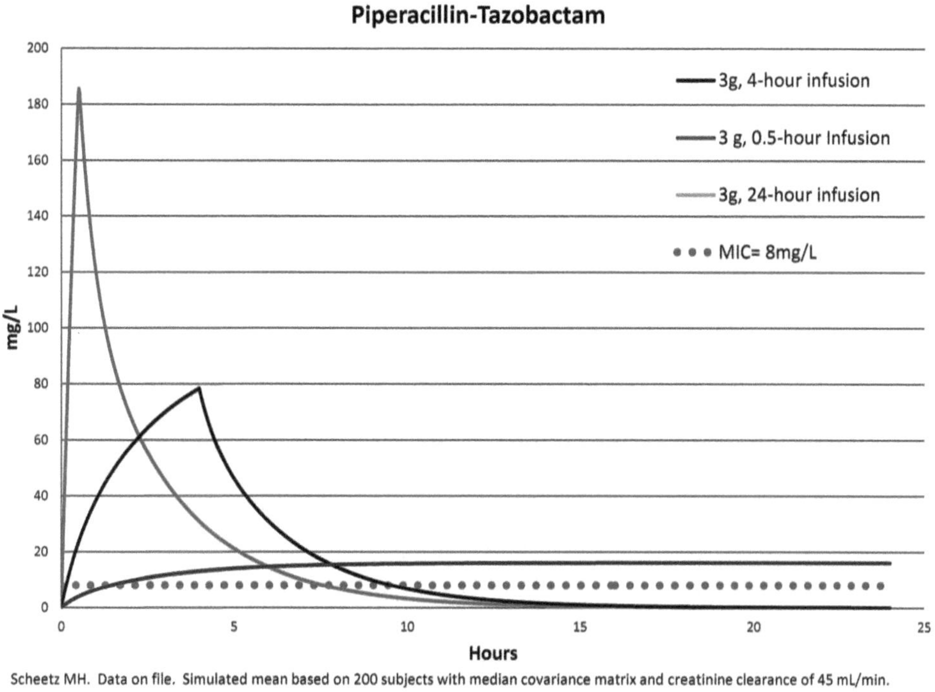

Fig. 2 Effect of prolonged and continuous infusion piperacillin-tazobactam on the concentration-time curve as compared with traditional 0.5-h infusion. Scheetz MH. Data on file. Simulated mean based on 200 subjects with median covariance matrix and creatinine clearance of 45 mL/min

continue to monitor compliance after implementation to mitigate any regression to baseline noncompliance levels in order to control variability in the *f*T% > MIC patients' experience.

2.1.3 Ex Vivo (Monte Carlo Simulation) Data to Support CI/PI Beta-Lactams

Mathematical modeling strategies for prediction of clinical outcomes for beta-lactams have been frequently employed in recent years. These techniques have been termed "ex vivo" or "in silico" to differentiate that these analyses are being performed as computer simulations. As noted above, beta-lactams frequently exhibit predictable pharmacokinetic disposition owing to renal and hepatic clearance mechanisms and relatively modest tissue distribution profiles. Pharmacokinetic disposition is frequently characterized by a structural model in which pharmacokinetic parameters can be estimated [24]. Often a two-compartment model is utilized for beta-lactams if the goal is to describe serum concentrations, where the serum is represented by the central compartment and the peripheral space represents all other distributive spaces.

Once a structural model is fit to the patient data, estimates for the individual parameters can be obtained and potentially improved if patient covariates are included in the model. The values for the parameters and their associated variation and covariation can be

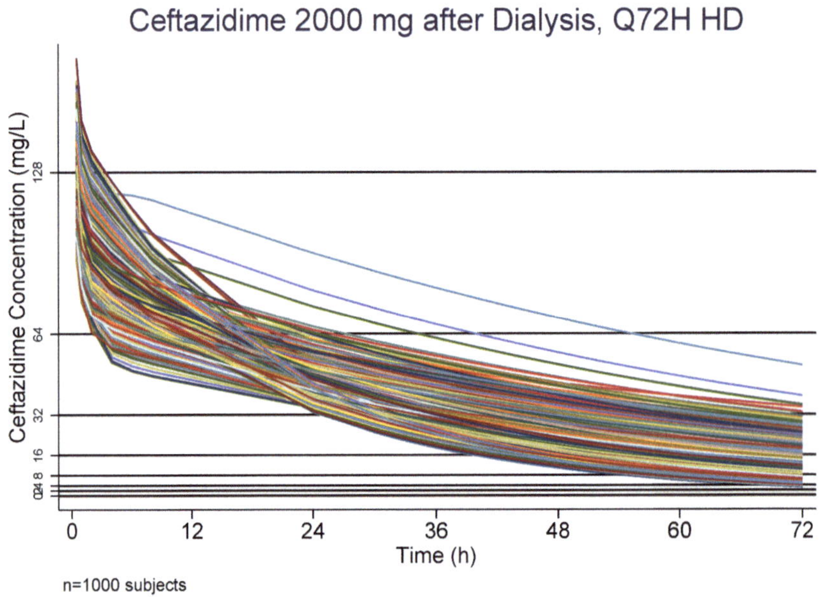

Fig. 3 One-thousand individual concentration-time profiles derived from mathematical modeling of ceftazidime 2000 mg post-dialysis. Scheetz MH. Unpublished data from: Antimicrob Agents Chemother. 2013 Dec; 57(12):5854–9

simulated to create a fictitious population that displays an amplification of the variability seen in the original sample group. For example, if 1000 patients are to be simulated, each patient in the simulation will be assigned parameter estimates based on known parameter variance and covariance. Once the fictitious population has parameters defined for each subject, this population is "given" a test dose and scheme for the beta-lactam in question. In this example, 1000 individual concentration time profiles are generated for the population (Fig. 3). Each individual patient pharmacokinetic exposure is then compared to the goal for the given beta-lactam for the organism in question (e.g., *f*T% > MIC of 40 %, see Chap. 1). That is, the probability that the target is attained (PTA) is calculated as a percentage of the number of subjects that exceeded the minimum *f*T% > MIC criterion (Fig. 4). To analyze these figures, one can determine the MIC at which the PTA becomes undesirable. By convention, this percentage is usually set at an arbitrary value of 90 % to provide acceptable efficacy for populations of patients. One can review Monte Carlo output and identify the highest MIC for which the PTA still exceeds 90 %. This MIC can generally be considered the PK-PD breakpoint for the drug-organism pair. That is, when treating patients with MICs above this value and the designated drug dosing scheme, clinical failure rates can be expected to increase. In the figure provided, 500 mg of ceftazidime for hemodialysis patients every 48 h could be

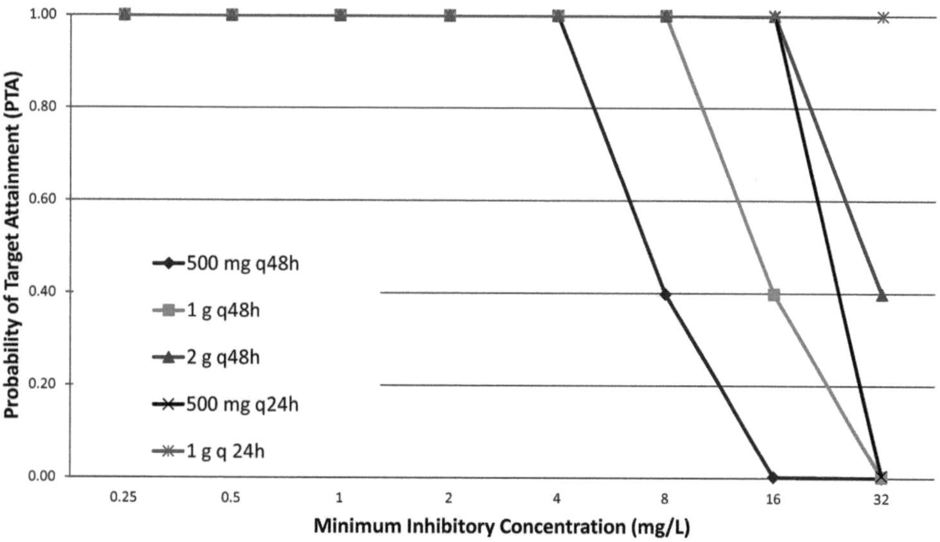

Fig. 4 Probability of target attainment (PTA) of ceftazidime in dialysis. Scheetz MH. Data from: Antimicrob Agents Chemother. 2013 Dec;57(12):5854–9

predicted as an efficacious regimen up to and including pathogen MICs of 4 mg/L. A large number of studies conducted using methods similar to those presented above have demonstrated the computer-simulated and theoretic benefits conferred by extended infusion to increase the *f*T% > MIC compared to intermittent infusion. The interested reader is referred to several articles that describe these processes in greater depth [24–36].

2.1.4 Clinical Studies Showing a Benefit for CI and PI Dosing and Relevant Methods

The predicted benefits of computer simulations have been borne out in several clinical studies, further providing proof for the principle of maximizing *f*T% > MIC. In one of the most impactful studies to date, Dulhunty and colleagues conducted a prospective trial evaluating the benefit of CI administration of beta-lactam antibiotics compared to traditional intermittent administration [5]. The authors compared clinical and pharmacokinetic outcomes among patients receiving piperacillin-tazobactam, meropenem, or ticarcillin-clavulanate administered by CI or traditional intermittent infusion. Patients in the CI group showed improvements in plasma antibiotic concentrations above the MIC (81.8 % vs. 28.6 %; $p = 0.001$), clinical cure on the test of cure date (76.7 % vs. 50 %; $p = 0.032$), and clinical cure on the test of cure date among patients not considered treatment failures (70 % vs. 43.3 %; $p = 0.037$). In another large prospective multinational study, Roberts and colleagues evaluated the impact of achievement of PK-PD indices among critically ill patients receiving beta-lactam antibiotics [37]. The authors evaluated the proportion of clinical cures without change or escalation in antibiotic therapy according to the achieved *f*T% > MIC of at least 50 % or at least

100 % of the dosing interval. Total infection-related mortality was observed in 8.9 % in the study population. Within the study population, 50 % $fT\% > MIC$ was achieved in 93 % of patients receiving PI dosing schemes but only 80 % of those receiving intermittent infusions. In their multivariate model, the authors found that increasing the achieved $fT\% > MIC$ between 50 and 100 % was associated with a 54 % improvement in the odds of achieving a positive clinical outcome adjusting for severity of illness measures (adjusted odds ratio [aOR] = 1.02; 95 % CI: 1.01–1.04 and aOR = 1.56; 95 % CI 1.15–2.13, respectively).

Lodise and colleagues conducted a retrospective cohort study of patients receiving either a standard infusion regimen (3.375 g intravenously over 30 minutes every 4 or 6 h) or a PI regimen (3.375 g intravenously over 4 h every 8 h) of piperacillin-tazobactam [1]. The authors identified a target beta-lactam, in this case piperacillin-tazobactam, which would be an ideal candidate for evaluation in a PI and CI paradigm. After implementing the PI program, they retrospectively reviewed the impact on clinical outcomes. The authors utilized binary recursive partitioning with classification and regression tree analysis (CART) to identify a difference in the binary outcome of 14-day mortality and length of stay (LOS) according to baseline predictors. A difference in 14-day mortality (5.2 % vs. 21.5 % mortality; $p = 0.001$) and LOS (median 18 days vs. 27.5 days; $p = 0.02$) was observed according to a difference in the subjects' APACHE II score, with the observed split identified between an APACHE II score of <17 and ≥17. Among patients with an APACHE II score <17, the authors did not find significant differences in the incidence of 14-day mortality or LOS. Among patients with an APACHE II score ≥17, the authors found a lower incidence of 14-day mortality (12.2 % vs. 31.6 %; $p = 0.04$) and a shorter median LOS (21 days vs. 38 days; $p = 0.02$) among patients receiving a PI compared to the standard infusion regimen.

Differences in clinical outcomes have also been observed with PI dosing of cefepime. Bauer and colleagues conducted a retrospective, quasi-experimental, study of patients receiving either a standard infusion regimen (2 g intravenously over 30 min every 8 h) or a PI regimen (2 g intravenously over 4 h every 8 h) of cefepime [4]. The authors selected a subset of the study population that had a documented respiratory or bloodstream infection with *Pseudomonas aeruginosa* in which to evaluate the outcomes of inpatient mortality, median hospital and intensive care unit (ICU) LOS, and median hospital cost during treatment with intravenous cefepime. Within the subgroup of patients with a positive clinical culture growing *Pseudomonas aeruginosa*, a lower incidence of inpatient mortality (3 % vs. 20 %; $p = 0.03$) and a shorter ICU LOS (8 days vs. 18.5 days; $p = 0.04$) were observed among patients receiving PI compared to standard infusion regimens. No significant differences were observed in median hospital LOS (14.5 days vs. 11 days; $p = 0.36$)

or median hospital costs (\$28,048 vs. \$51,231; $p=0.13$) between PI and standard infusion regimens. The authors conducted a multivariate logistic regression analysis to determine the confounder-adjusted risk of inpatient mortality. Candidate predictors significant in the univariate analysis included cefepime infusion type, ICU status at culture, and APACHE II score. The final multivariate model for inpatient mortality included cefepime infusion type (aOR = 0.06; 95 % confidence interval [95 % CI]: 0.001–0.64), ICU status at culture (aOR = 8.88; 95 % CI: 1.45–100.85), and APACHE II score (aOR = 1.13; 95 % CI: 1.03–1.27).

The benefits of PI beta-lactam administration have also been explored in a large, multicenter, retrospective cohort study by Yost and colleagues [38]. The authors aggregated data from 14 study centers for 359 patients receiving either a standard infusion regimen of a comparator agent or a PI regimen (3.375 g intravenously over 4 h every 8 h, dose adjusted if CrCl < 20 mL/min) of piperacillin-tazobactam. Comparator agents included standard infusions of intravenous cefepime, ceftazidime, imipenem-cilastatin, meropenem, doripenem, or piperacillin-tazobactam. While groups were not evenly balanced with EI patients receiving fewer aminoglycosides ($p=0.01$) and having fewer pseudomonal infections ($p=0.01$), the study demonstrated decreased in-hospital mortality in the EI piperacillin-tazobactam group vs. those receiving comparator antibiotics (9.7 % vs. 17.9 %, $p=0.02$).

Falagas and colleagues conducted a meta-analysis of clinical outcomes associated with CI and PI administration of carbapenems and piperacillin-tazobactam [39]. The authors aggregated data from 14 studies that included 1229 patients that received either standard infusion or CI or PI administration of piperacillin-tazobactam ($n=806$) or a carbapenem ($n=302$). Meropenem was the most frequently utilized carbapenem. The majority of included studies (8/14) included only patients with Gram-negative infections. The authors found a significant reduction in mortality in the pooled analysis among patients receiving CI and PI administration compared to standard infusion (relative risk [RR] = 0.59; 95 % CI: 0.41–0.83). This mortality benefit was observed among patients receiving CI administration (RR = 0.50; 95 % CI: 0.26–0.96) and PI administration (RR = 0.63; 95 % CI: 0.41–0.95) compared to standard infusion. The authors did not find a difference in clinical cure between standard infusion and CI and PI administration in the pooled analysis (RR = 1.13; 95 % CI: 0.99–1.28). A table summarizing several of the higher profile publications is included (Tables 1 and 2). In summary, many of the most notable publications point towards clinical benefits of CI/PI. Patients most likely to benefit are those with increased comorbidities and organisms with elevated MICs. The interested reader is referred to a more complete review of the published literature on clinical outcomes associated with CI and PI administration of beta-lactams [40, 41].

Table 1
Summary of design and results for clinical studies of continuous infusion (CI) of beta-lactams

Reference	Study design	Patients	Infection	Dosing regimen	CI findings
Bodey et al. [85]	RCT	235, cancer patients	Neutropenic fever	CMD 12 g/day CI vs. CMD 4 g q8h II	CI significantly higher cure rate (65 % vs. 21 %) only in subpopulation with persistent neutropenia (<100 neutrophils/mm^3)
Grant et al. [42]	Prospective, open-label controlled study	98, mixed infections	Gram-positive and -negative bacteria	TZP 8–12 g/day CI vs. TZP 3–4 g q6–8 h II	No difference in clinical (94 % vs. 82 %) or microbiological (89 % vs. 73 %) cure
Hanes et al. [86]	RCT	32, nosocomial pneumonia	Gram-negative bacteria	CAZ 60 mg/kg/day CI vs. CAZ 2 g q8h II	No difference in treatment outcomes
Lagast et al. [86]	RCT	45, septicemia	Gram-negative bacteria	CI CFP vs. II CFP	No difference in clinical response
Lau et al. [87]	Randomized, multicenter, open label	262, complicated intra-abdominal	Gram-positive and -negative bacteria	TZP 12 g/day CI vs. TZP 3 g q6h II	No difference in clinical (86.4 % vs. 88.4 %) or microbiological (83.9 % vs. 87.9 %) cure
Lorente et al. [88]	Retrospective, single center	89, VAP	Gram-negative bacteria	MEM 4 g/day CI vs. MEM 1 g q6h II	Significantly greater clinical cure rate (90.5 % vs. 59.6 %)
Lorente et al. [89]	Retrospective, single center	121, VAP	Gram-negative bacteria	CAZ 4 g/day CI vs. CAZ 2 g q12h II	Significantly greater clinical cure rate (89.3 % vs. 52.3 %)
Lorente et al. [90]	Retrospective, single center	83, VAP	Gram-negative bacteria	TZP 16 g/day CI vs. 4 g q6h II	Significantly greater clinical cure rate only when MIC of the pathogen is 8–16 mg/L
Nicolau et al. [91]	RCT	35, nosocomial pneumonia	Gram-positive and -negative bacteria	CAZ 3 g/day CI vs. CAZ 2 g q8h II	No difference in clinical (94 % vs. 83 %) and microbiological (76 % vs. 80 %) cure rates
Rafati et al. [92]	RCT	40, septic critically ill	Gram-negative bacteria	PIP 8 g/day CI vs. PIP 3 g q6h II	Significant reductions in the severity of illness (APACHE II)
Roberts et al. [93]	RCT	57, septic critically ill	Gram-positive and -negative bacteria	CRO 2 g/day CI vs. CRO 2 g q24h II	Significantly greater clinical and bacteriological cure rates only in patients receiving 4 or more days of treatment
Sakka et al. [94]	RCT	20, nosocomial pneumonia	Gram-positive and -negative bacteria	IMI 2 g/day CI vs. IMI 1 g q8h II	No difference in mortality
van Zanten et al. [95]	RCT	93, COPD exacerbation	Gram-positive and -negative bacteria	CTX 2 g/day CI vs. CTX 1 g q8h II	No difference in clinical cure rate (93 % vs. 93 %)

CAZ ceftazidime, *CFP* cefoperazone, *CI* continuous infusion, *CMD* cefamandole, *COPD* chronic obstructive pulmonary disease, *CRO* ceftriaxone, *CTX* cefotaxime, *II* intermittent infusion, *PIP* piperacillin, *TZP* piperacillin/tazobactam, *MEM* meropenem, *VAP* ventilator-associated pneumonia, *IMI* imipenem/cilastatin, *q6h* every 6 h, *q8h* every 8 h, *q12h* every 12 h, *q24h* every 24 h, *RCT* randomized controlled trial, *APACHE II* Acute Physiology and Chronic Health Evaluation II

Table 2
Summary of design and results for clinical studies of prolonged infusion (PI) of beta-lactams

Reference	Study design	Patients	Infection	Dosing regimen	PI findings
Chastre et al. [96]	Prospective, multicenter, randomized	531, VAP	Gram-positive and -negative bacteria	DOR 500 mg q8h 4-h inf. vs. IMI 500 mg q6h 30-min inf. or IMI 1 g q8h 1-h inf.	Comparable clinical (68.3 % vs. 64.8 %) and microbiological (73.3 % vs. 67.3 %) cure rates; no difference in mortality (10.8 % vs. 9.5 %)
Dow et al. [97]	Retrospective, single center	121, ICU	Gram-negative bacteria	TZP 3.375 g q8h or MEM 500 mg q6h 3- or 4-h inf. vs. TZP 3.375 g q6h or MEM 500 mg q6h 30-min inf.	No difference in mortality (12.4 % vs. 20.7 %)
Esterly et al. [98]	Retrospective, single center	71, bacteremia	*Acinetobacter baumannii*, *P. aeruginosa*, Enterobacteriaceae	IMI or MEM 3-h inf. vs. IMI or MEM 30-min inf.	No difference in mortality (28.6 % vs. 24.1 %)
Itabashi [99]	Prospective, single center	42, severe pneumonia	Gram-positive and -negative bacteria	MEM 500 mg q12h 4-h inf. vs. MEM 500 mg q12h 1-h inf.	Significantly lower mortality (5.6 % vs. 37.5 %)
Kollef et al. [100]	Prospective, multicenter, randomized	274, VAP	Gram-negative bacteria	DOR 1 g q8h 4-h inf. × 7 days vs. IMI 1 g q8h 1-h inf. × 10 days	Clinical cure (45.6 % vs. 56.8 %) numerically lower and 28-day mortality numerically higher (21.5 % vs. 14.8 %) in DOR treatment arm
Lee et al. [101]	Retrospective, multicenter	148, ICU	Gram-negative bacteria	TZP 3.375 g q8h 4-h inf. vs. TZP 2.25–4.5 g q6–8 h 30-min inf.	Significantly lower 30-day mortality (19 % vs. 38 %)
Nicasio et al. [46]	Prospective, single center	168, VAP	Gram-positive and -negative bacteria	Empirical VAP pathway with PI beta-lactam vs. empirical VAP therapy with TI beta-lactam	Significantly lower infection-related mortality (8.5 % vs. 21.6 %)
Patel et al. [102]	Retrospective, multicenter	129, mixed infections (mainly UTI and respiratory infection)	Gram-negative bacteria	TZP 3.375 g q8h 4-h inf. vs. TZP 3.375–4.5 g q6h or q8h 30-min inf.	No difference in mortality (5.7 % vs. 8.5 %)
Wang [44]	Retrospective, single center	30, HAP (ICU only)	*A. baumannii*	MEM 500 mg q6h 3-h inf. vs. MEM 1 g q8h 1-h inf.	No difference in clinical response

ICU intensive care unit, *FEP* cefepime, *TZP* piperacillin/tazobactam, *MEM* meropenem, *inf.* infusion, *q8h* every 8 h, *VAP* ventilator-associated pneumonia, *DOR* doripenem, *IMI* imipenem/cilastatin, *q6h* every 6 h, *CI* confidence interval, *EI* extended infusion, *RR* risk ratio, *q12h* every 12 h, *q4h* every 4 h, *APACHE* Acute Physiology and Chronic Health Evaluation, *TI* traditional infusion, *UTI* urinary tract infection, *HAP* hospital-acquired pneumonia

Adapted from MacVane SH, Kuti JL, Nicolau DP. Prolonging Beta-lactam infusion: A review of the rationale and evidence, and guidance for implementation. Int J Antimicrob Agents. 2014 Feb;43(2):105–13

2.1.5 Pharmacoeconomic Data to Support CI/PI Beta-Lactams

Favorable pharmacoeconomic outcomes are possible with CI and PI administration of beta-lactams. In fact, 29–52 % of institutions cite cost as a rationale for the use of CI and PI compared to standard infusion beta-lactam schemes [3]. In cost-benefit analyses, improvements can be realized by either decreasing the numerator (i.e., direct costs) or increasing positive outcomes in the denominator. Thus, pharmacoeconomic support for CI and PI beta-lactam infusion schemes can be divided into improvements in drug acquisition or administration costs and improvements in patient outcomes, which translate into favorable cost-benefit measures such as quality-adjusted life years (QALYS).

First, daily doses of beta-lactams can be decreased without decreasing attainment of pharmacodynamic parameters (e.g., fT% > MIC) as previously described. Optimal schemes not only retain similar target goals, but rather improve fT% > MIC while utilizing less drug. For instance, in one of the more commonly cited clinical efficacy studies for PI piperacillin-tazobactam [1], the authors were able to cut the number of 3.375 g piperacillin-tazobactam doses in half (i.e., cut from 6 doses per day to 3 doses per day) by increasing the infusion time from 30 min to 4 h. This less frequent PI administration improved the probability of target attainment (i.e., fT% > MIC of 50 %) from less than 50–100 % for MICs of 16 mg/L. This intervention alone was responsible for an estimated $68,000–135,000 reduction in drug acquisition cost during the first year of implementation at Albany Medical Center Hospital. As previously noted, mortality was also decreased with this scheme. Others have documented that PI schemes for piperacillin-tazobactam can be cost saving and efficacious [42]. In this study and others, costs were saved with CI and PI administration by decreasing pharmacist preparatory time and nursing administration time. In another example, CI administration of piperacillin-tazobactam decreased median labor costs (nursing administration and pharmacy preparation time) by 75 % [43]. Similarly for the carbapenems in the setting of hospital-acquired pneumonia, meropenem 500 mg every 6 h given as a 3-h infusion was associated with a 34 % cost decrease compared to 1 g every 8 h as a 1-h infusion (i.e., mean $684.06 vs. $1038.83, respectively) [44]. Clinical outcomes did not differ for these patients.

In other instances, using the most appropriate antimicrobial based on PK-PD principles may require more costly agents at higher doses than traditional infusions [45]. Particularly in settings where drug resistance is frequent, the use of higher doses of CI or PI may be necessary to achieve pharmacodynamic targets at a high rate. Due to the high prevalence of MDR *P. aeruginosa* in one hospital's ICUs, high-dosed PI cefepime, 2 g every 8 h as a 3-h infusion, was required to achieved the goal pharmacodynamic target (50 % fT > MIC) for the empiric therapy of VAP in their clinical pathway [46]. Although higher doses of more expensive antibiotics were used during Hartford Hospital's VAP clinical pathway, the attributable reduction in infection-related length of stay resulted in nearly $40,000 per patient reduction in the cost of care, with comparable overall antibiotic cost [47]. Reductions in length of stay and the utilization of healthcare resources have a greater impact on cost of care.

The ability to demonstrate an economic benefit certainly improves the sustainability for the program. However, achieving these measures should never adversely affect patient care. While decreased antibiotic expenditures, the so-called low-hanging fruit, may be the most obtainable measure and provide the initial justification for use of dose-optimized infusion schemes, quality measures that impact patient care and outcomes should always be investigated [48].

Cost-effectiveness analyses are a method of comparing two treatment strategies for both cost and efficacy simultaneously. Strong dominance is a principle that defines an intervention that is both more effective and less costly [49]. In these situations, selecting the most appropriate strategy does not require application of further principles. While we are not aware that cost-effectiveness analyses have been performed to compare CI and PI administration schemes to traditional intermittent infusions, the increased efficacy and decreased costs likely mean that CI and PI dosing schemes dominate intermittent infusions for beta-lactams and should be employed whenever possible. Such effects will hopefully be directly confirmed in the future.

2.2 Implementing a Continuous or Extended Infusion Beta-Lactam Program

2.2.1 Institution-Specific Needs

Continuous or prolonged infusions of beta-lactams are rational approaches to the optimal administration of these agents as previously described. However, little guidance exists on how to proceed with implementation of these dosing schemes into practice [50]. Such direction is only briefly outlined in the method's section of some research papers on the topic, leaving a significant knowledge gap for the first-time program implementer. Furthermore, the approach used to construct a dose-optimized program at a major academic medical center may be different and thus not applicable to a remote, critical-access community hospital. Taking the aforementioned challenges into account, it is no wonder that despite the recognized benefits, CI or PI beta-lactam dosing strategies are still not employed in most institutions.

As each institution may have varying needs and resources, an individualized approach is warranted to gather useful information on how the application of dose-optimized strategies will benefit one's hospital and its patients. For example, at institutions with significant rates of resistance to commonly utilized agents, prescribers may be forced to otherwise consider the use of older, more toxic antibiotics as the new standard of care. In this instance, the availability of CI or PI programs may provide additional treatment opportunities by improving the likelihood of achieving bactericidal exposure for beta-lactams in situations where traditional infusions would fail to provide adequate exposures. In contrast, CI and PI may also provide value in settings where standard beta-lactams infusions remain highly efficacious due to low levels of resistance [51]. In such a scenario, there is a theoretic possibility of decreased or slowed progression of resistance.

To effectively implement a CI or PI program first requires knowledge of relevant antibiotic susceptibility data for commonly isolated local pathogens, an appreciation of where the greatest benefit will be achieved (e.g., implementing hospital-wide vs. unit-specific vs. selected patient populations), an ability to interpret the pharmacokinetic and pharmacodynamic literature in order to identify the optimal antibiotic and dosing regimen for one's population, and a capacity to collaborate with a multidisciplinary team to implement the program. Heinrich and colleagues detailed a comprehensive example of their experience with developing and implementing a hospital-wide pharmacist-led piperacillin-tazobactam PI guideline at a 500-bed academic medical center [6]. These authors evaluated and considered their institution size, patient population (children were excluded at their institution due to lack of data in this population), medication workflow (ordering, distribution, dispensing, and documentation) process, technology level (CPOE, eMAR), and availability of resources (infusion pumps, etc.) when devising their rollout plan. With a better view of the scope of available resources and identifying barriers to implementation at one's facility, key contributors can be recruited to begin cohesive planning and development of the protocol.

Applying Local Resistance and MIC Distributions

It is the authors' advice to utilize local MIC data, when available, to make informed decisions regarding the appropriate application of dose-optimized infusion strategies. Information displayed on antibiograms is essential for the selection of empiric antimicrobial therapy as susceptibility patterns can vary considerably between countries, from hospital to hospital, and even among units or wards within the same hospital [52]. The importance of institution-specific data was elegantly shown by Rello and colleagues, who retrospectively compared the etiology of microorganisms collected from patients with VAP from three different institutions. Their examination revealed significant variations in the etiologies and susceptibility (inconsistent rates of MDR strains) among microorganisms implicated in VAP according to institution. Substantial differences were observed between sites for all groups of organisms, including drug-resistant bacteria such as MRSA, *Pseudomonas aeruginosa*, and *Acinetobacter baumannii* [52]. The authors suggested that antimicrobial therapy should be tailored based on institution-specific findings vs. general recommendations put forth in guidelines [52]. Therefore, while regional or national surveillance data may provide useful information on general trends of resistance over time, these resources should only be used to guide empirical therapy in the absence of institution-specific susceptibility, and preferably MIC data.

One hospital population that may benefit most from CI or PI regimens includes patients admitted to the ICU. It has been reported that antimicrobial resistance pathogens are more frequently seen in ICU rather than non-ICU locations [53]. An alternative approach to a single antibiogram for the entire institution is the construction of antibiograms from distinctive units within the institution targeting the most common pathogens. For example, distinguishing collection isolates based on hospital location (medical vs. surgical), acuity of illness (ICU vs. non-ICU), or disease-specific (cardiac vs. transplant vs. neurosurgery ICU) characteristics may offer additional information to be used for the best application of dose-optimized strategies. Use of unit-specific antibiograms has been proven superior at selecting appropriate empiric antimicrobial therapy as compared with hospital-wide antibiograms [53–55]. Binkley and colleagues compared susceptibility patterns over a 3-year period (a total of nearly 10,000 isolates) between unit-specific (general medicine and surgical wards, oncology, and medical and surgical ICU) and hospital-wide generated antibiograms [54]. They found that using a hospital-wide antibiogram substantially under-reported and over-reported the rates of resistant isolates compared with ICU- and non-ICU-specific antibiograms, respectively. For instance, rates of methicillin resistance were 20 % higher in the medical ICU than in the hospital overall, which would likely have a significant impact on the selection of empiric antimicrobials.

A similar scenario might influence the choice of the optimal beta-lactam antibiotic regimen. For example, a difference in the epidemiology and resistance patterns of *P. aeruginosa* isolates between three ICUs (medical, surgical, and neurosurgical) was described at one medical center [56]. This observation was the basis for the use of different prolonged infusion regimens depending on the patient's ICU location for the empiric treatment of VAP when developing a clinical pathway at this hospital. MICs were conducted by E-test methodology against *P. aeruginosa* isolates collected over the past 12 months and separated by ICU location. The difference in beta-lactam MICs against *P. aeruginosa* across the three ICUs required high-dose PI cefepime (2 g every 8 h as a 3-h infusion) for the surgical and neurotrauma ICU, because it produced the highest CFR against isolates collected in this unit. In contrast, for the medical ICU where cefepime MICs were higher due to resistance, a high-dose, prolonged infusion meropenem regimen (2 g every 8 h as a 3-h infusion) was selected for empiric therapy [46, 47]. Notably, CI or PI piperacillin-tazobactam resulted in lower CFRs among these ICUs; therefore, it was reserved for treatment once pathogen and susceptibility data were available on a patient-to-patient basis. As a result of this approach, the knowledge of susceptibility patterns on a unit-specific level allowed for informed decisions on the selection of empiric antimicrobial agent and dose(s), leading to significant reductions in infection-related mortality, length of stay, and overall costs without significantly increasing the drug budget [47]. A number of other studies have seen improved patient outcomes when utilizing a local antibiogram to guide antibiotic choice [57–59]. In the event that local MIC data is not available, the antibiogram along with published PTA literature can be used to estimate CFRs for the institution. This strategy assumes that the antibiotic MIC for against the target organism is equivalent to the respective susceptible, intermediate, and resistant breakpoints. For instance, if 65 %, 25 %, and 10 % of the *P. aeruginosa* are susceptible (≤8 mg/L), intermediate (≤16 mg/L), and resistant (≥32 mg/L) to cefepime at one's institution, respectively, the CFR can be calculated under the assumption that 65 %, 25 %, and 10 % of the population has cefepime MIC of 8 mg/L, 16 mg/L, and 32 mg/L, respectively. The least desirable approach is to assume that the local MIC distribution is comparable to the national data when extrapolating susceptibilities from surveillance studies to determine CFRs.

In certain scenarios, the application of CI and PI may fail to produce sufficient improvement in exposure for beta-lactams. This might be the case when the antibiotic MIC is very high (i.e., several dilutions above the resistance breakpoint), when the underlying comorbidities of a patient cause him or her to eliminate an antibiotic quicker than anticipated, or a combination of both [60, 61]. For instance, while PI piperacillin-tazobactam (3.375 g q8h as a 4-h infusion) can dramatically improve the PTA for organisms with a MIC of ≤16 mg/L as compared with traditional 30-min dosing regimens, PTAs are suboptimal at MICs of 32 and 64 mg/L, MICs for *P. aeruginosa*, which until recently were defined as susceptible to this antibiotic [62]. Additionally, recent data suggests that in patients with preserved or enhanced renal clearance (CrCl ≥ 100 mL/min), PI piperacillin-tazobactam (3.375 g q8h as a 4-h infusion) also provides suboptimal exposures at MICs of 16 mg/L (PTA = 0.73 for CrCl of 100 mL/min vs. PTA = 0.90 for CrCl of 60 mL/min), and thus a more aggressive dosing regimen (4 g of piperacillin administered for 3 h every 6 h) or an alternative agent should be considered [36, 63]. Thus, a one-size-fits-all approach may not be optimal for all hospitals and patients settings where alternative agents should be considered.

Hospital-Wide vs. Specific Population Use

Once MIC/susceptibility data have been considered and the specific antibiotic/dosing regimen selected for implementation, the protocol team should assess whether to implement the program hospital-wide, or only in specific units or patient populations. As the potential benefit of CI or PI regimens may vary depending on the patient population and the MIC of the infecting pathogen, dose-optimized regimens may not be applicable or appropriate for all patients, as many infections can be treated effectively with standard dosing regimens. Therefore, the greatest benefit of dose-optimized infusions may be realized in those with elevated morbidity and those most likely to be infected with the highest MIC organism [1]. This makes patients in the ICU and those with burns or cystic fibrosis an attractive target population for initial rollout of programs. Education can be focused towards caregivers of these populations, and compliance can be more easily tracked. Although targeted in its application, use of CI or PI beta-lactams only in very specific populations, however, may cause confusion and errors across the rest of the hospital. For instance, what happens when patients are transferred out of the ICU and are still receiving an optimized dosing regimen? The use of both standard and optimized dosing regimens may also complicate education of prescribers and nursing staff, particularly for those with overlapping coverage between different units in the hospital, or when patients are transferred to outside institutions [64]. Moreover, since a variety of organisms can unpredictably cause infection among a diverse population of patients, some patients that were not initially targeted may be excluded from the potential benefits of CI or PI. In contrast, a hospital-wide implementation requires significantly greater resources for education, availability of "smart" pumps (if utilized), and to ensure compliance across the entire institution. At Hartford Hospital, piperacillin-tazobactam is administered as a CI across the entire hospital population, with the exception of patients with severe renal dysfunction or those with intravenous line compatibility concerns. This decision was based on the antibiotic's popular use across medical and surgical wards and similarities in piperacillin-tazobactam MICs against *P. aeruginosa* between ICU and non-ICU populations. A similar approach is employed for PI doripenem. However, PI cefepime is only utilized in the ICUs because of only marginal increases in CFR against isolates collected outside of the ICU.

It may be reasonable to pilot the program in select units or floors within the institution, such as one or two ICUs, prior to implementing hospital-wide [23]. This strategy may identify barriers to the implementation process that may be informative to improving the plan for hospital-wide implementation. It is important to collect information during this pilot period to evaluate the compliance and identify problem areas with the program. Priority should be given to areas with adequate staffing to educate and direct the first-time users of the program.

Continuous vs. Prolonged Infusions

While both CI and PI administration can increase the likelihood of achieving the requisite pharmacodynamic target, both methods should be evaluated to determine their respective CFR using your own local MIC distributions [34]. In the event that prolonged and

Table 3
Pros and cons of dose-optimized infusion administration techniques

Type	Advantages	Disadvantages
Extended or prolonged infusions	• Less frequent administration (compared with intermittent) • Same dose/delivery package as intermittent doses • Daily antibiotic-free interval • Ambulatory patient	• Timing of administration for non-compatible drugs • Labor and supplies • Administration resources
Continuous infusions	• Reduced costs for labor, supplies, and administration • Once-daily administration	• Stability and drug waste • Dedicated line • Compatibility issues • Ambulatory patient

continuous infusions provide similar likelihoods of bactericidal exposure, the determining factor becomes dependent on the preference for once-daily administration (continuous) vs. availability of intravenous access (prolonged) [34]. There are advantages and limitations to each method of administration (Table 3). The primary disadvantages to administering beta-lactams via CI are that some agents, such as carbapenems and ampicillin, have limited stability at room temperature; furthermore, some agents are incompatible with other commonly used medications in the hospital (see section on "Practical Considerations" below). Additionally, the necessity for a dedicated IV line may make many institutions reluctant to employ continuous infusions. In contrast, PI regimens still require multiple daily doses and can also interfere with other drugs when compatibility is an issue. A continuous infusion may require the administration of a loading dose to get concentrations to steady state quickly, while PI is initiated as such with the initial dose. For instance in Fig. 2b, the time to first achieving a concentration of 8 mg/L for intermittent infusion, prolonged infusion, and continuous infusion is 2 min, 9 min, and 1.5 h, respectively. Regardless of the selected administration method, the inclusion and exclusion criteria for their use must be explicitly defined to minimize confusion and potentially serious complications if patients are given inappropriate regimens.

2.2.2 Protocol/Guideline Development

The focus of CI or PI antimicrobials is to maximize favorable clinical outcomes while minimizing adverse effects. While there is no "one way" to develop and implement dose-optimized infusion program, there are standard tactics that have successfully been used by many healthcare facilities [1, 6, 23]. To implement the program in an organized and proficient manner, it is recommended to consider the areas outlined under this section. Note that these principles are not specific to CI or PI of beta-lactams, but are universal global initiatives and pillars of patient care for most healthcare systems.

Key Personnel and Committees

When preparing to implement a dose-optimized infusion strategy, the buy-in should incorporate members throughout the institution, not solely infectious disease practitioners. One of the problems healthcare institutions often face in implementing effective dose-optimized regimens includes communicating their goals with hospital administrators. Buy-in from senior institutional leadership is a necessary key to success. Hospital administration provides the authority, payment, and infrastructure necessary for the program.

A core team should be responsible for establishing, drafting, and managing the dose optimization program. Potential members to include in the team are providers (infectious diseases, critical care, pulmonary, surgery, and emergency medicine), nursing, pharmacy, clinical microbiology, information technology, and administration, among other specialties. Each of these departments is vital to provide unified comprehension of the goals and implementation plan for the program. Team members should meet on a regular basis in an effort to direct and focus the program to ensure success. This team can also be responsible for addressing the feasibility of implementation and any technological or practical issues that may arise.

A member of the team should be designated as a "point" person that is dedicated to the supervision of the program, its development, and implementation. Since this program pertains to novel administration of an antibiotic, a pharmacist or physician with specific training or interest in infectious diseases often fulfils this role. Although a single representative may be branded as the "leader," infectious disease physicians, pharmacy, and administration must each pledge complete support and buy-in during the early phases of development. The program has limited chance of success without backing from essential personnel. Consideration may also be given to having other hospital committees that might be affected by implementation (e.g., infection control, stewardship, IV therapy, nursing education) offer comments or have the opportunity to ask questions. This universal approach maximizes the likelihood of approval at Pharmacy and Therapeutics Committee and minimizes opportunities for errors/protocol noncompliance during implementation.

The Role of Technology

When transitioning to CI or PI strategies, whether on an institutional or unit-specific basis, awareness of the technological capabilities can enhance the likelihood of a smooth conversion. Likewise, technologies such as computerized provider order entry (CPOE), electronic medical records (EMR), and computer-based surveillance can minimize errors related to prescribing, transcribing, and documenting of administration type.

Many institutions that have successfully implemented dose-optimized infusion programs obtained input and support from information technology during program development [1, 6, 23, 46]. CPOE can increase compliance by defaulting to the desired administration method (dose, frequency, and rate) for the specific approved use and can also decrease medical errors [65]. For example, if a PI regimen is only to be used for the treatment of infections in the ICU, then a specific critical order set can be designed that houses the PI line item, in essence preventing prescribers from ordering the dosing regimen for a patient outside of the ICU. Some CPOE systems can also generate electronic alerts to remind clinicians about dose-optimized regimens when they order select antimicrobials. The use of these computerized decision support programs has been associated with improved patient outcomes and reduced costs of care [66, 67].

The availability of infusion pumps equipped with medication libraries and other software to alert users of potential errors should also make for a simpler transition to CI or PI. Universally referred to as "smart pumps," this technology allows the operator to create a library of medications with dosing guidelines. By defining specific concentrations and dosages, these guidelines can be used with CI and PI to tailor antibiotic delivery to the exact requirements of certain patient populations based on various factors (location, severity of illness, bodyweight). This technology has been shown to improve the accuracy of IV infusions and reduce administration errors [68, 69]. However, these infusion pumps are not infallible, as the user can still potentially choose the wrong medication from the stock or the medication library [70]. Integration of smart pumps with other medication error aversion technologies such as barcode scanning and dosage limits can improve the accuracy of device programming and further reduce administration errors.

Practical Considerations

The physical and chemical characteristics of the antimicrobial must be considered before CI or PI can be applied. Patients undergoing antimicrobial therapy may concurrently be receiving a wide range of other drug treatments requiring intravenous access. While PI will occupy access for approximately 50 % of the dosing interval, continuous infusions will require either a dedicated line or consideration for the compatibility of concomitantly administered medications. Fortunately, a recent report showed that vancomycin and piperacillin-tazobactam, two of the three most commonly prescribed antimicrobials in US hospitals, are compatible during Y-site injection at concentrations commonly used during prolonged infusions [71].

An important consideration regarding CI and PI is the bag volume and pump settings, to ensure complete and precise administration. Dead space volume, from failing to flush the line following the antibiotic infusion, can result in a 40 % loss of the prescribed dose if prepared in 50 mL containers [64]. In response, one group of authors modified their extended infusion protocol to mandate a minimum container volume of 250 mL for non-ICU patients [64]. For patients in the ICU or requiring fluid restrictions, alternative pumps with less dead space can be used. Lam and colleagues calculated the residual tubing volumes for commonly used infusion pump models [72]. Use of microbore tubing to reduce infusion dead space, increasing the infusion volume to account for less than 10 mL of volume lost, or alternative pumps that can safely administer infusion line residuals were proposed solutions.

2.2.3 Disseminating the Program to Staff

Education

Education is considered an essential and important component of any program requiring a change in behavior of clinical practice [73, 74]. To do this effectively, the program must be straightforward, succinct, and easily accessible. Ideally, evidence-based medicine, as described above, should be provided. Print materials can augment your message and should be available to tackle common concerns and provide reinforcement. However, simply providing access to this information is unlikely to result in complete understanding [75]. Passive education on its own will only have a marginal effect [76]. Conducting in-service training to advise staff on the new procedure is recommended. Furthermore, the impact of CI and PI on clinical and economic outcomes should be provided in these education sessions. The better understanding the team has of the transition, the more likely protocol noncompliance will be minimized.

Knowing Your Audience

To communicate effectively, the message should be tailored to the audience and focused on areas that will influence their task. For instance, when introducing PI piperacillin-tazobactam at the Ohio State University Medical Center (OSUMC), Goff and colleagues envisioned that the nursing staff may be displeased that PI would require approximately 12 h of dedicated line access throughout the day [77]. Therefore, they emphasized the improved mortality rates seen with PI at other institutions, rather than the pharmacodynamic benefits, when presenting the PI method to nursing staff. This was in line with the nursing staffs' dedication to patient care. In contrast, a discussion on the influence of optimized regimens of the emergence of resistant subpopulations of bacteria may be better suited for the infectious disease practitioners and clinical microbiologists. Gearing your presentation towards the concerns of your audience can drastically improve your chances of earning their support. A well-illustrated example of the process of transitioning of alterative dosing schemes into practice was demonstrated at Albany Medical Center Hospital, where Lodise and colleagues applied dose-optimized infusion techniques to cefepime, meropenem, and piperacillin-tazobactam. The authors nicely highlight each step of the process from early idea generation to the eventual implementation [1, 29, 78].

3 Notes

3.1 Improving the Program through Reassessment and Modifications: The Role of Antibiotic Stewardship

Dose-optimized regimens are commonly utilized as a part of antimicrobial stewardship programs [45, 50, 77]. In line with other stewardship initiatives, periodic audits should be performed to evaluate compliance with the program, to track and identify unexpected issues, and to generate data in continued support of the dosing regimen.

3.1.1 Evaluating the Program: Process and Outcome Measures

A variety of methods and measures have been used to show value, including a number of process and outcome metrics [48]. Although process measures have repeatedly been shown to evaluate quality of care, they fail to explain the implications on patient outcomes. Likewise, outcome measures are not without shortcomings, as they do not reliably detect the effect on quality of care. Therefore, both process and outcome measures should be identified to determine the impact of the program intervention.

Selection of an appropriate and meaningful measure can be challenging. Demonstrating a link between process and outcome is crucial to assuring providers and administration that an observed benefit is attributed to the studied intervention. Despite the documented benefits of dose-optimized infusion strategies, unfortunately, endpoints are often chosen with nearly unobtainable goals, particularly in studies with a small number of observations and multiple infection types. The chief example is the endpoint of mortality, which is notably the clinical outcome of greatest importance. However, impact on mortality is usually multifactorial and difficult to show a causal relationship with a single intervention. Additionally, due to the complex nature of mortality, the difference is seldom large enough to reach statistical significance, even when making an effort to control for confounding factors. For example, the sickest patients who receive the highest quality care are still the most likely to die. Therefore, while mortality may still be an appropriate outcome measure for studying optimized beta-lactam therapy in ICU patients with MDR infections, it is also advantageous to select measures that are sensitive to changes in practice (i.e., antimicrobial resistance rates, adverse medication events, length of stay) [79]. Many programs have also focused on outcomes such as clinical response, length of stay, hospitalization costs, development of superinfections, as well as emergence and rates of resistance.

Common process measures include but are not limited to program compliance (number and percentage of use), antibiotic utilization (quantity used, duration of therapy), and antibiotic expenditures (cost savings). Note that antibiotic expenditures are considered process measures as they are directly related to the quantity of antibiotic prescribed, whereas total hospitalization costs are outcome measures because if a patient does better with an intervention, it can result in substantial, cross-departmental savings [48]. Pharmacy expenditures, particularly related to drug acquisition, are a budgetary item of high scrutiny for potential cost reductions. Under certain circumstances, CI or PI will require lower total daily doses than standard dosing regimens, reducing the cost of therapy. It is important to note that financial outcomes need to account for the change in cost over time and should adjust for the annual inflation rate [80]. Due to piperacillin-tazobactam's broad spectrum of activity and popular use, it is often the chosen antibiotic for the first attempt to prolong infusions for beta-lactams. However, similar observations have been described with the use of continuous infusions [42, 81, 82], and as previously noted less frequent dose administration and less pharmacy and nursing time may represent an additional cost savings by reducing their time requirements.

There are two common methods to evaluate drug consumption, defined daily doses (DDD) and days of therapy (DOT). DDD is calculated as the total number of grams of antibiotic consumed divided by the number of grams in an average daily dose, while DOT is simply the number of days the individual patient receives the antibiotic of interest. As the total amount of administered dose is reduced in PI regimens, corresponding reductions in DDDs will be observed. However, DOT will remain largely unchanged.

Lastly, although measuring the impact of PI on clinical and economic outcomes has been well described, the effect on the development of resistance is not as clearly defined due to the dynamic process and multifactorial nature of antimicrobial resistance. However, dosing regimens that are designed to attain pharmacodynamic targets will also likely reduce the probability of the emergence of resistance [51].

3.2 Potential Barriers and Proposed Solutions

Implementing a program for administering antimicrobial agents by continuous or extended infusion does not come without challenges. Several barriers exist to successful implementation [83]. These may include lack of provider participation or opposition, limited financial resources, personnel restraints, resistance for collaborative efforts from administration, and low perceived value compared to alternative efforts. The use of dose-optimized infusion strategies requires a change in traditionally prescribing practices. It may be difficult to change these practices; however, steps can be taken to alleviate concerns [84]. Possible solutions to overcome these obstacles are listed in Table 4.

Table 4
Challenges and possible solutions of continuous and prolonged infusion programs

Challenges of continuous and prolonged infusions	Solution strategies
• Limited resources	• Determine goals of the program and availability of resources • Present impact of potential clinical and economic benefits to administration
• Lack of interest and buy-in for providers	• Tailor your message towards the values of your audience • Provide evidence-based literature • Involve doubtful providers as team members of the program development
• Provider push-back and compliance issues	• Automatic substitution (Pharmacy and Therapeutics Committee) • Discuss opportunities to improve patient care and cost
• Inappropriate/improper use of the protocol	• Define inclusion and exclusion criteria of the population for use • Implement dosing protocols via computerized software
• Confusion with program procedure	• Conduct education prior to implementation • Devise an initial rollout plan with a "hotline" for questions and troubleshooting
• Errors	• Involve information technology to create electronic alerts • Incorporate into computerized provider order entry • Use reminders (product labels, standardized volumes, programmable infusion pumps)
• Challenges sustaining the program over time	• Plan continuing education sessions • Post reminders in newsletters and flyers • Reevaluate local MIC data to ensure optimal drug selection • Perform audits and collect outcome/process data to demonstrate benefit at your institution

4 Conclusion

Optimizing the administration of beta-lactam antibiotics through CI and PI administration is feasible and increasingly necessary as antimicrobial resistance increases. We have shown that institutions interested in implementing these protocols may find useful evidence and guidance in the literature. Local susceptibility data and institutional antimicrobial use guidelines are needed to select agents for appropriate empiric use. Implementation of a CI or PI protocol will require a multidisciplinary and multifaceted approach in order to assure successful and safe rollout. Measuring the impact of a protocol can be difficult, but minimally the observed cost differential should be presented to support the program's viability as clinical and microbiological outcome metrics are collected over time. Once the initial challenge of overcoming the inertia in a system has been met, vigilant monitoring will be needed to maintain and document improvements in patient care. Despite these challenges, CI and PI dosing regimens represent a straightforward intervention that may improve patient care and can readily be implemented by a champion user in essentially any institution.

References

1. Lodise TP Jr, Lomaestro B, Drusano GL (2007) Piperacillin-tazobactam for Pseudomonas aeruginosa infection: clinical implications of an extended-infusion dosing strategy. Clin Infect Dis 44(3):357–363. doi:10.1086/510590
2. Society for Healthcare Epidemiology of A, Infectious Diseases Society of A, Pediatric Infectious Diseases S (2012) Policy statement on antimicrobial stewardship by the Society for Healthcare Epidemiology of America (SHEA), the Infectious Diseases Society of America (IDSA), and the Pediatric Infectious Diseases Society (PIDS). Infect Control Hosp Epidemiol 33(4):322–327. doi:10.1086/665010
3. George JM, Colton BJ, Rodvold KA (2012) National survey on continuous and extended infusions of antibiotics. Am J Health Syst Pharm 69(21):1895–1904. doi:10.2146/ajhp110562
4. Bauer KA, West JE, O'Brien JM, Goff DA (2013) Extended-infusion cefepime reduces mortality in patients with Pseudomonas aeruginosa infections. Antimicrob Agents Chemother 57(7):2907–2912. doi:10.1128/AAC.02365-12
5. Dulhunty JM, Roberts JA, Davis JS, Webb SA, Bellomo R, Gomersall C, Shirwadkar C, Eastwood GM, Myburgh J, Paterson DL, Lipman J (2013) Continuous infusion of beta-lactam antibiotics in severe sepsis: a multicenter double-blind, randomized controlled trial. Clin Infect Dis 56(2):236–244. doi:10.1093/cid/cis856
6. Heinrich LS, Tokumaru S, Clark NM, Garofalo J, Paek JL, Grim SA (2011) Development and implementation of a piperacillin-tazobactam extended infusion guideline. J Pharm Pract 24(6):571–576. doi:10.1177/0897190011406984
7. Nichols KR, Knoderer CA, Cox EG, Kays MB (2012) System-wide implementation of the use of an extended-infusion piperacillin/tazobactam dosing strategy: feasibility of utilization from a children's hospital perspective. Clin Ther 34(6):1459–1465. doi:10.1016/j.clinthera.2012.05.005
8. Eagle H, Fleischman R, Musselman AD (1950) Effect of schedule of administration on the therapeutic efficacy of penicillin; importance of the aggregate time penicillin remains at effectively bactericidal levels. Am J Med 9(3):280–299
9. Andes D, Craig WA (2002) Animal model pharmacokinetics and pharmacodynamics: a critical review. Int J Antimicrob Agents 19(4):261–268
10. Craig WA (1998) Pharmacokinetic/pharmacodynamic parameters: rationale for antibacterial dosing of mice and men. Clin Infect Dis 26(1):1–10, quiz 11–12
11. Eagle H (1954) The binding of penicillin in relation to its cytotoxic action. I. Correlation between the penicillin sensitivity and combining activity of intact bacteria and cell-free extracts. J Exp Med 99(3):207–226
12. Eagle H (1954) The binding of penicillin in relation to its cytotoxic action. II. The reactivity with penicillin of resistant variants of streptococci, pneumococci, and staphylococci. J Exp Med 100(1):103–115
13. Eagle H (1954) The binding of penicillin in relation to its cytotoxic action. III. The binding of penicillin by mammalian cells in tissue culture (HeLa and L strains). J Exp Med 100(1):117–124
14. Highman B, Altland PD, Eagle H (1954) Experimental bacterial endocarditis in altitude rats; development and regression of cardiac lesions, including lesions in rats treated with penicillin. AMA Arch Pathol 58(3):241–257
15. Tam VH, McKinnon PS, Akins RL, Drusano GL, Rybak MJ (2003) Pharmacokinetics and pharmacodynamics of cefepime in patients with various degrees of renal function. Antimicrob Agents Chemother 47(6):1853–1861
16. Tam VH, McKinnon PS, Akins RL, Rybak MJ, Drusano GL (2002) Pharmacodynamics of cefepime in patients with Gram-negative infections. J Antimicrob Chemother 50(3):425–428

17. Craig WA (2003) Basic pharmacodynamics of antibacterials with clinical applications to the use of beta-lactams, glycopeptides, and linezolid. Infect Dis Clin North Am 17(3):479–501
18. Howie V (1992) Eradication of bacterial pathogens from middle ear infections. Clin Infect Dis 14(suppl 2):S209–S211
19. Li C, Du X, Kuti JL, Nicolau DP (2007) Clinical pharmacodynamics of meropenem in patients with lower respiratory tract infections. Antimicrob Agents Chemother 51:1725–1730
20. Muller AE, Punt N, Mouton JW (2013) Optimal exposures of ceftazidime predict the probability of microbiological and clinical outcome in the treatment of nosocomial pneumonia. J Antimicrob Chemother 68(4):900–906
21. MacVane SH, Kuti JL, Nicolau DP (2014) Clinical pharmacodynamics of antipseudomonal cephalosporins in patients with ventilator-associated pneumonia. Antimicrob Agents Chemother 58(3):1359–1364
22. Nicolau DP, Quintiliani R, Nightingale CH (1995) Antibiotic kinetics and dynamics for the clinician. Med Clin North Am 79(3):477–495
23. Xamplas RC, Itokazu GS, Glowacki RC, Grasso AE, Caquelin C, Schwartz DN (2010) Implementation of an extended-infusion piperacillin-tazobactam program at an urban teaching hospital. Am J Health Syst Pharm 67(8):622–628. doi:10.2146/ajhp090447
24. Neely MN, van Guilder MG, Yamada WM, Schumitzky A, Jelliffe RW (2012) Accurate detection of outliers and subpopulations with Pmetrics, a nonparametric and parametric pharmacometric modeling and simulation package for R. Ther Drug Monit 34(4):467–476. doi:10.1097/FTD.0b013e31825c4ba6
25. Bayard DS, Jelliffe RW (2004) A Bayesian approach to tracking patients having changing pharmacokinetic parameters. J Pharmacokinet Pharmacodyn 31(1):75–107
26. Jelliffe R, Bayard D, Milman M, Van Guilder M, Schumitzky A (2000) Achieving target goals most precisely using nonparametric compartmental models and "multiple model" design of dosage regimens. Ther Drug Monit 22(3):346–353
27. Jelliffe RW, Schumitzky A, Bayard D, Milman M, Van Guilder M, Wang X, Jiang F, Barbaut X, Maire P (1998) Model-based, goal-oriented, individualised drug therapy. Linkage of population modelling, new 'multiple model' dosage design, Bayesian feedback and individualised target goals. Clin Pharmacokinet 34(1):57–77. doi:10.2165/00003088-199834010-00003
28. Jelliffe RW, Schumitzky A, Van Guilder M, Liu M, Hu L, Maire P, Gomis P, Barbaut X, Tahani B (1993) Individualizing drug dosage regimens: roles of population pharmacokinetic and dynamic models, Bayesian fitting, and adaptive control. Ther Drug Monit 15(5):380–393
29. Lodise TP, Lomaestro BM, Drusano GL, Society of Infectious Diseases P (2006) Application of antimicrobial pharmacodynamic concepts into clinical practice: focus on beta-lactam antibiotics: insights from the Society of Infectious Diseases Pharmacists. Pharmacotherapy 26(9):1320–1332. doi:10.1592/phco.26.9.1320
30. Sheiner LB, Beal S, Rosenberg B, Marathe VV (1979) Forecasting individual pharmacokinetics. Clin Pharmacol Ther 26(3):294–305
31. Tatarinova T, Neely M, Bartroff J, van Guilder M, Yamada W, Bayard D, Jelliffe R, Leary R, Chubatiuk A, Schumitzky A (2013) Two general methods for population pharmacokinetic modeling: non-parametric adaptive grid and non-parametric Bayesian. J Pharmacokinet Pharmacodyn 40(2):189–199. doi:10.1007/s10928-013-9302-8
32. Courter JD, Kuti JL, Girotto JE, Nicolau DP (2009) Optimizing bactericidal exposure for beta-lactams using prolonged and continuous infusions in the pediatric population. Pediatr Blood Cancer 53(3):379–385. doi:10.1002/pbc.22051
33. Kim A, Kuti JL, Nicolau DP (2009) Probability of pharmacodynamic target attainment with standard and prolonged-infusion antibiotic regimens for empiric therapy in adults with hospital-acquired pneumonia. Clin Ther 31(11):2765–2778. doi:10.1016/j.clinthera.2009.11.026
34. Kim A, Sutherland CA, Kuti JL, Nicolau DP (2007) Optimal dosing of piperacillin-tazobactam for the treatment of Pseudomonas aeruginosa infections: prolonged or continuous infusion? Pharmacotherapy 27(11):1490–1497. doi:10.1592/phco.27.11.1490
35. Patel N, Scheetz MH, Drusano GL, Lodise TP (2010) Determination of antibiotic dosage adjustments in patients with renal impairment: elements for success. J Antimicrob Chemother 65(11):2285–2290. doi:10.1093/jac/dkq323
36. Patel N, Scheetz MH, Drusano GL, Lodise TP (2010) Identification of optimal renal dosage adjustments for traditional and extended-infusion piperacillin-tazobactam dosing regimens in hospitalized patients.

Antimicrob Agents Chemother 54(1):460–465. doi:10.1128/aac.00296-09

37. Roberts JA, Paul SK, Akova M, Bassetti M, De Waele JJ, Dimopoulos G, Kaukonen KM, Koulenti D, Martin C, Montravers P, Rello J, Rhodes A, Starr T, Wallis SC, Lipman J, Authors DS (2014) DALI: Defining Antibiotic Levels in Intensive care unit patients: are current beta-lactam antibiotic doses sufficient for critically ill patients? Clin Infect Dis 58:1072. doi:10.1093/cid/ciu027
38. Yost RJ, Cappelletty DM, group RS (2011) The Retrospective Cohort of Extended-Infusion Piperacillin-Tazobactam (RECEIPT) study: a multicenter study. Pharmacotherapy 31(8):767–775. doi:10.1592/phco.31.8.767
39. Falagas ME, Tansarli GS, Ikawa K, Vardakas KZ (2013) Clinical outcomes with extended or continuous versus short-term intravenous infusion of carbapenems and piperacillin/tazobactam: a systematic review and meta-analysis. Clin Infect Dis 56(2):272–282. doi:10.1093/cid/cis857
40. Macvane SH, Kuti JL, Nicolau DP (2013) Prolonging beta-lactam infusion: a review of the rationale and evidence, and guidance for implementation. Int J Antimicrob Agents 43:105. doi:10.1016/j.ijantimicag.2013.10.021
41. Abdul-Aziz MH, Dulhunty JM, Bellomo R, Lipman J, Roberts JA (2012) Continuous beta-lactam infusion in critically ill patients: the clinical evidence. Ann Intensive Care 2(1):37. doi:10.1186/2110-5820-2-37
42. Grant EM, Kuti JL, Nicolau DP, Nightingale C, Quintiliani R (2002) Clinical efficacy and pharmacoeconomics of a continuous-infusion piperacillin-tazobactam program in a large community teaching hospital. Pharmacotherapy 22(4):471–483
43. DeRyke CA, Kuti JL, Mansfield D, Dana A, Nicolau DP (2006) Pharmacoeconomics of continuous versus intermittent infusion of piperacillin-tazobactam for the treatment of complicated intraabdominal infection. Am J Health Syst Pharm 63(8):750–755. doi:10.2146/ajhp050323
44. Wang D (2009) Experience with extended-infusion meropenem in the management of ventilator-associated pneumonia due to multidrug-resistant Acinetobacter baumannii. Int J Antimicrob Agents 33(3):290–291. doi:10.1016/j.ijantimicag.2008.09.012
45. Goff DA, Nicolau DP (2013) When pharmacodynamics trump costs: an antimicrobial stewardship program's approach to selecting optimal antimicrobial agents. Clin Ther 35(6):766–771. doi:10.1016/j.clinthera.2013.05.004
46. Nicasio AM, Eagye KJ, Nicolau DP, Shore E, Palter M, Pepe J, Kuti JL (2010) Pharmacodynamic-based clinical pathway for empiric antibiotic choice in patients with ventilator-associated pneumonia. J Crit Care 25(1):69–77. doi:10.1016/j.jcrc.2009.02.014
47. Nicasio AM, Eagye KJ, Kuti EL, Nicolau DP, Kuti JL (2010) Length of stay and hospital costs associated with a pharmacodynamic-based clinical pathway for empiric antibiotic choice for ventilator-associated pneumonia. Pharmacotherapy 30(5):453–462. doi:10.1592/phco.30.5.453
48. Khadem TM, Dodds Ashley E, Wrobel MJ, Brown J (2012) Antimicrobial stewardship: a matter of process or outcome? Pharmacotherapy 32(8):688–706. doi:10.1002/j.1875-9114.2012.01154.x
49. Health Economics Resource Center (HERC) A1. What is cost-effectiveness analysis? U.S. Department of Veterans Affairs. Accessed 12 Jan 2014
50. Dellit TH, Owens RC, McGowan JE Jr, Gerding DN, Weinstein RA, Burke JP, Huskins WC, Paterson DL, Fishman NO, Carpenter CF, Brennan PJ, Billeter M, Hooton TM, Infectious Diseases Society of A, Society for Healthcare Epidemiology of A (2007) Infectious Diseases Society of America and the Society for Healthcare Epidemiology of America guidelines for developing an institutional program to enhance antimicrobial stewardship. Clin Infect Dis 44(2):159–177. doi:10.1086/510393
51. Drusano GL (2003) Prevention of resistance: a goal for dose selection for antimicrobial agents. Clin Infect Dis 36(Suppl 1):S42–S50. doi:10.1086/344653
52. Rello J, Sa-Borges M, Correa H, Leal SR, Baraibar J (1999) Variations in etiology of ventilator-associated pneumonia across four treatment sites: implications for antimicrobial prescribing practices. Am J Respir Crit Care Med 160(2):608–613. doi:10.1164/ajrccm.160.2.9812034
53. Kaufman D, Haas CE, Edinger R, Hollick G (1998) Antibiotic susceptibility in the surgical intensive care unit compared with the hospital-wide antibiogram. Arch Surg 133(10):1041–1045
54. Binkley S, Fishman NO, LaRosa LA, Marr AM, Nachamkin I, Wordell D, Bilker WB, Lautenbach E (2006) Comparison of unit-specific and hospital-wide antibiograms: potential implications for selection of empirical antimicrobial therapy. Infect Control Hosp Epidemiol 27(7):682–687. doi:10.1086/505921

55. Pogue JM, Alaniz C, Carver PL, Pleva M, Newton D, DePestel DD (2011) Role of unit-specific combination antibiograms for improving the selection of appropriate empiric therapy for gram-negative pneumonia. Infect Control Hosp Epidemiol 32(3):289–292. doi:10.1086/658665
56. Eagye KJ, Shore E, Dobkin E et al (2006) Differing epidemiology and resistance patterns of respiratory isolates (RI) from three intensive care units (ICUs) within the same institution. Poster [abstract K-259] presented at the 46th Interscience Conference on Antimicrobial Agents and Chemotherapy, San Francisco, CA, 27–30 September 2006
57. Ibrahim EH, Ward S, Sherman G, Schaiff R, Fraser VJ, Kollef MH (2001) Experience with a clinical guideline for the treatment of ventilator-associated pneumonia. Crit Care Med 29(6):1109–1115
58. Soo Hoo GW, Wen YE, Nguyen TV, Goetz MB (2005) Impact of clinical guidelines in the management of severe hospital-acquired pneumonia. Chest 128(4):2778–2787. doi:10.1378/chest.128.4.2778
59. Lancaster JW, Lawrence KR, Fong JJ, Doron SI, Garpestad E, Nasraway SA, Devlin JW (2008) Impact of an institution-specific hospital-acquired pneumonia protocol on the appropriateness of antibiotic therapy and patient outcomes. Pharmacotherapy 28(7):852–862. doi:10.1592/phco.28.7.852
60. Udy AA, Varghese JM, Altukroni M, Briscoe S, McWhinney BC, Ungerer JP, Lipman J, Roberts JA (2012) Subtherapeutic initial beta-lactam concentrations in select critically ill patients: association between augmented renal clearance and low trough drug concentrations. Chest 142(1):30–39. doi:10.1378/chest.11-1671
61. Claus B, Colpaert K, Hoste EA et al (2010) Increased glomerular filtration in the critically ill patient receiving anti-infective treatment. Crit Care 14(suppl 1):S170–S171
62. Lodise TP Jr, Lomaestro B, Rodvold KA, Danziger LH, Drusano GL (2004) Pharmacodynamic profiling of piperacillin in the presence of tazobactam in patients through the use of population pharmacokinetic models and Monte Carlo simulation. Antimicrob Agents Chemother 48(12):4718–4724. doi:10.1128/AAC.48.12.4718-4724.2004
63. Felton TW, Hope WW, Lomaestro BM, Butterfield JM, Kwa AL, Drusano GL, Lodise TP (2012) Population pharmacokinetics of extended-infusion piperacillin-tazobactam in hospitalized patients with nosocomial infections. Antimicrob Agents Chemother 56(8):4087–4094. doi:10.1128/aac.00521-12
64. Claus B, Buyle F, Robays H, Vogelaers D (2010) Importance of infusion volume and pump characteristics in extended administration of ss-lactam antibiotics. Antimicrob Agents Chemother 54(11):4950. doi:10.1128/AAC.00754-10
65. Kuperman GJ, Bobb A, Payne TH, Avery AJ, Gandhi TK, Burns G, Classen DC, Bates DW (2007) Medication-related clinical decision support in computerized provider order entry systems: a review. J Am Med Inform Assoc 14(1):29–40. doi:10.1197/jamia.M2170
66. Pestotnik SL, Classen DC, Evans RS, Burke JP (1996) Implementing antibiotic practice guidelines through computer-assisted decision support: clinical and financial outcomes. Ann Intern Med 124(10):884–890
67. Evans RS, Pestotnik SL, Classen DC, Clemmer TP, Weaver LK, Orme JF Jr, Lloyd JF, Burke JP (1998) A computer-assisted management program for antibiotics and other antiinfective agents. N Engl J Med 338(4):232–238. doi:10.1056/NEJM199801223380406
68. Wilson K, Sullivan M (2004) Preventing medication errors with smart infusion technology. Am J Health Syst Pharm 61(2):177–183
69. Manrique-Rodriguez S, Sanchez-Galindo AC, Lopez-Herce J, Calleja-Hernandez MA, Martinez-Martinez F, Iglesias-Peinado I, Carrillo-Alvarez A, Sanjurjo Saez M, Fernandez-Llamazares CM (2013) Impact of implementing smart infusion pumps in a pediatric intensive care unit. Am J Health Syst Pharm 70(21):1897–1906. doi:10.2146/ajhp120767
70. Trbovich PL, Cafazzo JA, Easty AC (2013) Implementation and optimization of smart infusion systems: are we reaping the safety benefits? J Healthc Qual 35(2):33–40. doi:10.1111/j.1945-1474.2011.00175.x
71. Leung E, Venkatesan N, Ly SC, Scheetz MH (2013) Physical compatibility of vancomycin and piperacillin sodium-tazobactam at concentrations typically used during prolonged infusions. Am J Health Syst Pharm 70(13):1163–1166. doi:10.2146/ajhp120409
72. Lam WJ, Bhowmick T, Gross A, Vanschooneveld TC, Weinstein MP (2013) Using higher doses to compensate for tubing residuals in extended-infusion piperacillin-tazobactam. Ann Pharmacother 47(6):886–891. doi:10.1345/aph.1R721
73. Charani E, Edwards R, Sevdalis N, Alexandrou B, Sibley E, Mullett D, Franklin BD, Holmes A (2011) Behavior change strategies to influence antimicrobial prescribing in acute care: a systematic review. Clin Infect Dis 53(7):651–662. doi:10.1093/cid/cir445

74. Armstrong D, Reyburn H, Jones R (1996) A study of general practitioners' reasons for changing their prescribing behaviour. BMJ 312(7036):949–952
75. Grol R, Grimshaw J (2003) From best evidence to best practice: effective implementation of change in patients' care. Lancet 362(9391):1225–1230. doi:10.1016/S0140-6736(03)14546-1
76. Oxman AD, Thomson MA, Davis DA, Haynes RB (1995) No magic bullets: a systematic review of 102 trials of interventions to improve professional practice. CMAJ 153(10):1423–1431
77. Goff DA (2011) Antimicrobial stewardship: bridging the gap between quality care and cost. Curr Opin Infect Dis 24(Suppl 1):S11–S20. doi:10.1097/01.qco.0000393484.17894.05
78. Lodise TP, Butterfield J (2011) Use of pharmacodynamic principles to inform beta-lactam dosing: "S" does not always mean success. J Hosp Med 6(Suppl 1):S16–S23. doi:10.1002/jhm.869
79. Drew RH, White R, MacDougall C, Hermsen ED, Owens RC Jr, Society of Infectious Diseases P (2009) Insights from the Society of Infectious Diseases Pharmacists on antimicrobial stewardship guidelines from the Infectious Diseases Society of America and the Society for Healthcare Epidemiology of America. Pharmacotherapy 29(5):593–607. doi:10.1592/phco.29.5.593
80. Griffith MC, Postelnick M, Scheetz MH (2012) Antimicrobial stewardship programs: methods of operation and suggested outcomes. Expert Rev Anti Infect Ther 10(1):66–73
81. Ambrose PG, Quintiliani R, Nightingale CH et al (1998) Continuous vs intermittent infusion of cefuroxime for the treatment of community-acquired pneumonia. Infect Dis Clin Pract 7:463–470
82. McNabb JJ, Nightingale CH, Quintiliani R, Nicolau DP (2001) Cost-effectiveness of ceftazidime by continuous infusion versus intermittent infusion for nosocomial pneumonia. Pharmacotherapy 21(5):549–555
83. Bal AM, Gould IM (2011) Antibiotic stewardship: overcoming implementation barriers. Curr Opin Infect Dis 24(4):357–362. doi:10.1097/QCO.0b013e3283483262
84. Kuti JL, Shore E, Palter M, Nicolau DP (2009) Tackling empirical antibiotic therapy for ventilator-associated pneumonia in your ICU: guidance for implementing the guidelines. Semin Respir Crit Care Med 30(1):102–115. doi:10.1055/s-0028-1119814
85. Bodey GP, Ketchel SJ, Rodriguez V (1979) A randomized study of carbenicillin plus cefamandole or tobramycin in the treatment of febrile episodes in cancer patients. Am J Med 67(4):608–616
86. Hanes SD, Wood GC, Herring V, Croce MA, Fabian TC, Pritchard E, Boucher BA (2000) Intermittent and continuous ceftazidime infusion for critically ill trauma patients. Am J Surg 179(6):436–440
87. Lau WK, Mercer D, Itani KM, Nicolau DP, Kuti JL, Mansfield D, Dana A (2006) Randomized, open-label, comparative study of piperacillin-tazobactam administered by continuous infusion versus intermittent infusion for treatment of hospitalized patients with complicated intra-abdominal infection. Antimicrob Agents Chemother 50(11):3556–3561. doi:10.1128/AAC.00329-06
88. Lorente L, Lorenzo L, Martin MM, Jimenez A, Mora ML (2006) Meropenem by continuous versus intermittent infusion in ventilator-associated pneumonia due to gram-negative bacilli. Ann Pharmacother 40(2):219–223. doi:10.1345/aph.1G467
89. Lorente L, Jimenez A, Palmero S, Jimenez JJ, Iribarren JL, Santana M, Martin MM, Mora ML (2007) Comparison of clinical cure rates in adults with ventilator-associated pneumonia treated with intravenous ceftazidime administered by continuous or intermittent infusion: a retrospective, nonrandomized, open-label, historical chart review. Clin Ther 29(11):2433–2439. doi:10.1016/j.clinthera.2007.11.003
90. Lorente L, Jimenez A, Martin MM, Iribarren JL, Jimenez JJ, Mora ML (2009) Clinical cure of ventilator-associated pneumonia treated with piperacillin/tazobactam administered by continuous or intermittent infusion. Int J Antimicrob Agents 33(5):464–468. doi:10.1016/j.ijantimicag.2008.10.025
91. Nicolau DP, McNabb J, Lacy MK, Quintiliani R, Nightingale CH (2001) Continuous versus intermittent administration of ceftazidime in intensive care unit patients with nosocomial pneumonia. Int J Antimicrob Agents 17(6):497–504
92. Rafati MR, Rouini MR, Mojtahedzadeh M, Najafi A, Tavakoli H, Gholami K, Fazeli MR (2006) Clinical efficacy of continuous infusion of piperacillin compared with intermittent dosing in septic critically ill patients. Int J Antimicrob Agents 28(2):122–127. doi:10.1016/j.ijantimicag.2006.02.020
93. Roberts JA, Boots R, Rickard CM, Thomas P, Quinn J, Roberts DM, Richards B, Lipman J (2007) Is continuous infusion ceftriaxone better than once-a-day dosing in intensive care? A randomized controlled pilot study. J Antimicrob Chemother 59(2):285–291. doi:10.1093/jac/dkl478

94. Sakka SG, Glauner AK, Bulitta JB, Kinzig-Schippers M, Pfister W, Drusano GL, Sorgel F (2007) Population pharmacokinetics and pharmacodynamics of continuous versus short-term infusion of imipenem-cilastatin in critically ill patients in a randomized, controlled trial. Antimicrob Agents Chemother 51(9):3304–3310. doi:10.1128/AAC.01318-06
95. van Zanten AR, Oudijk M, Nohlmans-Paulssen MK, van der Meer YG, Girbes AR, Polderman KH (2007) Continuous vs. intermittent cefotaxime administration in patients with chronic obstructive pulmonary disease and respiratory tract infections: pharmacokinetics/pharmacodynamics, bacterial susceptibility and clinical efficacy. Br J Clin Pharmacol 63(1):100–109. doi:10.1111/j.1365-2125.2006.02730.x
96. Chastre J, Wunderink R, Prokocimer P, Lee M, Kaniga K, Friedland I (2008) Efficacy and safety of intravenous infusion of doripenem versus imipenem in ventilator-associated pneumonia: a multicenter, randomized study. Crit Care Med 36(4):1089–1096. doi:10.1097/CCM.0b013e3181691b99
97. Dow R, Rose W, Fox B (2011) Retrospective study of prolonged versus intermittent infusion piperacillin-tazobactam and meropenem in Intensive Care Unit Patients at an Academic Medical Center. Infect Dis Clin Pract 19:413–417
98. Esterly JS, Wagner J, McLaughlin MM, Postelnick MJ, Qi C, Scheetz MH (2012) Evaluation of clinical outcomes in patients with bloodstream infections due to Gram-negative bacteria according to carbapenem MIC stratification. Antimicrob Agents Chemother 56(9):4885–4890. doi:10.1128/AAC.06365-11
99. Itabashi S (2007) Clinical efficacy of prolonged (4 hour) drip infusion of meropenem against severe pneumonia. Jpn J Antibiot 60(3):161–170
100. Kollef MH, Chastre J, Clavel M, Restrepo MI, Michiels B, Kaniga K, Cirillo I, Kimko H, Redman R (2012) A randomized trial of 7-day doripenem versus 10-day imipenem-cilastatin for ventilator-associated pneumonia. Crit Care 16(6):R218. doi:10.1186/cc11862
101. Lee GC, Liou H, Yee R, Quan CF, Neldner K (2012) Outcomes of extended-infusion piperacillin-tazobactam: a retrospective analysis of critically ill patients. Clin Ther 34(12):2297–2300. doi:10.1016/j.clinthera.2012.11.005
102. Patel GW, Patel N, Lat A, Trombley K, Enbawe S, Manor K, Smith R, Lodise TP Jr (2009) Outcomes of extended infusion piperacillin/tazobactam for documented Gram-negative infections. Diagn Microbiol Infect Dis 64(2):236–240. doi:10.1016/j.diagmicrobio.2009.03.002

Chapter 21

Pharmacodynamic Considerations in Critically Ill Patients

Mahipal G. Sinnollareddy and Jason A. Roberts

Abstract

Sepsis and related changes lead to an array of physiological changes in critically ill patients. As with all other interventional measures, early and appropriate antibiotic regimen is important for control of sepsis-related changes. Antibiotic dosing based on the information from less severely patients results in suboptimal dosing. Therefore, it is important to consider ICU patients as a separate cohort for drug dosing. It is important to understand the variability and quantitatively determine doses required to improve clinical and microbiological outcomes.

Key words Pharmacokinetics, Pharmacodynamics, Dosing, Antibiotics, Sepsis, Septic shock, Hypoalbuminemia, Acute kidney injury, Renal replacement therapy, Augmented renal clearance

1 Introduction

Infections and related sepsis are few of the most prevalent issues in critically ill patients [1–3]. Sepsis occurs as a result of complex interactions of pathogenic microorganisms and a subsequent plethora of host responses that cumulatively cause mortality rates up to 25–30 % for severe sepsis and 40–70 % for septic shock [4]. At any one time, 50 % of patients in intensive care units (ICU) are diagnosed with an infection and are receiving treatment with antibiotics [5]. Source control of the pathogen and early and appropriate broad-spectrum antibiotics along with other measures are vital clinical interventions for sepsis [6]. One of the essential components of the effective antibiotic therapy that can be modified by the clinician is optimization of dose. Adequate dosing in critically ill patients is of paramount importance not only because early and appropriate antibiotic therapy is proven to improve clinical outcomes but also because inadequate dosing will lead to emergence of resistance [7–9]. Due to an escalation of the incidence of bacteria resistant to currently available antibiotics and lack of development of new antibiotics with novel mechanisms to overcome resistance, optimal use of the current armamentarium is essential.

John C. Rotschafer et al. (eds.), *Antibiotic Pharmacodynamics*, Methods in Pharmacology and Toxicology,
DOI 10.1007/978-1-4939-3323-5_21, © Springer Science+Business Media New York 2016

Rational development and dosing of antibiotics could be achieved, especially in critically ill, with the application of pharmacokinetic (PK) and pharmacodynamic (PD) concepts. This chapter aims to discuss the PK/PD issues in relation to antibiotics relevant to ICU patients.

2 Altered Pathophysiology and Pharmacokinetics

Antibiotic dosing in the critically ill is generally based on the PK data obtained in healthy volunteers or moderately ill patients. These regimens do not generally account for various pathophysiological changes that occur in critically ill patients with sepsis and/or septic shock [10, 11]. Altered pathophysiology leads to significant changes in primary PK parameters—clearance (CL) and volume of distribution (Vd)—which in turn affect the plasma and infection site concentrations. As shown in Fig 1, PK changes in critically ill patients can occur with or without organ dysfunction and depend on both pathophysiological and drug-related (hydrophilicity and protein binding) factors as well as patient factors.

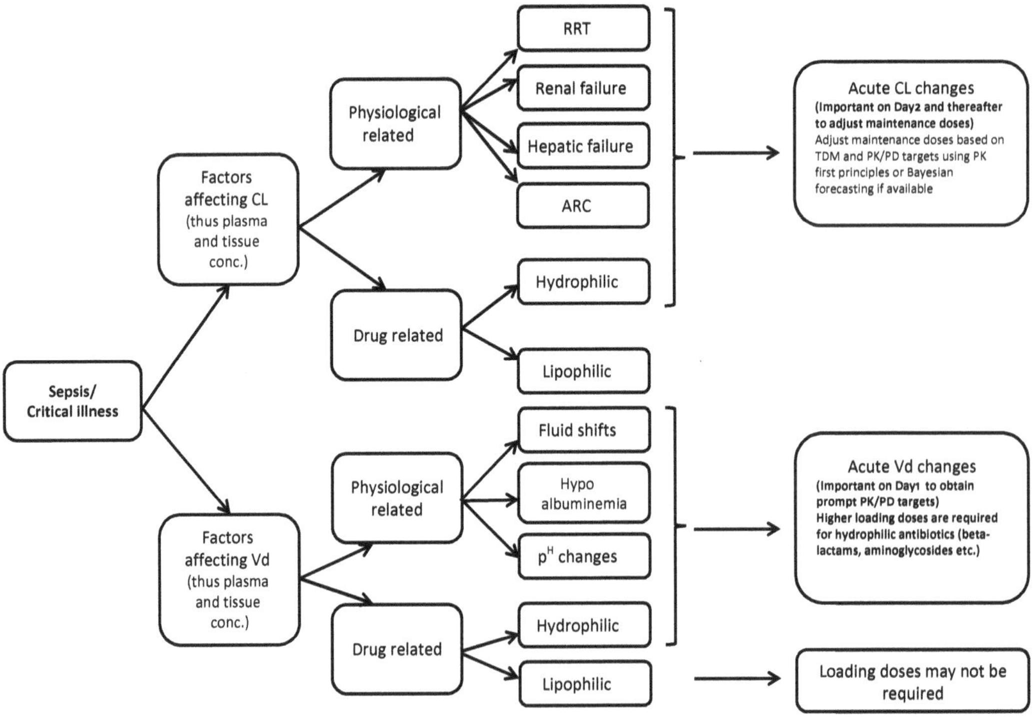

Fig. 1 Physiological and drug-related factors leading to PK changes that affect drug dosing and suggested dosing strategies. *CL* clearance, *Vd* volume of distribution, *RRT* renal replacement therapy, *ARC* augmented renal clearance, *TDM* therapeutic drug monitoring, *PK* pharmacokinetics, *PD* pharmacodynamics

3 Distribution Changes

3.1 Fluid Shifts and Changes in Volume of Distribution

The toxins released during the pathogenesis of sepsis can cause endothelial damage, increased capillary permeability, and maldistribution of blood flow. This capillary leak results in fluid shifts from the intravascular to the interstitial space. These changes result in an increased Vd leading to lower plasma and infection site concentrations of hydrophilic antibiotics (e.g., beta-lactams, aminoglycosides) which in general have lower Vd and intracellular penetration than that of lipophilic antibiotics. This has been demonstrated for beta-lactam antibiotics with many critically ill patients not achieving desired PK/PD targets with conventional doses [12, 13]. On the other hand, antibiotics with greater lipophilicity (e.g., fluoroquinolones, macrolides) have a higher volume of distribution and intracellular penetration as a characteristic feature and are not greatly affected by the fluid shifts [14]. Therefore, it is a feature of critically ill patients that higher loading doses may be required for hydrophilic antimicrobials to reach PK/PD targets promptly.

3.2 Tissue Hypoperfusion and Subtherapeutic Tissue Concentrations

Critical illness results in reduced microvascular perfusion leading to impaired distribution of antibiotics into the interstitial fluid. Reduced perfusion will affect different organs differently depending on the phase of the sepsis [15]. Since most of the bacterial and fungal infections are extracellular, diminished perfusion may result in suboptimal interstitial fluid (ISF) exposures of antimicrobials. This has been demonstrated in a few studies comparing the plasma and ISF concentrations of beta-lactams using the microdialysis technique where several fold decreases in ISF concentrations have been observed in critically ill patients compared to healthy volunteers [16, 17].

3.3 Hypoalbuminemia

Reduced serum albumin concentrations are frequently observed in critically ill patients. This will result in increased free drug concentrations in plasma and thus also in tissue ISF. However, because of the dilutional effect caused by fluid shifts and free drug available for clearance, ISF concentrations remain low. This effect is considered significant, in particular, for highly protein-bound hydrophilic antimicrobials like ceftriaxone and flucloxacillin [16–18].

4 Clearance Changes

4.1 Acute Kidney Injury and Renal Replacement Therapy

Acute kidney injury (AKI) is a common complication in critically ill patients with an incidence as high as 42 % reported in patients with severe sepsis or septic shock [19]. Two-thirds of these patients require renal replacement therapy (RRT) resulting in hospital mortality rates as high as 60 % [20]. Changes in Vd during AKI could be due to one of the three reasons—because of the sepsis-related changes as discussed above, secondly because of increased extravascular fluid volume secondary to reduced urinary output, and thirdly displacement of drug molecules by accumulated uremic molecules. Higher loading doses may be required for hydrophilic drugs to account for this increased Vd [20]. As the fluid overload is corrected, drug doses may need to be adjusted accordingly.

Renal excretion of a drug can occur through a combination of three processes—glomerular filtration, tubular secretion, and tubular reabsorption. AKI is not only associated with decreased glomerular filtration but also with impairment of tubular secretion and reabsorption. Therefore, it is important to consider the effects of tubular secretion and reabsorption in deciding the dosing regimens. For example, approximately 80 % of fluconazole is reabsorbed in the proximal tubule in patients with normal renal function. In critically ill patients undergoing RRT, reabsorption might be reduced leading to greater clearance, thus requiring higher or at least standard doses (not dose adjusted for renal dysfunction) of fluconazole [20, 21].

Accurate estimation of renal function is critical in ICU setting for optimal drug dosing. Due to non-steady-state concentrations of creatinine in critically ill, traditional methods (Cockroft-Gault and Modification of Diet in Renal Disease equations) may lead to inaccurate estimation of renal function. Urinary creatinine clearance (CrCL) should be used to estimate renal function, where possible. If not, the Jelliffe equation should be considered instead of traditional equations [22]. The product information is useful for the dosing recommendations but care must be taken to assess renal function accurately.

4.2 Renal Replacement Therapy

RRT is the commonly employed therapeutic measure for the treatment of severe AKI in critically ill patients. RRT has evolved over the years to meet the needs of individual patients. Continuous renal replacement therapy (CRRT) is more commonly used in the management of AKI patients in the critical care setting because of a greater hemodynamic intolerance of these patients to the traditional intermittent hemodialysis (IHD) [23]. CRRT includes three primary modalities—continuous veno-venous hemodialysis (CVVHD), continuous veno-venous hemofiltration (CVVHF), and continuous veno-venous hemodiafiltration (CVVHDF). A hybrid technique called sustained low-efficiency daily dialysis/diafiltration (SLED/SLED-*f*), also known as slow low-efficiency dialysis and extended daily dialysis, has been developed recently and combines the advantages of both intermittent hemodialysis and CRRT [24]. Drug clearance during RRT is influenced by the patient, drug, and the RRT settings [25].

In general the daily efficiency of solute removal depends on the type of technique used and could be ranked as follows:

CVVHDF > CVVHF > CVVHD > SLED > IHD

Although IHD has the greatest clearance per unit of time, the short duration means that over the course of 24 h, the total solute removed is the least with this mode.

Accurate drug dosing in critically ill patients on RRT is extremely difficult because of the concurrent changes that occur in critical illness as well as changes associated with RRT [26]. It is further complicated by the fact that the approach to use RRTs varies across different ICUs leading to variability in drug clearances. Moreover, a recent systematic review concluded that published PK studies using various RRT modalities did not report sufficient data to guide effective drug dosing [27]. The empirical approach to dosing in CRRT failed to achieve required trough concentrations in almost 25 % dosing intervals in a recent multicenter PK study [26]. Rational approaches based on the PK/PD of antibiotics and first principles of PK have been suggested until more robust studies encompassing different RRT settings and PK variability are conducted [25].

4.3 Augmented Renal Clearance

On the other hand, increased cardiac output due to various interventions to maintain hemodynamic stability in the early phases of severe sepsis/septic shock could lead to enhanced excretion of renally eliminated antibiotics leading to subtherapeutic concentrations [28, 29]. This phenomenon is termed augmented renal clearance (ARC) and has been increasingly recognized in subsets of critically ill patients. These patients have an apparent normal serum creatinine concentration and are most commonly young patients presenting with trauma and without any prior comorbidities or organ dysfunction [30–32].

4.4 Hepatic Clearance

Hepatic impairment in the critically ill could result from infectious causes, hypoperfusion or drug toxicity. Unlike renal function, methods to quantitate hepatic impairment in acute clinical setting do not exist. Thus evaluation of residual hepatic function is mainly based on clinical parameters. As discussed above, a reduction in albumin concentrations due to hepatic impairment can lead to PK changes of highly protein-bound drugs. Because of the subjective nature of drug dosing in acute liver impairment, it may be necessary to choose an alternative antibiotic if in doubt about the effect of hepatic dysfunction and when drug toxicity is anticipated.

5 Antibacterial Classes

Different antibiotic classes have different bacterial kill characteristics. These relationships have been determined from in vitro studies and describe the antibiotic exposure required for maximal activity [33]. Sometimes, these in vitro study findings have been replicated in animal in vivo studies as well as in clinical PD studies including studies in critically ill patients. For each antibiotic, it is the free (or unbound) concentration that is responsible for antibiotic effect. The beta-lactam group of antibiotics exhibit a time-dependent activity with the time the free (or unbound) antibiotic concentration remains above the minimum inhibitory concentration (MIC) of the pathogen ($fT_{>MIC}$) which is the best predictor of efficacy [34]. In contrast, aminoglycosides have a concentration-dependent activity where bacterial killing is determined by the ratio of maximum concentration to MIC (C_{max}/MIC) [35]. In the case of fluoroquinolones, the ratio of free antibiotic area under the concentration-time curve to MIC ($fAUC_{0-24}$/MIC), which is a function of both concentration- and time-dependent activity, is predictive of efficacy [36]. Below, the specific PK/PD characteristics for antibiotic classes that are likely to be altered in critically ill patients are discussed. Table 1 outlines the PK/PD indices, expected changes with critical illness, and dosing strategies for antibiotics commonly used in ICUs. For more detailed discussions about PD for each class of antibiotic, refer to the corresponding chapters.

5.1 Beta-Lactam Antibiotics

5.1.1 Optimal Beta-Lactam Exposures

Beta-lactams are probably the most studied antibiotics in critically ill patients given their broad spectrum of activity. Given that $fT_{>MIC}$ is the optimal PD index for beta-lactams, maintaining free drug concentrations above the MIC should be the aim of treatment. Several clinical studies have sought to confirm the findings from the dynamic in vitro and animal in vivo data but have described different %$fT_{>MIC}$ values for maximal clinical effects [37–43]. Most of these studies have looked at the clinical PD of beta-lactams against Gram-negative pathogens. Some have reported that $T_{>4-6\times MIC}$ has to be maintained for the 100 % of the dosing interval [39, 44] whereas others have suggested a target of 60 % $fT_{>MIC}$ depending on the outcome sought (clinical cure versus decreased bacterial resistance) [43]. It is unlikely that the actual %$fT_{>MIC}$ from the preclinical studies is incorrect, rather than that the clinical studies include a broad range of isolates where accurate MIC data may not be available, or may include patients with infection site PK that is not well represented by plasma PK.

Of the available studies, two in particular have evaluated PK/PD specifically in critically ill patients in ICU and will be highlighted here. McKinnon et al. [38] found that both AUC_{0-24}/MIC and $T_{>MIC}$ were predictive of clinical and bacteriological success for ceftazidime and cefepime. A $T_{>MIC}$ of 100 % (measured as total concentration, not unbound concentration) was found to be associated with higher rates of bacteriological eradication and clinical cure compared to a $T_{>MIC}$ less than 100 % (97 % vs. 44 % and 82 % vs. 33 %, respectively). In a more recent Defining Antibiotic Levels

Table 1
PK/PD indices, expected PK changes, and dosing strategies for commonly used antibiotics in ICUs

	PK/PD target	Expected PK changes: Increased Vd	Expected PK changes: ARC	LD required	Maintenance doses
Penicillin antibiotics		Yes	Yes[a]	Only with CI	Adjust based on renal function
Vancomycin	Total AUC_{0-24}/MIC > 400	Yes	Yes[a]	Yes	Adjust based on renal function using TDM approach
Gentamicin	C_{max}/MIC 8–10	Yes	Yes[b]	Yes	Adjust based on renal function using TDM approach
Ciprofloxac in	Total AUC_{0-24}/MIC > 125	No	Yes[c]	No	Dose reduction may not be necessary
Linezolid	Total AUC_{0-24}/MIC of 80–120 and 100 % $T_{>MIC}$	No	Yes[c]	No	Dose reduction is not necessary
Daptomycin	Total AUC_{0-24}/MIC 788–1460	Yes	Yes[a]	May be useful	Adjust based on renal function and toxic effects
Colistin	$fAUC_{0-24}$/MIC 37–46[d]	Yes	May be[c]	Yes	Adjust based on renal function and nephrotoxicity

See discussion for loading doses in the corresponding section
LD loading dose
[a]Demonstrated
[b]Likely
[c]Poorly understood
[d]No clinical data

in ICU patients (DALI) study—a multicenter prospective point-prevalence PK study—higher PK/PD target of 100 % $fT_{>MIC}$ was associated with a higher likelihood of a positive clinical outcome compared to 50 % $fT_{>MIC}$ (odds ratio: 1.02; 95 % CI: 1.01, 1.04, and 1.56; 95 % CI: 1.15, 2.13, respectively). This hypothesis-generating study also raises an interesting question whether achieving higher magnitude of PK/PD ratios at 50 % $fT_{>MIC}$ will improve clinical outcomes in less severely ill patients (Acute Physiology and Chronic Health Evaluation [APACHE] II scores < 14) [45].

In agreement with the PK/PD index, continuous infusion (CI) has been proposed as a mode of administration for beta-lactams to increase %$fT_{>MIC}$. Mouton and den Hollander [46] using an in vitro infection model have shown that doses administered by CI that achieve concentrations near the MIC did not provide bacteriological advantages in the absence of immune function. However, when concentrations are maintained at 4 × MIC, CI is associated with more extensive bacteriological eradication. Others have confirmed this finding, i.e., steady-state concentration has to be maintained at 4 × MIC with CI in the absence of immune function or with higher inoculum size [47–51]. These levels may not be safely achievable in patients with highly resistant pathogens (MIC 64 μg/ml) due to concerns about the toxicity [52].

In summary, the beta-lactam PK/PD target exposures for critically ill patients are yet to be clearly defined. Indeed, different targets for CI and bolus dosing therapy are likely to be necessary. Until further clinical validation data is available, for bolus dosing 100 % $fT_{>MIC}$ is suggested and 100 % $fT_{>4\times MIC}$ for CI therapy. In less critically ill patients, targets of higher ratios of 50 % $fT_{>MIC}$ appear likely to produce acceptable positive clinical outcomes.

5.1.2 Dosing Strategies and PK/PD Target Attainment

Beta-lactams exhibit wide variations in PK among critically ill patients. Prolonged infusion (PI) has (CI and extended infusion, EI) been proposed as a way to maximize the PK/PD target attainment while minimizing the PK variations. A few studies have been conducted in critically ill patients that have compared beta-lactam PK by PI and bolus dosing [53, 54]. With the use of PI strategy, the percentage of the time above the MIC for beta-lactams could be maintained for longer durations at the same time avoiding the higher peak concentrations which appear to offer no clinical benefit with the beta-lactams.

The DALI study authors have reported that patients in PI group are three times more likely to achieve the predefined PK/PD target (50 % $fT_{>MIC}$) compared to bolus group [45]. A few studies have used population PK modeling combined with Monte Carlo simulations (MCS) to compare the PK/PD target attainment among CI, EI, and bolus dosing in critically ill—sepsis, surgical, neutropenic, and ventilator-associated pneumonia patients. It should be noted that the chosen PK/PD targets have not been consistent across the studies. Rafati et al. [55] have reported a 100 % $T_{>MIC}$ with CI of piperacillin/tazobactam (8 g/day) compared to 62 % $T_{>MIC}$ with bolus dosing (3 g tds) against Gram-negative pathogens with an MIC of 16 mg/L. Another study comparing the CI, EI, and bolus dosing of piperacillin/tazobactam against *P. aeruginosa* found that EI and CI attained 90 % $T_{>MIC}$ for an MIC of 32 mg/L whereas bolus dosing only achieved 90 % $T_{>MIC}$ for a lower MIC of 8 mg/L [56]. Both EI and CI have attained similar higher PD targets compared to bolus dosing in this study demonstrating the equivalence of EI and CI. Similarly, in critically ill patients with nosocomial pneumonia, Sakka et al. [57] reported that CI of imipenem/cilastatin would achieve PK/PD targets (40 % $fT_{>MIC}$) for 90 % of organisms with an MIC of 2–4 mg/L whereas for bolus dosing the corresponding MIC would be 1–2 mg/L. This improved PK/PD target attainment was despite the use of 33 % lower doses in CI group. Similarly others have reported a better PK/PD target attainment with EI compared to bolus dosing [58, 59].

Given that most infections occur in the ISF of tissue, CI may provide a favorable beta-lactam exposure at the target site of infection compared with bolus dosing. Roberts et al. [60, 61] reported that both piperacillin/tazobactam and meropenem have a better PK/PD exposure in subcutaneous tissue with CI compared to bolus dosing. Similarly, Buijk et al. [62] have shown that CI (4.5 g/day) of ceftazidime achieved >90 % $T_{>4\times\text{MIC}}$ in peritoneal fluid compared to 44 % $T_{>4\times\text{MIC}}$ with bolus dosing (1.5 g tds) in patients with severe intra-abdominal infections. Boselli et al. [63] have shown that bolus dosing of piperacillin/tazobactam 4/0.5 g given every 8 h or CI of 12/1.5 g/day was not enough to achieve target alveolar antibiotic concentrations for ventilator-associated pneumonia in critically ill patients and suggested that a higher dose of 16/2 g/day is required to reach the target concentrations. It should be noted that there are no prospective studies evaluating the beta-lactam infection site concentrations and clinical outcomes.

In general, CI and EI of beta-lactams will provide superior achievement of PK/PD targets in plasma and ISF for less susceptible bacteria than bolus dosing avoiding the high peak concentrations, which are thought not to be advantageous.

5.1.3 Clinical Outcome

Based on the PK/PD index associated with beta-lactam activity, time dependency, using PI, either CI or EI, has been advocated as a strategy to increase the $fT_{>\text{MIC}}$. Preclinical (in vitro and animal in vivo) and PK/PD studies conducted in humans to date have shown that PI of beta-lactam antibiotics would provide an increased likelihood of achieving target $fT_{>\text{MIC}}$ compared with bolus dosing [64–67]. To date, 11 randomized controlled trials have compared the clinical outcome benefits of PI (all were CI) and the bolus dosing of beta-lactams in critically ill patients [55, 68–77]. In addition, observational and retrospective cohort studies have also been conducted and together demonstrate that PI strategy is likely to be beneficial in certain patient groups, in particular the critically ill [42, 78–82]. Three papers have meta-analyzed the available randomized control trials (RCT) (including critically ill and non-critically ill patients) for clinical and mortality benefits of antibiotics by CI and bolus dosing [83–85]. Recent meta-analyses have focused on beta-lactams alone and found no difference in clinical cure or mortality between CI and bolus dosing in hospitalized patients [83, 84]. However, these meta-analyses did have wide confidence intervals suggesting that a clinically relevant difference between the two administration strategies may still exist.

Methodological issues with RCTs included in the above meta-analyses [86, 87] and mortality and clinical cure benefits observed in a specific subset of critically ill patients in observational cohort studies have led to conduct of two recent meta-analyses [88, 89] that included RCTs as well as observational studies. One of them specifically looked at piperacillin-tazobactam and carbapenems whereas the other analyzed all penicillin class antibiotics as well as vancomycin and linezolid with subgroup analysis for piperacillin-tazobactam and carbapenems. It is important to highlight that both analyses largely comprised of critically ill patients with comparable doses in both arms in contrast to previous meta-analyses. Both analyses pointed towards improved clinical benefits with PI concluding the need for a well-designed multicenter RCT powered enough to detect outcome benefits. No serious adverse effects have been reported in the clinical studies to date [84].

5.2 Vancomycin

Vancomycin is commonly used for methicillin-resistant *S. aureus* (MRSA) infections. Consensus from in vitro, animal, and human PD studies is that AUC_{0-24}/MIC is the PK/PD index associated with clinical efficacy [90]. Current Infectious Diseases Society of America (IDSA) consensus guidelines recommend to target trough concentrations of 15–20 mg/L with intermittent 12-hourly i.v. dosing in order to achieve an $AUC_{0-24}/MIC \geq 400$ for vancomycin for pathogens with an MIC ≤ 1 mg/L [91]. This particular AUC_{0-24}/MIC was derived from a cohort of hospitalized patients with *S. aureus* pneumonia (methicillin-sensitive *S. aureus* and MRSA; largely ventilator-associated pneumonia patients). Patients with an $AUC_{0-24}/MIC \geq 345$ and $AUC_{0-24}/MIC \geq 866$ (MIC determined using broth micro-dilution method, BMD) had superior clinical and microbiological response, respectively [92]. This study excluded patients with endocarditis, osteomyelitis, and central nervous system infections. A few other studies have examined this relationship but included different infections and MIC determination methods and reported slightly different cutoff AUC_{0-24}/MIC values. One study has reported that an $AUC_{0-24}/MIC > 373$ (MIC using BMD) is associated with improved attributable mortality in *S. aureus* bacteremia patients [93] whereas another reported an $AUC_{0-24}/MIC > 211$ (MIC using E-test method) with improved attributable mortality in patients with bacteremia and infective endocarditis [94].

Vancomycin PK studies in ICU patients have reported a Vd twice that observed in normal patients (0.7–0.8 L/kg) [95–97]. Standard traditional doses (1 g every 12 h) would achieve the target AUC_{0-24}/MIC only if the MIC is ≤ 0.5 in a patient with CrCL >100 ml/min and an average weight (defined as 80 kg) [91]. This may be similar or even worse in ICU patients considering the possible PK changes that occur in these patients. Two studies have described the doses necessary to achieve the recommended PK/

PD targets in ICU patients [95, 96]. One of them suggested doses in the range of ≥3 g to achieve a high probability for target attainment (PTA) for *S. aureus* with an MIC 1 mg/L in patients with conserved renal function [95]. In the other study, standard doses were able to reach the target AUC_{0-24}/MIC in only 30 % of patients younger than 65 years and with a CrCL >60 ml/min for *S. aureus* with an MIC of 1 mg/L. However, in older patients with a CrCL < 60 ml/min, 96 % will achieve the targets. Doses up to, and exceeding, 5 g would be necessary to achieve approximately a 90 % probability of attaining PK/PD targets in patients <65 years while doses up to 4 g are required in patients older than 65 years that have a CrCL >60 ml/min [96]. These data highlight the need for the use of higher than traditional doses, particularly when dosing in patients with suspected ARC [98].

With the need for considerably higher doses in some patients, there is renewed interest in exposure-toxicity relationship of vancomycin. A recent meta-analysis has concluded that higher trough concentrations ≥15 mg/L were associated with increased risk of nephrotoxicity relative to low troughs (<15 mg/L) (OR, 3.12; 95 % CI, 1.81–5.37; $p < 0.01$) with greatest risk when concentrations were ≥20 mg/L. This highlights the need for more careful monitoring of at-risk patients with high trough concentrations. Critically ill patients receiving therapy for ≥7 days or on concomitant nephrotoxic drugs are at increased risk of renal injury [99].

In critically ill patients, loading doses of vancomycin were first proposed in 2001 to rapidly achieve PK/PD targets [100]. Consensus guidelines have recommended a loading dose of 25–30 mg/kg to achieve target trough concentration promptly which is necessary in critically ill patients [91]. However, it is not universally practiced across ICUs worldwide. Moreover, loading doses required to achieve prompt PK/PD targets are not well established in critically ill patients. In a study by Li et al. a median loading dose of 20 mg/kg has helped achieve a median AUC_{0-24}/MIC of 366 in the first 24 h in a cohort of ICU patients [101]. It is likely that loading doses as recommended by consensus guidelines would achieve the target trough concentration in ICU patients. CI of vancomycin has been proposed as a strategy to optimize attainment of PK/PD targets because of this drug's time-dependent kill characteristics. Although it was not shown to be clinically superior to bolus dosing [102], CI could be useful to maintain steady concentrations and provide better tissue penetration in difficult-to-treat infections [102]. A loading dose of 30–35 mg/kg and a maintenance dose of at least 35 mg/kg have been suggested to rapidly achieve and maintain a trough concentration of 20 mg/L in a patient with CrCl of 100 ml/min/1.73 m^2 [103]. Dosage regimens need to be carefully adjusted, in patients with renal impairment, following the loading dose due to expected longer half-life.

Evidence is emerging for improved survival if PK/PD targets are maintained and need for higher doses in critically ill patients to achieve those targets [93, 94]. With increased risk of nephrotoxicity at such high concentrations, PK/PD-guided dosing would be an invaluable tool while carefully monitoring renal function in at-risk patients.

5.3 Gentamicin

Gentamicin is a concentration-dependent antibiotic widely used for severe Gram-negative infections in critically ill patients. Two PK/PD parameters have been associated with gentamicin efficacy. Human PD studies have shown that an AUC_{0-24}/MIC of 80–120 or a C_{max}/MIC of 8–10 is associated with improved outcomes [104]. High-dose extended interval dosing regimens are now widely accepted in clinical practice, except for endocarditis, in order to reduce nephrotoxicity associated with aminoglycosides whilst improving PK/PD target attainment [105]. Furthermore, Kashuba et al. have shown, using logistic regression, that achieving a $C_{max}/MIC \geq 10$ within the first 48 h of treatment in patients with nosocomial pneumonia has led to a 90 % probability of clinical cure [106, 107].

Significantly increased Vd (0.4–0.8 L/kg) has been observed in critically ill patients with sepsis and septic shock. Cardiac index, APACHE II score, body weight, and female gender have been associated with an increased Vd [108–111]. These changes in Vd tend to decrease over time in critically ill patients as disease severity decreases and may return to values reported in non-ICU patients. Accordingly, Goncalves-Pereira et al. [110] have reported that only 66 % and 31 % of patients were able to attain a C_{max} of at least 16 mg/L and above 20 mg/L, respectively, with a median first dose of 7.4 mg/kg. Similar findings have been reported in a retrospective study [111]. The authors have shown, using MCS, that only 20 % of patients were able to achieve a C_{max}/MIC (MIC 2) of 10 with a dose of 7 mg/kg. This study has reported a mean Vd of 0.8 L/kg. One study in surgical trauma patients reported Vd similar to other hospitalized patients (0.3 L/kg) and a dose of 7 mg/kg was sufficient to achieve a C_{max} of 22.4 ± 5.9 mg/L [112]. Buijk et al. [108] in a cohort of septic shock patients have reported a mean C_{max} of 18.5 mg/L. However, statistically significant differences in Vd (0.4 ± 0.1 L/kg vs. 0.3 ± 0.1 L/kg, $p = 0.004$) and C_{max} (18.5 ± 5.6 mg/L vs. 21.3 ± 7.2 mg/L, $p = 0.03$) were observed between septic shock and non-shock patients. Therefore, evidence is conflicting as to whether critically ill patients will require higher loading doses to increase the probability of target attainment with MICs ≥1. However, it is clear from studies that doses ≥7 mg/kg may be required in a cohort of critically ill patients with larger Vd to attain the target PK/PD index. However, it will be a challenge in clinical practice, without any readily available measures to identify such patients.

5.4 Ciprofloxacin

Ciprofloxacin is a lipophilic antibiotic with activity against Gram-negative pathogens. It is widely used in ICUs as an empirical therapy in combination with beta-lactams. Ciprofloxacin is a concentration-dependent antibiotic with some time-dependent activity. Early studies have suggested a C_{max}/MIC around 8–10 for bacterial eradication. However, Forrest et al. [36] in a cohort of seriously ill patients with lower respiratory tract infections have reported that an AUC_{0-24}/MIC > 125 was associated with better clinical and microbiological outcomes (80 % vs. 42 % and 82 % vs. 26 %, respectively). Higher AUC_{0-24}/MICs were associated with rapid microbiological eradication and prevent the emergence of bacterial resistance, particularly in the critical care environment [113].

Unlike hydrophilic antibiotics, ciprofloxacin Vd was not increased in critically ill patients with severe sepsis and intra-abdominal infections [14, 114–116]. On the contrary, except in poly-trauma patients, it is interesting to note that Vd was smaller compared to non-ICU patients. The reasons for this remain unknown. Lipman et al. [114] have studied PK of ciprofloxacin in severe sepsis patients on days D0, D2, and D7 and reported that 1200 mg/day was able to achieve an AUC_{0-24}/MIC > 125 for bacteria with an MIC up to 0.3 mg/L. There was no evidence of significant accumulation over 7 days in patients with CrCL > 60 ml/min. Forrest et al. [36] have also raised the same concern that 1200 mg/day may not be able to achieve an AUC_{0-24}/MIC > 125 for organisms with MIC of 0.5 mg/L. Higher doses or combination therapy will be required if treating an organism with MIC ≥ 0.5 mg/L. More recent studies [115, 116] using MCS have echoed the earlier results published by Lipman et al. and Forrest et al. Some authors have suggested that in view of maintaining clinical efficacy and observed variations in AUC_{0-24}, dose reduction is not necessary in renal impairment as higher doses have been used without any significant adverse effects and significant accumulation has not been reported.

5.5 Linezolid

Linezolid is a hydrophilic antibiotic with Vd close to total body water (≈50 L) with 31 % protein binding and good distribution into major tissues including epithelial lining fluid, central nervous system, bone, muscle, and synovial fluid [117]. The clinical PD of linezolid were studied by Rayner et al. [118] in patients enrolled in a compassionate-use program. One-third of the patients were treated in ICU and had significantly reduced serum albumin concentrations. Consistent with in vitro and in vivo studies, authors have reported that linezolid efficacy is associated with both AUC_{0-24}/MIC and $T_{>MIC}$. An AUC_{0-24}/MIC of 80–120 and 100 % $T_{>MIC}$ have been proposed to attain high probability of bacterial eradication and clinical cure in bacteremia, skin and skin structure infections, and lower respiratory tract infections. The authors have highlighted that $T_{>MIC}$ has to be 100 % for higher success rate and correlation was present between AUC_{0-24}/MIC and $T_{>MIC}$ (r^2 = 0.87).

The linezolid Vd has been reported to be similar to non-ICU patients across all studies involving critically ill patients [119–123]. Thus, it can be concluded that linezolid may not require a loading dose. However, it should be noted that the reported Vd has wider standard deviations indicating large variability among patients. Whitehouse et al. [120] have reported that 600 mg given twice a day is adequate enough to achieve C_{min} above 4 mg/L for the entire dosing interval and PK was not significantly different from healthy volunteers. However, interindividual variability was very high at 70 % in the population PK model. Dong et al. [119] have observed similar interindividual variability in a study involving critically ill patients. Thallinger et al. [121] and Buerger et al. [123] have examined the effect of severe sepsis and septic shock on interstitial fluid (ISF) penetration in adipose and subcutaneous tissue. Thallinger et al. [121] have reported the effects after a single dose whereas Buerger et al. [123] have monitored concentrations up to 72 h (days 1 and 3). It is interesting to note that in the former study, 600 mg dose is sufficient to achieve 100 % $T_{>MIC}$ in both plasma and ISF whereas in the latter only 40 % of patients have achieved more than 80 % $fT_{>MIC}$ and none of the patients have achieved the required $fAUC_{0-24}$/MIC. It was suggested that 600 mg given three-times-a-day dosing would be required to meet the targets for an organism with an MIC 4 mg/L.

In accordance with PK/PD index associated with efficacy, CI of linezolid has been proposed and compared with bolus dosing. Adembri et al. [122] have compared both regimens (600 g BD vs. 300 mg bolus followed by CI of 900 mg/day 1 and 1200 mg/day from day 2) in septic patients and monitored concentrations for 72 h. In bolus group, 50 % of the patients were reported to have a $C_{min} < 1$ mg/L. In CI group starting from 6 h, concentrations were significantly higher than bolus group and above 4 mg/L. The 6-h delay may be due to use of an inadequate loading dose. Similarly, attainment of AUC_{0-24}/MIC targets was significantly higher with CI than bolus dosing. Similarly, Boselli et al. [124, 125] have studied plasma and epithelial lining fluid concentrations in ventilator-associated pneumonia patients with both bolus and CI regimens. They have reported that bolus dosing was able to achieve the required targets ($C_{min} > 4$ mg/L) for only about 75 % of the 12-h dosing interval whereas it was 100 % with CI. From the above results, it may be the case that CI or more frequent dosing would be required in the initial phases of severe sepsis or septic shock to achieve required PK/PD targets and infection site concentrations.

5.6 Daptomycin

Daptomycin is a hydrophilic antibiotic with Vd close to 0.1 L/kg with approximately 92 % protein binding. In vivo PD studies have revealed that either AUC_{0-24}/MIC or C_{max}/MIC is the PK/PD parameter associated with optimal outcomes. Soon et al. [126] have analyzed the data from phase 1, 2, and 3 studies, using MCS, and reported that an AUC_{0-24}/MIC of 388–537, 588–750, and 788–1460 was associated with bacteriostasis, 1-log kill, and bactericidal activity, respectively, against four strains of *S. aureus* with an MIC of 0.5 mg/L, which are in close agreement with in vivo PD studies.

Prospective PK studies of daptomycin in ICU patients with sepsis have not been conducted to date. However, two studies involving neutropenic and other hospitalized patients (40 % were present in ICU with severe sepsis or septic shock) have observed a Vd at least twice as much as healthy volunteers and as high as 0.5 L/kg with large interindividual variability [127, 128]. Few other studies have supported this finding [29, 129]. Therefore, critically ill patients with severe sepsis or septic shock may have a significantly increased Vd. Three studies have examined daptomycin PK/PD in hospitalized patients [127–129]. Bubalo et al. [127] have studied neutropenic patients and concluded that 6 mg/kg was only sufficient to achieve concentrations required for bacteriostatic effect of daptomycin with organisms up to MIC of 0.5 mg/L. Only 34 % of patients have reached concentrations required for bactericidal effect with 6 mg/kg dose. Di Paolo et al. [129] have reported that 90 % and 75 % of patients have achieved AUC_{0-24}/MIC targets required for bacteriostatic and bactericidal effects, respectively, higher than reported by Bubalo et al. However, Di Paolo et al. have not reported MICs in their study and almost two-thirds of the patients have received doses >6 mg/kg. Combining the data from phase 1, 2, and 3 studies, Soon et al. have shown that 6 mg/kg doses are only able to achieve bacteriostatic activity and up to 12 mg/kg doses were required for bactericidal activity for pathogens with an MIC of 1 mg/L. These differences among Soon et al. [126] and other studies mentioned above for bacteriostasis may be due to different levels of sickness severity of patients involved in phase 1 and 2 studies. It should be mentioned that Bubalo et al. and Di Paolo et al. studies involved a small subset of critically ill patients. However, these findings may not be generalized to ICU patients with severe sepsis and septic shock. The probability of target attainment may be much lower in ICU patients if standard doses are used.

A recent study by Falcone et al. [29] including sepsis and non-sepsis patients (unknown whether present in ICU or not) has shown that daptomycin doses at 6 or 8 mg/kg lead to lower exposure in patients with MRSA bacteremia. Interesting finding from this study was that a higher proportion of patients with sepsis have augmented CL compared to non-sepsis patients (100 % vs. 24 %; CL—1.81 ± 0.409 L/h vs. 0.75 ± 0.17 L/h). It is already known that a group of ICU patients (younger patients with trauma and normal organ function) exhibit this phenomenon called ARC. However, in Falcone et al. study, mean age was 68 ± 14 years with a mean estimated CrCL of 63.7 ml/min. They have suggested, based on MCS, a fixed dose of 750 mg in sepsis patients rather than a dose of 10 mg/kg based on the incidence of estimated differences in toxicity (% probability of $C_{min}>24.3$ mg/L—1.26 vs. 2.64) as both regimens have yielded a similar cumulative fraction response. Fixed dose simulations were conducted based on the observation that body weight is not a predictor of variability for daptomycin CL. Considering the delay in attaining the steady-state (approximately 3 days) and significantly larger Vd in above studies, loading doses may be of utility for daptomycin. However, studies looking at differences in day 1 and later concentrations have not been conducted which may demonstrate whether loading doses are required. Higher doses up to 12 mg/kg have been used safely without any increase in creatinine kinase and peripheral neuropathy [130–132].

5.7 Colistin

Colistin is a hydrophilic polymyxin antibiotic active against Gram-negative bacteria. It was discovered in 1940s; its clinical use declined and was then phased out in 1970s due to a high incidence of nephrotoxicity and neurotoxicity. Due to emergence of multidrug-resistant bacteria and a lack of emerging antibiotics with novel mechanisms of activity, polymyxins have reemerged as a last resource or salvage therapy in critically ill patients. Colistin is a concentration-dependent antibiotic and $fAUC_{0-24}$/MIC is the best PK/PD parameter associated with efficacy. Magnitude of PK/PD index is variable depending on the bacteriostatic or bactericidal effect, bacterial species, and site of infection. In general, a value of 16–23 is required for bacteriostatic and 37–46 is required for bactericidal effect [133, 134]. However, clinical studies have focused on maintaining concentrations above the MIC. For detailed information on terminology used for colistimethate sodium (CMS, prodrug of colistin) and colistin dosing units refer to Li et al. [135].

Colistin and CMS PK/PD have been studied extensively over the last decade [136, 137]. Colistin Vd was significantly increased in critically ill patients compared to young healthy volunteers (0.17 L/kg vs. 0.3–2.0 L/kg) [138–145]. This is consistent with its limited distribution to extracellular fluid based on its physicochemical properties. In contrast, its half-life was prolonged, probably due to an increased Vd, compared to healthy volunteers (3 ± 0.6 h vs. 4–18.5 h).

Early PK studies [142, 143, 145] in critically ill patients using 2–3 million IU of CMS every 8–12 h have resulted in steady-state C_{max} around 2–3 mg/L and obtained steady-state after 2–3 days. This, along with slow conversion of CMS to colistin, has led to suboptimal exposure (below 2 mg/L, MIC breakpoint) in majority of critically ill patients. Based upon these considerations, using population PK and MCS approach, Plachouras et al. [145], Mohamed et al. [144], and Garonzik et al. [140] have suggested higher maintenance doses along with loading dose to achieve desired plasma steady-state concentrations of formed colistin. Plachouras et al. have suggested a loading dose of 9 or 12 million IU followed by 4.5 million IU of CMS given twice daily whereas

Mohamed et al. have recommended a loading dose of 6–9 million IU. A more recent population PK study [140] involving 105 critically ill patients (16 on RRT) with varying renal function has developed dosing guidelines to achieve desired steady-state plasma concentrations of formed colistin. Average steady-state concentrations ranged from 0.5 to 9.4 mg/L with a median concentration of 2.4 mg/L in the study patients. CrCL has been identified as an important covariate for the clearance of CMS as well as formed colistin. Loading and maintenance dosing nomogram was developed using body weight and CrCl as covariates, respectively, for patients receiving RRTs and not receiving RRTs. The authors have pointed out that with the current recommended doses, it is unlikely to achieve desired concentrations especially in patients with CrCl > 70 ml/min/1.73 m^2 and MIC ≥1 mg/L. It was recommended to use colistin as part of a combination therapy in such situations. Caution must be exercised when dosing colistin since incidence of nephrotoxicity is approximately 50 % with the currently recommended doses [146, 147].

It is important to note that the dosing recommendations suggested by Plachouras et al. [145] were validated in a preliminary study by Dalfino et al. [148] in a cohort of 28 critically ill patients. The authors have reported a clinical cure rate of 82 % and nephrotoxicity rate of 18 %. Despite a few limitations, this study has demonstrated that PK/PD-based dose optimization would improve the outcomes while minimizing toxicity.

6 Conclusion

PK/PD of antibiotics can be highly variable in critically ill patients. It is necessary to adjust dosing during initial stages of treatment to account for physiological changes that leads to increased Vd and augmented clearances. Maintenance doses need to be adjusted based on organ function to maximize efficacy and minimize toxicity. It may be necessary in some cases to utilize prolonged infusion strategies to improve PK/PD target attainment and infection site concentrations.

References

1. Angus DC, Linde-Zwirble WT, Lidicker J, Clermont G, Carcillo J, Pinsky MR (2001) Epidemiology of severe sepsis in the United States: analysis of incidence, outcome, and associated costs of care. Crit Care Med 29(7):1303–1310
2. Martin GS, Mannino DM, Eaton S, Moss M (2003) The epidemiology of sepsis in the United States from 1979 through 2000. N Engl J Med 348(16):1546–1554
3. Vincent JL, Sakr Y, Sprung CL, Ranieri VM, Reinhart K, Gerlach H et al (2006) Sepsis in European intensive care units: results of the SOAP study. Crit Care Med 34(2):344–353
4. Russell JA (2006) Management of sepsis. N Engl J Med 355(16):1699–1713

5. Vincent JL, Rello J, Marshall J, Silva E, Anzueto A, Martin CD et al (2009) International study of the prevalence and outcomes of infection in intensive care units. JAMA 302(21):2323–2329
6. Dellinger RP, Levy MM, Carlet JM, Bion J, Parker MM, Jaeschke R et al (2008) Surviving Sepsis Campaign: international guidelines for management of severe sepsis and septic shock: 2008. Crit Care Med 36(1):296–327
7. Kumar A, Roberts D, Wood KE, Light B, Parrillo JE, Sharma S et al (2006) Duration of hypotension before initiation of effective antimicrobial therapy is the critical determinant of survival in human septic shock. Crit Care Med 34(6):1589–1596
8. Roberts JA, Kruger P, Paterson DL, Lipman J (2008) Antibiotic resistance--what's dosing got to do with it? Crit Care Med 36(8):2433–2440
9. Drusano GL (2003) Prevention of resistance: a goal for dose selection for antimicrobial agents. Clin Infect Dis 36(Suppl 1):S42–S50
10. Roberts JA, Lipman J (2006) Antibacterial dosing in intensive care: pharmacokinetics, degree of disease and pharmacodynamics of sepsis. Clin Pharmacokinet 45(8):755–773
11. Roberts JA, Lipman J (2009) Pharmacokinetic issues for antibiotics in the critically ill patient. Crit Care Med 37(3):840–851
12. Roberts JA, Ulldemolins M, Roberts MS, McWhinney B, Ungerer J, Paterson DL et al (2010) Therapeutic drug monitoring of beta-lactams in critically ill patients: proof of concept. Int J Antimicrob Agents 36(4):332–339
13. Taccone FS, Laterre P-F, Dugernier T, Spapen H, Delattre I, Wittebole X et al (2010) Insufficient beta-lactam concentrations in the early phase of severe sepsis and septic shock. Crit Care 14(4):R126
14. Gous A, Lipman J, Scribante J, Tshukutsoane S, Hon H, Pinder M et al (2005) Fluid shifts have no influence on ciprofloxacin pharmacokinetics in intensive care patients with intra-abdominal sepsis. Int J Antimicrob Agents 26(1):50–55
15. Ulldemolins M, Roberts JA, Lipman J, Rello J (2011) Antibiotic dosing in multiple organ dysfunction syndrome. Chest 139(5):1210–1220
16. Ulldemolins M, Roberts JA, Wallis SC, Rello J, Lipman J (2010) Flucloxacillin dosing in critically ill patients with hypoalbuminaemia: special emphasis on unbound pharmacokinetics. J Antimicrob Chemother 65(8):1771–1778
17. Ulldemolins M, Roberts JA, Rello J, Paterson DL, Lipman J (2011) The effects of hypoalbuminaemia on optimizing antibacterial dosing in critically ill patients. Clin Pharmacokinet 50(2):99–110
18. Joynt GM, Lipman J, Gomersall CD, Young RJ, Wong EL, Gin T (2001) The pharmacokinetics of once-daily dosing of ceftriaxone in critically ill patients. J Antimicrob Chemother 47(4):421–429
19. Schrier RW, Wang W (2004) Acute renal failure and sepsis. N Engl J Med 351(2):159–169
20. Eyler RF, Mueller BA (2011) Antibiotic dosing in critically ill patients with acute kidney injury. Nat Rev Nephrol 7(4):226–235
21. Jezequel SG (1994) Fluconazole: interspecies scaling and allometric relationships of pharmacokinetic properties. J Pharm Pharmacol 46(3):196–199
22. Martin JH, Fay MF, Udy A, Roberts J, Kirkpatrick C, Ungerer J et al (2011) Pitfalls of using estimations of glomerular filtration rate in an intensive care population. Int Med J 41(7):537–543
23. Prowle JR, Bellomo R (2010) Continuous renal replacement therapy: recent advances and future research. Nat Rev Nephrol 6(9):521–529
24. Baldwin I, Bellomo R, Naka T, Koch B, Fealy N (2007) A pilot randomized controlled comparison of extended daily dialysis with filtration and continuous veno-venous hemofiltration: fluid removal and hemodynamics. Int J Artif Organs 30(12):1083–1089
25. Choi G, Gomersall CD, Tian Q, Joynt GM, Freebairn R, Lipman J (2009) Principles of antibacterial dosing in continuous renal replacement therapy. Crit Care Med 37(7):2268–2282
26. Roberts DM, Roberts JA, Roberts MS, Liu X, Nair P, Cole L et al (2012) Variability of antibiotic concentrations in critically ill patients receiving continuous renal replacement therapy: a multicentre pharmacokinetic study. Crit Care Med 40(5):1523–1528
27. Li AM, Gomersall CD, Choi G, Tian Q, Joynt GM, Lipman J (2009) A systematic review of antibiotic dosing regimens for septic patients receiving continuous renal replacement therapy: do current studies supply sufficient data? J Antimicrob Chemother 64(5):929–937
28. Udy AA, Varghese JV, Altukroni M, Briscoe S, McWhinney B, Ungerer J et al (2011) Subtherapeutic initial β-lactam concentrations in select critically ill patients: association between augmented renal clearance and low trough drug concentrations. Chest 42(1):30–39
29. Falcone M, Russo A, Venditti M, Novelli A, Pai MP (2013) Considerations for higher doses of daptomycin in critically ill patients

with methicillin-resistant Staphylococcus aureus bacteremia. Clin Infect Dis 57(11):1568–1576
30. Udy AA, Putt MT, Shanmugathasan S, Roberts JA, Lipman J (2010) Augmented renal clearance in the Intensive Care Unit: an illustrative case series. Int J Antimicrob Agents 35(6):606–608
31. Udy AA, Roberts JA, Boots RJ, Paterson DL, Lipman J (2010) Augmented renal clearance: implications for antibacterial dosing in the critically ill. Clin Pharmacokinet 49(1):1–16
32. Udy AA, Roberts JA, Lipman J (2011) Implications of augmented renal clearance in critically ill patients. Nat Rev Nephrol 7(9):539–543
33. Nicolau DP (2003) Optimizing outcomes with antimicrobial therapy through pharmacodynamic profiling. J Infect Chemother 9(4):292–296
34. Craig WA (1998) Pharmacokinetic/pharmacodynamic parameters: rationale for antibacterial dosing of mice and men. Clin Infect Dis 26(1):1–10
35. Moore RD, Smith CR, Lietman PS (1984) Association of aminoglycoside plasma levels with therapeutic outcome in gram-negative pneumonia. Am J Med 77(4):657–662
36. Forrest A, Nix DE, Ballow CH, Goss TF, Birmingham MC, Schentag JJ (1993) Pharmacodynamics of intravenous ciprofloxacin in seriously ill patients. Antimicrob Agents Chemother 37(5):1073–1081
37. Lee SY, Kuti JL, Nicolau DP (2007) Cefepime pharmacodynamics in patients with extended spectrum beta-lactamase (ESBL) and non-ESBL infections. J Infect 54(5):463–468
38. McKinnon PS, Paladino JA, Schentag JJ (2008) Evaluation of area under the inhibitory curve (AUIC) and time above the minimum inhibitory concentration (T > MIC) as predictors of outcome for cefepime and ceftazidime in serious bacterial infections. Int J Antimicrob Agents 31(4):345–351
39. Tam VH, McKinnon PS, Akins RL, Rybak MJ, Drusano GL (2002) Pharmacodynamics of cefepime in patients with Gram-negative infections. J Antimicrob Chemother 50(3):425–428
40. Li C, Du X, Kuti JL, Nicolau DP (2007) Clinical pharmacodynamics of meropenem in patients with lower respiratory tract infections. Antimicrob Agents Chemother 51(5):1725–1730
41. Ariano RE, Nyhlén A, Donnelly JP, Sitar DS, Harding GK, Zelenitsky SA (2005) Pharmacokinetics and pharmacodynamics of meropenem in febrile neutropenic patients with bacteremia. Ann Pharmacother 39(1): 32–38
42. Lodise TP, Lomaestro B, Drusano GL (2007) Piperacillin-tazobactam for Pseudomonas aeruginosa infection: clinical implications of an extended-infusion dosing strategy. Clin Infect Dis 44(3):357–363
43. Crandon JL, Bulik CC, Kuti JL, Nicolau DP (2010) Clinical pharmacodynamics of cefepime in patients infected with Pseudomonas aeruginosa. Antimicrob Agents Chemother 54(3):1111–1116
44. Manduru M, Mihm LB, White RL, Friedrich LV, Flume PA, Bosso JA (1997) In vitro pharmacodynamics of ceftazidime against Pseudomonas aeruginosa isolates from cystic fibrosis patients. Antimicrob Agents Chemother 41(9):2053–2056
45. Roberts JA, Paul SK, Akova M, Bassetti M, De Waele JJ, Dimopoulos G et al (2014) DALI: Defining Antibiotic Levels in Intensive care unit patients: are current beta-lactam antibiotic doses sufficient for critically ill patients? Clin Infect Dis 58:1072. doi:10.1093/cid/ciu027
46. Mouton JW, den Hollander JG (1994) Killing of Pseudomonas aeruginosa during continuous and intermittent infusion of ceftazidime in an in vitro pharmacokinetic model. Antimicrob Agents Chemother 38(5):931–936
47. Cappelletty DM, Kang SL, Palmer SM, Rybak MJ (1995) Pharmacodynamics of ceftazidime administered as continuous infusion or intermittent bolus alone and in combination with single daily-dose amikacin against Pseudomonas aeruginosa in an in vitro infection model. Antimicrob Agents Chemother 39(8):1797–1801
48. Tessier PR, Nicolau DP, Onyeji CO, Nightingale CH (1999) Pharmacodynamics of intermittent- and continuous-infusion cefepime alone and in combination with once-daily tobramycin against Pseudomonas aeruginosa in an in vitro infection model. Chemotherapy 45(4):284–295
49. Alou L, Aguilar L, Sevillano D, Giménez MJ, Echeverría O, Gómez-Lus ML et al (2005) Is there a pharmacodynamic need for the use of continuous versus intermittent infusion with ceftazidime against Pseudomonas aeruginosa? An in vitro pharmacodynamic model. J Antimicrob Chemother 55(2):209–213
50. Robaux MA, Dube L, Caillon J, Bugnon D, Kergueris MF, Navas D et al (2001) In vivo efficacy of continuous infusion versus intermittent dosing of ceftazidime alone or in combination with amikacin relative to human kinetic profiles in a Pseudomonas aeruginosa rabbit endocarditis model. J Antimicrob Chemother 47(5):617–622
51. Navas D, Caillon J, Gras-Le Guen C, Jacqueline C, Kergueris MF, Bugnon D et al

(2004) Comparison of in vivo intrinsic activity of cefepime and imipenem in a Pseudomonas aeruginosa rabbit endocarditis model: effect of combination with tobramycin simulating human serum pharmacokinetics. J Antimicrob Chemother 54(4):767–771
52. Moriyama B, Henning SA, Childs R, Holland SM, Anderson VL, Morris JC et al (2010) High-dose continuous infusion beta-lactam antibiotics for the treatment of resistant Pseudomonas aeruginosa infections in immunocompromised patients. Ann Pharmacother 44(5):929–935
53. Abdul-Aziz M, Staatz C, Kirkpatrick CM, Lipman J, Roberts JA (2011) Continuous infusion vs. bolus dosing: implications for beta-lactam antibiotics. Minerva Anestesiol 78(1):94–104
54. Kasiakou SK, Lawrence KR, Choulis N, Falagas ME (2005) Continuous versus intermittent intravenous administration of antibacterials with time-dependent action: a systematic review of pharmacokinetic and pharmacodynamic parameters. Drugs 65(17):2499–2511
55. Rafati MR, Rouini MR, Mojtahedzadeh M, Najafi A, Tavakoli H, Gholami K et al (2006) Clinical efficacy of continuous infusion of piperacillin compared with intermittent dosing in septic critically ill patients. Int J Antimicrob Agents 28(2):122–127
56. Kim A, Sutherland CA, Kuti JL, Nicolau DP (2007) Optimal dosing of piperacillin-tazobactam for the treatment of Pseudomonas aeruginosa infections: prolonged or continuous infusion? Pharmacotherapy 27(11):1490–1497
57. Sakka SG, Glauner AK, Bulitta JB, Kinzig-Schippers M, Pfister W, Drusano GL et al (2007) Population pharmacokinetics and pharmacodynamics of continuous versus short-term infusion of imipenem-cilastatin in critically ill patients in a randomized, controlled trial. Antimicrob Agents Chemother 51(9):3304–3310
58. Jaruratanasirikul S, Sudsai T (2009) Comparison of the pharmacodynamics of imipenem in patients with ventilator-associated pneumonia following administration by 2 or 0.5 h infusion. J Antimicrob Chemother 63(3):560–563
59. Jaruratanasirikul S, Sriwiriyajan S, Punyo J (2005) Comparison of the pharmacodynamics of meropenem in patients with ventilator-associated pneumonia following administration by 3-hour infusion or bolus injection. Antimicrob Agents Chemother 49(4):1337–1339
60. Roberts JA, Kirkpatrick CM, Roberts MS, Robertson TA, Dalley AJ, Lipman J (2009) Meropenem dosing in critically ill patients with sepsis and without renal dysfunction: intermittent bolus versus continuous administration? Monte Carlo dosing simulations and subcutaneous tissue distribution. J Antimicrob Chemother 64(1):142–150
61. Roberts JA, Roberts MS, Robertson TA, Dalley AJ, Lipman J (2009) Piperacillin penetration into tissue of critically ill patients with sepsis--bolus versus continuous administration? Crit Care Med 37(3):926–933
62. Buijk SL, Gyssens IC, Mouton JW, Van Vliet A, Verbrugh HA, Bruining HA (2002) Pharmacokinetics of ceftazidime in serum and peritoneal exudate during continuous versus intermittent administration to patients with severe intra-abdominal infections. J Antimicrob Chemother 49(1):121–128
63. Boselli E, Breilh D, Cannesson M, Xuereb F, Rimmelé T, Chassard D et al (2004) Steady-state plasma and intrapulmonary concentrations of piperacillin/tazobactam 4 g/0.5 g administered to critically ill patients with severe nosocomial pneumonia. Intensive Care Med 30(5):976–979
64. Craig WA (2003) Basic pharmacodynamics of antibacterials with clinical applications to the use of beta-lactams, glycopeptides, and linezolid. Infect Dis Clin North Am 17(3):479–501
65. MacGowan A (2011) Revisiting Beta-lactams - PK/PD improves dosing of old antibiotics. Curr Opin Pharmacol 11(5):470–476
66. Mouton JW, Vinks AA (2007) Continuous infusion of beta-lactams. Curr Opin Crit Care 13(5):598–606
67. Drusano GL (2004) Antimicrobial pharmacodynamics: critical interactions of 'bug and drug'. Nat Rev Microbiol 2(4):289–300
68. Angus BJ, Smith MD, Suputtamongkol Y, Mattie H, Walsh AL, Wuthiekanun V et al (2000) Pharmacokinetic-pharmacodynamic evaluation of ceftazidime continuous infusion vs intermittent bolus injection in septicaemic melioidosis. Br J Clin Pharmacol 50(2):184–191
69. Georges B, Conil JM, Cougot P, Decun JF, Archambaud M, Seguin T et al (2005) Cefepime in critically ill patients: continuous infusion vs. an intermittent dosing regimen. Int J Clin Pharmacol Ther 43(8):360–369
70. Hanes SD, Wood GC, Herring V, Croce MA, Fabian TC, Pritchard E et al (2000) Intermittent and continuous ceftazidime infusion for critically ill trauma patients. Am J Surg 179(6):436–440
71. Kojika M, Sato N, Hakozaki M, Suzuki Y, Takahasi G, Endo S et al (2005) A preliminary study of the administration of carbape-

nem antibiotics in sepsis patients on the basis of the administration time. Jpn J Antibiot 58(5):452–457
72. Lagast H, Meunier-Carpentier F, Klastersky J (1983) Treatment of gram-negative bacillary septicemia with cefoperazone. Eur J Clin Microbiol 2(6):554–558
73. Lau WK, Mercer D, Itani KM, Nicolau DP, Kuti JL, Mansfield D et al (2006) Randomized, open-label, comparative study of piperacillin-tazobactam administered by continuous infusion versus intermittent infusion for treatment of hospitalized patients with complicated intra-abdominal infection. Antimicrob Agents Chemother 50(11):3556–3561
74. Nicolau DP, McNabb J, Lacy MK, Quintiliani R, Nightingale CH (2001) Continuous versus intermittent administration of ceftazidime in intensive care unit patients with nosocomial pneumonia. Int J Antimicrob Agents 17(6):497–504
75. Roberts JA, Boots R, Rickard CM, Thomas P, Quinn J, Roberts DM et al (2007) Is continuous infusion ceftriaxone better than once-a-day dosing in intensive care? A randomized controlled pilot study. J Antimicrob Chemother 59(2):285–291
76. Chastre J, Wunderink R, Prokocimer P, Lee M, Kaniga K, Friedland I (2008) Efficacy and safety of intravenous infusion of doripenem versus imipenem in ventilator-associated pneumonia: a multicenter, randomized study. Crit Care Med 36(4):1089–1096
77. Dulhunty JM, Roberts JA, Davis JS, Webb SA, Bellomo R, Gomersall C et al (2013) Continuous infusion of beta-lactam antibiotics in severe sepsis: a multicenter double-blind, randomized controlled trial. Clin Infect Dis 56(2):236–244
78. Patel GW, Patel N, Lat A, Trombley K, Enbawe S, Manor K et al (2009) Outcomes of extended infusion piperacillin/tazobactam for documented Gram-negative infections. Diagn Microbiol Infect Dis 64(2):236–240
79. Patel N, Scheetz MH, Drusano GL, Lodise TP (2010) Determination of antibiotic dosage adjustments in patients with renal impairment: elements for success. J Antimicrob Chemother 65(11):2285–2290
80. Patel N, Scheetz MH, Drusano GL, Lodise TP (2010) Identification of optimal renal dosage adjustments for traditional and extended-infusion piperacillin-tazobactam dosing regimens in hospitalized patients. Antimicrob Agents Chemother 54(1):460–465
81. Lorente L, Lorenzo L, Martín MM, Jiménez A, Mora ML (2006) Meropenem by continuous versus intermittent infusion in ventilator-associated pneumonia due to gram-negative bacilli. Ann Pharmacother 40(2):219–223
82. Lorente L, Jiménez A, Martín MM, Iribarren JL, Jiménez JJ, Mora ML (2009) Clinical cure of ventilator-associated pneumonia treated with piperacillin/tazobactam administered by continuous or intermittent infusion. Int J Antimicrob Agents 33(5):464–468
83. Roberts JA, Webb S, Paterson D, Ho KM, Lipman J (2009) A systematic review on clinical benefits of continuous administration of beta-lactam antibiotics. Crit Care Med 37(6):2071–2078
84. Tamma PD, Putcha N, Suh YD, Van Arendonk KJ, Rinke ML (2011) Does prolonged β-lactam infusions improve clinical outcomes compared to intermittent infusions? A meta-analysis and systematic review of randomized, controlled trials. BMC Infect Dis 11:181
85. Kasiakou SK, Sermaides GJ, Michalopoulos A, Soteriades ES, Falagas ME (2005) Continuous versus intermittent intravenous administration of antibiotics: a meta-analysis of randomised controlled trials. Lancet Infect Dis 5(9):581–589
86. Sinnollareddy MG, Roberts MS, Lipman J, Roberts JA (2012) beta-lactam pharmacokinetics and pharmacodynamics in critically ill patients and strategies for dose optimization: a structured review. Clin Exp Pharmacol Physiol 39(6):489–496
87. Drusano GL, Lodise TP (2013) Saving lives with optimal antimicrobial chemotherapy. Clin Infect Dis 56(2):245–247
88. Falagas ME, Tansarli GS, Ikawa K, Vardakas KZ (2013) Clinical outcomes with extended or continuous versus short-term intravenous infusion of carbapenems and piperacillin/tazobactam: a systematic review and meta-analysis. Clin Infect Dis 56(2):272–282
89. Chant C, Leung A, Friedrich JO (2013) Optimal dosing of antibiotics in critically ill patients by using continuous/extended infusions: a systematic review and meta-analysis. Crit Care 17(6):R279
90. Vandecasteele SJ, De Vriese AS, Tacconelli E (2013) The pharmacokinetics and pharmacodynamics of vancomycin in clinical practice: evidence and uncertainties. J Antimicrob Chemother 68(4):743–748
91. Rybak M, Lomaestro B, Rotschafer JC, Moellering R Jr, Craig W, Billeter M et al (2009) Therapeutic monitoring of vancomycin in adult patients: a consensus review of the American Society of Health-System Pharmacists, the Infectious Diseases Society of America, and the Society of Infectious Diseases Pharmacists. Am J Health Syst Pharm 66(1):82–98

92. Moise PA, Forrest A, Bhavnani SM, Birmingham MC, Schentag JJ (2000) Area under the inhibitory curve and a pneumonia scoring system for predicting outcomes of vancomycin therapy for respiratory infections by Staphylococcus aureus. Am J Health Syst Pharm 57(Suppl 2):S4–S9
93. Holmes NE, Turnidge JD, Munckhof WJ, Robinson JO, Korman TM, O'Sullivan MV et al (2013) Vancomycin AUC/MIC ratio and 30-day mortality in patients with Staphylococcus aureus bacteremia. Antimicrob Agents Chemother 57(4): 1654–1663
94. Brown J, Brown K, Forrest A (2012) Vancomycin AUC24/MIC ratio in patients with complicated bacteremia and infective endocarditis due to methicillin-resistant Staphylococcus aureus and its association with attributable mortality during hospitalization. Antimicrob Agents Chemother 56(2):634–638
95. del Mar Fernandez de Gatta Garcia M, Revilla N, Calvo MV, Dominguez-Gil A, Sanchez Navarro A (2007) Pharmacokinetic/pharmacodynamic analysis of vancomycin in ICU patients. Intensive Care Med 33(2): 279–85
96. Revilla N, Martin-Suarez A, Perez MP, Gonzalez FM, Fernandez de Gatta Mdel M (2010) Vancomycin dosing assessment in intensive care unit patients based on a population pharmacokinetic/pharmacodynamic simulation. Br J Clin Pharmacol 70(2):201–212
97. Llopis-Salvia P, Jimenez-Torres NV (2006) Population pharmacokinetic parameters of vancomycin in critically ill patients. J Clin Pharm Ther 31(5):447–454
98. Baptista JP, Sousa E, Martins PJ, Pimentel JM (2012) Augmented renal clearance in septic patients and implications for vancomycin optimisation. Int J Antimicrob Agents 39(5):420–423
99. van Hal SJ, Paterson DL, Lodise TP (2013) Systematic review and meta-analysis of vancomycin-induced nephrotoxicity associated with dosing schedules that maintain troughs between 15 and 20 milligrams per liter. Antimicrob Agents Chemother 57(2):734–744
100. Wang JT, Fang CT, Chen YC, Chang SC (2001) Necessity of a loading dose when using vancomycin in critically ill patients. J Antimicrob Chemother 47(2):246
101. Li J, Udy AA, Kirkpatrick CM, Lipman J, Roberts JA (2012) Improving vancomycin prescription in critical illness through a drug use evaluation process: a weight-based dosing intervention study. Int J Antimicrob Agents 39(1):69–72
102. Cataldo MA, Tacconelli E, Grilli E, Pea F, Petrosillo N (2012) Continuous versus intermittent infusion of vancomycin for the treatment of Gram-positive infections: systematic review and meta-analysis. J Antimicrob Chemother 67(1):17–24
103. Roberts JA, Taccone FS, Udy AA, Vincent JL, Jacobs F, Lipman J (2011) Vancomycin dosing in critically ill patients: robust methods for improved continuous-infusion regimens. Antimicrob Agents Chemother 55(6):2704–2709
104. Turnidge J (2003) Pharmacodynamics and dosing of aminoglycosides. Infect Dis Clin North Am 17(3):503–528, v
105. Munckhof WJ, Grayson ML, Turnidge JD (1996) A meta-analysis of studies on the safety and efficacy of aminoglycosides given either once daily or as divided doses. J Antimicrob Chemother 37(4):645–663
106. Kashuba ADM, Bertino JS, Nafziger AN (1998) Dosing of aminoglycosides to rapidly attain pharmacodynamic goals and hasten therapeutic response by using individualized pharmacokinetic monitoring of patients with pneumonia caused by gram-negative organisms. Antimicrob Agents Chemother 42(7):1842–1844
107. Kashuba ADM, Nafziger AN, Drusano GL, Bertino JS (1999) Optimizing aminoglycoside therapy for nosocomial pneumonia caused by gram-negative bacteria. Antimicrob Agents Chemother 43(3):623–629
108. Buijk SE, Mouton JW, Gyssens IC, Verbrugh HA, Bruining HA (2002) Experience with a once-daily dosing program of aminoglycosides in critically ill patients. Intensive Care Med 28(7):936–942
109. Tang GJ, Tang JJ, Lin BS, Kong CW, Lee TY (1999) Factors affecting gentamicin pharmacokinetics in septic patients. Acta Anaesthesiol Scand 43(7):726–730
110. Goncalves-Pereira J, Martins A, Povoa P (2010) Pharmacokinetics of gentamicin in critically ill patients: pilot study evaluating the first dose. Clin Microbiol Infect 16(8):1258–1263
111. Rea RS, Capitano B, Bies R, Bigos KL, Smith R, Lee H (2008) Suboptimal aminoglycoside dosing in critically ill patients. Ther Drug Monit 30(6):674–681
112. Finnell DL, Davis GA, Cropp CD, Ensom MH (1998) Validation of the Hartford nomogram in trauma surgery patients. Ann Pharmacother 32(4):417–421
113. Thomas JK, Forrest A, Bhavnani SM, Hyatt JM, Cheng A, Ballow CH et al (1998) Pharmacodynamic evaluation of factors associated with the development of bacterial resistance in acutely ill patients during therapy.

Antimicrob Agents Chemother 42(3):521–527
114. Lipman J, Scribante J, Gous AG, Hon H, Tshukutsoane S (1998) Pharmacokinetic profiles of high-dose intravenous ciprofloxacin in severe sepsis. The Baragwanath Ciprofloxacin Study Group. Antimicrob Agents Chemother 42(9):2235–2239
115. van Zanten AR, Polderman KH, van Geijlswijk IM, van der Meer GY, Schouten MA, Girbes AR (2008) Ciprofloxacin pharmacokinetics in critically ill patients: a prospective cohort study. J Crit Care 23(3):422–430
116. Conil JM, Georges B, de Lussy A, Khachman D, Seguin T, Ruiz S et al (2008) Ciprofloxacin use in critically ill patients: pharmacokinetic and pharmacodynamic approaches. Int J Antimicrob Agents 32(6):505–510
117. Dryden MS (2011) Linezolid pharmacokinetics and pharmacodynamics in clinical treatment. J Antimicrob Chemother 66(Suppl 4):iv7–iv15
118. Rayner CR, Forrest A, Meagher AK, Birmingham MC, Schentag JJ (2003) Clinical pharmacodynamics of linezolid in seriously ill patients treated in a compassionate use programme. Clin Pharmacokinet 42(15):1411–1423
119. Dong H, Wang X, Dong Y, Lei J, Li H, You H et al (2011) Clinical pharmacokinetic/pharmacodynamic profile of linezolid in severely ill intensive care unit patients. Int J Antimicrob Agents 38(4):296–300
120. Whitehouse T, Cepeda JA, Shulman R, Aarons L, Nalda-Molina R, Tobin C et al (2005) Pharmacokinetic studies of linezolid and teicoplanin in the critically ill. J Antimicrob Chemother 55(3):333–340
121. Thallinger C, Buerger C, Plock N, Kljucar S, Wuenscher S, Sauermann R et al (2008) Effect of severity of sepsis on tissue concentrations of linezolid. J Antimicrob Chemother 61(1):173–176
122. Adembri C, Fallani S, Cassetta MI, Arrigucci S, Ottaviano A, Pecile P et al (2008) Linezolid pharmacokinetic/pharmacodynamic profile in critically ill septic patients: intermittent versus continuous infusion. Int J Antimicrob Agents 31(2):122–129
123. Buerger C, Plock N, Dehghanyar P, Joukhadar C, Kloft C (2006) Pharmacokinetics of unbound linezolid in plasma and tissue interstitium of critically ill patients after multiple dosing using microdialysis. Antimicrob Agents Chemother 50(7):2455–2463
124. Boselli E, Breilh D, Caillault-Sergent A, Djabarouti S, Guillaume C, Xuereb F et al (2012) Alveolar diffusion and pharmacokinetics of linezolid administered in continuous infusion to critically ill patients with ventilator-associated pneumonia. J Antimicrob Chemother 67(5):1207–1210
125. Boselli E, Breilh D, Rimmele T, Djabarouti S, Toutain J, Chassard D et al (2005) Pharmacokinetics and intrapulmonary concentrations of linezolid administered to critically ill patients with ventilator-associated pneumonia. Crit Care Med 33(7):1529–1533
126. Soon RL, Turner SJ, Forrest A, Tsuji BT, Brown J (2013) Pharmacokinetic/pharmacodynamic evaluation of the efficacy and safety of daptomycin against Staphylococcus aureus. Int J Antimicrob Agents 42(1):53–58
127. Bubalo JS, Munar MY, Cherala G, Hayes-Lattin B, Maziarz R (2009) Daptomycin pharmacokinetics in adult oncology patients with neutropenic fever. Antimicrob Agents Chemother 53(2):428–434
128. Falcone M, Russo A, Cassetta MI, Lappa A, Tritapepe L, d'Ettorre G et al (2013) Variability of pharmacokinetic parameters in patients receiving different dosages of daptomycin: is therapeutic drug monitoring necessary? J Infect Chemother 19(4):732–739
129. Di Paolo A, Tascini C, Polillo M, Gemignani G, Nielsen EI, Bocci G et al (2013) Population pharmacokinetics of daptomycin in patients affected by severe Gram-positive infections. Int J Antimicrob Agents 42(3):250–255
130. Gould IM, Miro JM, Rybak MJ (2013) Daptomycin: the role of high-dose and combination therapy for Gram-positive infections. Int J Antimicrob Agents 42(3):202–210
131. Parra-Ruiz J, Duenas-Gutierrez C, Tomas-Jimenez C, Linares-Palomino JP, Garrido-Gomez J, Hernandez-Quero J (2012) Safety analysis of high dose (>6 mg/kg/day) daptomycin in patients with concomitant statin therapy. Eur J Clin Microbiol Infect Dis 31(8):1771–1774
132. Lai CC, Sheng WH, Wang JT, Cheng A, Chuang YC, Chen YC et al (2013) Safety and efficacy of high-dose daptomycin as salvage therapy for severe gram-positive bacterial sepsis in hospitalized adult patients. BMC Infect Dis 13:66
133. Dudhani RV, Turnidge JD, Coulthard K, Milne RW, Rayner CR, Li J et al (2010) Elucidation of the pharmacokinetic/pharmacodynamic determinant of colistin activity against Pseudomonas aeruginosa in murine thigh and lung infection models. Antimicrob Agents Chemother 54(3):1117–1124
134. Dudhani RV, Turnidge JD, Nation RL, Li J (2010) fAUC/MIC is the most predictive pharmacokinetic/pharmacodynamic index of colistin against Acinetobacter baumannii in murine thigh and lung infection models. J Antimicrob Chemother 65(9):1984–1990

135. Li J, Nation RL, Turnidge JD, Milne RW, Coulthard K, Rayner CR et al (2006) Colistin: the re-emerging antibiotic for multidrug-resistant Gram-negative bacterial infections. Lancet Infect Dis 6(9):589–601
136. Bergen PJ, Landersdorfer CB, Lee HJ, Li J, Nation RL (2012) 'Old' antibiotics for emerging multidrug-resistant bacteria. Curr Opin Infect Dis 25(6):626–633
137. Bergen PJ, Landersdorfer CB, Zhang J, Zhao M, Lee HJ, Nation RL et al (2012) Pharmacokinetics and pharmacodynamics of 'old' polymyxins: what is new? Diagn Microbiol Infect Dis 74(3):213–223
138. Bergen PJ, Li J, Nation RL (2011) Dosing of colistin-back to basic PK/PD. Curr Opin Pharmacol 11(5):464–469
139. Bode-Boger SM, Schopp B, Troger U, Martens-Lobenhoffer J, Kalousis K, Mailander P (2013) Intravenous colistin in a patient with serious burns and borderline syndrome: the benefits of therapeutic drug monitoring. Int J Antimicrob Agents 42(4):357–360
140. Garonzik SM, Li J, Thamlikitkul V, Paterson DL, Shoham S, Jacob J et al (2011) Population pharmacokinetics of colistin methanesulfonate and formed colistin in critically ill patients from a multicenter study provide dosing suggestions for various categories of patients. Antimicrob Agents Chemother 55(7):3284–3294
141. Imberti R, Cusato M, Accetta G, Marino V, Procaccio F, Del Gaudio A et al (2012) Pharmacokinetics of colistin in cerebrospinal fluid after intraventricular administration of colistin methanesulfonate. Antimicrob Agents Chemother 56(8):4416–4421
142. Imberti R, Cusato M, Villani P, Carnevale L, Iotti GA, Langer M et al (2010) Steady-state pharmacokinetics and BAL concentration of colistin in critically Ill patients after IV colistin methanesulfonate administration. Chest 138(6):1333–1339
143. Markou N, Markantonis SL, Dimitrakis E, Panidis D, Boutzouka E, Karatzas S et al (2008) Colistin serum concentrations after intravenous administration in critically ill patients with serious multidrug-resistant, gram-negative bacilli infections: a prospective, open-label, uncontrolled study. Clin Ther 30(1):143–151
144. Mohamed AF, Karaiskos I, Plachouras D, Karvanen M, Pontikis K, Jansson B et al (2012) Application of a loading dose of colistin methanesulfonate in critically ill patients: population pharmacokinetics, protein binding, and prediction of bacterial kill. Antimicrob Agents Chemother 56(8):4241–4249
145. Plachouras D, Karvanen M, Friberg LE, Papadomichelakis E, Antoniadou A, Tsangaris I et al (2009) Population pharmacokinetic analysis of colistin methanesulfonate and colistin after intravenous administration in critically ill patients with infections caused by gram-negative bacteria. Antimicrob Agents Chemother 53(8):3430–3436
146. Hartzell JD, Neff R, Ake J, Howard R, Olson S, Paolino K et al (2009) Nephrotoxicity associated with intravenous colistin (colistimethate sodium) treatment at a tertiary care medical center. Clin Infect Dis 48(12):1724–1728
147. Akajagbor DS, Wilson SL, Shere-Wolfe KD, Dakum P, Charurat ME, Gilliam BL (2013) Higher incidence of acute kidney injury with intravenous colistimethate sodium compared with polymyxin B in critically ill patients at a tertiary care medical center. Clin Infect Dis 57(9):1300–1303
148. Dalfino L, Puntillo F, Mosca A, Monno R, Spada ML, Coppolecchia S et al (2012) High-dose, extended-interval colistin administration in critically ill patients: is this the right dosing strategy? A preliminary study. Clin Infect Dis 54(12):1720–1726

Chapter 22

Pharmacodynamic Considerations and Special Populations: Pediatrics

Jennifer Le and John S. Bradley

Abstract

The complexity of infectious disease pharmacotherapy intensifies in pediatric patients since two pertinent elements must be accounted for—the immunologic and physiologic developmental processes that occur with age. Physiologic development may alter the pharmacokinetics of a drug with enhanced clearance to potentially result in subtherapeutic responses, while overexposure may have consequences for adverse events, especially in young, rapidly growing neonates and infants. Understanding the pharmacokinetic variability stemming from age-related physiologic maturation and the pharmacodynamic target effect (or desired response) can assist the clinician in selecting the ideal antimicrobial agent and dosing regimen. This chapter presents the following: (1) the factors (including physiologic maturation, organ function, and size) that contribute to pharmacokinetic alterations that occur with age; (2) the impact of immunologic development on microbiologic and clinical outcomes; (3) the unique exposure-response relationship, or the pharmacodynamic index for antimicrobial agents in pediatrics; (4) critical review of specific antibacterial agents with recent information in the literature (including beta-lactams, aminoglycosides, and vancomycin); and (5) overcoming challenges to pharmacokinetic-pharmacodynamic studies in pediatrics.

Key words Pharmacokinetic, Pharmacodynamic, Pediatrics, Neonates, Antimicrobials, Vancomycin, Monte Carlo simulation, Beta-lactams, Vancomycin, Aminoglycosides, Antibiotics

1 Introduction

The amalgamation of information pertaining to the antimicrobial agent (drug), pathogen (bug), and patient is critical in optimizing pharmacotherapy for infectious diseases. In addition to appropriate antimicrobial selection based on the susceptibility of the pathogen and the site of infection, the complexity of infectious disease pharmacotherapy intensifies in pediatric patients since two other pertinent elements must be accounted for—the immunologic and physiologic developmental processes that occur with age. Compared with adults with intact immune system, the immune system of neonates and infants is immature, potentially altering the observed response to antimicrobial therapy. Physiologic development may alter the pharmacokinetics (PK) of a drug to potentially

John C. Rotschafer et al. (eds.), *Antibiotic Pharmacodynamics*, Methods in Pharmacology and Toxicology,
DOI 10.1007/978-1-4939-3323-5_22, © Springer Science+Business Media New York 2016

Table 1
Pediatric age groups

Group	Age range
Premature neonate	<37 weeks' gestation
Neonates	<1 month of life
Infants	1–12 months old
Children	1–12 years old
Adolescents	13–18 years old
Pediatrics	Birth to 18 years old

result in subtherapeutic responses. Understanding the PK variability stemming from age-related physiologic maturation and the pharmacodynamic (PD) target effect (or desired response) can assist the clinician in selecting the ideal antimicrobial agent and dosing regimen [1].

Pediatric drug dosing is generally individualized to the child based on age and body size; therefore, appreciating age and weight is an imperative step towards dosing any drug in a child. Both age and weight are demographic indicators of growth and development that are tangible and easily retrievable. In particular, age confers information on physiologic maturation and organ function. The broad age spectrum within the pediatric population contributes to a considerable variation in a drug's PK, with disparities detected even between the five distinct pediatric age groups (Table 1). This underscores the intricacy in drug dosing (usually by altering the actual dose and/or frequency depending on the drug's PD exposure target) and the unequivocal need for age-specific dosing in the pediatric population. In this chapter, the PK-PD principles that affect different pediatric age groups and specific antimicrobial agents are presented.

2 Age-Specific Pharmacokinetic Variability

Physiologic maturation, organ function, and size are the principle contributors to PK variability. Maturation and organ function are largely determined by age in the pediatric population (assuming the absence of disease conditions that may be associated with altered organ function such as cystic fibrosis). The physiologic maturation that affects a drug's PK occurs mainly during the neonatal and infant periods, albeit some age-related changes continue into childhood (Table 2). Per se, age correlates reasonably well with the maturation of drug clearance, and significantly contributes to appropriate drug dosing in neonates, infants, and young children, but becomes less helpful in late childhood and adolescence.

Table 2
Age-related physiologic changes affecting drug pharmacokinetics

Variable	Neonate	Infant	Child	Adolescent
Absorption				
Gastric pH	↑ (pH >5)	↑ (pH 2–4)	↔ (pH 2–3)	↔
Gastric and intestinal emptying time	↑	↑	↔	↔
Biliary function, pancreatic function, and gut microbial colonization	↓	↔	↔	↔
Intramuscular absorption	↓	↑	↑ to ↔	↔
Skin permeability and percutaneous absorption	↑	↑	↔	↔
Distribution				
Total body water and extracellular water	↑	↑	↔ (by 12–13 years)	↔
Total body fat and muscle mass	↓	↓	Increases by 5–15 years	↔
Total plasma proteins	↓	↓ or ↔	↔ (by 2 years)	↔
Metabolism				
CYP 1A2	↓	↓ (50 % of adult activity by 1 year)	↔ (after 1 year)	↔
CYP 2C9	↓ (30 % of adult activity)	↔ (by 1–6 months)	↑ (peak activity 3–10 years)	↔ (decreases to adult value at puberty)
CYP 2C19	↓ (30 % of adult activity)	↔ by 6 months	↑ (peak activity 3–4 years)	↔ (decreases to adult value at puberty)

(continued)

Table 2 (continued)

Variable	Neonate	Infant	Child	Adolescent
CYP 2D6	↓ (30 % of adult activity)	↔ by 1 year	↔	↔
CYP 2E1	No data	↓ (30–40 % of adult activity)	↔ (by 10 years)	↔
CYP 3A4	↓ (30–40 % of adult activity)	↔ by 1 year	↑ (1–4 years, then progressively decreases)	↔ (at puberty)
Uridine 5-diphosphate glucuronyl transferase	↓	↓ (25 % by 3 months)	↔ (by 6 months–3 years)	↔
N-acetyl transferase 2	↓	↓	↔ (past 1 year)	↔
Methyltransferase	↑	↔	↔	↔
Sulfotransferase	↓	↑ for specific drugs	↑ for specific drugs	↔
Renal elimination				
Glomerular filtration	↓	↔	↔	↔
Tubular secretion and reabsorption	↓	↔	↔	↔

↔ = same as adult activity; ↓ = decreased activity compared to adults; ↑ = increased activity compared to adults

Adapted with permission from Vinita BP and Nahata MC. Drug Dosing in Pediatric Patients (Chapter 4). In: Murphy JE. ed. Clinical Pharmacokinetics, 5e. Bethesda: American Society of Health-System Pharmacists; 2012

The most striking developmental changes occur within the first year of life, which involves a rapid surge in renal function due to an increase in renal blood flow within the first 2 weeks of life [2, 3]. Notably, this developmental process does not occur linearly with age, resulting in a plateau of drug dosing expressed in milligram or gram per kilogram (e.g., increasing drug dosages up to a certain age when it then decreases). Furthermore, a drug's PK may not be solely dependent on postnatal age, particularly in the extremely premature neonates, because nephrogenesis, which contributes to increasing glomerular filtration rate in utero, requires completion of 36 weeks' gestation [2, 3]. The use of postnatal age alone, as compared to postmenstrual age which incorporates both gestational and postnatal age, as an indicator for the maturation of drug elimination is therefore unacceptable for premature neonates [4].

Analogous to the maturation of renal function, hepatic function also advances with age. Two exceptions are the enhanced activities of methyltransferase and sulfotransferase in the neonate and infant, respectively (Table 2). Maturation of various hepatic clearance pathways occurs at different rates for the first months to years of life, further complicating any calculations of dosages for drugs metabolized by the liver. In addition to the maturation of renal and hepatic function, significant developmental alteration in body composition occurs during the first few months of life. Compared to adults, the total body water content in full-term neonates and infants is higher (75 % versus 60 %), thus leading to enhanced distribution of water-soluble drugs like gentamicin (0.5 L/kg vs. 0.3 L/kg) [5, 6].

As an indicator of body size, total body weight is a common and appropriate measure to use for drug dosing in normal-sized children. Pediatric drug doses cannot be normalized directly from an adult dose using total body weight (i.e., adult dose in milligram per kilogram) since drug elimination, particularly via the renal route, is nonlinear to weight [7]. This nonlinear relationship between weight and drug CL underestimates CL in children and yet overestimates it in adults. However, a child's body size can be referenced to a 70-kg adult using allometric scaling with a coefficient of 1 for volume (Vd) and 0.75 for clearance (CL; Eqs. (1) and (2)) [4]. The accuracy of this allometric method for the prediction of CL appears to be suboptimal in neonates and young infants, but reasonable for application in children >5 years of age, including those with cystic fibrosis [8, 9]. Improved accuracy for CL prediction has been suggested by using an exponent of 1 (or no exponent) in neonates and infants ≤1 year old, and referencing by age (instead of weight) to 20-year-old adult in children between 1 and 5 years old (Eq. (3)) [10]. Nonetheless, the optimal allometric scaling (i.e., exponent value) should be derived for each individual drug through population-based PK-PD studies, which are essential for age-specific dosing in the various pediatric age groups:

$$V_{\text{Child}} = V_{\text{Adult}} \times (\text{Weight}_{\text{Child}} / 70\text{kg}) \quad (1)$$

$$\text{CL}_{\text{Child}} = \text{CL}_{\text{Adult}} \times (\text{Weight}_{\text{Child}} / 70\text{kg})^{0.75} \quad (2)$$

$$\text{CL}_{\text{Child}} = \text{CL}_{\text{Adult}} \times (\text{Age}_{\text{Child}} / 20\text{years})^{X} \quad (3)$$

X is the exponent obtained from the log-log plot of clearance and age for a given drug.

Obesity has become a global public health challenge, with an estimated 45 million affected children under 5 years of age in 2010 [11]. Despite exhibiting minimal metabolic activity, excessive amounts of adipose tissue can significantly influence body size to inflict changes in a drug's PK and therefore its dosing [12]. Using total body weight is not always acceptable for drug dosing in overweight or obese children since the excess weight is disproportional in amounts of lean body and fat mass [13]. With this extensive deviation in fat affecting body composition, other measurements are necessary to improve drug dosing specifically in obese children. Indirect measures of body composition consist of body surface area, body mass index (BMI), ideal body weight, and adjusted body weight (Table 3). These measures can be applied to an obese child (although its selection is dependent on the drug's properties) and easily estimated by the clinician using a child's height, weight, or girth. Great interest in lean body mass (which is a measure of fat-free mass that incorporates vital organs, extracellular fluid, bones, and muscles) has emerged in recent years, but its application is encumbered by the need to estimate BMI-for-age Z-scores and population ancestry (Table 3) [14]. The application of these indirect measures is limited in neonates and infants.

For systemic drugs, PK alterations are represented by two primary physiologic-based parameters that govern dosing—Vd and CL. The Vd correlates to the total amount of drug distributed throughout the body (including tissues), and determines the initial or loading dose. It is driven by the characteristics of the drug as well as body composition. For example, a drug's hydrophilicity, which is the affinity to concentrate in water, will dictate the extent of drug distribution into tissues. Hydrophilic drugs (e.g., aminoglycosides and linezolid) distribute mainly in the extracellular fluid compartment and thus generally have small Vd compared with drugs that also distribute intracellularly.

Table 3
Measures of body composition

Weight measure	Equation	Unit	Age category
Adjusted body weight (AdjBW)	AdjBW = IBW (kg) + 0.4 [TBW (kg) − IBW (kg)]	kg	Adult
Body mass index (BMI)	$BMI = \frac{TBW(kg)}{Height(m)^2}$ Adjust for age and gender by growth charts	Percentile	Child and adolescent
Body surface area (BSA)[a]	$BSA = [TBW\ (kg)^{0.5378} \times Height\ (cm)^{0.3964}] \times 0.024265$	m^2	Infant, child, and adult
	$BSA = \sqrt{\frac{[Height(cm) \times TBW(kg)]}{3600}}$	m^2	Child and adult
Ideal body weight (IBW)[b]	$IBW = \frac{(Height\ in\ cm)^2(1.65)}{1000}$	kg	Child or adolescent 1–18 years
	$IBW = 2.396 \times e^{0.01863\ (Height\ in\ cm)}$	kg	Child or adolescent 1–17 years
	IBW = 39 kg + 2.27 kg per inch over 5 ft	kg	Male child ≥5 ft
	IBW = 42.2 kg + 2.27 kg per inch over 5 ft	kg	Female child ≥5 ft
Lean body weight (LBW)	$\ln[LBW] = -2.9585 + 0.8208 \times \ln[height\ (cm)] + 0.5607 \times \ln[TBW\ (kg)] + 0.0000184 \times TBW\ (kg)^2 - 0.0159 \times BMIz^2 + 0.0135 \times age\ (year) + 0.0225 \times African\ American$	kg	Boys >5 years, including population ancestry
	$\ln[LBW] = -2.8990 + 0.8064 \times \ln[height\ (cm)] + 0.5674 \times \ln[TBW\ (kg)] + 0.0000185 \times TBW\ (kg)^2 - 0.0153 \times BMIz^2 + 0.0132 \times age\ (year)$	kg	Boys >5 years excluding population ancestry [14]
	$\ln[LBW] = -3.9361 + 0.9786 \times \ln[height\ (cm)] + 0.6431 \times \ln[TBW\ (kg)] - 0.0118 \times BMIz^2 + 0.0290 \times African\ American$	kg	Girls >5 years including population ancestry
	$\ln[LBW] = -3.8345 + 0.954 \times \ln[height\ (cm)] + 0.6515 \times \ln[TBW\ (kg)] - 0.0102 \times BMIz^2$	kg	Girls >5 years excluding population ancestry

TBW = total (or actual) body weight
[a]West nomogram can also be used to determine BSA
[b]Traub nomogram can also be used to determine IBW for drug dosing. Methods that utilize growth charts (e.g., McLaren and Moore) are used to determine nutritional status

Neonates and young infants have increased total body and extracellular water content; therefore, the Vd of aminoglycosides and linezolid are enhanced and consequently higher loading doses (in mg/kg) are required to achieve peak concentrations similar to those targeted in adults [15, 16].

In addition to total body water content, plasma protein binding affects the Vd. Neonates, infants, and young children have decreases in both the concentration and the affinity of certain proteins (e.g., albumin and alpha-1-acid glycoprotein) to bind to drugs. Accordingly, the amount of free drug (which is the pharmacologically active) may increase, particularly if the drug undergoes saturable elimination. This reduction in plasma protein binding becomes clinically relevant when interpreting measured drug concentrations, with normal total drug concentrations yet increased unbound concentrations.

Albumin binds to endogenous substances (like bilirubin) and certain antibiotics (including sulfonamides, ceftriaxone, and other beta-lactams). With decreased albumin binding, sulfonamides and ceftriaxone compete and displace bilirubin from albumin binding, resulting in a toxic effect called kernicterus observed only in neonates and young infants [17].

Clearance accounts for both metabolism and elimination of a drug from the body, and is the main determinant for maintenance doses. Unaffected directly by a drug's chemical property, CL is regulated by the metabolic capacity and perfusion to certain organs responsible for drug elimination, primarily the liver and kidneys. The liver is the body's primary source for drug metabolism. While most microsomal cytochrome P450 enzymes responsible for metabolism are present at birth, the activities of these enzymes are reduced during infancy and require time for maturation (Table 2). Consequently, the metabolic CL is lower in neonates and infants than adults. The immature hepatic metabolism, particularly the glucuronidation reaction, is responsible for the reduced CL of chloramphenicol, resulting in toxic drug accumulation and a condition called "gray baby syndrome" observed exclusively in preemies and infants when doses exceed 50–100 mg/kg [18]. The immature metabolic CL parallels renal elimination, including reduced glomerular filtration, tubular secretion, and reabsorption (Table 2). Many antibiotics, including beta-lactams, aminoglycosides, and vancomycin, are eliminated primarily via glomerular filtration (Table 4). For example, the lack of mature renal function decreases CL of gentamicin, prolonging its expected half-life from ~2 h reported in adults to ~10 h in premature infants and resulting in higher trough concentrations to potentially increase the risk for toxicity if dosing intervals remain unadjusted [16].

Table 4
Pharmacokinetic and pharmacodynamic properties of antimicrobial agents for neonates, infants, older children, and adolescents

Agent	Pharmacokinetics						Pharmacodynamics [65, 101]		
	Oral bioavailability	Protein binding	Body distribution and CSF penetration	Metabolism	Excretion	Elimination ($t_{1/2}$)[a]	Mechanism	Index	Dose optimization
Aminoglycosides									
Gentamicin and tobramycin Amikacin Kanamycin	Poorly absorbed	<25 %	Primarily to extracellular fluids and vascularized tissues, fetus, ascitic, synovial, and amniotic fluid; minimally into CSF	None	Renal	Neonates <1 week, 5–14 h (varies inversely with birth weight) Neonates >1 week and infants, 3–5 h Children/adults, ~2 h	Concentration dependent with moderate post-antibiotic effect	Cmax/MIC, AUC_{24}/MIC	Increase dose to maximize Cmax or AUC_{24}
Streptomycin	Poorly absorbed	35 %	Same as gentamicin	10–30 % at unknown site	Renal	Neonates, 4–10 h Adults, 2–3 h			
Beta-lactams									
Penicillin G	Erratic, 15–80 % Not available in oral formulation	60–65 %	Penetrates most tissues, fetus, and amniotic fluid; poorly into CSF[b]	Hepatic <30 %	Renal	Neonates, 1–3 h varies inversely with (postnatal age) Infants/children, 0.5–1.2 h	Time dependent with no to minimal post-antibiotic effect	$fT > MIC$	Increase duration of infusion, or frequency of administration
Penicillin V	60 %	80 %	Penetrates most tissues; poorly into CSF, not used to treat meningitis	Same as penicillin G with additional gut inactivation (metabolized) of 35–70 % of an oral dose	Same as penicillin G	Adults, 0.5 h			
Penicillinase-resistant penicillins									
Dicloxacillin	35–76 % Give on empty stomach	98 %	Penetrates most tissues, fetus, and amniotic fluid; poorly into CSF	Hepatic 10 %	Renal	Adults, 30–40 min	Time dependent with no to minimal post-antibiotic effect	$fT > MIC$	Increase duration of infusion, or frequency of administration
Oxacillin	No oral form available	94 %	Penetrates most tissues, fetus, and amniotic fluid; poorly into CSF[b]	Hepatic ~50 %	Renal	Neonates and infants, 1–2 h Adults, 30–60 min			
Nafcillin	Not administered orally	90 %	Penetrates most tissues, fetus, and amniotic fluid; poorly into CSF[b]	Hepatic 60 %	Biliary (with enterohepatic recirculation); renal 10–30 %	Neonates, 2.2–5.5 h Infants, 1–2 h Children and adults, 30–90 min			

(continued)

Table 4
(continued)

Agent	Pharmacokinetics						Pharmacodynamics [65, 101]		
	Oral bioavailability	Protein binding	Body distribution and CSF penetration	Metabolism	Excretion	Elimination ($t_{1/2}$)[a]	Mechanism	Index	Dose optimization
Aminopenicillins									
Amoxicillin	85 %	20 %	Penetrates most tissues, fetus, and amniotic fluid; poorly into CSF[b]	Hepatic 10 %	Renal	Neonates, 3.7 h Children, 1–2 h Adults, 1–1.5 h	Time dependent with no to minimal post-antibiotic effect	$fT>MIC$	Increase duration of infusion, or frequency of administration
Clavulanate (amoxicillin pharmacokinetics not affected by clavulanate)	Well absorbed	25 %	Penetrates most tissues, fetus, and amniotic fluid; poorly into CSF	Hepatic extensive	Renal 25–40 %	Adults, 1 h			
Ampicillin	50 %	22 % 10 % in neonates	Penetrates most tissues, fetus, and amniotic fluid; poorly into CSF[b]	Hepatic 10 %	Renal	Neonates, <1 week, 3–6 h Neonates, >1 week, 2–4 h Children, 1–2 h Adults, 1–1.5 h			
Sulbactam	Not administered orally	38 %	Penetrates most tissues, fetus, and amniotic fluid; poorly into CSF[b]	Hepatic 10 %	Renal	Adults 1–1.5 h			
Extended-spectrum penicillins									
Ticarcillin	Not administered orally	45 %	Penetrates most tissues, fetus, and amniotic fluid; poorly into CSF[b]	Hepatic 10 %	Renal	Neonates <1 week, 4–5 h Neonates >1 week, ~2 h Infants/children, ~1 h	Time dependent with no to minimal post-antibiotic effect	$fT>MIC$	Increase duration of infusion, or frequency of administ ration
Piperacillin	Not administered orally	15–20 %	Penetrates most tissues, fetus, and amniotic fluid; poorly into CSF[b]	Hepatic minimal	Renal; biliary <20 %	Neonates, 2–3 h Infants/children, 0.5–1 h Adults, 0.5 h (increases to 1–1.5 h for high dose due to saturation of hepatobiliary excretion (dose-dependent $t_{1/2}$))			
Tazobactam (piperacillin kinetics are unaffected by tazobactam)	Not administered orally	20–23 %	Penetrates most tissues, fetus, and amniotic fluid; poorly into CSF[b]	Hepatic minimal	Renal	Infants, 1.6 h Children/adults, 45 min–1 h			

Cephalosporins								
First generation								
Cefadroxil	Well absorbed	20 %	Penetrates most tissues, fetus, and amniotic fluid; minimally into CSF	None	Renal (slower excretion rate than cephalexin)	Adult, 1–2 h	Time dependent $fT>MIC$ with no to minimal post-antibiotic effect	Increase du ration of infusion, or frequency of admini stration
Cefazolin	Not administered orally	80 %	Penetrates most tissues, fetus, and amniotic fluid; minimally into CSF	None	Renal	Neonates, 3–5 h Adult, 1.5–2.5 h		
Cephalexin	Well absorbed; ↓ with food	6 %	Penetrates most tissues, fetus, and amniotic fluid; minimally into CSF	None	Renal; some biliary	Neonates, 5 h Infants, 2.5 h Children/adults, 1 h		
Cephradine	Well absorbed; ↓ with food	10 %	Penetrates most tissues, fetus, and amniotic fluid; minimally into CSF	None	Renal; some biliary	Children/adults, ~1 h		
Second generation								
Cefaclor	Well absorbed	25 %	Penetrates most tissues; unknown fetal, amniotic, and CSF distribution	Unknown	Renal (nonrenal: elimination at unknown site in renal failure)	Adults, 0.5–1 h	Time dependent $fT>MIC$ with no to minimal post-antibiotic effect	Increase duration of infusion, or frequency of admini stration
Cefprozil	95 %	36 %	Penetrates middle-ear fluids and tonsillar, adenoidal, skin, and soft tissues well; unknown fetal, amniotic and CSF distribution	Unknown	Renal; nonrenal 30 %	Infants/children, 1.5–2 h Adults, 1–1.5 h		
Cefuroxime	37 % (as axetil); ↑ to 52 % when given with food	50 %	Penetrates most tissues, fetus, and amniotic fluid; minimally into CSF	None	Renal	Neonates, 3–6 h Infants/children, 1.5–2 h Adults, 1.2 h		
Cefoxitin	Not administered orally	75 %	Penetrates most tissues, fetus, and amniotic fluid; minimally into CSF[a]	Hepatic minimal	Renal	Neonates, 1.4 h Infants/children/ adults, ~45 min		

(continued)

Table 4
(continued)

Agent	Pharmacokinetics						Pharmacodynamics [65, 101]		
	Oral bioavailability	Protein binding	Body distribution and CSF penetration	Metabolism	Excretion	Elimination ($t_{1/2}$)[a]	Mechanism	Index	Dose optimization
Third generation									
Cefdinir	16–21 % cap; 25 % suspension	60–70 %	Penetrates most tissues; unknown fetal, amniotic and CSF distribution	None	Renal	Adults, 1.7 h	Time dependent with no to minimal post-antibiotic effect	$fT > MIC$	Increase duration of infusion, or frequency of administration
Cefixime	40–50 %	65–70 %	Not well studied	Unknown	Renal, biliary	Adults, 3–4 h			
Cefoperazone	Not administered orally	90 %	Penetrates most tissues, fetus, and amniotic fluid; minimally into CSF[b]	Hepatic <20 %	Biliary, renal 20–30 %	Neonates, 6–10 h (varies inversely with postnatal age) Infants/children, 2.2–2.3 h Adults, ~2 h			
Cefotaxime	Not administered orally	35–40 %	Penetrates most tissues, fetus, and amniotic fluid; adequately into CSF[b]	Hepatic	Renal	Neonates, 2–6 h (varies inversely with gestational and postnatal age) Infants/children, 1–1.5 h Older children/adults, 45 min–1 h			
Cefpodoxime	50 %	20–30 %	Penetrates most tissues, unknown fetal, amniotic, and CSF distribution	None	Renal	Adults, 2–3 h			
Ceftazidime	Not administered orally	<10 %	Penetrates most tissues, fetus, and amniotic fluid; adequately into CSF[b]	None	Renal	Neonates, 4–7 h (varies inversely with gestational age) Adults, 1.4–2 h			
Ceftibuten	>90 %	65–77 %	Penetrates most tissues, unknown fetal, amniotic, and CSF distribution	Hepatic minimal	Renal	Children/adults, 1.5–2.5 h			
Ceftizoxime	Not administered orally	31 %	Penetrates most tissues, fetus, and amniotic fluid; minimally into CSF[b]	None	Renal	Neonates, 2–4 h Adults, 1–2 h			
Ceftriaxone	Not administered orally	95 %	Penetrates most tissues, fetus, and amniotic fluid; adequately into CSF[b]	None	Renal; biliary	Neonates, 9–19 h Children, 4–7 h Adults, 6–9 h			

Fourth generation									
Cefepime	Not administered orally	20 %	Penetrates most tissues, fetus, and amniotic fluid; adequately into CSF[b]	Hepatic minimal	Renal	Neonates, 3–7 h Children/adults, ~2 h	Time dependent with no to minimal post-antibiotic effect	$fT > MIC$	Increase duration of infus ion, or fre quency of adminis tration
Other beta-lactams, monobactams									
Aztreonam	Not administered orally	50–70 %	Penetrates most tissues, fetus, and amniotic fluid; minimally into CSF[b]	Minimal hydrolysis at unknown site	Renal; biliary minor	Neonates <1 week, 6–10 h (varies inversely with birth weight) Neonates >1 week, ~3 h Children/adults, 1.5–2 h	Time dependent with no to minimal post-antibiotic effect	$fT > MIC$	Increase duration of infus ion, or fre quency of administ ration
Carbapenems									
Meropenem	Not administered orally	Minimal	Penetrates most tissues, fetus, and amniotic fluid; adequately into CSF[b]	Renal, serum, hepatic 20–25 %	Renal; biliary minor	Neonates, 2–3 h Infants, 1.5 h Adults, 1 h	Time dependent with no to minimal post-antibiotic effect	$fT > MIC$	Increase duration of infu sion, or freque ncy of adm inistration
Imipenem (I) + cilastatin (C)	Not administered orally	20 % (I) 40 % (C)	Penetrates most tissues, fetus, and amniotic fluid; adequately into CSF[b] but relatively contraindicated for meningitis	Renal, serum, hepatic 20–25 %	Renal; biliary minor	Neonates, 1.5–2.5 h (cilastatin 3–8 h) Infants/children, 1–1.4 h Adults, ~1 h			
Ertapenem	Not administered orally	95 %	Penetrates interstitial fluids; unknown fetal, amniotic, and CSF distribution	Renal 20 %, hepatic minor	Renal; biliary minor	Infants/children, 2.5 h Adolescents/adults, 4 h			
Amphenicols									
Chloramphenicol succinate (injection)	PO forms (base and palmitate salt) not available	~50 %	Widely distributed including fetal, amniotic, and CSF	Hepatic	Renal (as succinate salt and glucuronide metabolite) biliary minimal	Highly variable; see text	Time dependent with some post-antibiotic effect against Gram-positive bacteria [102]	AUC_{24}/MIC	Increase dose, frequency of administr ation or duration of infusion

(continued)

Table 4 (continued)

Agent	Pharmacokinetics						Pharmacodynamics [65, 101]		
	Oral bioavailability	Protein binding	Body distribution and CSF penetration	Metabolism	Excretion	Elimination ($t_{1/2}$)[a]	Mechanism	Index	Dose optimization
Fluoroquinolones and quinolones									
Ciprofloxacin	60–80 %; >90 % in adolescents with CF	20–40 %	Penetrates most tissues, fetus, amniotic fluid; minimally into CSF[b]	Hepatic <20 %	Renal, feces	Neonates/infants/children/adults, ~3–5 h	Concentration dependent with moderate post-antibiotic effect	Cmax/MIC, AUC_{24}/MIC	Increase dose to maximize Cmax or AUC_{24}
Levofloxacin	99 %	24–38 %	Penetrates most tissues, fetus, amniotic fluid, CSF	Minimal	Renal	Infants/children, 4–7 h Adults, 6–8 h			
Norfloxacin	30–40 %	10–15 %	Penetrates GU and GI, fetus, and amniotic fluid; CSF unknown	Hepatic extensive	Renal, biliary	Adults, 3–4 h			
Nalidixic acid	>90 %	90–95 %	Not widely distributed; penetrates renal tissue well; crosses placenta	Hepatic, renal	Renal (85 % as inactive form)	Adults, 1.5 h			
Lincosamides									
Clindamycin	90 %	94 %	Penetrates most tissues, fetus, amniotic fluid; minimally into uninflamed CSF, but adequately into inflamed CSF or brain abscess	Hepatic	Biliary; renal minor	Neonates, 3.6–8.7 h (inversely related to gestational age and birth weight) Infants/children/adults, ~2–3.5 h	Time dependent with moderate to prolonged post-antibiotic effect	AUC_{24}/MIC	Increase dose, frequency of administration or duration of infusion
Lipopeptides									
Daptomycin	Not administered orally	~90 %	Limited distribution; fetal, amniotic, and CSF penetration unknown	Renal	Renal	Adults, 7–10 h	Concentration dependent with moderate post-antibiotic effect	AUC_{24}/MIC	Increase dose to maximize Cmax or AUC_{24}

Macrolides and azalides									
Azithromycin	37 %	20–50 %	Widely distributed including fetus, amniotic fluid; minimally into CSF[b]	Hepatic	Biliary; renal, minimal	Infants/children, >50 h Adults, 35–40 h	Time dependent with moderate to prolonged post-antibiotic effect	AUC_{24}/MIC	Increase dose, frequency of admin istration or duration of infusion
Clarithromycin	50–55 %	60–70 %	Penetrates most tissues, fetus; CSF penetration unknown	Hepatic	Renal 40–50 % (as drug and active metabolite)	Infants/children/adults, 3–7 h (dose dependent)			
Erythromycin	Poor, 25–65 % depending on salt and form	80–90 %	Penetrates most tissues, fetus, amniotic fluid; minimally into CSF[b]	Hepatic	Biliary, renal minimal	Adult, 1–2 h (estolate 3–8 h)			
Nitroimidazoles									
Metronidazole	100 %	<20 %	Widely distributed, including fetus, amniotic fluid, CSF	Hepatic	Renal (60–80 % with 10–20 % as unchanged drug); biliary minor	Neonates, 17–109 h (varies inversely with post-menstrual or gestational age) [103] Children/adults, 6–14 h	Concentration dependent with moderate post-antibiotic effect	AUC_{24}/MIC	Increase dose to maximize Cmax or AUC_{24}
Urinary anti-infectives									
Nitrofurantoin	Well | absorbed	90 %	Mainly urinary tract, prostate, and placenta	Tissues	Renal, biliary	Adults, 20 min	Time dependent for *E. coli*, concentration dependent against *S. saprophyticus* and *E. faecium*	$fT>MIC$, AUC_{24}/MIC	Increase dose, freq uency of administra tion or duration of infusion
Oxazolidinones									
Linezolid	100 %	31 %	Penetrates most tissues, including CSF; fetus, amniotic fluid unknown	Hepatic	Renal	Neonates, 1.5–10 h (varies inversely with gestational age) Infants/children, 2–3 h Adults, 3–6 h	Time dependent with moderate to prolonged post-antibiotic effect	AUC_{24}/MIC, $fT>MIC$	Increase dose, frequency of admin istration, or duration of infusion

(continued)

Table 4
(continued)

	Pharmacokinetics						Pharmacodynamics [65, 101]		
Agent	**Oral bioavailability**	**Protein binding**	**Body distribution and CSF penetration**	**Metabolism**	**Excretion**	**Elimination ($t_{1/2}$)[a]**	**Mechanism**	**Index**	**Dose opti mization**
Polymyxins									
Colistimethate (injection)	Not administered orally	Minimal	Penetrates most tissues, fetus and amniotic fluid; minimal to pleural or joint cavities or to CSF	Tissue minor and slow	Renal	Children, 2–3 h Adults, 1.5–3 h	Concentration dependent with moderate post-antibiotic effect [104]	AUC_{24}/MIC	Increase dose to maximize Cmax or AUC_{24}
Rifamycins									
Rifampin	90–95 %	60–90 %	Widely distributed including fetus, amniotic fluid; minimally into CSF[b]	Hepatic	Biliary, renal	Infants/children/adults, ~2–4 h	Concentration dependent with moderate post-antibiotic effect at ≥16×MIC [105]	Cmax/MIC, AUC_{24}/MIC	Increase dose to maximize Cmax or AUC_{24}
Rifaximin	Poorly absorbed	N/A	Minimal systemic distribution due to poor oral bioavailability, but high intraluminal GI concentrations	Hepatic minimal	Feces absorption	Minimal systemic			
Sulfonamides and trimethoprim									
Sulfadiazine	100 %	20 %	Widely distributed, including fetus, amniotic fluid, CSF	Hepatic wide individual variation	Renal (free and conjugated forms)	Adults, 7–17 h	Concentration dependent with moderate post-antibiotic effect [106, 107]	Cmax/MIC, AUC_{24}/MIC	Increase dose to maximize Cmax or AUC_{24}
Sulfamethoxazole	100 %	65 %	Widely distributed, including fetus, amniotic fluid, CSF	Hepatic wide individual variation	Renal (free and conjugated forms)	Adults, 9–12 h			
Sulfisoxazole	100 %	85 %	Widely distributed, including fetus, amniotic fluid, CSF	Hepatic wide individual variation	Renal (free and conjugated forms)	Adults, 5–8 h			
Trimethoprim	100 %	~45 %	Widely distributed, including fetus, amniotic fluid, CSF	Hepatic <20 %	Renal	Infants/children, 3–5.5 h Adults, 8–10 h			

Tetracyclines and glycylcyclines									
Doxycycline	90–100 %	82 %	Widely distributed including fetus, amniotic fluid; minimally into CSF[b]	Hepatic	Renal, biliary	Adults, ~20 h	Time dependent with moderate to prolonged post-antibiotic effect	AUC_{24}/MIC	Increase dose, frequency of adminis tration, or duration of infusion
Minocycline	90–100 %	76 %	Widely distributed including fetus, amniotic fluid; minimally into CSF[b]	Hepatic minimal	Biliary, renal	Adults, 11–22 h			
Tetracycline	75–80 %; decreases significantly with food	65 %	Widely distributed including fetus, amniotic fluid; minimally into CSF[b]	Hepatic minimal	Renal, biliary	Adults, 7–10 h			
Tigecycline	Not administered orally	70–90 %	Widely distributed; fetal, amniotic fluid and CSF unknown	Hepatic 5–20 %	Biliary, renal	Adults, 40 h	Time dependent with moderate to prolonged post-antibiotic effect	AUC_{24}/MIC	Increase dose, frequency of admini stration, or duration of infusion
Glycopeptides									
Vancomycin	Negligible	30 %	Penetrates most tissues, fetus, amniotic fluid; adequately but erratically into CSF[b]	None	Renal; biliary minimal	Neonates, 4–11 h (varies inversely with gestational age) Infants, 2–4 h Children, 2–2.5 h Adults, 4–6 h	Time dependent with moderate to prolonged post-antibiotic effect	AUC_{24}/MIC	Increase dose, frequency of admini stration, or duration of infusion

AUC_{24}, area under the concentration–time curve over a 24-h period; CF, cystic fibrosis; Cmax, maximum serum concentration; CSF, cerebrospinal fluid; GI, gastrointestinal; GU, genitourinary; IM, intramuscular; IV, intravenous; MIC, minimum inhibitory concentration; PO, orally; $fT > MIC$, fraction or percentage of the dosing interval above the MIC

[a]Agents with primarily renal excretion will have a prolonged $t_{1/2}$ in a patient with renal impairment

[b]Concentration of drug in CSF significantly increased with inflamed meninges

Reproduced with revisions from Bradley JS and Sauberan JB. Antimicrobial Agents. In: Long: Principles and Practice of Pediatric Infectious Diseases, 4th ed. B. Saunders, An Imprint of Elsevier, Maryland Heights, MO; 2012

3 Immunologic Development Impact on Microbiologic and Clinical Outcomes

The innate and adaptive immune responses are indispensible in supporting the eradication of microbiologic pathogens causing infections. Comprised of physical barriers (i.e., skin and mucosal surfaces), antimicrobial peptides, phagocytes (e.g., neutrophils and macrophages), the complement enzymatic system, natural killer cells, and other cells or proteins, the innate immune system embodies the first line of host defense against infection. Components of the innate immune system form throughout the different stages of fetal development, with maturation ensuing birth [19, 20]. For example, the bone marrow commences production of phagocytic cells during the first trimester of pregnancy and antimicrobial peptides that possess activity against Gram-negative bacteria and fungal pathogens originate from the vernix caseosa during the third trimester [20]. In neonates at full-term birth, the peripheral neutrophil count is elevated, resulting in levels even higher than those of adults. However, this neutrophil elevation is accompanied by reduced phagocytic and bactericidal functional capacity, which hinders response to active infection and potentially increases susceptibility to pneumonia, cellulitis, and multifocal infections [21–23]. In addition, the underdeveloped skin of infants with very low birth weights (i.e., <1000 g) contributes to their vulnerability to infections due to decreased function as a barrier to invasive infection.

The complement system provides innate immunity through direct binding to nonspecific pathogenic surfaces. However, it can also enhance specific humoral immunity and facilitate phagocytosis. While formation initiates during third trimester, most serum proteins of the complement system (except for C7) take 18 months from birth to reach adult concentrations, and their concentrations, including those of C9, correlate with gestational age [24]. Low levels of C9 and C5a have been associated with ineffective bactericidal activity against *E. coli* and increased risk of infection to group B streptococcus in neonates, respectively [25, 26].

Lymphocyte function development is also delayed in neonates, increasing susceptibility to viral infections including herpes viruses and enteroviruses. Cytotoxic natural killer cells, also part of innate immunity, develop during the first trimester. Prematurity before 36 weeks contributes to the diminished activity of natural killer cells, although corticosteroid treatment for preterm labor increases their rate of maturation [27, 28]. The cytotoxic activity of these cells matures by 6 months of age and 10 % of peripheral blood lymphocytes in adults are composed of natural killer cells [29]. With their antiviral activity, natural killer cells protect infants against herpes simplex virus infection and human immunodeficiency virus transmission. In addition, mutation in natural killer cells has resulted in a form of severe combined immunodeficiency with defects in both natural killer cells and T lymphocytes [27].

The deficiencies evident in the innate immunity of neonates and infants, especially if premature, make them vulnerable to infections that can lead to significant morbidity and mortality. Upon incomplete or inadequate protection to infection by the innate immunity, the adaptive immune system subsequently responds by activating effector B- and T-lymphocytes to facilitate production of pathogen-specific antibodies and immunologic memory, respectively. These are two very crucial functions of the adaptive immune response.

Although B-lymphocytes are fully developed at birth, the gamut of antibodies in neonates is only fractional due to their limited exposure to pathogens early in life. As such, transplacental transfer of passively acquired maternal antibodies, which initiates during second trimester but ensues primarily during third trimester, is a critical accompaniment to this narrow gamut [27]. In contrast to neonates born at full term, the levels of serum immunoglobulin G (IgG) antibodies (which protect against group B streptococcal infection) in preemies are low due to the decreased transplacental transfer that peaks in the third trimester [30]. Another component of humoral (or antibody-mediated) immunity is the active production of antibodies (including IgG, IgM, and lastly IgA) that begins during gestation but does not achieve maturation until 6–8 years of age [27]. If exposed, term infants can produce antibodies within the first few days of life, although their response is attenuated with lower levels than adults [31].

Despite its abundance, the naïve population of T-lymphocytes in neonates exhibits limited functional capacity, including decreased development of immunologic memory and cytokine production. These immature T-lymphocytes contribute to the increased susceptibility to infections caused by viruses and other intracellular pathogens, such as *Toxoplasma gondii* and *Listeria*. Maturation of T-lymphocytes occurs by 7 years of age [32].

In addition to the immature immunity evident in premature neonates and infants, congenital abnormalities and immune deficiencies (including those acquired by medication use) contribute to the vulnerability of children to infections. Immunosuppression may occur in children with hematologic/oncologic cancers, rheumatologic conditions, and inflammatory bowel disease with the use of chemotherapeutic agents, tumor necrosis factors, and other immune modulators. For any of the conditions noted above in which the host component of response to infection is decreased, the drug exposure that is expected to result in a microbiologic and clinical cure may be greater than that demonstrated in normal hosts.

4 Pharmacodynamics and Monte Carlo Simulation

To successfully treat or cure an infection, which is the desired effect for infectious disease pharmacotherapy, utilizing the PD property of an antimicrobial agent can facilitate optimization of therapy by maximizing drug exposure to inhibit or eradicate the pathogens, or to potentially suppress the development of resistance [33]. Depending on the antibiotic, the drug concentration of interest (specifically, the active unbound moiety) can be the peak, trough, or average concentration, or exposure over a period of time (i.e., area-under-time-concentration curve over 24 h [AUC_{24}]) (refer to Chaps. 8, 9, and 11–17). In addition to free drug concentrations, PD exposure calculations most often incorporate a pathogen-specific susceptibility component via the minimum inhibitory concentration (MIC).

The predictability of the exposure-response relationship for an antimicrobial agent differs between pediatrics and adults. Although underlying genetic and clinical factors may alter response, a standard antibiotic dose will generally provide a baseline exposure to elicit a predictable clinical response in adults. In contrast, substantial variability exists in exposure to an antibiotic across the pediatric age spectrum since it is largely affected by the child's stage of physiologic and immunologic maturation. These physiologic and immunologic differences make a drug's exposure less predictable in a child than an adult [2]. Once the exposure is adjusted in children to achieve equivalence to adults, antimicrobial effects (microbiologic and clinical cure) can be assumed to be similar in pediatrics.

A PD exposure target or index for microbiologic and clinical cure (or even for resistance suppression) must be explicitly defined in order to identify the best dosing regimen derived from Monte Carlo simulations that incorporate age-specific PK data. The PD indices incorporate drug exposure and microbiologic susceptibility and consist of peak concentration over MIC (Cmax/MIC), area-under-time-concentration curve within 24 h over MIC (AUC_{24}/MIC), and time that free drug concentrations remain above the MIC (*f*T > MIC) (refer to Chaps. 8, 9, and 11–17). Unfortunately, the derivation of PD exposure targets has been primarily from pre-clinical models and limited clinical studies [33]. Even amongst the few human clinical investigations, most data were collected retrospectively, and in adult patients rather than in children. There are no well-designed, published studies to date in the USA that validate PD targets for antimicrobial agents in actual pediatric patients. While the number of pediatric PK studies is increasing, it is also important to document the PD target and consequent dose required for cure over the entire spectrum of pediatric ages. The PD targets will ideally account for protein binding and immunologic developmental changes that occur with age.

5 Antibacterial Agents

In the sections that follow, specific antibacterial agents are presented to illustrate the application of PK-PD properties to optimize infectious disease pharmacotherapy. The selection of the specific antibiotic was based on its PD features, including concentration-dependent, time-dependent, and post-antibiotic effects. Only antibiotics with adequate number of PK-PD evaluations in pediatrics were critically reviewed. Otherwise, the PD properties of antibiotics with absent to limited PK-PD studies are described in Table 4.

5.1 Beta-Lactams

The most extensively studied class of antibiotics that have been evaluated for their PK-PD properties in pediatrics is the beta-lactam, primarily because of their long-standing safety profile and their mixed spectrum of antibacterial activity (i.e., some agents possess broad activity while others have a narrow spectrum). Exhibiting time-dependent bactericidal effects with minimal post-antibiotic activity and increasing the infusion time or the dosing frequency optimize the use of beta-lactams (Table 4). While both strategies exploit the PD property of time-dependent killing, extending the infusion time (even towards continuous infusion) has been evaluated more than increased dosing frequency (i.e., from every 6–4 h) for its practicality in the clinical setting, especially in certain pediatric patients with prematurity, cystic fibrosis, or hematologic/oncologic disorders that necessitate the use of multiple other medications.

Using the Monte Carlo method to assess how often the required exposure can be achieved with various dosing regimens against pathogens with varying susceptibilities, simulations were performed in children between 1 and 12 years of age using beta-lactams active against *Pseudomonas aeruginosa* (including cefepime, ceftazidime, imipenem/cilastatin, meropenem, and piperacillin/tazobactam) [34–36]. For bactericidal exposures, the PD targets based on the $fT > MIC$ were ≥40 % for carbapenems and ≥50 % for penicillins or cephalosporins. Lower thresholds of ≥20 % $fT > MIC$ for carbapenems and ≥30 % $fT > MIC$ for penicillins or cephalosporins may be appropriate PD targets for bacteriostatic activity. These studies demonstrated that prolongation of infusion time from 30 min to 3 h significantly improved the probability of target attainment (PTA) to >90 % to achieve the bactericidal $fT > MIC$ target for all studied antibiotics [35, 36]. Similar results were observed for continuous infusion. Specifically in critically ill children 1–6 years old, piperacillin/tazobactam 400 mg/kg/day administered as a 3-h infusion in four divided doses, or as a 24-h continuous infusion was required to achieve optimal PTA against all susceptible Gram-negative bacteria [36]. Although CL was similar, these critically ill young children had increased Vd of piperacillin (0.51 L/kg versus ~0.28 L/kg in non-critically ill children), potentially due to their underlying disease states and third-fluid spacing (i.e., increased extracellular fluids observed in third-fluid spacing increases the Vd, especially for water-soluble drugs) [36, 37].

Increasing the dose alone, without optimizing the PD property by increasing infusion time, may not always achieve adequate drug exposure, depending on the susceptibilities of the pathogen that are based on the distribution of MICs in the population of pathogens that is expected to cause the infection. For example, increasing the meropenem dose from 20 to 40 mg/kg, administered every 8 h using 30-min infusions, resulted in a low PTA of 58 % at one institution with elevated MICs amongst the *P. aeruginosa* isolates [34]. In this scenario, increasing the dose alone is not recommended for serious resistant infections. In contrast, the rich capillary bed and small volume of the interstitial fluid of the middle ear facilitate access of antibiotics, resulting in blunted peaks and high trough concentrations, and delayed CL from the middle ear [38]. Consequently, increased doses of amoxicillin at 75–90 mg/kg/day administered twice daily and ceftriaxone 50 mg/kg as a single intramuscular dose achieve adequate antibiotic concentrations in the middle ear to successfully treat acute otitis media caused by penicillin-resistant *S. pneumoniae* [38–40]. This highlights the importance of incorporating the PD property of the drug, institution-specific MIC data, and PK of the drug at the site of infection to optimize empiric antimicrobial therapy to achieve the desired response.

In recent years, emerging interest in elucidating age-related PK alterations, with the most extreme differences in preterm infants and neonates, has resulted in several population-based PK-PD evaluations in this population [41–46]. One central theme from these studies was the construction of dosing strategies prudently based on gestational and postnatal age to account for the pronounced age-related PK alterations that exist in neonates [42, 43, 45, 46]. In addition, higher PD targets (i.e., >60 % *f*T > MIC for meropenem and >75 % *f*T > MIC for ampicillin and piperacillin) were employed by study investigators who assumed that this degree of antibiotic exposure was necessary for microbiologic and clinical efficacy in neonates who possess deficiencies in their immune response system [41, 43, 46].

Meropenem was evaluated in two studies for its bactericidal effect against nosocomial Gram-negative pathogens, including *P. aeruginosa*, in preterm and full-term neonates <2 months old with gestational ages of 23–42 weeks [43, 44]. Post-conceptional or post-menstrual age, weight, and serum creatinine were identified as important covariates for predicting meropenem CL, which increased in neonates who were older by gestational age and chronologic age. Meropenem 20 mg/kg every 8 h, infused over 30 min, achieved >90 % PTA [43]. For less susceptible organisms with MIC of 4–8 μg/mL, meropenem 40 mg/kg every 8 h, using prolonged 4-h infusions, was preferable [43, 44]. For the treatment of meningitis in neonates, meropenem concentrations in the cerebrospinal fluid (CSF) vary from 4.1 to 34.6 μg/mL (which is 70 % [range 5–148 %] penetration) [45]. These CSF concentrations were obtained during routine clinical care as "test-of-cure" samples without accounting for the time after infusion. As such, data are not available to construct CSF concentration-time curves during the dosing interval. However, in experimental animal models, the peak CSF concentrations of beta-lactam antibiotics were less than and were delayed a few hours after the peak serum concentrations. Furthermore, failure in the treatment of pathogens that are susceptible in vitro has not been routinely reported in neonates. This CSF range of concentrations will be different for older infants and children, and specifically timed CSF collections following an IV dose have also not been available in studies of pediatric meningitis.

Meropenem and piperacillin were evaluated in premature and term infants ≤90 days old with suspected or complicated intra-abdominal infections [41, 45]. Approximately 85 % of 200 infants treated with meropenem 20–30 mg/kg every 8 or 12 h (exact dose based on gestational age and postnatal age) experienced therapeutic success. Overall, meropenem was well tolerated [42]. While 50 % of infants experienced adverse events (including 6 % sepsis, 5 % seizures, 5 % elevated conjugated bilirubin, and 5 % hypokalemia), none were probably or definitely related to meropenem [45]. Similar to meropenem, piperacillin CL increased with advancing gestational age at birth, but decreased by 60 % when serum creatinine was ≥1.2 mg/dL [41]. Administration of piperacillin 80–100 mg/kg every 8 h did not meet PD target for *P. aeruginosa* in ~70 % of infants, implying that the current dosing per standard of care is inadequate and further studies are warranted [41].

In addition to premature infants, children with cystic fibrosis have altered PK that may necessitate different dosing strategies. In fact, patients with cystic fibrosis have increased CL (e.g., aztreonam 100 mL/min versus 76 mL/min in healthy subjects, $p < 0.01$), albeit Vd appears to remain constant [9, 47]. The application of the PD property of antimicrobial agents is especially pertinent in this population to prevent subtherapeutic dosing. In one study that demonstrated the importance of optimizing the PD property of beta-lactams, prolonged infusion by 4 or 5 h or continuous infusion of ceftazidime 6 g per day (weight-adjusted for 70 kg) significantly improved the PTA of ≥65 % *f*T > MIC. In contrast to a 30-min infusion that achieved ≥90 % PTA for only pathogens with MIC ≤ 1 μg/mL, extended or continuous infusions increased the MIC attainment to ≤8–12 μg/mL [9]. Enhanced MIC attainment proves invaluable in patients with cystic fibrosis who are frequently exposed to antibiotics for both acute and chronic respiratory infections, and have increased antibiotic resistance rates [48, 49].

In another study of patients with cystic fibrosis, ticarcillin-clavulanate 100 mg/kg every 6 h (which was higher than the approved package labeling by Food and Drug Administration) achieved bactericidal and bacteriostatic activity against *P. aeruginosa* at MICs of 16 μg/mL and 32 μg/mL, respectively [50]. Drug safety did not appear to be an issue at this dose. In addition, aztreonam 1000 mg every 8 h achieved 50–60 % *f*T > MIC at MIC of 4 mg/L and 1–2 mg/L for healthy subjects and patients with cystic fibrosis, respectively [47]. Due to the increased CL, patients with cystic fibrosis should be monitored closely for therapeutic response, with the potential need to adjust the dosing regimen based on the antibiotic PD feature.

One aggressive proposed PD target, that is not supported by animal model or human clinical data, for *P. aeruginosa* infections specifically in patients with immune-compromised status is maintaining drug concentrations at 100 % *f*T > 6 times the MIC [51, 52]. Using this unvalidated PD target, piperacillin/tazobactam 350–400 mg/kg/day infused continuously, after a loading dose of 100 mg/kg, was necessary to achieve >99 % PTA at MIC of 4 mg/L in adolescents with febrile neutropenia [51]. Notably, piperacillin/tazobactam at the standard dose of 300 mg/kg/day achieved only ~85 % PTA, which was deemed inappropriate for patients at high risk for serious infections (e.g., recent intensive chemotherapy, predicted prolonged and profound neutropenia, or fever >39 °C) and potentially treatment failure. Some studies in adults have evaluated 100 % *f*T > MIC as the PD target to improve clinical cure and microbiologic eradication using cefepime, piperacillin/tazobactam, meropenem, and ceftobiprole [53, 54].

In summary, the studies in different pediatric groups have demonstrated an enhancement of PD target attainment using frequent dosing, and extended or continuous infusions of beta-lactams, which may be advantageous for patients who are critically ill (including premature neonates), are immunocompromised, have cystic fibrosis, or are infected with pathogens exhibiting high MICs. Nonetheless, more well-designed prospective clinical trials in pediatrics are necessary since one systematic review concluded that limited clinical evidence exists to support the use of extended or continuous infusion of beta-lactam antibiotics [55]. Furthermore, the correlation between achievement of the PD target and clinical outcomes in pediatrics is limited. One Phase 3 study conducted in Japanese pediatric patients demonstrated that meropenem 40 mg/kg, administered as 4-h infusions, every 8 h, was effective against *P. aeruginosa* with MIC ≥ 2 μg/mL. In this study, the 97 % PTA for 50 % *f*T > MIC was correlated to both microbiological and clinical efficacy at 97 % and 96 %, respectively [56]. This is the only study, to our knowledge, that directly connected a PD target to microbiological and clinical outcomes in pediatrics. In another study of children with bacteremia caused by *P. aeruginosa*, those with elevated MICs experienced a threefold increase in mortality [57]. This compellingly suggests consideration for an alternative antibiotic administration strategy or perhaps therapy, especially when piperacillin MIC is ≥32 μg/mL since standard dosing recommendations administered as 30-min infusions do not successfully achieve bactericidal PTA of ≥50 % *f*T > MIC [36, 57].

Confronted with insufficient pediatric studies, adult data must be extrapolated to formulate a recommendation for the use of extended or continuous infusions of beta-lactam antibiotics. The use of adult data assumes that the PK-PD targets and the interplay between the bacteria and the antibiotic are consistent in pediatrics. One study in adults documented clinical and economic benefits associated with a 4-h infusion of cefepime for *P. aeruginosa* bacteremia and pneumonia [58]. Significant reductions in mortality (20 % versus 3 %, $p = 0.03$) and stay in the intensive care unit (18.5 days versus 8 days, $p = 0.04$) were observed in those who received extended infusion. In addition, a trend towards decreases in both the length of hospital stay by 3.5 days and hospital costs by $23,183 per patient was reported with extended infusion.

5.2 Aminoglycosides

The aminoglycosides that have been most examined in pediatrics are gentamicin and tobramcyin. Displaying concentration-dependent bactericidal activity with substantial post-antibiotic sub-MIC and post-antibiotic leukocyte enhancement effects, clinical response to these antibiotics in adults is enhanced when the maximum or peak concentration (Cmax)/MIC ratio is 8–10 using traditional multiple-daily dosing (Table 4) [59, 60]. Optimizing these PD features and potentially minimizing adaptive resistance by complete elimination of the drug before the subsequent dose, the extended-interval (or once-daily) dosing strategy has been evaluated in children with cystic fibrosis, febrile neutropenia, and neonates [60–64]. Extended-interval dosing of aminoglycosides permits administration of large doses, as single daily doses, to achieve peak concentrations high enough to augment efficacy against certain bacteria (including those that are less susceptible with MIC > 1 μg/mL) [65, 66]. Capitalizing on the post-antibiotic effects, integrating a drug-free interval allows serum aminoglycoside concentrations to fall below the MIC of susceptible organisms, usually <1 μg/mL, and yet preserve bacterial growth inhibition. Furthermore, the extended-interval strategy may reduce nephrotoxicity since it allots sufficient time for complete elimination of the drug prior to re-administration [62, 66]. However, compared to once-daily dosing, traditional multiple-daily dosing has been associated with decreased resistance patterns, albeit resistance suppression of *P. aeruginosa* has been observed with increased Cmax/MIC target at 30 for gentamicin [64, 67].

Patients with cystic fibrosis experience pulmonary infections frequently caused by *P. aeruginosa* throughout their lifetime that necessitate the repeated use of intravenous aminoglycosides, either as monotherapy or in combination therapy. Theoretically, extended-interval dosing is a rational strategy for patients with cystic fibrosis for the following reasons: they have increased drug Vd and CL requiring higher doses; adequate antibiotic concentrations are difficult to achieve in the epithelial lining fluid and mucosal surfaces where the infection is present; and the bacteria that infect this population often have decreased antibiotic susceptibility owing to frequent exposure [64].

In a meta-analysis evaluating four randomized, controlled studies consisting of a total of 328 pediatric and adult subjects with cystic fibrosis, the efficacy and safety of traditional thrice-daily dosing of tobramycin at 10 or 15 mg/kg/day (or the dose last known to give satisfactory concentrations) were compared to extended-interval dosing [63]. The lack of significant differences in pulmonary function, nutritional status, time to first pulmonary exacerbation after treatment course, and ototoxicity between the two dosing strategies may have been confounded by the use of concurrent antibiotics, primarily ceftazidime. However, less nephrotoxicity (defined by a smaller rise in concentrations of serum creatinine and urinary renal biomarkers, such as N-acetyl-β-d glucosaminidase and α-1-microglobulin) was demonstrated in children receiving the extended-interval dosing strategy.

The Cystic Fibrosis Foundation supports extended-interval dosing as the preferred strategy for aminoglycosides [68]. Tobramycin 10 mg/kg/day administered once daily can be used empirically to achieve Cmax of 20–40 μg/mL, trough concentrations of <1 μg/mL, and AUC_{24} of 60–120 mg h/L; and amikacin 30–35 mg/kg/day, to target Cmax of 80–120 μg/mL, trough concentrations of <1 μg/mL, and AUC_{24} of 235 ± 110 mg h/L (total drug concentrations reported) [64]. These once-daily dosing regimens achieve the PD index of Cmax/MIC ≥ 10 for high MICs, specifically of at least 2 μg/mL for tobramycin and at least 4 μg/mL for amikacin. The clinical significance of targeted AUC monitoring for aminoglycosides requires further investigation. Dose fractionation studies indicate that AUC/MIC may be correlated to resistance development among *P. aeruginosa* isolates [60, 67].

While tobramycin and amikacin are the primary aminoglycosides used to treat pulmonary infections caused by *P. aeruginosa* in cystic fibrosis, gentamicin is more widely used for the treatment of suspected or proven bacterial sepsis in neonates. Gentamicin is bactericidal against Gram-negative bacteria, with synergy in combination with beta-lactams that can be documented in vitro (although the defined clinical benefit to combination therapy is not well established). Gentamicin acts synergistically both in vitro and in vivo against most enterococci when combined with beta-lactam antibiotics. The PK of gentamicin in neonates are influenced by multiple factors, including age (gestational and postnatal, or post-conceptional), weight, and renal function. Individualized dosing strategies are especially advantageous in premature neonates since their drug PK are not always predictable and can be highly variable depending on gestational and postnatal age. In a multicenter study of neonatal intensive care units, individualized dose optimization, along with therapeutic drug monitoring, subjugated nomogram-based dosing in rapidly achieving therapeutic concentrations with reduction in both the need for gentamicin concentrations and dosing adjustments [69].

The PD targets for gentamicin in neonates are Cmax of 5–10 μg/mL for efficacy (assuming MIC ≤ 1 μg/mL) and trough concentrations <1–2 μg/mL to minimize toxicity [62]. "Once-a-day" dosing in neonates (or even 36–48 h in preemies) is logical since gentamicin's half-life is prolonged due largely to their immature renal function and, to a lesser extent, increased Vd [61]. If once-a-day dosing achieves therapeutic peak concentrations while minimizing toxic trough concentrations, the need for frequent dosing and drug monitoring may be circumvented, which is convenient for neonates who usually receive gentamicin for sepsis pending culture results for a limited 48–72 h. One meta-analysis of 11 randomized or quasi-randomized controlled trials (N = 574) compared once-a-day versus multiple-daily dosing strategies, both with initial loading doses, in neonates <28 days of life [62]. Although the efficacy for proven sepsis was similar, once-a-day dosing significantly improved attainment of peak concentrations ≥5 μg/mL and trough concentrations <2 μg/mL in neonates, especially those >32 weeks' gestation. Ototoxicity and nephrotoxicity, with the latter determined by changes in serum creatinine and renal biomarkers (including urinary beta-2-microglobulin and aminopeptidase), were also comparable between the once-a-day versus multiple-daily dosing strategies.

In children with febrile neutropenia due to cancer chemotherapy or stem cell transplantation, gentamicin or tobramycin doses of 6–10.5 mg/kg/day, depending on age, were required to achieve Cmax/MIC ~ 10 to treat infections caused by *P. aeruginosa* [70–72]. Significant findings from these studies underscore the importance of age-based dosing (with higher mg/kg dose for younger children), the preference for once-daily (versus thrice-daily) administration to maximize efficacy and minimize nephrotoxicity, and the utility of loading doses to achieve therapeutic peak concentrations early in the course of therapy (which may be beneficial in this population with minimal post-antibiotic leukocyte enhancement due to their immunocompromised status).

The most concerning adverse effects that limit the clinical use of aminoglycosides are nephrotoxicity and ototoxicity. Nephrotoxicity occurs through the internalization and subsequent accumulation of aminoglycosides in the proximal renal tubular epithelial cells. Exposure to high, intermittent drug concentrations using once-daily dosing, in contrast to the frequent exposure at low concentrations with multiple-daily dosing, elicits saturation of the uptake process to thereby increase excretion of the drug products that have not been internalized [60, 62]. Consequently, once-daily dosing decreases nephrotoxicity. This advantage of once-daily has been documented in prospective randomized trials and in one study that suggested a slower rate of increase in the urinary N-acetyl-d-glucosaminidase:creatinine ratio, which is a sensitive indicator of nephrotoxicity, using once-daily gentamicin dosing in neonates [60, 73, 74]. Furthermore, individualized PK dosing with therapeutic monitoring and drug discontinuation within 9 days of therapy also minimizes the risk of nephrotoxicity [66, 73, 75]. The occurrence of ototoxicity, which is caused by irreversible damage of cochlear and vestibular hair cells from the production of free radicals, is independent of the frequency of aminoglycoside administration [60, 76].

5.3 Vancomycin

Vancomycin exhibits time-dependent bactericidal activity similar to beta-lactam antibiotics (Table 4). In contrast, vancomycin also inhibits bacterial growth after serum concentrations fall below the MIC, with this so-called post-antibiotic effect (PAE) lasting 0.7–2.6 h for *Staphylococcus aureus* and 4.3–6.5 h for *Staphylococcus epidermidis* [77]. Using the PK-PD properties of vancomycin, improved clinical outcomes for invasive methicillin-resistant *S. aureus* (MRSA) infections have been correlated to an AUC/MIC ratio ≥ 400, which is a minimum concentration of 15–20 μg/mL when the MIC is 1 μg/mL in adults [78, 79]. However, two independent studies using Bayesian estimation and Monte Carlo simulations suggest lower trough concentrations of 8–10 μg/mL when the MIC is ≤1 μg/mL (evaluated using broth microdilution and E-test methods) for pediatrics >3 months of age [80, 81]. This reiterates the fact that “kids are not just small adults” and the urgent need for additional PK-PD studies specific for this vulnerable population. In particular, PD data to associate improved outcomes with attainment of vancomycin AUC/MIC ≥ 400 in pediatrics are insufficient [82].

Based on a population-based PK study evaluating sparse sampling in a large cohort of 702 pediatric subjects >3 months old, important covariates contributing to vancomycin CL were weight, age, and serum creatinine, which cumulatively account for developmental and renal maturation [81]. The study investigators uncovered two significant findings: (1) vancomycin 60–70 mg/kg/day was necessary to achieve 75 % PTA for AUC/MIC ≥ 400, depending on age, serum creatinine, and MIC distribution (which was determined using E-tests); and (2) targeted exposure using vancomycin AUC/MIC, compared with trough concentrations, is a more realistic target in children. Since vancomycin is eliminated primarily via glomerular filtration with some active tubular secretion, a less frequent dosing at 15 mg/kg every 8 h (i.e., 45 mg/kg/day) may be more appropriate as empiric dosing for older children with acute renal insufficiency, who may require close monitoring since recovery of renal function may occur during therapy [83, 84]. Higher doses of 90–100 mg/kg/day did not achieve 90 % PTA when >30 % of MRSA isolates had MICs > 1 μg/mL evaluated by E-tests, and produced excessively high AUCs of 840–940 mg-h/L with concentrations exceeding 20 μg/mL [81]. This unwarranted and potentially toxic exposure is concerning in light of recent evidence to suggest the increased risks of nephrotoxicity when trough concentrations are ≥15 μg/mL and doses are ≥10 mg/kg in children [85, 86]. Incorporating age-related developmental changes and MIC data are crucial to optimize vancomycin use since PK studies in pediatrics (excluding neonates) correlated lower trough concentrations to achieve AUC/MIC ≥ 400 and PD data linking to clinical outcomes are minuscule.

Several population-based PK studies with Bayesian estimation have evaluated dose optimization of vancomycin in preterm and full-term neonates [87–89]. Depending on serum creatinine and post-menstrual age, maintenance doses ranging from 15 to 60 mg/kg/day administered intermittently every 8–24 h, or as continuous infusions, have been suggested to achieve trough concentrations of 15–20 μg/mL (up to 25 μg/mL targeted in some studies) [87–90]. Notably, these studies did not evaluate PTA by AUC/MIC ≥ 400, which is the PD target best linked to successful treatment outcomes in adults based on limited data. The correlation between AUC/MIC and trough concentrations, with assessment of clinical benefits, should be evaluated in neonates, especially with recent evidence to suggest lower trough concentrations to achieve AUC/MIC ≥ 400 in pediatrics >3 months of age. Furthermore, the incidence of nephrotoxicity in neonates at higher trough concentrations has not been studied, albeit the risk appears minimal with low exposure [84]. While efficacy appears comparable to intermittent administration, continuous infusion has been investigated in neonates in several studies and may offer a few advantages that have been reported in adults, including decreased risk of nephrotoxicity, early attainment of target concentrations, and reduced variability in the total daily dose [91, 92].

The inherent feasibility of monitoring trough concentrations in clinical practice is challenged by recent PK data to suggest that trough concentrations needed to achieve the PD vancomycin exposure target of AUC/MIC ≥ 400 in children differ from adults

[80, 81]. With little evidence to support targeting trough concentrations for treatment success in children, it is prudent to monitor vancomycin exposure by AUC (with MIC when available) since it is a more achievable target, and to prevent excessive dosing, frequent dosing adjustments, and potentially adverse effects [80, 81, 93]. The performance of the one-sample strategy (i.e., trough concentrations) for therapeutic drug monitoring to estimate AUC has not been well studied in children, despite its frequent use at pediatric hospitals [94]. Using Bayesian analysis, a recent study of 138 pediatric subjects demonstrated improved accuracy and precision using the two-sample strategy (i.e., both peak and trough concentrations), compared to trough concentrations alone, for AUC estimations [95].

6 Overcoming Challenges to Pharmacokinetic-Pharmacodynamic Studies

The most conspicuous, inherent challenge of pediatric PK-PD studies surrounds the ethnics and logistics of obtaining blood samples (encompassing both the number and volume) sufficient enough to accurately estimate and validate PK-PD parameters in this vulnerable population. Several measures may be implemented to overcome this challenge: sparse sampling, dried blood spot technique, and opportunistic study design. In contrast to the traditional intensive approach, sparse sampling reduces the number of blood draws, and, with the application of population-based modeling, still derive both individual and population PK estimates with inter-subject, intra-subject, and unexplained residual variabilities [96]. Sparse sampling is more appropriate and practical in pediatrics, with its reduced blood sampling albeit a requirement for a larger sample size; its application is appearing more in recently published studies [41, 46, 81, 95, 97].

Dried blood spot is a sampling technique that utilizes an ultralow volume (i.e., 30 μL of whole blood, which is 20 times lower than traditional venous or arterial samples) to evaluate the PK of drugs that are stable in this medium. In addition, dried blood spots eliminate the need for centrifugation or freezing of samples and measure drug concentration in whole blood. Using this technique, the estimates and precision of metronidazole PK parameters for premature infants were similar between plasma and dried blood spot samples [98]. Furthermore, the dried blood spot samples were 15 % lower than plasma. Limited pediatric PK studies currently utilize this technique [98, 99]. Future studies should explore this sampling strategy.

The opportunistic study design is attractive in pediatric research since it capitalizes on several aspects of standard clinical care. The opportunistic design may (1) employ a drug that is already prescribed by clinical indication, (2) coincide blood collection for PK samples with routine labs to minimize pricking, (3) utilize scavenged samples to maximize the use of drawn blood which would otherwise be wasted, and (4) obtain data on drug concentrations already measured by the clinical laboratory. In aggregate, this design curtails research-related costs, and improves parental consent since these activities are part of routine care and thus perceived as minimal risk. Opportunistic studies can provide preliminary data critical to the design of Phase I–III trials and enhance the dosing of currently marketed antimicrobial agents in children [46, 81, 100].

7 Conclusion

The fundamental physiologic and immunologic differences between pediatrics and adults produce variability in responses to antimicrobial agents, thereby potentially leading to undesired subtherapeutic and unanticipated toxic effects in pediatrics. This underscores the importance of understanding the physiologic and immunologic changes that occur with growth and development. Regulatory agencies are requiring more advanced antimicrobial PK-PD data for investigational drugs. Minimally, PK data are now required for pediatrics for any agent that seeks approval from the FDA for use in adults. However, PK/PD outcome data are virtually nonexistent in children. This dearth of PK-PD studies in pediatrics is a serious challenge for rational drug dosing, emphasizing that adequate pediatric research is essential for the future.

Acknowledgments

Drs. Bradley and Le have no personal financial involvement with any company that creates, develops, markets, or sells antimicrobial agents. Their employer, the University of California, has contracts with many companies to develop and test antimicrobial agents.

References

1. Bradley JS, Garonzik SM, Forrest A, Bhavnani SM (2010) Pharmacokinetics, pharmacodynamics, and Monte Carlo simulation: selecting the best antimicrobial dose to treat an infection. Pediatr Infect Dis J 29(11):1043–1046. doi:10.1097/INF.0b013e3181f42a53
2. Kearns GL, Abdel-Rahman SM, Alander SW, Blowey DL, Leeder JS, Kauffman RE (2003) Developmental pharmacology--drug disposition, action, and therapy in infants and children. N Engl J Med 349(12):1157–1167. doi:10.1056/NEJMra035092
3. van den Anker JN, Schwab M, Kearns GL (2011) Developmental pharmacokinetics. Handb Exp Pharmacol 205:51–75. doi:10.1007/978-3-642-20195-0_2
4. Anderson BJ, Holford NH (2008) Mechanism-based concepts of size and maturity in pharmacokinetics. Annu Rev Pharmacol Toxicol 48:303–332. doi:10.1146/annurev.pharmtox.48.113006.094708
5. Reed MD, Besunder JB (1989) Developmental pharmacology: ontogenic basis of drug disposition. Pediatr Clin North Am 36(5):1053–1074

6. Hayani KC, Hatzopoulos FK, Frank AL, Thummala MR, Hantsch MJ, Schatz BM, John EG, Vidyasagar D (1997) Pharmacokinetics of once-daily dosing of gentamicin in neonates. J Pediatr 131(1 Pt 1):76–80
7. Anderson BJ, Holford NH (2013) Understanding dosing: children are small adults, neonates are immature children. Arch Dis Child 98(9):737–744. doi:10.1136/archdischild-2013-303720
8. Mahmood I (2007) Prediction of drug clearance in children: impact of allometric exponents, body weight, and age. Ther Drug Monit 29(3):271–278. doi:10.1097/FTD.0b013e318042d3c4
9. Bulitta JB, Landersdorfer CB, Huttner SJ, Drusano GL, Kinzig M, Holzgrabe U, Stephan U, Sorgel F (2010) Population pharmacokinetic comparison and pharmacodynamic breakpoints of ceftazidime in cystic fibrosis patients and healthy volunteers. Antimicrob Agents Chemother 54(3):1275–1282. doi:10.1128/AAC.00936-09
10. Mahmood I (2006) Prediction of drug clearance in children from adults: a comparison of several allometric methods. Br J Clin Pharmacol 61(5):545–557. doi:10.1111/j.1365-2125.2006.02622.x
11. World Health Organization. Childhood overweight and obesity. http://www.who.int/dietphysicalactivity/childhood/en/index.html. Accessed on 31 Dec 2013
12. Anderson BJ, Holford NH (2011) Tips and traps analyzing pediatric PK data. Paediatr Anaesth21(3):222–237.doi:10.1111/j.1460-9592.2011.03536.x
13. Mulla H, Johnson TN (2010) Dosing dilemmas in obese children. Arch Dis Child Educ Pract Ed 95(4):112–117. doi:10.1136/adc.2009.163055
14. Foster BJ, Platt RW, Zemel BS (2012) Development and validation of a predictive equation for lean body mass in children and adolescents. Ann Hum Biol 39(3):171–182. doi:10.3109/03014460.2012.681800
15. Vinita BP, Nahata MC (2012) Drug dosing in pediatric patients, Chapter 3. In: Murphy JE (ed) Clinical pharmacokinetics, 5th edn. American Society of Health-System Pharmacists, Bethesda, MD
16. Nielsen EI, Sandstrom M, Honore PH, Ewald U, Friberg LE (2009) Developmental pharmacokinetics of gentamicin in preterm and term neonates: population modelling of a prospective study. Clin Pharmacokinet 48(4):253–263. doi:10.2165/00003088-200948040-00003
17. Walker PC (1987) Neonatal bilirubin toxicity. A review of kernicterus and the implications of drug-induced bilirubin displacement. Clin Pharmacokinet 13(1):26–50
18. Craft AW, Brocklebank JT, Hey EN, Jackson RH (1974) The ‘grey toddler’. Chloramphenicol toxicity. Arch Dis Child 49(3):235–237
19. Petrikin JE, Gaedigk R, Leeder JS, Truog WE (2010) Selective Toll--like receptor expression in human fetal lung. Pediatr Res 68(4):335–338.doi:10.1203/PDR.0b013e3181ed1134, 10.1203/00006450-201011001-00656
20. Yoshio H, Tollin M, Gudmundsson GH, Lagercrantz H, Jornvall H, Marchini G, Agerberth B (2003) Antimicrobial polypeptides of human vernix caseosa and amniotic fluid: implications for newborn innate defense. Pediatr Res 53(2):211–216. doi:10.1203/01.PDR.0000047471.47777.B0
21. Christensen RD, MacFarlane JL, Taylor NL, Hill HR, Rothstein G (1982) Blood and marrow neutrophils during experimental group B streptococcal infection: quantification of the stem cell, proliferative, storage and circulating pools. Pediatr Res 16(7):549–553. doi:10.1203/00006450-198207000-00011
22. Laver J, Duncan E, Abboud M, Gasparetto C, Sahdev I, Warren D, Bussel J, Auld P, O’Reilly RJ, Moore MA (1990) High levels of granulocyte and granulocyte-macrophage colony-stimulating factors in cord blood of normal full-term neonates. J Pediatr 116(4):627–632
23. Mease AD (1990) Tissue neutropenia: the newborn neutrophil in perspective. J Perinatol 10(1):55–59
24. Wolach B, Dolfin T, Regev R, Gilboa S, Schlesinger M (1997) The development of the complement system after 28 weeks’ gestation. Acta Paediatr 86(5):523–527
25. Anderson DC, Hughes BJ, Edwards MS, Buffone GJ, Baker CJ (1983) Impaired chemotaxigenesis by type III group B streptococci in neonatal sera: relationship to diminished concentration of specific anticapsular antibody and abnormalities of serum complement. Pediatr Res 17(6):496–502. doi:10.1203/00006450-198306000-00015
26. Lassiter HA, Wilson JL, Feldhoff RC, Hoffpauir JM, Klueber KM (1994) Supplemental complement component C9 enhances the capacity of neonatal serum to kill multiple isolates of pathogenic Escherichia coli. Pediatr Res 35(4 Pt 1):389–396
27. de la Morena M (2012) Immunologic development and susceptibility to infection. In:

Long SS, Pickering LK, Prober CG (eds) Long: principles and practice of pediatric infectious diseases, vol 4, 4th edn. W. B. Saunders, An Imprint of Elsevier, Maryland Heights, MO

28. Kavelaars A, van der Pompe G, Bakker JM, van Hasselt PM, Cats B, Visser GH, Heijnen CJ (1999) Altered immune function in human newborns after prenatal administration of betamethasone: enhanced natural killer cell activity and decreased T cell proliferation in cord blood. Pediatr Res 45(3):306–312. doi:10.1203/00006450-199903000-00003
29. Yabuhara A, Kawai H, Komiyama A (1990) Development of natural killer cytotoxicity during childhood: marked increases in number of natural killer cells with adequate cytotoxic abilities during infancy to early childhood. Pediatr Res 28(4):316–322. doi:10.1203/00006450-199010000-00002
30. Kohler PF, Farr RS (1966) Elevation of cord over maternal IgG immunoglobulin: evidence for an active placental IgG transport. Nature 210(5040):1070–1071
31. Smith RT, Eitzman DV (1964) The development of the immune response. Characterization of the response of the human infant and adult to immunization with salmonella vaccines. Pediatrics 33:163–183
32. Wilson CB, Penix L, Weaver WM, Melvin A, Lewis DB (1992) Ontogeny of T lymphocyte function in the neonate. Am J Reprod Immunol 28(3-4):132–135
33. Drusano GL (2007) Pharmacokinetics and pharmacodynamics of antimicrobials. Clin Infect Dis 45(Suppl 1):S89–S95. doi:10.1086/518137
34. Ellis JM, Kuti JL, Nicolau DP (2005) Use of Monte Carlo simulation to assess the pharmacodynamics of beta-lactams against Pseudomonas aeruginosa infections in children: a report from the OPTAMA program. Clin Ther 27(11):1820–1830. doi:10.1016/j.clinthera.2005.11.007
35. Courter JD, Kuti JL, Girotto JE, Nicolau DP (2009) Optimizing bactericidal exposure for beta-lactams using prolonged and continuous infusions in the pediatric population. Pediatr Blood Cancer 53(3):379–385. doi:10.1002/pbc.22051
36. Cies JJ, Shankar V, Schlichting C, Kuti JL (2013) Population pharmacokinetics of piperacillin/tazobactam in critically ill young children. Pediatr Infect Dis J 33:168. doi:10.1097/INF.0b013e3182a743c7
37. Reed MD, Goldfarb J, Yamashita TS, Lemon E, Blumer JL (1994) Single-dose pharmacokinetics of piperacillin and tazobactam in infants and children. Antimicrob Agents Chemother 38(12):2817–2826
38. Craig WA, Andes D (1996) Pharmacokinetics and pharmacodynamics of antibiotics in otitis media. Pediatr Infect Dis J 15(3):255–259
39. Canafax DM, Yuan Z, Chonmaitree T, Deka K, Russlie HQ, Giebink GS (1998) Amoxicillin middle ear fluid penetration and pharmacokinetics in children with acute otitis media. Pediatr Infect Dis J 17(2):149–156
40. Seikel K, Shelton S, McCracken GH Jr (1998) Middle ear fluid concentrations of amoxicillin after large dosages in children with acute otitis media. Pediatr Infect Dis J 17(10):969–970
41. Cohen-Wolkowiez M, Benjamin DK Jr, Ross A, James LP, Sullivan JE, Walsh MC, Zadell A, Newman N, White NR, Kashuba AD, Ouellet D (2012) Population pharmacokinetics of piperacillin using scavenged samples from preterm infants. Ther Drug Monit 34(3):312–319. doi:10.1097/FTD.0b013e3182587665
42. Cohen-Wolkowiez M, Poindexter B, Bidegain M, Weitkamp JH, Schelonka RL, Randolph DA, Ward RM, Wade K, Valencia G, Burchfield D, Arrieta A, Mehta V, Walsh M, Kantak A, Rasmussen M, Sullivan JE, Finer N, Rich W, Brozanski BS, van den Anker J, Blumer J, Laughon M, Watt KM, Kearns GL, Capparelli EV, Martz K, Berezny K, Benjamin DK Jr, Smith PB, Meropenem Study T (2012) Safety and effectiveness of meropenem in infants with suspected or complicated intra-abdominal infections. Clin Infect Dis 55(11):1495–1502. doi:10.1093/cid/cis758
43. Bradley JS, Sauberan JB, Ambrose PG, Bhavnani SM, Rasmussen MR, Capparelli EV (2008) Meropenem pharmacokinetics, pharmacodynamics, and Monte Carlo simulation in the neonate. Pediatr Infect Dis J 27(9):794–799. doi:10.1097/INF.0b013e318170f8d2
44. van den Anker JN, Pokorna P, Kinzig-Schippers M, Martinkova J, de Groot R, Drusano GL, Sorgel F (2009) Meropenem pharmacokinetics in the newborn. Antimicrob Agents Chemother 53(9):3871–3879. doi:10.1128/aac.00351-09
45. Smith PB, Cohen-Wolkowiez M, Castro LM, Poindexter B, Bidegain M, Weitkamp JH, Schelonka RL, Ward RM, Wade K, Valencia G, Burchfield D, Arrieta A, Bhatt-Mehta V, Walsh M, Kantak A, Rasmussen M, Sullivan JE, Finer N, Brozanski BS, Sanchez P, van den Anker J, Blumer J, Kearns GL, Capparelli EV, Anand R, Benjamin DK Jr, Meropenem Study T (2011) Population pharmacokinetics of meropenem in plasma and cerebrospinal fluid of infants with suspected or complicated

intra-abdominal infections. Pediatr Infect Dis J 30(10):844–849. doi:10.1097/INF.0b013e31822e8b0b

46. Tremoulet A, Le J, Poindexter B, Sullivan JE, Laughon M, Delmore P, Salgado A, Chong SI, Melloni C, Gao J, Benjamin DK Jr, Capparelli EV, Cohen-Wolkowiez M, on behalf of the Administrative Core Committee of the Best Pharmaceuticals for Children Act - Pediatric Trials N (2014) Characterization of the population pharmacokinetics of ampicillin in neonates using an opportunistic study design. Antimicrob Agents Chemother 58(6):3013–3020. doi:10.1128/AAC.02374-13
47. Vinks AA, van Rossem RN, Mathot RA, Heijerman HG, Mouton JW (2007) Pharmacokinetics of aztreonam in healthy subjects and patients with cystic fibrosis and evaluation of dose-exposure relationships using monte carlo simulation. Antimicrob Agents Chemother 51(9):3049–3055. doi:10.1128/aac.01522-06
48. Ashish A, Shaw M, Winstanley C, Ledson MJ, Walshaw MJ (2012) Increasing resistance of the Liverpool Epidemic Strain (LES) of Pseudomonas aeruginosa (Psa) to antibiotics in cystic fibrosis (CF)--a cause for concern? J Cyst Fibros 11(3):173–179. doi:10.1016/j.jcf.2011.11.004
49. Spencker FB, Staber L, Lietz T, Schille R, Rodloff AC (2003) Development of resistance in Pseudomonas aeruginosa obtained from patients with cystic fibrosis at different times. Clin Microbiol Infect 9(5):370–379
50. Zobell JT, Stockmann C, Young DC, Cash J, McDowell BJ, Korgenski K, Sherwin CM, Spigarelli M, Chatfield BA, Ampofo K (2011) Population pharmacokinetic and pharmacodynamic modeling of high-dose intermittent ticarcillin-clavulanate administration in pediatric cystic fibrosis patients. Clin Ther 33(11):1844–1850. doi:10.1016/j.clinthera.2011.09.010
51. Delvallee M, Mazingue F, Abouchahla W, Delebarre M, Wallet F, Courcol R, Kipnis E, Dessein R (2013) Optimization of continuous infusion of piperacillin-tazobactam in children with fever and neutropenia. Pediatr Infect Dis J 32(9):962–964. doi:10.1097/INF.0b013e318298dfb8
52. Kuti JL, Nightingale CH, Quintiliani R, Nicolau D (2002) Pharmacodynamic profiling of continuously infused piperacillin/tazobactam against Pseudomonas aeruginosa using Monte Carlo analysis. Diagn Microbiol Infect Dis 44(1):51–57
53. Tam VH, McKinnon PS, Akins RL, Rybak MJ, Drusano GL (2002) Pharmacodynamics of cefepime in patients with Gram-negative infections. J Antimicrob Chemother 50(3):425–428
54. Zelenitsky SA, Ariano RE, Zhanel GG (2011) Pharmacodynamics of empirical antibiotic monotherapies for an intensive care unit (ICU) population based on Canadian surveillance data. J Antimicrob Chemother 66(2):343–349. doi:10.1093/jac/dkq348
55. Walker MC, Lam WM, Manasco KB (2012) Continuous and extended infusions of beta-lactam antibiotics in the pediatric population. Ann Pharmacother 46(11):1537–1546. doi:10.1345/aph.1R216
56. Ohata Y, Tomita Y, Nakayama M, Kozuki T, Sunakawa K, Tanigawara Y (2011) Optimal dosage regimen of meropenem for pediatric patients based on pharmacokinetic/pharmacodynamic considerations. Drug Metab Pharmacokinet 26(5):523–531
57. Tamma PD, Turnbull AE, Milstone AM, Hsu AJ, Carroll KC, Cosgrove SE (2012) Does the piperacillin minimum inhibitory concentration for Pseudomonas aeruginosa influence clinical outcomes of children with pseudomonal bacteremia? Clin Infect Dis 55(6):799–806. doi:10.1093/cid/cis545
58. Bauer KA, West JE, O'Brien JM, Goff DA (2013) Extended-infusion cefepime reduces mortality in patients with Pseudomonas aeruginosa infections. Antimicrob Agents Chemother 57(7):2907–2912. doi:10.1128/AAC.02365-12
59. Moore RD, Lietman PS, Smith CR (1987) Clinical response to aminoglycoside therapy: importance of the ratio of peak concentration to minimal inhibitory concentration. J Infect Dis 155(1):93–99
60. Pagkalis S, Mantadakis E, Mavros MN, Ammari C, Falagas ME (2011) Pharmacological considerations for the proper clinical use of aminoglycosides. Drugs 71(17):2277–2294. doi:10.2165/11597020-000000000-00000
61. Mohamed AF, Nielsen EI, Cars O, Friberg LE (2012) Pharmacokinetic-pharmacodynamic model for gentamicin and its adaptive resistance with predictions of dosing schedules in newborn infants. Antimicrob Agents Chemother 56(1):179–188. doi:10.1128/AAC.00694-11
62. Rao SC, Srinivasjois R, Hagan R, Ahmed M (2011) One dose per day compared to multiple doses per day of gentamicin for treatment of suspected or proven sepsis in neonates.

Cochrane Database Syst Rev (11): CD005091. doi: 10.1002/14651858.CD005091.pub3

63. Smyth AR, Bhatt J (2012) Once-daily versus multiple-daily dosing with intravenous aminoglycosides for cystic fibrosis. Cochrane Database Syst Rev (2): CD002009. doi: 10.1002/14651858.CD002009.pub4
64. Young DC, Zobell JT, Stockmann C, Waters CD, Ampofo K, Sherwin CM, Spigarelli MG (2013) Optimization of anti-pseudomonal antibiotics for cystic fibrosis pulmonary exacerbations: V. Aminoglycosides. Pediatr Pulmonol 48(11):1047–1061. doi:10.1002/ppul.22813
65. Downes KJ, Hahn A, Wiles J, Courter JD, Vinks AA (2013) Dose optimisation of antibiotics in children: application of pharmacokinetics/pharmacodynamics in paediatrics. Int J Antimicrob Agents 43:223. doi:10.1016/j.ijantimicag.2013.11.006
66. Drusano GL, Louie A (2011) Optimization of aminoglycoside therapy. Antimicrob Agents Chemother 55(6):2528–2531. doi: 10.1128/AAC.01314-10
67. Tam VH, Ledesma KR, Vo G, Kabbara S, Lim TP, Nikolaou M (2008) Pharmacodynamic modeling of aminoglycosides against Pseudomonas aeruginosa and Acinetobacter baumannii: identifying dosing regimens to suppress resistance development. Antimicrob Agents Chemother 52(11):3987–3993. doi:10.1128/AAC.01468-07
68. Flume PA, Mogayzel PJ Jr, Robinson KA, Goss CH, Rosenblatt RL, Kuhn RJ, Marshall BC, Clinical Practice Guidelines for Pulmonary Therapies C (2009) Cystic fibrosis pulmonary guidelines: treatment of pulmonary exacerbations. Am J Respir Crit Care Med 180(9):802–808. doi:10.1164/rccm.200812-1845PP
69. Glover ML, Shaffer CL, Rubino CM, Cuthrell C, Schoening S, Cole E, Potter D, Ransom JL, Gal P (2001) A multicenter evaluation of gentamicin therapy in the neonatal intensive care unit. Pharmacotherapy 21(1):7–10
70. Dupuis LL, Sung L, Taylor T, Abdolell M, Allen U, Doyle J, Taddio A (2004) Tobramycin pharmacokinetics in children with febrile neutropenia undergoing stem cell transplantation: once-daily versus thrice-daily administration. Pharmacotherapy 24(5):564–573
71. Inparajah M, Wong C, Sibbald C, Boodhan S, Atenafu EG, Naqvi A, Dupuis LL (2010) Once-daily gentamicin dosing in children with febrile neutropenia resulting from antineoplastic therapy. Pharmacotherapy 30(1): 43–51. doi:10.1592/phco.30.1.43
72. Sung L, Dupuis LL, Bliss B, Taddio A, Abdolell M, Allen U, Rolland M, Tong A, Taylor T, Doyle J (2003) Randomized controlled trial of once- versus thrice-daily tobramycin in febrile neutropenic children undergoing stem cell transplantation. J Natl Cancer Inst 95(24):1869–1877
73. van Lent-Evers NA, Mathot RA, Geus WP, van Hout BA, Vinks AA (1999) Impact of goal-oriented and model-based clinical pharmacokinetic dosing of aminoglycosides on clinical outcome: a cost-effectiveness analysis. Ther Drug Monit 21(1):63–73
74. de Alba RC, Gomez Castillo E, Manzanares Secades C, Rodriguez Lopez J, Arreaza Lopez L, Saenz Valiente P (1998) Once daily gentamicin dosing in neonates. Pediatr Infect Dis J 17(12):1169–1171
75. Bartal C, Danon A, Schlaeffer F, Reisenberg K, Alkan M, Smoliakov R, Sidi A, Almog Y (2003) Pharmacokinetic dosing of aminoglycosides: a controlled trial. Am J Med 114(3): 194–198
76. Beaubien AR, Desjardins S, Ormsby E, Bayne A, Carrier K, Cauchy MJ, Henri R, Hodgen M, Salley J, St Pierre A (1989) Incidence of amikacin ototoxicity: a sigmoid function of total drug exposure independent of plasma levels. Am J Otolaryngol 10(4):234–243
77. Lowdin E, Odenholt I, Cars O (1998) In vitro studies of pharmacodynamic properties of vancomycin against Staphylococcus aureus and Staphylococcus epidermidis. Antimicrob Agents Chemother 42(10):2739–2744
78. Kullar R, Davis SL, Levine DP, Rybak MJ (2011) Impact of vancomycin exposure on outcomes in patients with methicillin-resistant Staphylococcus aureus bacteremia: support for consensus guidelines suggested targets. Clin Infect Dis 52(8):975–981. doi:10.1093/cid/cir124
79. Rybak M, Lomaestro B, Rotschafer JC, Moellering R Jr, Craig W, Billeter M, Dalovisio JR, Levine DP (2009) Therapeutic monitoring of vancomycin in adult patients: a consensus review of the American Society of Health-System Pharmacists, the Infectious Diseases Society of America, and the Society of Infectious Diseases Pharmacists. Am J Health Syst Pharm 66(1):82–98. doi:10.2146/ajhp080434
80. Frymoyer A, Guglielmo BJ, Hersh AL (2013) Desired vancomycin trough serum concentration for treating invasive methicillin-resistant Staphylococcal infections. Pediatr Infect Dis J 32(10):1077–1079. doi:10.1097/INF.0b013e318299f75c

81. Le J, Bradley JS, Murray W, Romanowski GL, Tran TT, Nguyen N, Cho S, Natale S, Bui I, Tran TM, Capparelli EV (2013) Improved vancomycin dosing in children using area under the curve exposure. Pediatr Infect Dis J 32(4):e155–e163. doi:10.1097/INF.0b013e318286378e
82. Welsh KJ, Abbott AN, Lewis EM, Gardiner JM, Kruzel MC, Lewis CT, Mohr JF, Wanger A, Armitige LY (2010) Clinical characteristics, outcomes, and microbiologic features associated with methicillin-resistant Staphylococcus aureus bacteremia in pediatric patients treated with vancomycin. J Clin Microbiol 48(3):894–899. doi:10.1128/JCM.01949-09
83. Le J, Vaida F, Nguyen E, Adler-Shohet FC, Romanowski GL, Kim J, Vo T, Capparelli EV (2014) Population-based pharmacokinetic modeling of vancomycin in children with renal insufficiency. J Pharmacol Clin Toxicol 2(1):1017–1026
84. Jacqz-Aigrain E, Zhao W, Sharland M, van den Anker JN (2013) Use of antibacterial agents in the neonate: 50 years of experience with vancomycin administration. Semin Fetal Neonatal Med 18(1):28–34. doi:10.1016/j.siny.2012.10.003
85. McKamy S, Hernandez E, Jahng M, Moriwaki T, Deveikis A, Le J (2011) Incidence and risk factors influencing the development of vancomycin nephrotoxicity in children. J Pediatr 158(3):422–426. doi:10.1016/j.jpeds.2010.08.019
86. Myers AL, Gaedigk A, Dai H, James LP, Jones BL, Neville KA (2012) Defining risk factors for red man syndrome in children and adults. Pediatr Infect Dis J 31(5):464–468. doi:10.1097/INF.0b013e31824e10d7
87. Mehrotra N, Tang L, Phelps SJ, Meibohm B (2012) Evaluation of vancomycin dosing regimens in preterm and term neonates using Monte Carlo simulations. Pharmacotherapy 32(5):408–419. doi:10.1002/j.1875-9114.2012.01029.x
88. Zhao W, Kaguelidou F, Biran V, Zhang D, Allegaert K, Capparelli EV, Holford N, Kimura T, Lo YL, Peris JE, Thomson A, van den Anker JN, Fakhoury M, Jacqz-Aigrain E (2013) External evaluation of population pharmacokinetic models of vancomycin in neonates: the transferability of published models to different clinical settings. Br J Clin Pharmacol 75:1068. doi:10.1111/j.1365-2125.2012.04406.x
89. Zhao W, Lopez E, Biran V, Durrmeyer X, Fakhoury M, Jacqz-Aigrain E (2013) Vancomycin continuous infusion in neonates: dosing optimisation and therapeutic drug monitoring. Arch Dis Child 98(6):449–453. doi:10.1136/archdischild-2012-302765
90. Patel AD, Anand D, Lucas C, Thomson AH (2013) Continuous infusion of vancomycin in neonates. Arch Dis Child 98(6):478–479. doi:10.1136/archdischild-2012-303197
91. Cataldo MA, Tacconelli E, Grilli E, Pea F, Petrosillo N (2012) Continuous versus intermittent infusion of vancomycin for the treatment of Gram-positive infections: systematic review and meta-analysis. J Antimicrob Chemother 67(1):17–24. doi:10.1093/jac/dkr442
92. Wysocki M, Delatour F, Faurisson F, Rauss A, Pean Y, Misset B, Thomas F, Timsit JF, Similowski T, Mentec H, Mier L, Dreyfuss D (2001) Continuous versus intermittent infusion of vancomycin in severe Staphylococcal infections: prospective multicenter randomized study. Antimicrob Agents Chemother 45(9):2460–2467
93. Gordon CL, Thompson C, Carapetis JR, Turnidge J, Kilburn C, Currie BJ (2012) Trough concentrations of vancomycin: adult therapeutic targets are not appropriate for children. Pediatr Infect Dis J 31(12):1269–1271. doi:10.1097/INF.0b013e31826a3eaf
94. Moffett BS, Edwards MS (2013) Analysis of vancomycin therapeutic drug monitoring trends at pediatric hospitals. Pediatr Infect Dis J 32(1):32–35. doi:10.1097/INF.0b013e31826fd98d
95. Le J, Ngu B, Bradley JS, Murray W, Nguyen A, Nguyen L, Romanowski GL, Vo T, Capparelli EV (2014) Vancomycin monitoring in children using Bayesian estimation. Ther Drug Monit 36:510. doi:10.1097/FTD.0000000000000039
96. Barker CI, Standing JF, Turner MA, McElnay JC, Sharland M (2012) Antibiotic dosing in children in Europe: can we grade the evidence from pharmacokinetic/pharmacodynamic studies - and when is enough data enough? Curr Opin Infect Dis 25(3):235–242. doi:10.1097/QCO.0b013e328353105c
97. Meibohm B, Laer S, Panetta JC, Barrett JS (2005) Population pharmacokinetic studies in pediatrics: issues in design and analysis. AAPS J 7(2):E475–E487. doi:10.1208/aapsj070248
98. Cohen-Wolkowiez M, Sampson M, Bloom BT, Arrieta A, Wynn JL, Martz K, Harper B, Kearns GL, Capparelli EV, Siegel D, Benjamin DK Jr, Smith PB, Best Pharmaceuticals for Children Act-Pediatric Trials N (2013) Determining population and developmental pharmacokinetics of metronidazole using plasma and dried blood spot samples from premature infants. Pediatr Infect Dis J 32(9):956–961. doi:10.1097/INF.0b013e3182947cf8
99. Suyagh M, Collier PS, Millership JS, Iheagwaram G, Millar M, Halliday HL, McElnay JC (2011)

Metronidazole population pharmacokinetics in preterm neonates using dried blood-spot sampling. Pediatrics 127(2):e367–e374. doi:10.1542/peds.2010-0807

100. Wade KC, Wu D, Kaufman DA, Ward RM, Benjamin DK Jr, Sullivan JE, Ramey N, Jayaraman B, Hoppu K, Adamson PC, Gastonguay MR, Barrett JS, National Institute of Child H, Development Pediatric Pharmacology Research Unit N (2008) Population pharmacokinetics of fluconazole in young infants. Antimicrob Agents Chemother 52(11):4043–4049. doi:10.1128/AAC.00569-08
101. Rubino CM, Bradley JS (2007) Optimizing therapy with antibacterial agents: use of pharmacokinetic-pharmacodynamic principles in pediatrics. Paediatr Drugs 9(6):361–369
102. Burgess DS, Frei CR, Lewis Ii JS, Fiebelkorn KR, Jorgensen JH (2007) The contribution of pharmacokinetic-pharmacodynamic modelling with Monte Carlo simulation to the development of susceptibility breakpoints for Neisseria meningitidis. Clin Microbiol Infect 13(1):33–39. doi:10.1111/j.1469-0691.2006.01617.x
103. Cohen-Wolkowiez M, Ouellet D, Smith PB, James LP, Ross A, Sullivan JE, Walsh MC, Zadell A, Newman N, White NR, Kashuba AD, Benjamin DK Jr (2012) Population pharmacokinetics of metronidazole evaluated using scavenged samples from preterm infants. Antimicrob Agents Chemother 56(4):1828–1837. doi:10.1128/AAC.06071-11
104. Michalopoulos AS, Falagas ME (2011) Colistin: recent data on pharmacodynamics properties and clinical efficacy in critically ill patients. Annals Intens Care 1(1):30. doi:10.1186/2110-5820-1-30
105. Gumbo T, Louie A, Deziel MR, Liu W, Parsons LM, Salfinger M, Drusano GL (2007) Concentration-dependent Mycobacterium tuberculosis killing and prevention of resistance by rifampin. Antimicrob Agents Chemother 51(11):3781–3788. doi:10.1128/AAC.01533-06
106. Close SJ, McBurney CR, Garvin CG, Chen DC, Martin SJ (2002) Trimethoprim-sulfamethoxazole activity and pharmacodynamics against glycopeptide-intermediate Staphylococcus aureus. Pharmacotherapy 22(8):983–989
107. Rodvold KA (2001) Pharmacodynamics of antiinfective therapy: taking what we know to the patient's bedside. Pharmacotherapy 21(11 Pt 2):319S–330S

Chapter 23

Pharmacodynamics and Obesity

Manjunath P. Pai

Abstract

Five hundred million adults meet the current definition of obesity worldwide. This high global prevalence of obesity offers unique challenges to the selection of the optimal antimicrobial dose. Early phase clinical trials tend to exclude obese healthy volunteers, while late phase clinical trials are not adequately powered to identify potential differences in the clinical outcomes in this population. The interaction of obesity on antimicrobial directed pathogen–host response is also not well described. Hence, dose selection in this population relies on the desire to achieve pharmacokinetic bioequivalence across the clinical body weight distribution. Pharmacodynamic data supporting well-defined doses that optimize outcomes in the obese population are limited. Specific recommendations for antimicrobial dosing should be established through consensus guidance with endorsement from international societies that advocate for the appropriate use of antimicrobials.

Key words Allometry, Antibiotic, Antimicrobial, Body mass index, Dosing, Infection, Weight, Obese, Overweight, Pharmacokinetics

1 Definition and Prevalence of Obesity

Obesity is currently defined based on a body mass index (BMI) ≥ 30 kg/m^2, which is the weight of the person in kilograms divided by their height in squared meters [1]. An estimated 500 million (60 % female) adults meet this definition of obesity worldwide [1]. Figure 1 illustrates the top ten countries/regions of the world with the highest prevalence of obesity [2]. As evident from this chart, obesity is no longer a disease that is limited to developed nations. The Micronesian nations of Nauru, Tonga, Samoa, Cook Islands, Palau, and other federated states within this region have an adult prevalence of obesity that exceeds 50 % of their population. Egypt, Kuwait, Saudi Arabia, and the United Arab Emirates have rates of obesity that impact a quarter to a third of their adult population [2]. Sedentary lifestyles and access to energy-dense foods are recognized to be primary contributors to this explosion in the prevalence of obesity over the past generation [1]. In the USA, the adult prevalence of obesity appears to have stabilized at 35 % over the

John C. Rotschafer et al. (eds.), *Antibiotic Pharmacodynamics*, Methods in Pharmacology and Toxicology,
DOI 10.1007/978-1-4939-3323-5_23,

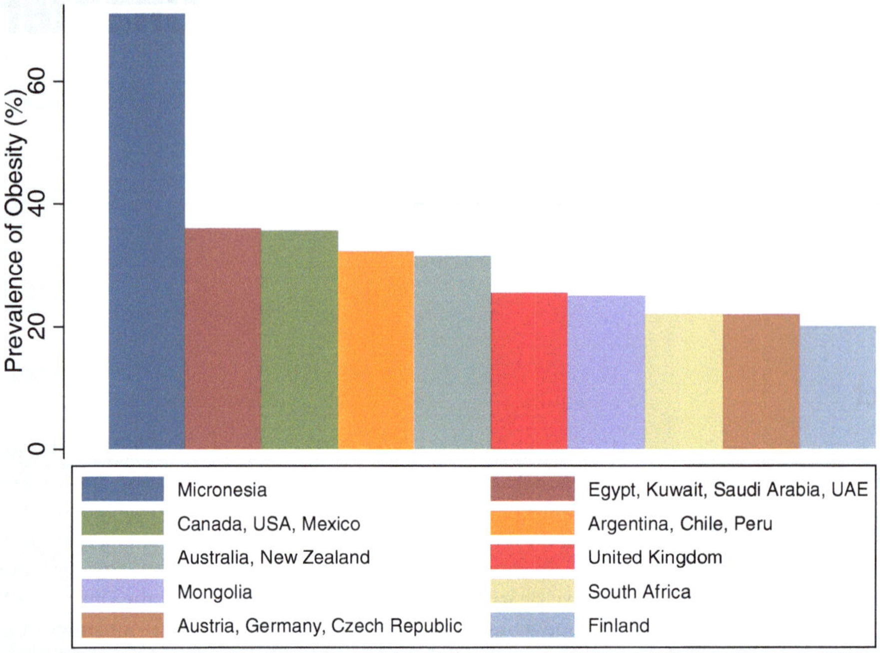

Fig. 1 Prevalence of obesity among select regions of the world recognized to have the highest rates of obesity among individuals ≥15 years of age

past decade though the proportion of patients with extreme obesity (BMI ≥ 40 kg/m^2) continues to rise [3]. This later term "extreme obesity" is also referred to as "morbid obesity," categorically defined as Class III obesity, and has taken additional definitions such as "super obesity" (BMI ≥ 50 kg/m^2) [1, 4, 5]. This shift in the adult weight distribution has clear consequences to our current methods of dose translation across body size. The average adult in the USA weighs 81 kg, and most adults are expected to exist within a 50–100 kg weight range [6]. To date, the heaviest human on record weighed 635 kg (1400 lb) [7]. So from a clinical perspective, the potential need to select the right dose of an antimicrobial for an infected patient that is up to eightfold larger than the average is a clear possibility but still an extreme reality. The more likely scenario in the clinical setting is to expect extremely obese adults between an approximately 100–250 kg range that are 1.2–3.1-fold larger than the average adult.

2 Association of Obesity and Infection

Obesity is associated with comorbidities such as type 2 diabetes ("diabesity") that can predispose these patients to worse clinical outcomes secondary to infection [8]. However, this correlation between obesity and diabetes makes identification of the independent effects of obesity and infection difficult to tease out. Epidemiologic studies have found obesity to be a significant risk factor of post-surgical skin and skin structure infections (SSTIs) [9–16]. Case–control studies have demonstrated that the risk of developing cellulitis increase in patients that are obese [17, 18]. Pregnant obese women are more likely to have a Caesarean section for delivery and have a higher risk for developing a post-surgical SSTI [9]. Disrupted macrocirculation and microcirculation, decreased wound healing, and lymphedema are key physiological factors that may influence this association between SSTIs and obesity [18]. Physical factors of high adiposity with skin-folding can lead to intertriginous skin barrier disruptions that provide a route for bacterial invasion [19].

Extreme obesity compromises the ability to obtain vascular access and respiratory intubation that may be required emergently [20, 21]. This is particularly problematic during acute trauma where an emergent venous "cut down" procedure may be required to establish vascular access [22]. Obese patient require greater elevation of their head, neck and shoulders to permit laryngoscope viewing during intubation [22]. These factors may contribute to the observation that critically ill trauma patients who are obese have a twofold increased risk of developing bloodstream and respiratory tract infections [23]. Although this is the case, obesity may not be a negative risk factor for sepsis-related outcomes and mortality. Trends for a lower risk of mortality have been seen as a function of increasing BMI strata [24–26]. However, an explanation for this improved probability of survival is unclear and is part of the commonly referred to "obesity paradox" [27].

Despite this lack of clear association between obesity and sepsis-related mortality, the adipose tissue is increasingly recognized to contribute to the formation of various inflammatory mediators such as the adipokines [28]. Leptin, adipokine, resistin, omentin, and visfatin are key adipokines that have been shown to contribute to tissue-level cross talk between adipocytes and leucocytes [29]. Altered T-cell proliferation, reduced macrophage differentiation, decreased natural killer cell activity, and decreased antigen presentation of dendritic cells have been documented as potential consequence of altered adipokine secretion [28]. The potential pro-inflammatory effects of obesity and resultant poor outcomes were documented during the 2009 H1N1 influenza pandemic [30]. Approximately 50 % of adults hospitalized in California during the 2009 H1N1 influenza pandemic were obese [31]. Additional studies have demonstrated obese patients hospitalized with the H1N1 influenza strain had longer lengths of stay when admitted to the intensive care unit [32]. A potential age-dependent effect has been suggested by one epidemiologic study, where obesity was identified as a risk factor for poor H1N1 influenza related outcomes among adults <60 years of age [33]. An animal model of diet-induced obesity has also demonstrated higher rates of mortality in obese relative to lean animals infected with the H1N1 strain [34]. Similar to this poor-prognostic profile between obesity and influenza, the prognosis is worse in obese patients with chronic Hepatitis C virus (HCV) infection [35]. Hepatic steatosis and fibrosis is more common in obese nondiabetic compared to normal weight patients with HCV [36]. Response to antiviral therapy has also been shown to be impaired in obese relative to nonobese patients with HCV [36]. Taken together, we are unlikely to establish a clear correlation between obesity and all forms of infection related morbidity and mortality. There are likely to be disease-related, sex-related, age-related, and potentially polymorphic differences in the adipokine-related genes that contribute to obesity-related effects on infection outcomes [37]. In addition to these pathogen and host related factors, potential alterations in antimicrobial pharmacology could impact the outcomes of obese individuals with active infections.

3 Current Antimicrobial Dosing Paradigm in Obesity

Antimicrobials are currently dosed by three major approaches when considering body size [38]. The underlying basis for dose modification for body size (if necessary) is the achievement of bioequivalent exposure of the antimicrobial across the body size distribution [38]. From this perspective, let us consider the dosing paradigms. The first is the use of fixed-based dosing that does not include dose modification for body-size, an example of such an approach would be the dosing of levofloxacin (e.g., 750 mg/day) [39]. The second is the application of a weight-stratified fixed-dosing approach, such as the use of 1000 mg dose of ribavirin in patients <75 kg and 1200 mg in patients ≥75 kg [40]. The third is weight based dosing that can include a fixed mg/kg dosing recommendation irrespective of body size, such as use of 10 mg/kg of telavancin based on total body weight [41]. From a drug dosing paradigm perspective, use of a fixed-dose could theoretically lead to under dosing and weight-based (mg/kg) dosing could lead to over dosing in extremely obese patients [38]. Table 1, includes a summary of key antimicrobial classes and agents that are dosed on a fixed and weight basis in adults.

Some drugs have both weight and fixed dosing recommendations that can be a cause of confusion in clinical practice. A key example of this dosing paradigm contradiction is vancomycin. The vancomycin product label recommends doses that are on a fixed-dose basis, 500 mg every 6 h or 1000 mg every 12 h [42]. However, treatment guidelines recommend that vancomycin doses should be based on a 15–20 mg/kg per dose basis [43]. The fortunate

Table 1
Summary of the typical dosing paradigm for major antimicrobial classes and individual drugs for drug classes with limited representative agents

Fixed doses	Fixed and weight based doses	Weight based doses
Beta-lactams	Vancomycin	Aminoglycosides
Tetracyclines	Trimethoprim/sulfamethoxazole	Polymyxin (B and E)
Glycyclines	Antituberculosis agents	Teicoplanin
Macrolides	Voriconazole	Quinupristin-Dalfopristin
Lincosamides	Acyclovir	Daptomycin
Nitroimidazole	Ganciclovir	Telavancin
Oxazolidinone	Ribavirin	Polyenes
Dalbavancin		Flucytosine
Dapsone		Foscarnet
Fluoroquinolones		
Nitrofurantoin		
Fosfomycin		
Triazoles		
Valacyclovir		
Valganciclovir		
Oseltamivir		
NRTIs		
NNRTIs		
Protease inhibitors		

availability of therapeutic drug monitoring (TDM) to modify this empiric recommendation makes this contradiction less of an issue for vancomycin compared to drugs that do not have accessible TDM. The more important issue at hand is whether obesity leads to alterations in the concentration–time profile that will adversely affect the pharmacodynamic profile of the antimicrobial.

4 Obesity and Pharmacodynamic Bioequivalence

The antimicrobial concentration–time profile is often characterized through measurement of plasma or serum concentrations after the administration of single or multiple intravenous or oral antimicrobial doses. Chapter 1 reviews the general pharmacokinetic and pharmacodynamic (PK-PD) principles that are used to optimize drug dose selection by antimicrobial class. We broadly expect antimicrobials to follow concentration-dependent or time-dependent PK-PD [44]. Concentration-dependent antimicrobials are optimized by ensuring that the maximum-concentration (C_{max}) and the closely correlated parameter of area under the curve (AUC) achieve a certain target value. Time-dependent antimicrobials are optimized by ensuring that the concentration profile remains above a concentration threshold for a specified duration of the dosing interval. Classification of specific antimicrobials based on these PK-PD indices is detailed in an excellent review [45].

From this perspective, an increase in the volume of distribution of a drug in an obese person without a resultant change in drug clearance will lead to a lowering of the C_{max} but no significant change in the AUC. This aforementioned change in Vd but not CL will lead to an extension in the elimination half-life. Figure 2 illustrates the expected serum concentration–time profile in a normal (60 kg) and obese (120 kg) individual if the Vd doubles but the CL does not change. So, in the case of a time-dependent antimicrobial, the percent time above a threshold may actually increase in the setting of extreme obesity. Figure 2 includes an arbitrary

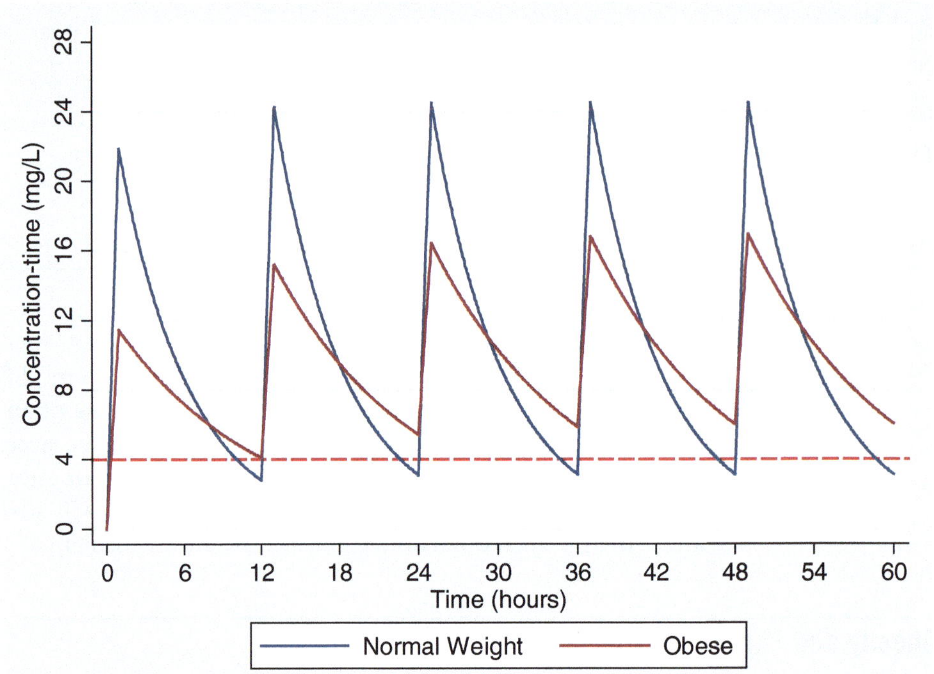

Fig. 2 Simulated serum concentration–time profile of a normal weight (60 kg) individual compared to an obese (120 kg) individual if the volume of distribution doubles with weight (25–50 L) but no change in drug clearance occurs. Based on simulation of a 600 mg dose administered every 12 h as a 1 h infusion

threshold of 4 mg/L, which shows concentrations above this value for 100 % of dosing interval in the obese individual but not the normal weight individual. This may not be apparent with single dose administration but will be the case with multiple dose administration. Studies that have looked at the use of beta-lactams for surgical prophylaxis have shown lower concentrations that necessitate doubling the dose for example [46–49]. Although this may be reasonable because surgical prophylaxis often includes a single dose or limited term use, these perceived pharmacodynamic benefits may not extend to multiple dose administration. Alternatively, the potential role of a loading dose in obese individual followed by the same maintenance dose (as normal weight) could achieve pharmacodynamic bioequivalence.

Alternatively, Fig. 3 illustrates the similar type of case as Fig. 2 but now assumes the Vd remains the same, while the CL increases by 50 % (typical scenario). Under this scenario the time below the threshold concentration declines and the AUC is lower in the obese compared to the normal weight scenario. This scenario represents a potential dosing problem for both concentration-dependent and time-dependent antimicrobials. Under this scenario, pharmacodynamic bioequivalence between the obese and normal weight individual can be achieved by increasing the dose

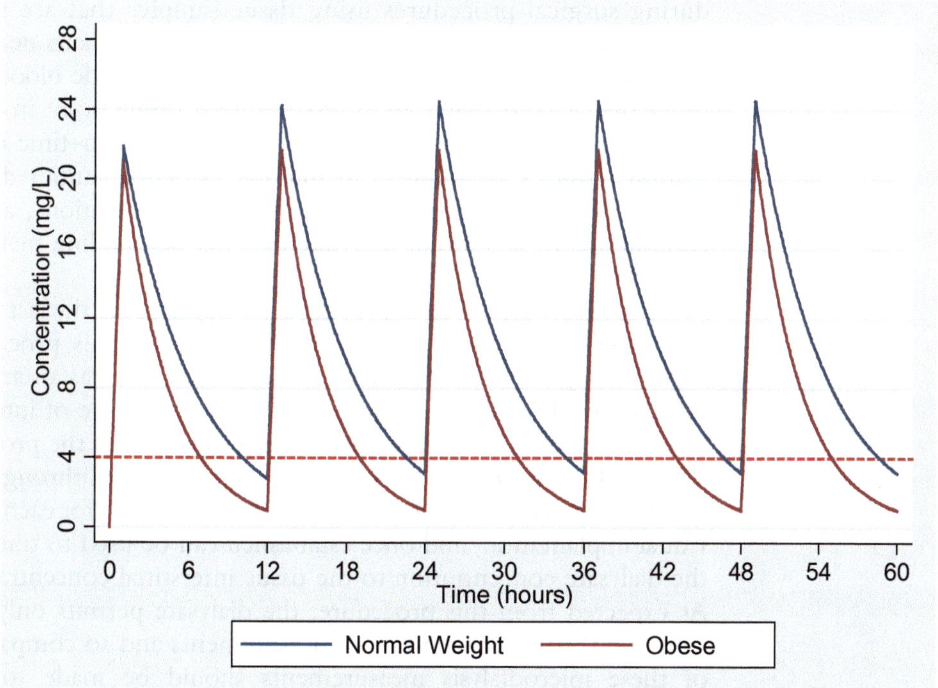

Fig. 3 Simulated serum concentration–time profile of a normal weight (60 kg) individual compared to an obese (120 kg) individual if no change in volume of distribution occurs but the clearance increases by 50 % (4.69–7.03 L/h). Based on simulation of a 600 mg dose administered every 12 h as a 1 h infusion

from 600 to 900 mg (50 % increase) and maintain the dosing interval (every 12 h) that may be desirable for a concentration-dependent agent. Alternatively, the dose could be maintained at 600 mg and the frequency of administration increased to every 8 h for a time-dependent agent. The integrated serum concentration–time profile (i.e., AUC) will be correlated to the tissue concentration–time profile. However, a key limitation of this form of assessment of pharmacodynamic bioequivalence is that it assumes that the serum concentration profile reflects the tissue-concentration profile. The shape of the tissue concentration–time profile in poorly perfused tissue like the adipose may not be similar to concentrations in the bloodstream [50, 51]. This is relevant because the optimal drug PK-PD profile must be achieved at the target site(s) of infection.

5 Obesity and Antimicrobial Tissue Concentrations

Collection of samples to measure tissue concentrations of antimicrobial at the site of infection is not easy to accomplish in the clinical setting. The most accessible tissue for such evaluation includes the skin and skin structure tissue, adipose tissue and muscle. Direct tissue collections from such sources may include sample collection during surgical procedures using tissue samples that are to be discarded [52]. These discarded samples may represent necrotic material that has been excised, or samples that include blood and other tissues, and represent evaluation for a single point in time. Hence, direct soft tissue evaluation for concentration–time information requires sampling from multiple patients, cannot distinguish tissue form vascular and interstitial concentrations, and is confounded by significant heterogeneity in the sampling methodology [52].

The most viable alternative that has emerged over the last three decades includes the use of microdialysis [53]. This procedure requires surgical implantation of a microprobe that has a semipermeable membrane of variable porosity into the tissue of interest. Dialysis fluid can then be passed through the inlet of the probe at a relatively slow rate of infusion and sample collected through the outlet. Multiple protocols exist to calibrate the probe for each individual implantation, and once established can be used to translate the dialysate concentration to the tissue interstitial concentration. As expected from this procedure, the dialysate permits only free (unbound) drug concentration measurements and so comparison of these microdialysis measurements should be made to free serum/plasma concentrations for fair comparison. This approach has been used to characterize the tissue concentration time profile antimicrobials in the skin and skin structure of obese and diabetic patients.

Brill and colleague recently completed a noteworthy study of subcutaneous pharmacokinetics of cefazolin in eight morbidly obese (107–175 kg) and seven nonobese patients (72–109 kg) who received a single 2 g intravenous bolus injection dose prior to surgery [54]. A subcutaneous microdialysis catheter was implanted and calibrated 3 h prior to the surgery and used to sample the interstitial space for 4 h post cefazolin dosing. The area under the time-unbound concentration curve ($fAUC_{0\text{–}4\ h}$) was significantly lower in the microdialysate samples but not the plasma samples when comparing the morbidly obese to normal weight subjects. As a consequence the subcutaneous tissue penetration ratio ($fAUC_{0\text{–}4\ h\ tissue}/fAUC_{0\text{–}4\ h\ plasma}$) was 0.70 (0.68–0.83) in the morbidly obese compared to 1.02 (0.85–1.41) in the nonobese patients [54]. These results suggest that potential bioequivalence demonstrated by measurement of plasma concentrations may not be reflective of target tissue concentrations that are relevant for the effective surgical prophylactic use of cefazolin. The clinical implications of these results remain to be defined. However, modeling and simulations generated from these data suggest that the probability of target attainment declines sharply against potential pathogens with MIC values >2 mg/L especially if surgical procedures are likely to exceed a 3 h duration of time. A review of the population pharmacokinetic model parameters suggests that the CL is not dependent on weight, while weight impacts the Vd. However, this relationship between Vd and weight is not proportionate such that a 150 kg patient is expected to have an approximately 50 % higher value than a 75 kg patient. Hence this change in the PK profile of cefazolin may more closely match the scenario illustrated in Fig. 2. The impact of obesity may be relevant with the first dose (surgical prophylaxis) but may not be clinically relevant with multiple doses (treatment of SSTI). Thus, clinical practice guideline recommendations to consider use of a 3 g dose of cefazolin in patients' ≥120 kg and consideration for redosing after 4 h from the initial dose is well founded [55].

Similar to this study, evaluations of cefoxitin abdominal subcutaneous tissue concentrations are lower in obese relative to nonobese volunteers and patients [47]. Microdialysis data demonstrate superimposable subcutaneous cefoxitin concentration–time profiles in obese versus nonobese volunteers even though obese patients received twice the dose (2 g versus 1 g). Furthermore, direct tissue sampling at the time of surgical incision and closure were lower in the obese relative to nonobese patients [47]. These data support the use of a 2 g dose of cefoxitin in obese adult patients for surgical prophylaxis. Contrary to these findings, the tissue concentration–time profile of ertapenem has not been shown to be vastly affected in obese versus nonobese patients [56]. Dose recommendations above 1 g has been suggested for moderately susceptible strains associated with diabetic foot infections but have not been recommended by guidelines for surgical prophylaxis [57].

Antimicrobial tissue concentrations for non-skin and skin structure sites have not been evaluated systematically among obese patients. As an example, a literature search for key terms "epithelial lining fluid" and "obese" revealed no relevant results using "PubMed" or "Google" as key search engines. Hence the potential effects of obesity on pulmonary tissue penetration of antimicrobials have not been characterized. This is relevant because extreme obesity is known to adversely impact the mechanics of breathing [58]. Severely obese patients have been shown to have reduced end-tidal functional residual capacity and expiratory reserve volume in the upright and supine positions [58]. These altered mechanics can contribute to an increased risk of aspiration pneumonia especially post-surgically for gastric bypass or lap-band procedures that are performed as surgical weight-loss intervention [59]. Thus there is a paucity of target-site tissue concentration data in the extremely obese population. Hence dose selection based on inference from serum/plasma concentration–time data for non-bacteremia related infections should recognize this potential limitation when comparing obese to nonobese patients.

6 Obesity and Initial Dose Selection

We expect obese patients to require larger doses than average sized patients but that these doses are not necessarily proportionate to their total body weight [38]. So the empiric approach to initial dose selection may occur through consideration of body size. Weight and height are the measured body size parameters that can be translated into alternate body size descriptors such as adjusted body weight, lean body weight, or body surface area [38]. These alternate body size descriptors are semantically different but serve a singular purpose as scalars. They prevent the computation of values that are more than 2.5-fold different between a 50 kg patient and a 250 kg patient (that is fivefold different) [38, 60]. These body size descriptors prevent computation of doses that would be erroneously high in an obese individual if they were dosed on total body weight. For example, a 150 kg (69 in.) male patient would have an adjusted body weight of approximately 100 kg. So dosing a 75 kg patient based on a 10 mg/kg basis would yield a dose of 750 mg, and 1000 mg in the 150 kg patient (dosed on 100 kg adjusted body weight basis). So the 150 kg patient will receive a dose that is 33 % higher than the average dose calculated in a 75 kg patient.

This alternate body size descriptor method of dose scaling would be comparable to calculating the dose by allometry [61], where the dose could be computed based on:

Obese Patient Dose = Average Dose × (Obese Patient Weight/ Average Weight)β

Where β is often a value of 0.5–0.75 [38]. So in the above scenario an average dose of 750 mg (75 kg patient) would be translated to an initial dose of 1060–1260 mg. For an orally administered drug, the dosage will likely be based on the available formulation, while for intravenously administered drugs the vial size and drug cost (use two 500 mg vials instead of wasting a third vial to deliver the 60 mg marginal dose) will be factored into the dose selection. The third alternative is to create dosing recommendations that include a range such as 7.5–10 mg/kg with the caveat that lower mg/kg doses are required in bigger patients. So if 7.5 mg/kg were selected instead of 10 mg/kg, the dose in the 150 kg patient would be computed as 1125 mg (well within the expected range).

As shown above, a reasonable approach would be to use the empiric population average dose (that is expected to be based on a 60–90 kg individual) and increase that dose by at least 50 % (40–70 %) for an individual that is up to twice that size (120–180 kg). So an average initial antimicrobial dose of 500 mg could be empirically and reasonably translated to 750 mg in an extremely obese patient. If a patient is up to three times (180–270 kg) the size of an average patient then doubling the average dose (1000 mg) would be reasonable. The aforementioned dose increment of cefazolin from 2 to 3 g is a clear example of this principle [56]. The subsequent maintenance doses require consideration of physiologic clearance mechanisms that may be patient and extrinsic factor dependent. Ultimately, body size may explain some but not all of the interindividual variability of a given PK parameter [62]. However, in the absence of alternate objective clinical measures, initial dose selection based on this general approach is not an unreasonable starting point.

7 Obesity and Maintenance Dose Selection

Selection of an optimal maintenance dose of an antimicrobial is dependent on individual drug CL. Interindividual variability in drug CL is a function of numerous variables such as age, sex, weight, kidney function, liver function, drug–drug interactions, drug–food interactions, and pharmacogenomic polymorphisms [63]. More recently, the gut microbiome (or more broadly the metagenome) is recognized to influence drug metabolism and body size that may impact dose selection [64, 65]. As listed above, these covariates can be delineated as modifiable (e.g., kidney function) and non-modifiable (age, sex, pharmacogenomics polymorphisms, etc.) parameters. Estimates of kidney function incorporate the parameters of age, sex, and weight and so serve as composite variable that often predicts the CL of antimicrobials that are eliminated by the kidneys [62]. Liver function is a more difficult parameter to objectively quantify and so closer attention is required when considering the antimicrobial metabolic pathway. To date, obesity has primarily been shown to affect the cytochrome P450 (CYP) 2E1 isoenzymes system that is not a major pathway of drug metabolism [66, 67]. Higher drug CL values have been documented with other CYP systems but this average change is not substantially above that expected from simple allometric scaling [67]. Higher drug CL values have been shown for substrates of CYP2C9 and CYP2C19 in obese subjects [67]. However, these isoenzymes systems are known to demonstrate significant genetic polymorphisms that make the association between obesity and the function of CYP2C9 and CYP2C19 spurious [68].

Let us take the example of the antifungal voriconazole, an agent with highly unpredictable PK that is metabolized in part by CYP2C19 [69]. Several loss of function (LoF *1 to *10) alleles and a one gain of function (GoF *17) allele has been reported in the literature to date [70]. Recent surveillance of the "normal" or the population dominant profile among white ($n = 357$), African American ($n = 149$), Hispanic ($n = 346$), and Ashkenazi Jewish ($n = 342$) patients indicated that 39–58 % have the CYP2C19*1/*1 genotype [70]. About 24 % of individuals in this survey carried a *17 allele (extensive metabolizers) and 3.1 % carried two *17 alleles with no deficiency alleles (ultrarapid metabolizers) [70]. As expected, the exposure of voriconazole for a given dose will be significantly lower in individuals with CYP2C19 GoF alleles relative to those with LoF alleles. Population PK analysis of voriconazole has shown that current dosing regimens result in subtherapeutic exposures in patients that do not have CYP2C19 LoF alleles [71]. The dosing of this agent is currently recommended based on weight and as a fixed dose regimen [72]. Body size has no direct relationship to the CYP2C19 phenotype hence dosing on this parameter cannot ensure adequate exposure. Obese patients should not have dose adjustments made to voriconazole simply on body size [72]. Similarly, simply characterizing an individual genotype does not guarantee a predictable phenotype in the clinical milieu of drug–drug interactions. As an example, omeprazole is a potent inhibitor of CYP2C9 and CYP2C19 that can boost the concentrations of voriconazole in patients that may have CYP2C19 GoF alleles to essentially have a profile that is consistent with the "normal" wild-type phenotype [73]. Hence, the "essential role of TDM" is now recognized as the only way to ensure that the maintenance dose of voriconazole is correct in any given patients irrespective of their body size [71].

In contrast to liver function assessment, kidney function can be objectively quantified to provide an estimate of the glomerular filtration rate (GFR). Drug clearance mechanisms are also dependent on renal tubular secretion and reabsorption [74]. Various renal tubular transporters of the solute like carrier and ATPase Binding Cassette families have been identified but their role and functional changes in the setting of obesity are not well known [75, 76]. To date limited influence of obesity on renal tubular transport has been shown relative to the more easily measurable effects of obesity on GFR [68, 69]. Tubular secretion (organic anion transporter) of the activated form of the antiviral agent oseltamivir (carboxylate metabolite) plays a major role in the elimination of this agent through urine [77]. Several studies have now shown that the CL of this agent is not enhanced in obese adults [78–81]. This is consistent with the observation in animal models of diet induced obesity that have shown reduced organic anion transport in the liver but not the kidneys [82]. Kidney biopsy data from obese (non-diabetic) subjects show a 94 % higher Bowman's space volume, and a 33 % higher cross-sectional area of the proximal tubular epithelium [83]. These changes in renal histology can be attributed to glomerular hyperfiltration in the extremely obese population. In these comparisons the average GFR is 1.62-fold higher despite an approximately twofold change in body size (137 kg versus 70 kg adult) that is consistent with allometry [84]. Hence scaling kidney function to total body weight will overestimate the GFR in obese patients [60].

Similar to selection of alternate body size descriptors to dose antimicrobials, these descriptors have been used to scale the estimate of kidney function [60]. A single point measurement of the endogenous biomarker serum creatinine is used to estimate GFR (staging disease) or creatinine clearance (CLcr) for drug dosing. The critical point to recognize is that use of serum creatinine in this manner leads to a cross-sectional "estimate" of kidney function even if urine is collected to "measure" CLcr. Measurement and translation of serum creatinine to CLcr relies on the major assumption that the rate of production and rate of elimination of this byproduct of skeletal muscle metabolism is under homeostasis. Patients that are acutely infected or have had traumatic injuries are not under a stable homeostatic state. As a consequence translation of serum creatinine to CLcr is fundamentally limited. This point estimate of kidney function is a snapshot in time of an estimate of kidney function that may or may not reflect the evolving kidney function in an acutely ill patient.

With this point in mind, clinical trials that ultimately define the dose of an antimicrobial rely on a population level defined dose that should maximize the probability of effect and minimize the probability of toxicity. Dose modification for kidney function is typically based on the PK evaluation of a cohort of non-infected individual with renal impairment [74]. This method of study leads to the dose recommendations that may suggest dose reduction when the point estimate of CLcr is below a specific threshold such as <60 mL/min. So as an example a dose of 250 mg may be recommended in patients with CLcr <60 mL/min to match the average AUC in adults with CLcr ≥60 mL/min dosed with 500 mg/day [74]. The mathematical model that often relates CLcr to drug CL can be a nonlinear (power function) or a linear function (slope and intercept). The relationship of CLcr to drug CL is continuous but is stratified into categories by PK modelers to simplify the dose selection process [74]. Unfortunately, these models are not used to project doses above the average range, i.e., should the dose be increased for a sub-population of patients with CLcr >120 mL/min as an example? If obese patients have higher GFR or if this renal function augmented during acute illness should they not require higher doses [85, 86]? The answer is obviously yes [87–89]. The problem is that we lack clinical tools such as TDM or systems to measure (and not estimate) GFR with exogenous substrates to make that judgment for an individual patient.

As a consequence the maintenance dose that is selected for a given patient should be based on the acuity of illness, type of infection, and clinical judgment on the evolving nature of the medical case. If the patient is critically ill, then the risk of preventing underexposure outweighs the risk of overexposure. The potential degree of renal function augmentation could be discerned through alternate means. Research groups have shown that aminoglycoside CL closely reflects GFR [90, 91]. Because TDM is widely applied to dose aminoglycosides, the information gained from this assessment could serve as a pharmacologic biomarker of augmented kidney function. This approach has recently been applied to improve the dosing of beta-lactams by using information gained from TDM of amikacin in patients treated in the Intensive Care Unit setting [92]. In the absence of TDM, pharmacologic biomarkers, easily measurable responses, or product label guidance, the selection of the maintenance dose in an obese individual is left to clinical intuition.

In the case of an SSTI such as cellulitis, a lack of clear response within 48–72 h of therapy would prompt clinical consideration of the use of higher maintenance dose or an alternate agent. As an example, selection of a 600 mg every 8 h regimen of linezolid is reasonable if an obese adult does not appear to be responding after 48 h of therapy at an acceptable rate with the standard 600 mg every 12 h regimen. We do not perform TDM to optimize the dose of linezolid because an assay to measure this agent is not readily available (as is the case for most drugs). Ironically, population PK models that have evaluated linezolid have demonstrated that the interindividual variability in the PK of this agent is far greater than that observed with vancomycin and aminoglycosides that suggests TDM may be necessary [93]. Similarly, selection of higher weight based regimens of agents such as daptomycin will in theory lead to higher exposures in obese patients [87]. Recent data suggest that the CL of daptomycin may be augmented and return to a "normal" state over time in the critically ill [87–89]. The presence of such a physiologic phenomenon would imply that the maintenance dose should be temporarily increased for the first 72–96 h and then returned to normal doses after this period [88, 89]. Evaluation of this titrated maintenance dosing strategy is often not studied through prospective clinical trial design. However, it represents an important consideration for drug dosing that is independent of body size as the sole consideration of antimicrobial dose selection.

8 Obesity and Specifying Antimicrobial Dosage Recommendations

Obesity is not recognized by regulatory bodies as a "special population" to mandate Phase I pharmacokinetic studies in this population to ensure that the dosing paradigm is correct [38, 94]. Additionally, specific guidelines to mandate post hoc analysis of Phase 3 studies that likely include obese relative to nonobese study participants do not currently exist [38]. Hence a potential signal for poor outcomes (safety or efficacy) in this population may not be apparent until the antimicrobial is used in the general population of obese patients. This should be unacceptable to the public because at least a third of the adult population meet the definition of obesity [3]. This issue is not limited to antimicrobials and perhaps is of greater concern for agents with a low therapeutic index such as cancer chemotherapy agents and anticoagulants [38]. Hence specific dose recommendations that may be derived from small pharmacokinetic studies are useful to identify a "signal" but cannot reflect the full picture that would be derived from large prospective randomized controlled trials.

Given that this review is focused on antimicrobials, we should reflect on the key point that few novel antibiotics have been introduced in the USA since 1980. These novel antibiotics include linezolid, telithromycin, ertapenem, daptomycin, doripenem, tigecycline, telavancin, ceftaroline fosamil, fidaxomicin, and bedaquiline [95].

Currently, product label recommendations for dosing of these newer agents in obesity only exist for daptomycin, where no specific adjustment for obesity is recommended. However, the population PK model that is the basis of the dosing of this agent at a 4 mg/kg basis did not demonstrate an independent relationship between drug CL and weight [96]. The clearance of daptomycin was higher in patients with active infection relative to healthy volunteers and this relationship was modeled in part as a function of body temperature. Literature generated post-approval of this agent has shown: (1) the CL of this agent to not increase in proportion to total body weight; (2) the CL of this agent may be altered during acute illness; and (3) use of a fixed dose may reduce interindividual variability in daptomycin AUC than weight based dosing [89]. The natural solution to correct this potential mislabeled approach to dosing daptomycin would be the prospective comparison of a fixed dosing regimen to weight based dosing. However, there is no incentive to a manufacturer to retract a specific dosing paradigm especially when the patent life of that agent is likely to sunset before this information enters the public space.

Very similar to this discordant dosing scenario is the case of telavancin dosing. In preclinical trials of telavancin, doses of ≥50 mg/kg/day in rats and of ≥25 mg/kg/day in dogs were associated with renal injury [97]. These doses in animals represented a human dose equivalent of 8 mg/kg/day (allometry based on the rat) and 13.5 mg/kg/day (allometry based on the dog) that is well within the currently approved human dose of 10 mg/kg/day. These projections led the US FDA clinical pharmacology reviewer to conclude, "The significant nonclinical toxicity findings (renal, hepatic, and reproductive toxicities) observed with systemic exposure levels to the drug similar to those seen in clinical studies suggest that clinical use of the drug may not be safe" [97] Given that this drug is dosed on body weight, dosing obese patients on a 10 mg/kg/day basis should lead to higher exposures because drug CL does not increase in proportion to total body weight. Post hoc analysis demonstrated that renal events occurred at a rate that was approximately threefold higher in patients with SSTI treated with telavancin if their BMI ≥ 35 kg/m^2 compared to patients with BMI < 35 kg/m^2 [98]. Higher rates of renal adverse events have also been observed in clinical practice, and the potential basis for this observation has been published [99, 100]. Despite clear evidence to suggest that telavancin dosing may not be PD bioequivalent when dosed on a weight basis in obese adults, no further studies or changes in the labeling of this agent have occurred since its regulatory approval. An incentive to mandate a labeling change or further studies can only occur through public advocacy or from societies responsible for establishing guidelines for drug dosing in the public interest [38].

Several reviews exist in the literature on the dosing of drugs in obesity including specific reviews on antimicrobials [66, 67, 101–103]. Over the past decade, specific studies have been performed to characterize the PK of antimicrobials in this population [66, 67]. These studies have involved the evaluation of small cohorts of healthy volunteers and have in large part supported and in some cases challenged the existing dosing paradigm. Whether or not these studies are sufficient to be translatable from healthy obese volunteers to infected obese patients is less clear. Further work in this domain is clearly needed to ensure that dosing recommendations that are suggested in this population are based on a systematic evaluation of the data to date that integrate outcome related information [104]. A specific consensus panel of experts that can critically review the available literature in this domain should be convened to establish dosage recommendations for specific antimicrobials in this now common population of obese patients.

9 Summary and Future Directions

Obesity is a global phenomenon that has exploded in prevalence due to increased access to energy rich diets and sedentary lifestyles. This modification in the human weight distribution has directly impacted our dosing paradigm which in the case of antimicrobials has in part been based on weight. We expect obese patients to require larger doses but recognize that defining maintenance doses on total body weight to not be bioequivalent by PK-PD analysis. An array of alternate body size descriptors have been developed over time to correct for this overestimation problem with total body weight dosing. These body size descriptors obey principles that are aligned with simple allometry. A universal approach to antimicrobial dosing cannot be established because the pharmacodynamic characteristics of the agent may or may not be significantly impacted by body size. Most product labels do not provide guidance for antimicrobial dosing in obesity. Clinical trials with newer antimicrobial agents are likely to include or have included obese patients that create an opportunity to model and simulate alternate dosing approaches in this population. Specific recommendations for antimicrobial dosing can only be established through consensus guidance with endorsement from international societies that advocate for the appropriate use of antimicrobials.

References

1. World Health Organization Media Centre (2013) Obesity and overweight. http://www.who.int/mediacentre/factsheets/fs311/en/. Accessed 25 Apr 2014
2. WHO Global Infobase: data on overweight and obesity, mean BMI, healthy diets and physical inactivity (2011). https://apps.who.int/infobase/. Accessed 25 Apr 2014
3. Ogden CL, Carroll MD, Kit BK, Flegal KM (2014) Prevalence of childhood and adult obesity in the United States, 2011–2012. JAMA 311:806–814. doi:10.1001/jama.2014.732
4. Clinical guidelines on the identification, evaluation, and treatment of overweight and obesity in adults: the evidence report (1998). http://www.nhlbi.nih.gov/guidelines/obesity/ob_gdlns.htm. Accessed 25 Apr 2014
5. Obesity (2014). http://en.wikipedia.org/wiki/Obesity. Accessed 25 Apr 2014
6. Ogden CL, Fryar CD, Carroll MD et al (2004) Mean body weight, height, and body mass index, United States 1960–2002. Adv Data 347:1–17
7. Guinness World Records (2014). http://www.guinnessworldrecords.com/world-records/3000/heaviest-man. Accessed 25 Apr 2014
8. From the NIH: Successful diet and exercise therapy is conducted in Vermont for "diabesity" (1980). JAMA 243:519–520

9. Marrs CC, Moussa HN, Sibai BM, Blackwell SC (2014) The relationship between primary cesarean delivery skin incision type and wound complications in women with morbid obesity. Am J Obstet Gynecol 210:319.e1–e4. doi:10.1016/j.ajog.2014.01.018
10. Mehta AI, Babu R, Sharma R, Karikari IO, Grunch BH, Owens TR et al (2013) Thickness of subcutaneous fat as a risk factor for infection in cervical spine fusion surgery. J Bone Joint Surg Am 95:323–328. doi:10.2106/JBJS.L.00225
11. Early GJ, Seifried SE (2012) Risk factors for community-associated *Staphylococcus aureus* skin infection in children of Maui. Hawaii J Med Public Health 71:218–223
12. Thornburg LL, Linder MA, Durie DE, Walker B, Pressman EK, Glantz JC (2012) Risk factors for wound complications in morbidly obese women undergoing primary cesarean delivery. J Matern Fetal Neonatal Med 25:1544–1548. doi:10.3109/14767058.2011.653422
13. Mehta AI, Babu R, Karikari IO, Grunch B, Agarwal VJ, Owens TR et al (2012) 2012 Young Investigator Award winner: The distribution of body mass as a significant risk factor for lumbar spinal fusion postoperative infections. Spine (Phila Pa 1976) 37:1652–1656. doi:10.1097/BRS.0b013e318241b186
14. Patel GA, Wiederkehr M, Schwartz RA (2009) Tinea cruris in children. Cutis 84:133–137
15. Araco A, Zaccheddu R, Araco F, Gravante G (2008) Methicillin-resistant superinfection of the wound after body-contouring abdominal surgery. Aesthetic Plast Surg 32:681–683. doi:10.1007/s00266-008-9177-z
16. Karppelin M, Siljander T, Vuopio-Varkila J, Kere J, Huhtala H, Vuento R, Jussila T, Syrjänen J (2010) Factors predisposing to acute and recurrent bacterial non-necrotizing cellulitis in hospitalized patients: a prospective case-control study. Clin Microbiol Infect 16:729–734. doi:10.1111/j.1469-0691.2009.02906
17. Bartholomeeusen S, Vandenbroucke J, Truyers C, Buntinx F (2007) Epidemiology and comorbidity of erysipelas in primary care. Dermatology 215:118–122
18. Yosipovitch G, DeVore A, Dawn A (2007) Obesity and the skin: skin physiology and skin manifestations of obesity. J Am Acad Dermatol 56:901–916
19. Janniger CK, Schwartz RA, Szepietowski JC, Reich A (2005) Intertrigo and common secondary skin infections. Am Fam Physician 72:833–838
20. Sebbane M, Claret PG, Lefebvre S, Mercier G, Rubenovitch J, Jreige R et al (2013) Predicting peripheral venous access difficulty in the emergency department using body mass index and a clinical evaluation of venous accessibility. J Emerg Med 44:299–305. doi:10.1016/j.jemermed.2012.07.051
21. Dargin JM, Emlet LL, Guyette FX (2013) The effect of body mass index on intubation success rates and complications during emergency airway management. Intern Emerg Med 8:75–82. doi:10.1007/s11739-012-0874-x
22. Lewis GC, Crapo SA, Williams JG (2013) Critical skills and procedures in emergency medicine: vascular access skills and procedures. Emerg Med Clin North Am 31:59–86. doi:10.1016/j.emc.2012.09.006
23. Dossett LA, Dageforde LA, Swenson BR, Metzger R, Bonatti H, Sawyer RG, May AK (2009) Obesity and site-specific nosocomial infection risk in the intensive care unit. Surg Infect (Larchmt) 10:137–142. doi:10.1089/sur.2008.028
24. Prescott HC, Chang VW, O'Brien JM Jr, Langa KM, Iwashyna T (2014) Obesity and 1-year outcomes in older Americans with severe sepsis. Crit Care Med 42(8):1766–1774
25. Tremblay A, Bandi V (2003) Impact of body mass index on outcomes following critical care. Chest 123:1202–1207
26. Kuperman EF, Showalter JW, Lehman EB, Leib AE, Kraschnewski JL (2013) The impact of obesity on sepsis mortality: a retrospective review. BMC Infect Dis 13:377
27. Nie W, Zhang Y, Jee SH, Jung KJ, Li B, Xiu Q (2014) Obesity survival paradox in pneumonia: a meta-analysis. BMC Med 12:61
28. de Heredia FP, Gómez-Martínez S, Marcos A (2012) Obesity, inflammation and the immune system. Proc Nutr Soc 71:332–338. doi:10.1017/S0029665112000092
29. Al-Suhaimi EA, Shehzad A (2013) Leptin, resistin and visfatin: the missing link between endocrine metabolic disorders and immunity. Eur J Med Res 18:12. doi:10.1186/2047-783X-18-12
30. Almond MH, Edwards MR, Barclay WS, Johnston SL (2013) Obesity and susceptibility to severe outcomes following respiratory viral infection. Thorax 68:684–686. doi:10.1136/thoraxjnl-2012-203009
31. Louie JK, Acosta M, Samuel MC, Schechter R, Vugia DJ, Harriman K, Matyas BT,

California Pandemic (H1N1) Working Group (2011) A novel risk factor for a novel virus: obesity and 2009 pandemic influenza A (H1N1). Clin Infect Dis 52:301–312. doi:10.1093/cid/ciq152

32. Díaz E, Rodríguez A, Martin-Loeches I, Lorente L, del Mar Martín M, Pozo JC, H1N1 SEMICYUC Working Group et al (2011) Impact of obesity in patients infected with 2009 influenza A (H1N1). Chest 139:382–386. doi:10.1378/chest.10-1160

33. Yu H, Feng Z, Uyeki TM, Liao Q, Zhou L, Feng L, Ye M, Xiang N, Huai Y, Yuan Y, Jiang H, Zheng Y, Gargiullo P, Peng Z, Feng Y, Zheng J, Xu C, Zhang Y, Shu Y, Gao Z, Yang W, Wang Y (2011) Risk factors for severe illness with 2009 pandemic influenza A (H1N1) virus infection in China. Clin Infect Dis 52:457–465. doi:10.1093/cid/ciq144

34. Karlsson EA, Sheridan PA, Beck MA (2010) Diet-induced obesity impairs the T cell memory response to influenza virus infection. J Immunol 184:3127–3133. doi:10.4049/jimmunol.0903220

35. Zakhari S (2013) Bermuda Triangle for the liver: alcohol, obesity, and viral hepatitis. J Gastroenterol Hepatol 28(Suppl 1):18–25. doi:10.1111/jgh.12207

36. Negro F, Clément S (2009) Impact of obesity, steatosis and insulin resistance on progression and response to therapy of hepatitis C. J Viral Hepat 16:681–688. doi:10.1111/j.1365-2893.2009.01186.x

37. Ahasic AM, Zhao Y, Su L, Sheu CC, Thompson BT, Christiani DC (2014) Adiponectin genepolymorphisms and acute respiratory distress syndrome susceptibility and mortality. PLoS One 9(2):e89170. doi:10.1371/journal.pone.0089170

38. Pai MP (2012) Drug dosing based on weight and body surface area: mathematical assumptions and limitations in obese adults. Pharmacotherapy 32:856–868. doi:10.1002/j.1875-9114.2012.01108.x

39. Drugs@FDA Database. US Food and Drug Administration (2014) Levaquin label. http://www.accessdata.fda.gov/scripts/cder/drugsatfda/index.cfm. Accessed 25 Apr 2014

40. Drugs@FDA Database. US Food and Drug Administration (2014) Copegus label. http://www.accessdata.fda.gov/scripts/cder/drugsatfda/index.cfm. Accessed 25 Apr 2014

41. Drugs@FDA Database. US Food and Drug Administration (2014) Vibativ label. http://www.accessdata.fda.gov/scripts/cder/drugsatfda/index.cfm. Accessed 25 Apr 2014

42. Drugs@FDA Database. US Food and Drug Administration (2014) Vancomycin hydrochloride label. http://www.accessdata.fda.gov/scripts/cder/drugsatfda/index.cfm. Accessed 25 April 2014

43. Rybak MJ, Lomaestro BM, Rotschafer JC, Moellering R, Craig W, Billeter M et al (2009) Vancomycin therapeutic guidelines: a summary of consensus recommendations from the Infectious Diseases Society of America, the American Society of Health-System Pharmacists, and the Society of Infectious Diseases Pharmacists. Am J Health Syst Pharm 66:82–98

44. Craig WA (1998) Pharmacokinetic/pharmacodynamic parameters: rationale for antibacterial dosing of mice and men. Clin Infect Dis 26:1–10

45. Martinez MN, Papich MG, Drusano GL (2012) Dosing regimen matters: the importance of early intervention and rapid attainment of the pharmacokinetic/pharmacodynamic target. Antimicrob Agents Chemother 56:2795–2805. doi:10.1128/AAC.05360-11

46. Ho VP, Nicolau DP, Dakin GF, Pomp A, Rich BS, Towe CW, Barie PS (2012) Cefazolin dosing for surgical prophylaxis in morbidly obese patients. Surg Infect (Larchmt) 13:33–37. doi:10.1089/sur.2010.097

47. Toma O, Suntrup P, Stefanescu A, London A, Mutch M, Kharasch E (2011) Pharmacokinetics and tissue penetration of cefoxitin in obesity: implications for risk of surgical site infection. Anesth Analg 113:730–737. doi:10.1213/ANE.0b013e31821fff74

48. Pevzner L, Swank M, Krepel C, Wing DA, Chan K, Edmiston CE Jr (2011) Effects of maternal obesity on tissue concentrations of prophylactic cefazolin during cesarean delivery. Obstet Gynecol 117:877–882. doi:10.1097/AOG.0b013e31820b95e4

49. Barbour A, Schmidt S, Rout WR, Ben-David K, Burkhardt O, Derendorf H (2009) Soft tissue penetration of cefuroxime determined by clinical microdialysis in morbidly obese patients undergoing abdominal surgery. Int J Antimicrob Agents 34:231–235. doi:10.1016/j.ijantimicag.2009.03.019

50. Adams F, Jordan J, Schaller K, Luft FC, Boschmann M (2005) Blood flow in subcutaneous adipose tissue depends on skin-fold thickness. Horm Metab Res 37:68–73

51. Thallinger C, Buerger C, Plock N, Kljucar S, Wuenscher S, Sauermann R et al (2008)

Effect of severity of sepsis on tissue concentrations of linezolid. J Antimicrob Chemother 61:173–176

52. Rodvold KA, Gotfried MH, Cwik M, Korth-Bradley JM, Dukart G, Ellis-Grosse EJ (2006) Serum, tissue and body fluid concentrations of tigecycline after a single 100 mg dose. J Antimicrob Chemother 58:1221–1229
53. Plock N, Kloft C (2005) Microdialysis—theoretical background and recent implementation in applied life-sciences. Eur J Pharm Sci 25:1–24
54. Brill MJ, Houwink AP, Schmidt S, Van Dongen EP, Hazebroek EJ, van Ramshorst B et al (2014) Reduced subcutaneous tissue distribution of cefazolin in morbidly obese versus non-obese patients determined using clinical microdialysis. J Antimicrob Chemother 69:715–723. doi:10.1093/jac/dkt444
55. Bratzler DW, Dellinger EP, Olsen KM, Perl TM, Auwaerter PG, Bolon MK, American Society of Health-System Pharmacists; Infectious Disease Society of America; Surgical Infection Society; Society for Healthcare Epidemiology of America et al (2013) Clinical practice guidelines for antimicrobial prophylaxis in surgery. Am J Health Syst Pharm 70:195–283. doi:10.2146/ajhp120568
56. de Werra C, Di Micco R, Pilone V, Formato A, Montella E, Lambiase A et al (2013) Serum in vivo and in vitro activity of single dose of ertapenem in surgical obese patients for prevention of SSIs. Obes Surg 23:911–919. doi:10.1007/s11695-013-0879-1
57. Sauermann R, Burian B, Burian A, Jäger W, Höferl M, Stella A et al (2013) Tissue pharmacokinetics of ertapenem at steady-state in diabetic patients with leg infections. J Antimicrob Chemother 68:895–899. doi:10.1093/jac/dks479
58. Steier J, Lunt A, Hart N, Polkey MI, Moxham J (2014) Observational study of the effect of obesity on lung volumes. Thorax. doi:10.1136/thoraxjnl-2014-205148
59. Avriel A, Warner E, Avinoach E, Avnon LS, Shteinberg M, Shteinberg D et al (2012) Major respiratory adverse events after laparoscopic gastric banding surgery for morbid obesity. Respir Med 106:1192–1198. doi:10.1016/j.rmed.2012.05.002
60. Pai MP (2010) Estimating the glomerular filtration rate in obese adult patients for drug dosing. Adv Chronic Kidney Dis 17(5):e53–e62. doi:10.1053/j.ackd.2010.05.010
61. Mahmood I (2010) Theoretical versus empirical allometry: facts behind theories and application to pharmacokinetics. J Pharm Sci 99:2927–2933. doi:10.1002/jps.22073
62. Bonate PL (2006) Nonlinear mixed effects models: practical issues. In: Bonate PL (ed) Pharmacokinetic-pharmacodynamic modeling and simulation. Springer, New York, pp 267–307
63. Guidance for Industry. Population Pharmacokinetics. U.S. Department of Health and Human Services (1999) http://www.fda.gov/downloads/ScienceResearch/SpecialTopics/WomensHealthResearch/UCM133184.pdf. Accessed 25 Apr 2014
64. Kang MJ, Kim HG, Kim JS, Oh do G, Um YJ, Seo CS et al (2013) The effect of gut microbiota on drug metabolism. Expert Opin Drug Metab Toxicol 9:1295–1308. doi:10.1517/17425255.2013.807798
65. Burcelin R, Serino M, Chabo C, Garidou L, Pomié C, Courtney M et al (2013) Metagenome and metabolism: the tissue microbiota hypothesis. Diabetes Obes Metab 15(Suppl 3):61–70. doi:10.1111/dom.12157
66. Hanley MJ, Abernethy DR, Greenblatt DJ (2010) Effect of obesity on the pharmacokinetics of drugs in humans. Clin Pharmacokinet 49:71–87. doi:10.2165/11318100-000000000-00000
67. Brill MJ, Diepstraten J, van Rongen A, van Kralingen S, van den Anker JN, Knibbe CA (2012) Impact of obesity on drug metabolism and elimination in adults and children. Clin Pharmacokinet 51:277–304. doi:10.2165/11599410-000000000-00000
68. Wijnen PA, Op den Buijsch RA, Drent M, Kuijpers PM, Neef C, Bast A et al (2007) Review article: The prevalence and clinical relevance of cytochrome P450 polymorphisms. Aliment Pharmacol Ther 26(Suppl 2):211–219. doi:10.1111/j.1365-2036.2007.03490.x
69. Theuretzbacher U, Ihle F, Derendorf H (2006) Pharmacokinetic/pharmacodynamic profile of voriconazole. Clin Pharmacokinet 45:649–663
70. Strom CM, Goos D, Crossley B, Zhang K, Buller-Burkle A, Jarvis M et al (2012) Testing for variants in CYP2C19: population frequencies and testing experience in a clinical laboratory. Genet Med 14:95–100. doi:10.1038/gim.0b013e3182329870
71. Dolton MJ, Mikus G, Weiss J, Ray JE, McLachlan AJ (2014) Understanding variability with voriconazole using a population pharmacokinetic approach: implications for optimal dosing. J Antimicrob Chemother 69:1633–1641

72. Pai MP, Lodise TP (2011) Steady-state plasma pharmacokinetics of oral voriconazole in obese adults. Antimicrob Agents Chemother 55:2601–2605. doi:10.1128/AAC.01765-10
73. Boyd NK, Zoellner CL, Swancutt MA, Bhavan KP (2012) Utilization of omeprazole to augment subtherapeutic voriconazole concentrations for treatment of Aspergillus infections. Antimicrob Agents Chemother 56:6001–6002. doi:10.1128/AAC.00700-12
74. Rowland Yeo K, Aarabi M, Jamei M, Rostami-Hodjegan A (2011) Modeling and predicting drug pharmacokinetics in patients with renal impairment. Expert Rev Clin Pharmacol 4:261–274. doi:10.1586/ecp.10.143
75. Pelis RM, Wright SH (2011) Renal transport of organic anions and cations. Compr Physiol 1:1795–1835. doi:10.1002/cphy.c100084
76. Perri D, Ito S, Rowsell V, Shear NH (2003) The kidney—the body's playground for drugs: an overview of renal drug handling with selected clinical correlates. Can J Clin Pharmacol 10(1):17–23
77. He G, Massarella J, Ward P (1999) Clinical pharmacokinetics of the prodrug oseltamivir and its active metabolite Ro 64-0802. Clin Pharmacokinet 37:471–484
78. Ariano RE, Sitar DS, Zelenitsky SA, Zarychanski R, Pisipati A, Ahern S et al (2010) Enteric absorption and pharmacokinetics of oseltamivir in critically ill patients with pandemic (H1N1) influenza. CMAJ 182:357–363. doi:10.1503/cmaj.092127
79. Thorne-Humphrey LM, Goralski KB, Slayter KL, Hatchette TF, Johnston BL, McNeil SA, 2009 OPTIMO Study Group (2011) Oseltamivir pharmacokinetics in morbid obesity (OPTIMO trial). J Antimicrob Chemother 66:2083–2091. doi:10.1093/jac/dkr257
80. Pai MP, Lodise TP Jr (2011) Oseltamivir and oseltamivir carboxylate pharmacokinetics in obese adults: dose modification for weight is not necessary. Antimicrob Agents Chemother 55:5640–5645. doi:10.1128/AAC.00422-11
81. Jittamala P, Pukrittayakamee S, Tarning J, Lindegardh N, Hanpithakpong W, Taylor WR et al (2014) Pharmacokinetics of orally administered oseltamivir in healthy obese and nonobese Thai subjects. Antimicrob Agents Chemother 58:1615–1621
82. More VR, Slitt AL (2011) Alteration of hepatic but not renal transporter expression in diet-induced obese mice. Drug Metab Dispos 39:992–999. doi:10.1124/dmd.110.037507
83. Tobar A, Ori Y, Benchetrit S, Milo G, Herman-Edelstein M, Zingerman B et al (2013) Proximal tubular hypertrophy and enlarged glomerular and proximal tubular urinary space in obese subjects with proteinuria. PLoS One 8:e75547. doi:10.1371/journal.pone.0075547
84. Chagnac A, Herman M, Zingerman B, Erman A, Rozen-Zvi B, Hirsh J, Gafter U (2008) Obesity-induced glomerular hyperfiltration: its involvement in the pathogenesis of tubular sodium reabsorption. Nephrol Dial Transplant 23:3946–3952. doi:10.1093/ndt/gfn379
85. Udy AA, Baptista JP, Lim NL, Joynt GM, Jarrett P, Wockner L, Boots RJ, Lipman J (2014) Augmented renal clearance in the ICU: results of a multicenter observational study of renal function in critically ill patients with normal plasma creatinine concentrations. Crit Care Med 42:520–527. doi:10.1097/CCM.0000000000000029
86. Udy AA, Roberts JA, Boots RJ, Paterson DL, Lipman J (2010) Augmented renal clearance: implications for antibacterial dosing in the critically ill. Clin Pharmacokinet 49:1–16. doi:10.2165/11318140-000000000-00000
87. Falcone M, Russo A, Venditti M, Novelli A, Pai MP (2013) Considerations for higher doses of daptomycin in critically ill patients with methicillin-resistant Staphylococcus aureus bacteremia. Clin Infect Dis 57:1568–1576
88. Di Paolo A, Polillo M, Tascini C, Lewis R, Menichetti F, Danesi R (2014) Different recommendations for daptomycin dosing over time in patients with severe infections. Clin Infect Dis 58:1788–1789
89. Falcone M, Russo A, Venditti M, Novelli A, Pai MP (2014) Reply to Di Paolo et al. Clin Infect Dis 58:1789–1790
90. Zarowitz BJ, Robert S, Peterson EL (1992) Prediction of glomerular filtration rate using aminoglycoside clearance in critically ill medical patients. Ann Pharmacother 26:1205–1210
91. Pai MP, Nafziger AN, Bertino JS Jr (2011) Simplified estimation of aminoglycoside pharmacokinetics in underweight and obese adult patients. Antimicrob Agents Chemother 55:4006–4011. doi:10.1128/AAC.00174-11
92. Delattre IK, Musuamba FT, Jacqmin P, Taccone FS, Laterre PF, Verbeeck RK et al (2012) Population pharmacokinetics of four β-lactams in critically ill septic patients come-

dicated with amikacin. Clin Biochem 45:780–786. doi:10.1016/j.clinbiochem.2012.03.030
93. Boak LM, Rayner CR, Grayson ML, Paterson DL, Spelman D, Khumra S et al (2014) Clinical population pharmacokinetics and toxicodynamics of linezolid. Antimicrob Agents Chemother 58(4):2334–2343. doi:10.1128/AAC.01885-13
94. Edholm M, Gil Berglund E, Salmonson T (2008) Regulatory aspects of pharmacokinetic profiling in special populations: a European perspective. Clin Pharmacokinet 47:693–701
95. Bassetti M, Merelli M, Temperoni C, Astilean A (2013) New antibiotics for bad bugs: where are we? Ann Clin Microbiol Antimicrob 12:22. doi:10.1186/1476-0711-12-22
96. Dvorchik B, Arbeit RD, Chung J, Liu S, Knebel W, Kastrissios H (2004) Population pharmacokinetics of daptomycin. Antimicrob Agents Chemother 48:2799–2807
97. Drugs@FDA Database. US Food and Drug Administration (2014) Vibativ drug approval package, pharmacology reviews. http://www.accessdata.fda.gov/drugsatfda_docs/nda/2009/022110s000_PharmR.pdf. Accessed 25 Apr 2014
98. Slover CM, Nkechi A, Barriere SL et al (2011) Telavancin for treatment of complicated skin and skin structure infections in obese patients. In: Abstracts of the Fifty-first Interscience Conference on Antimicrobial Agents and Chemotherapy, Chicago, IL, Abstract L1-1491. American Society for Microbiology, Washington, DC, USA
99. Marcos LA, Camins BC, Ritchie DJ, Casabar E, Warren DK (2012) Acute renal insufficiency during telavancin therapy in clinical practice. J Antimicrob Chemother 67:723–726. doi:10.1093/jac/dkr518
100. Pai MP (2012) Comment on: Acute renal insufficiency during telavancin therapy in clinical practice. J Antimicrob Chemother 67:1300–1301. doi:10.1093/jac/dks029, author reply 1301–1302
101. Janson B, Thursky K (2012) Dosing of antibiotics in obesity. Curr Opin Infect Dis 25:634–649. doi:10.1097/QCO.0b013e328359a4c1
102. Pai MP, Bearden DT (2007) Antimicrobial dosing considerations in obese adult patients. Pharmacotherapy 27:1081–1091
103. Wurtz R, Itokazu G, Rodvold K (1997) Antimicrobial dosing in obese patients. Clin Infect Dis 25:112–118
104. Clinical Practice Guidelines We Can Trust. Institute of Medicine of the National Academies (2011) http://www.iom.edu/Reports/2011/Clinical-Practice-Guidelines-We-Can-Trust.aspx. Accessed 25 Apr 2014

Chapter 24

Drug Development Process and Regulatory Science

Evelyn J. Ellis-Grosse and Jogarao Gobburu

Abstract

The pursuit of antimicrobial drug development has been met with reluctance by many large pharmaceutical companies. In part, this has been due to the enormous resources required to meet regulatory standards, the risk of failure, and the current perception of regulatory uncertainty. This comes at a time when rates of antimicrobial resistance are on the rise across the globe, and there is a critical need for antimicrobial therapy. In this review, emphasis has been placed on the regulatory incentives to enhance antimicrobial drug development, and the value of pharmacokinetics-pharmacodynamics (PK-PD) principles from early development of an antimicrobial agent through late stage and post-approval/life cycle management strategies in accordance with recent guidelines. This demonstrates the potential to not only streamline the development process, driving down costs and time, but also improve the likelihood of regulatory success, making antibiotic drug development more viable and these needed agents available to the therapeutic armamentarium.

Key words Antibiotic drug development, FDA, EMA/ICH, In vivo modeling, PK-PD, Pharmacometrics, Regulatory initiatives

1 Regulatory Initiatives Pertinent to PK-PD

1.1 Health Authority Guidance Documents

The Food and Drug Administration (FDA), European Medicines Agency (EMA), and International Conference on Harmonisation of Technical Requirements for Registration of Pharmaceuticals for Human Use (ICH) have issued a number of guidance documents for industry to clarify for sponsors how to implement the exposure–response paradigm. The 1999 FDA Guidance for Industry on Population Pharmacokinetics discusses how to design and execute collection of sparse pharmacokinetic (PK) data from late-phase clinical trials, as well as how to analyze population pharmacokinetic data using modeling applications [1]. EMA published Guidelines on Reporting the Results of Population Pharmacokinetic Analyses [2]. In contrast to the FDA guidance on how to conduct a population PK analyses, the EMA guidance provides points to consider when presenting the results in order to provide a level of detail to enable a secondary evaluation by a regulatory assessor.

John C. Rotschafer et al. (eds.), *Antibiotic Pharmacodynamics*, Methods in Pharmacology and Toxicology,
DOI 10.1007/978-1-4939-3323-5_24, © Springer Science+Business Media New York 2016

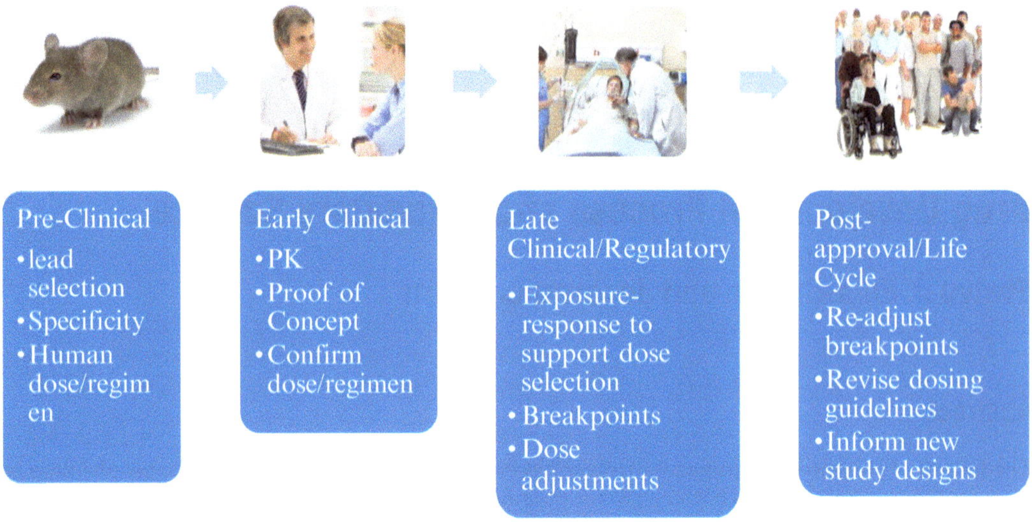

Fig. 1 Role and utility of PK-PD analyses in the various stages of drug development (preclinical through post-approval and life cycle management)

The value of understanding the exposure–response relationship has been acknowledged in several regulatory documents, such as the ICH E4: Dose Response Information to Support Drug Registration and the Guidance on Clinical Evidence of Effectiveness [3, 4]. However, it was not until 2003 that the FDA stressed the importance of exposure–response trials in regulatory decision making by issuing the Guidance for Industry on Exposure–Response Relationships [5]. Moreover, in a landmark report describing challenges and opportunities on the critical path to new medical products (the Critical Path Initiative), the FDA recognized the importance of model-based drug development as a way to improve decision making for effectiveness and safety [6]. Figure 1 presents the various phases of drug development and the role of PK-PD analyses.

1.2 Recent Initiatives

Recent initiatives and emerging regulatory considerations with respect to accelerating anti-infective drug development programs for important indications, for medical countermeasure needs, and to identify more efficient clinical endpoints are discussed in this section.

Antibiotics reflect a critical advancement in the medical arsenal not simply from a treatment point of view but also from routine surgical procedures to organ transplants and cancer treatment. Yet the pipeline of new antibiotics is abysmal. Antibiotics generate small revenue compared with "blockbuster" drugs such as those chronic therapies used for high blood pressure or cholesterol, which may be taken daily by millions of patients. Therefore, there is little incentive for manufacturers to develop new antibiotics. Many major pharmaceutical companies have abandoned their investment in developing new antibiotics and instead are focusing their resources on medicines with the potential of producing greater profits. Drug-resistant bacteria are spreading. According to a 2013 report by the Centers for Disease Control and Prevention (CDC), more than two million people develop resistant infections, and more than 23,000 die as a result [7].

The Food and Drug Administration Safety and Innovation Act (FDASIA), signed into law on July 9, 2012, expands the FDA's authorities to advance public health. Generating Antibiotic Incentives Now (GAIN), which is part of FDASIA, provides incentives for the development of antibacterial and antifungal drugs intended to treat serious and life-threatening infections [8]. Under GAIN, a sponsor may be granted a *qualified infectious disease product* (*QIDP*) designation for a drug that meets the criteria outlined in the statute. A drug that receives a QIDP designation is eligible for fast track designation and, upon submission of an NDA or supplement for that designated use, will receive a priority review. Upon approval of an application for a QIDP, a 5-year extension will be added to any exclusivity granted with that approval. This additional period of exclusivity increases the potential for profits from new antibiotics by giving innovative companies more time to recoup their investment costs. As of October 2013, there are 16 programs designated QIDP and two New Drug Applications (dalbavancin and tedizolid for acute bacterial skin and skin structure infections) submitted to FDA for review and were approved for clinical use.

FDASIA also provides FDA with a new expedited drug development tool, known as the "breakthrough therapy." This new designation helps FDA assist drug developers to expedite the development and review of new drugs with preliminary clinical evidence that indicates that the drug may offer a substantial improvement over available therapies for patients with serious or life-threatening diseases. A breakthrough therapy designation permits sponsors to engage FDA more frequently for timely advice as well as more intensive FDA guidance on an efficient drug development program. In our opinion, the latter is a more attractive offer to sponsor companies. The development program for the breakthrough therapy could be considerably shorter than for other drugs intended to treat the disease being studied. During these interactions, the agency may suggest, or a sponsor can propose, alternative clinical trial designs (e.g., adaptive designs, an enrichment strategy, use of historical controls) that may result in smaller trials or more efficient trials that require less time to complete. Such trial designs could also help minimize the number of patients exposed to a potentially less efficacious treatment (i.e., the control group treated with available therapy).

For the evaluation of new drug and biologic products as countermeasures for chemical, biological, radiological, and nuclear threats, an innovative regulatory approach was needed. The "Animal Rule" was published in 2002 which applies only "when adequate and well-controlled clinical studies in humans cannot be ethically conducted and field efficacy studies are not feasible" [9]. The importance of translational pharmacology and utility of PK-PD in this arena have been underscored by FDA for other emerging infections [10].

Efficacy endpoints for previous registrational trials of antimicrobials for acute bacterial skin and skin structure infections (ABSSSIs) and community-acquired bacterial pneumonia (CABP) were based on nonstandardized, clinician-based observations and decisions, as well as on patient reports. More quantifiable, reproducible, and externally verifiable endpoints could improve the design of future non-inferiority trials. The Foundation for the National Institutes of Health's scientific project team identified early response endpoints to anchor non-inferiority hypotheses in ABSSSI and CABP registrational trials [11]. The EMA has also shown a willingness to examine alternative methods, such as those based upon pharmacometrics, for evaluating no-treatment effect for the analysis of active comparator clinical studies: "Historical data are often used to estimate the no-treatment effect but the relevance of these data to current medical practise may be questionable. Sponsors are encouraged to explore alternative and emerging methods for estimating the no-treatment effect (e.g., using pharmacometric-based approaches)" [12]. This encourages an integrated drug development approach further underscoring a pivotal role for PK-PD approaches [13].

Traditionally, antibacterial agents have been studied in large non-inferiority clinical trials that focus on patient populations with a wide range of disease symptoms and severity. Clinical trials of disease state or site of infection (e.g., pneumonia, intra-abdominal infection) have been the focus to establish requisite safety and efficacy. However, recent alternative development and design approaches have been proposed that bring flexibility to sponsors' registrational data requirements by highlighting comprehensive pharmacologic understandings and PK-PD principles.

The four-tiered approach proposes a regulatory framework that allows either disease-based or pathogen-based label indications [14]. Such a framework is considered within the bounds of present FDA and EMA regulatory approaches, making it amenable to international harmonization [15, 16]. For this proposed approach, required data for registration would vary by tier:

- Tier A is a site of infection or disease-focused approach. Two large, well-controlled, adequately powered phase 3 clinical trials would be required for the initial indication, and data would be generated for a range of susceptible pathogens. This approach is consistent with the "traditional" paradigm for antibiotic drug development in which PK-PD is considered secondary to clinical trial data.

- Tier B intends to reduce the risks and limitations associated with smaller clinical datasets. One phase 3 study, plus small comparative and descriptive studies relying equally on the totality of data (pharmacology, microbiology, clinical trial, and PK-PD), would be generated. This approach would be well suited for broad-spectrum agents that work in a variety of mixed infection settings.
- Tier C is a pathogen-focused approach. The range of feasible studies for a less common pathogen or mechanism of resistance would be limited to small prospective comparative trials, open-label datasets, and historical data. This approach would rely equally on totality of data (pharmacology, microbiological, clinical trial, and PK-PD) and provides an approach that would be well suited for narrow-spectrum agents.
- Tier D encompasses the animal rule, as discussed previously, which is applied when acquisition of any clinical efficacy data pre-market is neither ethical nor feasible (e.g., anthrax) and there is reliance on PK-PD principles.

While this proposal brings the welcome step toward flexibility of development approaches, regulatory consensus is emerging. The recent draft guidance for industry entitled "Antibacterial Therapies for Patients With Unmet Medical Need for the Treatment of Serious Bacterial Diseases" acknowledges FDA's emerging considerations of limited data for a registrational approach [17]. Importantly, this draft guidance underscores FDA's flexibility to work with sponsors to achieve feasible studies and development programs utilizing the strengths of PK-PD to meet the urgent need of new antibiotics for the medical community.

Lastly, conduct of superiority trials for infections caused by highly antibiotic-resistant bacteria represents a new, and as yet, untested paradigm for antibacterial drug development [18, 19]. If all available therapies are inadequately effective, such as for extreme drug-resistant organisms or unacceptably toxic, superiority of an investigational agent to the comparator agent is ethical to study, since available effective therapy is not being denied to patients. Such advances in the selection of endpoints may facilitate more efficient trials and generation of better efficacy evidence.

2 Implementing a Prospective PK-PD Program

2.1 Evolution to Revolution

The regulatory environment is beginning to acknowledge that our understanding and application of PK-PD principles to that of antimicrobial drug development have evolved and grown exponentially into a reliable tool. This is largely due to the expanded utility

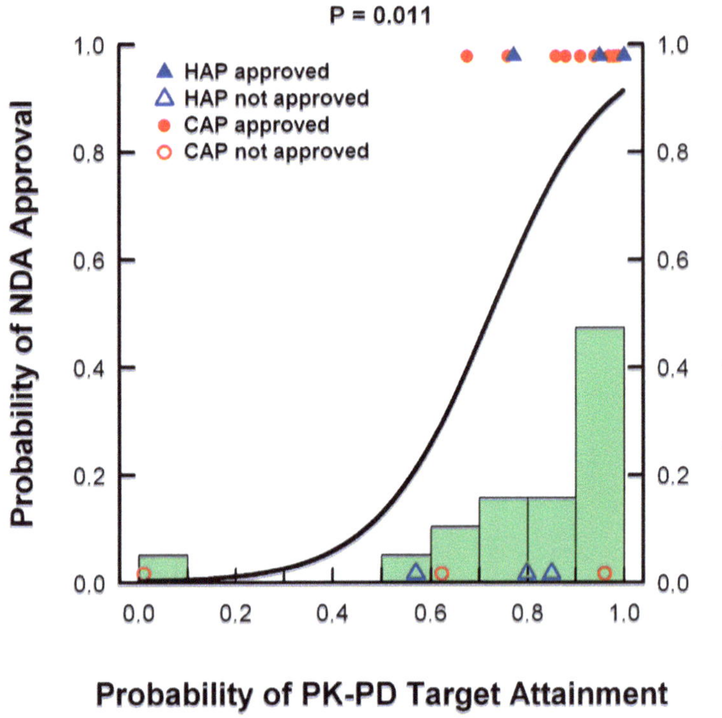

Fig. 2 Relationship between the regulatory approval and the probability of preclinical PK-PD target attainment (1996–2011) [24]

of in vitro data coupled with laboratory models of infection permitting early exploration of exposure–response relationships. A variety of laboratory evaluations exist to facilitate an understanding of the PK-PD index and the magnitude best associated with efficacy including in vitro time-kill, PAE studies, in vitro infection models, and in vivo infection models. As the major PD marker has relied on antimicrobial MIC data, these relationships have played an essential role in the identification of well-characterized PK-PD indices that are associated with efficacy for many classes of antibiotics [20–22]. Patient-derived data across multiple infectious disease indications has demonstrated concordance among relationships identified from the non-clinical studies. This knowledge evolution has led to a revolution in the application and regulatory acceptance of PK-PD analyses to antibacterial drug development [23].

PK-PD data derived from early animal models have indeed been shown to forecast the regulatory approval of an antimicrobial agent [24]. Figure 2 provides the relationship between the regulatory approval and the probability of preclinical PK-PD target attainment. In review of community- and hospital-acquired bacterial pneumonia, antibiotics were identified ($n = 17$) in which 14 received regulatory approval and 6 failed ($p = 0.011$).

Several examples of the utility of PK-PD throughout the drug development and regulatory process are available in the literature. This includes lead candidate selection and early characterization through regulatory approval and setting interpretive criteria (e.g., breakpoints), to an application for potential use of informing clinical study design. Table 1 provides a small sampling of such study exemplars demonstrating how key understandings of antimicrobial agents may evolve with the continued application throughout the different phases of antimicrobial drug development [25–40].

There has been a recent and growing appreciation of the potential value of incorporating the principles gained from nonclinical models of infection into all stages of clinical drug development for antimicrobial agents. As evidenced above, this appreciation has reached the attention of various regulatory authorities that now recommend investigations of the PK-PD relationship for antibacterial agents to be included as a driver of drug development programs. The integration of PK-PD relationships derived from

Table 1
PK-PD investigational exemplars during the phases of drug development

Phase/drug	Impact to development program
Preclinical (phase 0)	
Tigecycline [25]	Using an in vivo model (mouse thigh model), these data support the lead candidate selection and established estimates for the PK-PD indices (e.g., driver for efficacy) for future evaluation and dose selection.
Ceftolozane/ tazobactam [26]	The in vitro dose fractionation (e.g., hollow fiber model) study provided data to support the selection of ceftolozane-tazobactam dosing regimens that would minimize the potential for on-therapy drug resistance amplification.
Oritavancin [27]	Pharmacodynamic data suggested that a single dose of oritavancin at 1200 mg would be efficacious in humans. Simulation of this dose in neutropenic mice was highly effective in methicillin-sensitive *S. aureus* and MRSA thigh and bacteremia infections and pneumococcal lung infections.
P-873 [28]	From an in vivo animal infection model, these data support the lead candidate selection and established estimates for the PK-PD indices.
Early clinical	
Tigecycline [29]	These data provided estimates of the PK-PD relationship, bridging animal data to phase 1 PK obtained in healthy volunteers, underscoring the evaluation of covariates affecting the PK-PD relationship.
Fusidic acid [30]	PK-PD data provided a basis for the administration of front-loaded dosing regimens of sodium fusidate which would allow for effective concentrations to be achieved early in therapy, optimizing efficacy.
Ceftaroline [31]	Population PK data were integrated enabling a model to evaluate dose adjustments for patients with renal impairment and generate ceftaroline exposures for use in pharmacokinetic-pharmacodynamic assessments of efficacy in patients with ABSSSI or CABP.

(continued)

Table 1
(continued)

Phase/drug	Impact to development program
Late clinical/registration	
Ceftaroline [32]	These data utilized exposures in a murine infection model simulating the human dose of 600 mg i.v. every 12 h to demonstrate that the pharmacodynamic targets against MRSA and MSSA were achievable supporting the US FDA breakpoints.
Tigecycline [33]	This phase 3 exposure–response analysis supported registrational efficacy and the dosing justification for patients with complicated skin-skin structure Infections.
Linezolid [34]	This in vitro study established a pharmacodynamically optimized regimen for linezolid to treat *B. anthracis* and prevent resistance emergence at lower dosages. The authors concluded that the lower dosage for the pharmacodynamically optimized regimen may decrease drug toxicity and improve patient compliance.
Ceftaroline [35]	Results of these analyses, which suggested that in vitro susceptibility test interpretive criteria defining susceptibility, provide support for current FDA and CLSI breakpoints. Further, recommendations for dose adjustments for patients with renal impairment were also supported by the results of these analyses.
Post-approval/life cycle management	
Tigecycline [36]	These analyses demonstrate the utility of frequentist and Bayesian pharmacometric-based analyses for the determination of the estimation of "treatment effect" to inform study design using contemporary trial endpoints.
Tigecycline [37]	This analysis retrospectively focuses on the PK-PD data needed to guide dosing regimen decisions for patients with hospital-acquired bacterial pneumonia or ventilator-associated bacterial pneumonia. Early consideration of these data in development programs will reduce risk not only to sponsors but also, most importantly, to the patients enrolled in the clinical trials.
Carbapenem and ceftazidime [38]	Utilizing an in vivo infection model, data suggest carbapenems may not be a reliable treatment for treating the emerging problematic microorganisms (such as OXA-48, KPC, and NDM-1). The authors suggest that genotype may better predict the activity of the carbapenems than the phenotypic profile when selecting appropriate antimicrobial therapy.

preclinical infection models can be used to identify and select lead drug candidates and set initial efficacy targets [22, 24]. With the expansion of well-characterized models and the use of a variety of challenging bacterial strains, integration with phase 1 pharmacokinetic data provides an early opportunity to optimize antimicrobial dosing regimens for phase 2 and 3 studies [26, 36, 41, 42]. The early integration of such knowledge increases the probability of successfully selecting clinically efficacious dosing regimens for late-phase development [30] as well as an early opportunity for evaluation of patient covariates that may impact drug disposition [29] and/or the requirements for dosing modifications [31] to successfully position a phase 3 study.

A cohesive pharmacologic story utilizing PK-PD analyses of late-stage or clinical registration studies further allows for the refinement and validation of dose regimen selection decisions, including those in special patient groups (e.g., renal or hepatic impairment) [33, 34]. Importantly, the target attainment analyses have become a cornerstone for determining the susceptibility breakpoints relating outcome to the MIC of a microorganism treated in a clinical study, and also for those microorganisms anticipated in a disease state but sparsely procured [32, 35]. Indeed, for select agents (e.g., those of bioterrorism concern), no human testing may ethically be performed. Instead, animal models and PK-PD relationships are utilized to ascertain the dosing recommendations, effectiveness, and ultimate approval of a suitable antimicrobial agent [34].

Adequately positioned, PK-PD information gained throughout development programs continues to produce meaningful data. Continued reevaluation, application, and analyses from animal studies through registration studies can be utilized to support additional programs during life cycle management. In vivo infection models can renew an evaluation of existing antibiotic dosing regimens, particularly against emerging problematic organisms. This provides a cost-effective and a meaningful way to determine the continued utility of these antimicrobial agents [38]. Further, broader based applications have used PK-PD to improve the evaluation models to reduce risk associated with dosing variability in differing patient subtypes assisting drug developers in scrutinizing emerging data to improve dosing requirements in particular disease states [37]. Lastly, pharmacometric approaches are being considered of value in more contemporary study design issues. Application of Bayesian methods has demonstrated that value is the utility of PK-PD approaches to estimate a contemporary "treatment effect" to provide a more informed non-inferiority study design [36]. Further several key regulatory decisions driven by pharmacometrics strategy in the area of anti-infectives as well as other areas are well documented [37, 38] and continue to emerge [12, 17] enabling low-risk and streamlined development.

References

1. Food and Drug Administration (1999) Guidance for industry: population pharmacokinetics. www.fda.gov/downloads/Drugs/GuidanceComplianceRegulatoryInformation/Guidances/ucm072137.pdf
2. EMA (2008) Guideline on report the results of population pharmacokinetic analyses. Doc. Ref. CHMP/EWP/185990/06. http://www.ema.europa.eu/docs/en_GB/document_library/Scientific_guideline/2009/09/WC500003067.pdf
3. International Conference Harmonization (1994) E4: Dose-response information to support drug registration. www.ich.org/LOB/media/MEDIA480.pdf
4. Food and Drug Administration (1998) Guidance for industry: providing clinical evidence of effectiveness for human drug and biological products. www.fda.gov/downloads/Drugs/GuidanceComplianceRegulatoryInformation/Guidances/UCM078749.pdf

5. Food and Drug Administration (2003) Guidance for industry: exposure-response relationships – study design, data analysis, and regulatory applications. U.S. Department of Health and Human Services, Food and Drug Administration. www.fda.gov/downloads/Drugs/GuidanceComplianceRegulatoryInformation/Guidances/ucm072109.pdf
6. Food and Drug Administration (2004) FDA critical path initiatives white paper: innovation or stagnation? Challenge and opportunity on the critical path to new medical products. http://www.fda.gov/downloads/ScienceResearch/SpecialTopics/CriticalPathInitiative/CriticalPathOpportunitiesReports/UCM113411.pdf
7. U.S. Department of Health and Human Services (2013) Centers for disease control and prevention. Antibiotic resistance threats in the United States. http://www.cdc.gov/drugresistance/pdf/ar-threats-2013-508.pdf
8. Food and Drug Administration (2014) Food and drug administration safety and innovation act (FDASIA). http://www.fda.gov/RegulatoryInformation/Legislation/FederalFoodDrugandCosmeticActFDCAct/SignificantAmendmentstotheFDCAct/FDASIA/
9. Roberts R, McCune SK (2008) Animal studies in the development of medical countermeasures. Clin Pharmacol Ther 83:918–920
10. Bergman KL (2009) The animal rule and emerging infections: the role of clinical pharmacology in determining an effective dose. Clin Pharmacol Ther 86:328–331
11. Talbot GH, Powers JH, Fleming TR, Siuciak JA, Bradley J, Boucher H, on behalf of the CABP-ABSSSI Project Team (2012) Progress on developing endpoints for registrational clinical trials of community-acquired bacterial pneumonia and acute bacterial skin and skin structure infections: update from the biomarkers consortium of the foundation for the National Institutes of Health. Clin Infect Dis 55:1114–1121
12. European Medicines Agency (2011) Committee for Medicinal Products for Human Use. Guideline on the evaluation of medicinal products indicated for treatment of bacterial infections. http://www.ema.europa.eu/docs/en_GB/document_library/Scientific_guideline/2009/09/WC500003417.pdf
13. Ambrose PG, Bhavnani SM, Dudley MN, Ellis-Grosse EJ, Drusano GL (2012) New EMA guideline for antimicrobial development. Lancet Infect Dis 12:266–267
14. Rex JH, Eisenstine BI, Alder J, Goldberger M, Meyer R, Dane A, Friedland I, Knirsch C, Sanhai WR, Tomayko J, Lancaster C, Jackson J (2013) A comprehensive regulatory framework to address the unmet need for new antibacterial treatments. Lancet Infect Dis 13:269–275
15. Tomayko JF, Rex JH, Tenero DM, Goldberger M, Eisenstine BI (2014) New regulatory tools to support product development. Clin Pharmacol Ther 96:166–168
16. Rex JH, Goldberger M, Eisenstine BI, Harney C (2014) The evolution of the regulatory framework for antibacterial agents. Ann N Y Acad Sci 1323:11–21
17. Food and Drug Administration (2013) Draft guidance for industry antibacterial therapies for patients with unmet medical need for the treatment of serious bacterial diseases. http://www.fda.gov/downloads/drugs/guidancecomplianceregulatoryinformation/guidances/ucm359184.pdf
18. Infectious Disease Society of America (2012) White Paper: Recommendations on the conduct of superiority and organism-specific clinical trials of antibacterial agents for the treatment of infections caused by drug-resistant bacterial pathogens. Clin Infect Dis 55:1031–1046
19. Nambiar S, Laessig K, Toerner J, Farley J, Cox E (2014) Antibacterial drug development: challenges, recent developments, and future considerations. Clin Pharmacol Ther 96:147–149
20. Craig WA (1998) Pharmacokinetic/pharmacodynamic parameters: rationale for antibacterial dosing in mice and men. Clin Infect Dis 26:1–12
21. Andes D, Craig WA (2002) Animal model pharmacokinetics and pharmacodynamics: a critical review. Int J Antimicrob Agents 19:261–268
22. Mouton JW, Dudley MN, Cars O, Derendorf H, Drusano GL (2005) Standardization of pharmacokinetic/pharmacodynamic (PK/PD) terminology for anti-infective drugs: an update. J Antimicrob Chemother 55:601–607
23. Ambrose PG, Bhavnani SM, Rubino CM, Louie A, Gumbo T, Forrest A, Drusano GL (2007) Pharmacokinetics-pharmacodynamics of antimicrobial therapy: it's not just for mice anymore. Clin Infect Dis 44:79–86
24. Bulik CC, Bhavnani SM, Hammel JP, Forrest A, Dudley MN, Ellis-Grosse EJ, Drusano GL, Ambrose PG (2013) Evaluation of the probability of regulatory approval based on preclinical PK-PD target attainment for community-acquired and hospital-acquired pneumonia A-295. 53rd InterScience conference on antimicrobial agents and chemotherapy, Denver CO, 10–13 September

25. Van Ogtrop ML, Andes D, Stamstad TJ, Conklin B, Weiss WJ, Craig WA, Vesga O (2000) In vivo pharmacodynamic activities of two glycylcyclines against Gram-positive and Gram-negative bacteria. Antimicrob Agents Chemother 44:943–949
26. Vanscoy B, Mendes RE, Castanheira M, McCauley J, Bhavnani SM, Forrest A, Jones RN, Okusanya OO, Friedrich LV, Steenbergen J, Ambrose PG (2013) Relationship between ceftolozane-tazobactam exposure and drug resistance amplification in a hollow-fiber infection model. Antimicrob Agents Chemother 57:4134–4138
27. Ambrose PG, Drusano GL, Craig WA (2012) In vivo activity of oritavancin in animal infection models and rationale for a new dosing regimen in humans. Clin Infect Dis 54(Suppl 3):S220–S228
28. Lamb LM, Crandon JL, Nicolau DP (2013) Pharmacokinetic and pharmacodynamic evaluation of P-873 versus Klebsiella pneumoniae in a neutropenic murine thigh infection model. Antimicrob Agents Chemother 57:1971–1973
29. Meagher AK, Ambrose PG, Grasela TH, Ellis-Grosse EJ (2005) Pharmacokinetic/pharmacodynamic profile for tigecycline: a new glycylcycline antimicrobial agent. Diagn Microbiol Infect Dis 52:165–171
30. Bulitta JB, Okusanya OO, Forrest A, Bhavnani SM, Clark K, Still JG, Fernandes P, Ambrose PG (2013) Population pharmacokinetics of fusidic acid: rationale for front-loaded dosing regimens due to autoinhibition of clearance. Antimicrob Agents Chemother 57:498–507
31. Van Wart SA, Forrest A, Khariton T, Rubino CM, Bhavnani SM, Reynolds DK, Riccobene T, Ambrose PG (2013) Population pharmacokinetics of ceftaroline in patients with acute bacterial skin and skin structure infections or community-acquired bacterial pneumonia. J Clin Pharmacol 53:1155–1167
32. Bhalodi AA, Crandon JL, Biek D, Nicolau DP (2012) Efficacy of ceftaroline fosamil in a staphylococcal murine pneumonia model. Antimicrob Agents Chemother 56:6160–6165
33. Meagher AK, Passarell JA, Cirincione BB, Van Wart SA, Ellis-Grosse EJ, Ambrose PG (2007) Exposure-response analyses of tigecycline efficacy in patients with complicated skin and skin-structure infections. Antimicrob Agents Chemother 51:1939–1945
34. Louie A, Heine HS, Kim K, Brown DL, VanScoy B, Liu W, Kinzig-Schippers M, Sörgel F, Drusano GL (2008) Use of an in vitro pharmacodynamic model to derive a linezolid regimen that optimizes bacterial kill and prevents emergence of resistance in Bacillus anthracis. Antimicrob Agents Chemother 52:2486–2496
35. Van Wart SA, Ambrose PG, Rubino CM, Khariton T, Riccobene TA, Friedland HD, Critchley IA, Bhavnani SM (2014) Pharmacokinetic-pharmacodynamic target attainment analyses to evaluate in vitro susceptibility test interpretive criteria for ceftaroline against Staphylococcus aureus and Streptococcus pneumoniae. Antimicrob Agents Chemother 58:885–891
36. Ambrose PG, Hammel JP, Bhavnani SM, Rubino CM, Ellis-Grosse EJ, Drusano GL (2012) Frequentist and Bayesian pharmacometric-based approaches to facilitate critically needed new antibiotic development: overcoming lies, damn lies, and statistics. Antimicrob Agents Chemother 56: 1466–1470
37. Ambrose PG, Bhavnani SM, Ellis-Grosse EJ, Drusano GL (2010) Pharmacokinetic-pharmacodynamic considerations in the design of hospital-acquired or ventilator-associated bacterial pneumonia studies: look before you leap! Clin Infect Dis 51(Suppl 1):S103–S110
38. Wiskirchen DE, Nordmann P, Crandon JL, Nicolau DP (2013) Efficacy of humanized carbapenem and ceftazidime regimens against Enterobacteriaceae producing the OXA-48 carbapenemase in a murine infection model. Antimicrob Agents Chemother 2014:1678–1683
39. Jang SH, Colangelo PM, Gobburu JV (2010) Exposure-response of posaconazole used for prophylaxis against invasive fungal infections: evaluating the need to adjust doses based on drug concentrations in plasma. Clin Pharmacol Ther 88:115–119
40. Tornøe CW, Tworzyanski JJ, Imoisili MA, Alexander JJ, Korth-Bradley JM, Gobburu JV (2007) Optimising piperacillin/tazobactam dosing in paediatrics. Int J Antimicrob Agents 30:320–324
41. Drusano GL, Preston SL, Hardalo C, Hare R, Banfield C, Andes D, Vesga O, Craig WA (2001) Use of preclinical data for selection of a phase II/III dose for evernimicin and identification of a preclinical MIC breakpoint. Antimicrob Agents Chemother 45:13–22
42. Bhavnani SM, Hammel JP, Cirincione BB, Wikler MA, Ambrose PG (2005) Use of pharmacokinetic-pharmacodynamic target attainment analyses to support phase 2 and 3 dosing strategies for doripenem. Antimicrob Agents Chemother 49:3944–3947

Chapter 25

Antibiotic Stewardship and Applications of Pharmacodynamics

Elizabeth D. Hermsen and Lynne Fehrenbacher

Abstract

The need for antimicrobial stewardship is driven by a combination of increased antimicrobial resistance, frequent inappropriate use of antibiotics, and a sparse antibiotic pipeline. Antimicrobial stewardship programs (ASPs) are advocated as a mechanism to optimize the use of antibiotics and minimize the negative consequences of such use. Various resources are needed to support an ASP, and ASPs may use a combination of core and supplemental strategies to improve patient outcomes and public health. Pharmacodynamics can be applied in ASPs through the formulary decision-making process, patient-specific dosing recommendations, and institution-wide dosing protocols.

Key words Antimicrobial stewardship, Pharmacodynamics, Formulary, Dose optimization, Vancomycin, Aminoglycosides, Fluoroquinolones, Extended infusion

1 Introduction

Antimicrobial resistance is increasing and has detrimental effects on patients and healthcare systems [1, 2]. According to the World Health Organization, antimicrobial use is a primary driver of antimicrobial resistance [3]. Particularly troublesome is the fact that studies consistently report that up to half of all antibiotic use is inappropriate [4]. The problem of antimicrobial resistance and inappropriate antibiotic use is compounded by a reduction in the number of novel antimicrobials introduced to market over the last few decades, with no clear recovery predicted in the near future [5, 6]. This triad of increasing antimicrobial resistance, widespread inappropriate use of antibiotics, and lack of new antibiotics emphasizes the need for antimicrobial stewardship in order to preserve our current antimicrobial arsenal.

Antimicrobial stewardship is a systematic, rational approach to optimizing antimicrobial use in order to maximize clinical cure or prevention of infection and minimize unintended consequences of antimicrobial use, including antimicrobial resistance, adverse

John C. Rotschafer et al. (eds.), *Antibiotic Pharmacodynamics*, Methods in Pharmacology and Toxicology, DOI 10.1007/978-1-4939-3323-5_25, events, and cost [4]. An appreciation of antimicrobial pharmacodynamics in the context of antimicrobial stewardship efforts is of utmost importance in order to ensure appropriate antimicrobial selection and dosing. Pharmacodynamics can be applied by antimicrobial stewardship programs (ASPs) in a number of ways, including formulary decisions and dose optimization, on both a patient-specific and institution-wide level. This chapter addresses ASPs in the acute care hospital setting because this setting has been the primary focus for ASPs to date, although ASPs are now expanding into nontraditional settings such as skilled nursing facilities, ambulatory care clinics, and outpatient infusion centers, among others.

2 Development of an Antimicrobial Stewardship Program

2.1 Resources Needed

When designing and building an ASP, it is important to identify core members and an efficient process to develop and move initiatives forward. The Infectious Diseases Society of America (IDSA) and the Society for Healthcare Epidemiology of America (SHEA) Guidelines for Developing an Institutional Program to Enhance Antimicrobial Stewardship published in 2007 suggest that core team members include an infectious disease (ID) physician and an ID-trained pharmacist [4]. While the IDSA/SHEA guidelines state that the core members should be compensated for their time, in the cost-conscious environment of healthcare, the implementation of new ASPs often occurs despite limited resource allocation. In the 2012 policy statement on antimicrobial stewardship, IDSA, SHEA, and the Pediatric Infectious Diseases Society (PIDS) recognized that stewardship teams may vary in structure based upon institution size, organizational structure, and specialized personnel [7]. The policy statement recommends that core members include a physician, a pharmacist, an infection preventionist, and a clinical microbiologist, with at least one of the core members having stewardship training (*see* **Note 1**).

In addition to the core members, several supporting members and key collaborative relationships help optimize the ASP (*see* Table 1). The core personnel often develop an antimicrobial subcommittee to the Pharmacy & Therapeutics (P&T) Committee that helps to vet various antimicrobial-related initiatives, policies, and formulary requests. The ID physician typically serves as the committee chair with the ID pharmacist in a co-chair or secretary role. The composition of the subcommittee usually includes a multidisciplinary (e.g., medical, pharmacy, nursing, laboratory staff) group of those who are high antibiotic users and/or are likely to be affected by various ASP initiatives. In addition to development of an antimicrobial subcommittee, a clinical microbiologist can offer insight regarding incorporation of available laboratory

Table 1
Antimicrobial stewardship program team members

Essential core members	Ideal additional team members	Key adjunct relationships
(IDSA 2007) Infectious disease physician(s) Infectious disease pharmacist(s) (SHEA/IDSA/PIDS 2012)[a] Physician Pharmacist Infection preventionist Clinical microbiologist	Clinical microbiologist Hospital/health-system epidemiologist Infection preventionist Data analyst/IT support Administrative assistant support	Hospital/health-system administration Health-system communications team Pharmacy & Therapeutics Committee Medical staff Nursing staff Pharmacist staff

[a]At least one core member with stewardship training

technology, such as automated susceptibility testing and rapid diagnostic assays, into stewardship initiatives and also can assist with development of the antibiogram(s). Informatics support can help develop reports that the ASP can use to identify opportunities for initiative development, provide metrics to ensure that interventions are data driven, and assist in measuring the impact of the ASP on various outcomes. Since a key component of reducing antibiotic burden is avoiding hospital-acquired infections and nosocomial transmission of resistant organisms, an infection preventionist and hospital epidemiologist offer valuable insight into local epidemiology and the potential impact of the ASP on the antibiogram. If possible, allocation of administrative assistant, data analyst, and/or research assistant time will help increase the amount of time the ASP personnel have for planning, managing, and executing the clinical, educational, and investigational aspects of the ASP. While ASP personnel are the thought leaders and designers for optimizing antimicrobial use within an institution, best practice cannot be achieved without committed partnerships with medical, nursing, pharmacy, laboratory, and other supportive staff.

Recognizing that resources are often limited, and site-specific ASP design is imperative to the success of a program, the Centers for Disease Control and Prevention (CDC) published their recommended core elements of an ASP [8] (*see* Table 2). Designed to be a companion to the prior ASP guiding publications, the CDC document reflected on experiences of existing and successful ASPs to formulate the core elements. A checklist document included in the materials helps sites assess gaps in their existing ASP structure and focus, as well as provides a baseline assessment for sites looking to build a new ASP.

2.2 Core and Supplemental Strategies

A sense of urgency for antimicrobial stewardship is reiterated by the CDC Threat Report 2013, which discusses the detrimental effects of antibiotic resistance [1]. The CDC identifies

Table 2
CDC Core elements of hospital antimicrobial stewardship programs [8]

Leadership commitment	Dedicating necessary human, financial, and information technology resources.
Accountability	Appointing a single leader responsible for program outcomes. Experience with successful programs shows that a physician leader is effective.
Drug expertise	Appointing a single pharmacist leader responsible for working to improve antibiotic use.
Action	Implementing at least one recommended action, such as systemic evaluation of ongoing treatment need after a set period of initial treatment (i.e., "antibiotic time-out" after 48 h).
Tracking	Monitoring antibiotic prescribing and resistance patterns.
Reporting	Regular reporting information on antibiotic use and resistance to doctors, nurses, and relevant staff.
Education	Educating clinicians about resistance and optimal prescribing.

antimicrobial stewardship as one of the four core components to prevent antibiotic resistance. While ASP needs and goals will vary by institution, the IDSA/SHEA guidelines suggest two active core strategies for stewardship endeavors: (1) prospective audit and feedback and (2) formulary restriction and authorization [4]. There are several examples in the literature that illustrate reduced antimicrobial consumption and expenditures and decreased rates of *Clostridium difficile* infection and resistant pathogens after implementing these core strategies [9–13].

Prospective audit and feedback rely on review of patient information by ASP personnel to identify patient-specific opportunities for antimicrobial therapy optimization. This intervention is not to be considered a formal ID consult, rather a supporting service to enhance appropriate therapies. Patient review may be triggered by clinical decision support systems, established internal reports, and/or microbiology culture result review. The ASP personnel discuss the patient case and make suggestions to the managing medical team. Creating a collaborative environment for discussions that focus on evidence-based practice, patient safety, and minimization of collateral damage from antimicrobials helps keep this recommendation patient centered with a positive team effect. Barriers to this approach include the misconceptions that the ASP is attempting to take away the autonomy of the prescribing physician, generate consults for ID physicians, or serve as the "antibiotic police." It is important to remember that the suggestions being provided to the managing medical team are unsolicited, which lends to the potential for an antagonistic interaction. Polite persistence over time and offering physicians the opportunity to review ASP metrics, ask questions, or proactively participate in ASP initiatives can help engage providers and overcome negative perceptions surrounding this recommended core strategy.

In contrast to prospective audit and feedback, which tends to be dynamic and relies on concurrent patient review and personal interaction, formulary restriction and authorization are often incorporated into formal policy. Execution of these methods can vary considerably depending on resources, infrastructure, and institutional culture. With respect to antimicrobial formulary restriction, ASPs identify certain antimicrobials that are considered restricted and require authorization for use. The reasons for restriction may include a high frequency of or potential for inappropriate use or collateral damage, safety/toxicity concerns, or cost, among others. The use of such agents may be restricted to only the ASP personnel or may include selected specialty services (e.g., ID, critical care, oncology). ASP personnel develop agent- or class-specific prescribing criteria to outline what is deemed appropriate and inappropriate use within their institution. These criteria are typically endorsed by the P&T Committee and implemented as policy or clinical guidelines.

Because delays in the initiation of appropriate antimicrobial therapy can have detrimental effects on patient outcomes [14], most prescribing criteria include the ability for prescribers to order the agent with a time window (24–48 h) for review by the ASP personnel or clinical pharmacist and authorization. While this approach may be considered a form of concurrent audit and feedback, it formalizes what is deemed to be appropriate or inappropriate and may allow for autonomous action based on P&T-approved policies. In contrast, some restriction policies require preauthorization, meaning that no drug will be dispensed until authorized (usually by an ID physician or ASP personnel). This method relies on a structure that includes individuals who are (1) trained to evaluate whether using the agent in a selected patient is appropriate, (2) able to make recommendations on the spot for alternative agents if therapy is not appropriate, and (3) available to be reached in a timely manner at all hours and days of the week. The most common practice setting where preauthorization occurs is in academic teaching institutions where ID fellows are incorporated into call coverage. For smaller hospitals and those predominantly served by private practice ID physicians, this model becomes more difficult to support. In many cases, a single first dose will be dispensed before official preauthorization is received in order to avoid a delay in antibiotic administration.

When monitoring the effectiveness of formulary restriction and authorization, the ASP should assess whether restricting a certain antimicrobial agent or class results in an associated increase in use of alternate agents. As this occurs, the program should evaluate the potential impact on selective pressure that simply shifts from one agent to another as a result of restriction. Even when formulary restriction and authorization programs are optimized, timely reevaluation of therapy and targeted de-escalation are imperative. The CDC recommends taking an antibiotic "time-out" for this purpose [8]. Available data should be reviewed at hour 48 of therapy and the following key questions should be asked in order to more appropriately focus antimicrobial therapy: (1) Does this patient have an infection that will respond to antibiotics? (2) If so, is the patient on the right antibiotic(s), dose, and route of administration? (3) Can a more targeted antibiotic be used to treat the infection? (4) How long should the patient receive the antibiotic(s)? Incorporating time-outs into the culture of antimicrobial administration, in a fashion similar to many surgical and high-risk medication use procedures, also helps promote a sense of responsibility and awareness that all caregivers should be involved in optimizing antimicrobial use.

Several more passive, supplemental strategies are recommended to augment the active core strategies of successful ASPs. Education is essential for the required change of culture that is needed for a sustainable program. Providing educational opportunities with varied target audiences helps keep ASP initiatives a priority for all who are involved. Focusing education on areas that the ASP has identified as targets for practice improvement, presenting evidence-based practice guideline updates, patient case, and lessons learned discussions are all forums that will expand knowledge and engagement for caregivers. While important, education is not recommended as a sole stewardship intervention due to the variable and often temporary impact it yields. Likewise, in taking the lead to develop hospital or health-system-specific infection treatment protocols and clinical guidelines, the ASP can ensure that current organism trends, appropriate agents, and dose optimization considerations for special patient populations are incorporated. Avoiding redundant therapies, such as anaerobic double-coverage, developing parenteral to oral conversion programs, and streamlining the antimicrobial de-escalation process are also recommended arenas for ASP focus.

As part of the policy statement recommendations, IDSA/SHEA/PIDS identified two primary issues of importance: (1) benchmarking of antimicrobial use within and between institutions and (2) development of clear, well-defined, and validated process or outcome measures that may be utilized to assess clinical impact of ASPs [7]. The organizations call for standardized definitions of appropriate and inappropriate antimicrobial use, standardized data collection tools, and well-designed, patient-centered outcome research. Currently, IDSA and SHEA have again partnered to develop clinical practice guidelines on antimicrobial stewardship that focus on presenting different approaches to antimicrobial stewardship in various healthcare settings, with a focus on helping institutions individualize programs based on resources (projected publication 2015).

2.3 Steps for Developing an Antimicrobial Stewardship Program

The core and supplemental personnel and strategies must be considered by healthcare providers devising a plan for an ASP. The following steps should be taken when developing an ASP:

1. Identify key stakeholders at the institution. Examples include but are not limited to ID physicians, pharmacists, clinical microbiologists, infection preventionists, hospitalists, high users of antimicrobials (e.g., critical care, oncology), and hospital and pharmacy administrators.
2. Build buy-in among stakeholders. Garnering support should focus on patient outcomes and quality improvement. Hospital-specific data should be used whenever possible. For example, resistance rates at the hospital, according to the antibiogram or infection prevention databases, could be compared to published data.
3. Determine the core and supplemental strategies that will be used. Consideration must be given to the human and financial resources available and the information technology infrastructure, as this may dictate which strategies are most amenable to the institution.
4. Delineate the goals and outcome measures of the program. A variety of outcome measures may be evaluated by an ASP. Outcomes can typically be categorized into four central themes: improved patient outcomes, improved patient safety, reduced antimicrobial resistance, and reduced antimicrobial and overall cost.
5. Draft a formal proposal. The formal proposal should include the following sections: background, program goals and strategies, required up-front and anticipated future personnel, outcome measures, and financial justification (*see* **Note 2**).
6. Take the formal proposal to stakeholders for approval of program. After approval of the program is received, the implementation process can begin (*see* **Note 3**).

3 Considerations for Pharmacodynamics in Antimicrobial Stewardship

The core ASP personnel, as discussed above, include an ID physician and an ID pharmacist. Both of these individuals have specialized training in ID and antibiotics. This specialized training lends to the application of antibiotic pharmacodynamics in the conduct of an ASP through formulary decision making, patient-specific dose optimization, and institution-wide dose optimization protocols.

3.1 Formulary Decision Making

An example of how pharmacodynamics can be applied to formulary decision making is when considering the relevance of the potency of antimicrobials within the same class. More specifically, ciprofloxacin is generally regarded as more potent than levofloxacin against *Pseudomonas aeruginosa*. This purported advantage has the potential to influence the decision of which fluoroquinolone to include on an institutional formulary. However, when considering the pharmacodynamics of the two fluoroquinolones, the clinical relevance of this increased potency [i.e., lower minimum inhibitory concentration (MIC)] is minimal. Fluoroquinolones are concentration-dependent antibiotics with the area under the concentration curve (AUC) to MIC or peak-to-MIC ratios as the pharmacodynamic parameters that best correlate with outcome. AUC/MIC ratios of 100–125 or peak/MIC ratios of >10 are suggested for clinical and microbiological success and prevention of bacterial resistance [15]. Although the MIC of ciprofloxacin for *P. aeruginosa* is typically twofold lower than that of levofloxacin, the AUC is also typically twofold lower. Thus, using a hypothetical example of a *P. aeruginosa* isolate with a levofloxacin MIC of 0.5 mg/L and a ciprofloxacin MIC of 0.25 mg/L (twofold lower), and a levofloxacin-free AUC of 50 mg h/L versus a ciprofloxacin-free AUC of 22 mg h/L (twofold lower), the resulting AUC/MIC ratios are not appreciably different (100 versus 88, respectively). A simple table illustrating this concept can be constructed to inform the P&T Committee's decision (*see* Table 3).

Another example of how pharmacodynamics can be applied to formulary decision making is with regard to the dosing frequency of antimicrobials. Less frequent dosing may increase patient adherence and thus increase the likelihood of pharmacodynamic target attainment. This concept is more directly applicable to patients receiving antimicrobial therapy outside of the hospital setting because adherence should be 100 % while hospitalized, but is still relevant to hospital formularies as patients may be discharged from the hospital for continued administration of the inpatient antimicrobial.

Table 3
Illustrative example of AUC/MIC comparison of ciprofloxacin and levofloxacin

	Free AUC_{24} (mg h/L)	MIC (mg/L)				
Drug		**2**	**1**	**0.5**	**0.25**	**0.125**
Ciprofloxacin	22	11	22	44	**88**	177
Levofloxacin	50	25	50	**100**	200	400

3.2 Patient-Specific Dose Optimization

One pillar of antimicrobial stewardship is ensuring appropriate antibiotic dosing with consideration of infection-, patient-, and pathogen-specific factors. Authors of other chapters in this text have presented detailed information about the pharmacodynamics of antibacterial agents and have highlighted how they can be altered in special patient populations such as the critically ill, pediatric, and obese. The ASP often plays a role in bridging the data from in vitro/animal studies and Monte Carlo analyses to bedside clinical application.

3.2.1 Vancomycin and Aminoglycosides

Most hospitals and health systems have an established pharmacokinetic consult or dosing service for vancomycin and aminoglycosides. For vancomycin, an AUC/MIC ratio of ≥400 is suggested to optimize the chance for successful therapy outcomes. While this recommendation was originally based on a single study in pneumonia patients, it is used to justify trough targets in other disease states in the absence of randomized trials [16]. An additional site-specific analysis of bacteremia supported this target, while another correlated low AUC/MIC ratios (<211) with higher rates of attributable mortality [17, 18]. Since obtaining multiple vancomycin random levels in the clinical setting is expensive and often not operationally practical, trough monitoring is used as a surrogate marker for AUC [19]. Vancomycin trough levels of 15 mg/L correlate with an AUC/MIC ratio of 400 if the organism MIC is ≤1 mg/L. While widely used as a surrogate, more data are needed to know whether this is truly the optimal method of managing vancomycin therapy [20].

The ASP plays an important role in connecting microbiology trends that may impact probability of target attainment with clinical dosing protocols. For example, through trending vancomycin MIC distributions for an institution's *S. aureus* isolates, the ASP can assess for increasing MICs over time (MIC "creep") and identify cases where vancomycin may no longer be appropriate empiric therapy, despite optimized protocols, due to the inability to reach the pharmacodynamic target. A confounding variable in assessing vancomycin MIC trends is the discordance noted depending on the methodology used as well as incongruence in the literature. For example one recent study suggested that the Etest method overestimates the MIC when compared to automated susceptibility testing methods while another recent study suggests that this is not the case [21, 22]. Additional study is needed to further elucidate vancomycin MIC discordance and the potential clinical impact it may have when using AUC/MIC as an outcome predictor. Of note, the AUC/MIC threshold of 400 was established using broth microdilution for the MIC determination, and studies have shown that the threshold should be adjusted when using other susceptibility testing methods [17, 23]. The ASP should ascertain which methods are used locally and understand the potential impact of interpreting vancomycin MIC data from those methods.

With respect to aminoglycosides, a goal peak/MIC ratio of ≥10 is desired. Implementing and optimizing use of an extended interval dosing protocol (e.g., Hartford nomogram) for appropriate patient populations maximize the peak/MIC ratio [24]. When trending aminoglycoside MICs for *P. aeruginosa*, the ASP might direct empiric prescribing toward tobramycin if gentamicin MICs routinely approach 4 mcg/ml or greater as a peak/MIC ratio of ≥10 will be difficult to achieve even with extended interval dosing. Finally, in partnering with the pharmacy department, the ASP can serve as a supporting/reviewing body that tracks protocol adherence and target level achievement and can recommend ideas for protocol and process improvement.

3.3 Institution-Wide Dose Optimization

In contrast to patient-specific dosing recommendations, the ASP can also apply pharmacodynamics to the development and implementation of institution-wide dosing protocols, such as extended infusion of beta-lactams or renal dosage adjustments (*see* **Note 4**).

3.3.1 Extended Infusion of Beta-Lactams

The pharmacodynamic parameter that best correlates with optimal activity of beta-lactams is the proportion of the dosing interval that the free drug concentration remains above the MIC for the infecting organism (*T*>MIC). One mechanism to optimize the *T*>MIC is to extend the infusion of the drug. Monte Carlo simulations have shown that a piperacillin/tazobactam dose of 3.375 g every 8 h given via a 4-h infusion achieves over 90 % probability of target attainment against *P. aeruginosa* up to an MIC of 16 mg/L versus an MIC of only 1 mg/L for the standard dose of 3.375 g every 6 h given via a 30-min infusion [25]. However, the need for an extended infusion protocol should first be established by evaluating the MIC distribution of problematic pathogens, such as *P. aeruginosa*, in an individual institution. If the MICs seen in the local environment are not elevated, an extended infusion protocol may not be worth the logistical challenges often encountered during implementation and maintenance of an institution-wide policy, but rather extended infusion could be used on a case-by-case basis if the isolate's MIC is elevated.

Some of the logistical challenges of an institution-wide extended infusion protocol include quality of care considerations, such as ensuring infusions are given over the extended timeframe, residual volume in the infusion tubing, and compatibility issues. In the case of piperacillin/tazobactam, if the extended infusion dose of 3.375 g every 8 h is accidentally administered via the standard 30-min infusion, the patient will receive a subtherapeutic dose. Thus, building pre-programmed infusion times into libraries of infusion pumps when a particular drug is selected can help avoid this problem. Caregiver education, particularly of the nursing staff, is vital and should include background information supporting the need for the extended infusion protocol, the specific details of the protocol, and contact information for questions. The resources necessary for such education, both human and financial, should not be underestimated as the education must be provided to all staff, including full-time and part-time, during all shifts and must be enduring to allow for education of new employees. Additionally, consideration must be given to the residual volume in the infusion tubing at the end of the infusion. If the volume is significant and this is not accounted for, the patient will receive subtherapeutic dosing. In order to account for residual volume, the dose can be increased, or the line must be flushed. For example, when administering piperacillin/tazobactam with the Alaris® pump (CareFusion, San Diego, CA), approximately 20 mL remains in the tubing after the end of the infusion. If the dose is increased to 4.5 g rather than 3.375 g, given in 100 mL total volume, the patient will receive a dose of approximately 3.6 g when accounting for the residual volume of 20 mL [4.5 g − (4.5 g × 0.2) = 3.6 g]. Lastly, when administering a medication over an extended infusion, compatibility with other intravenous medications or fluids becomes an issue. Compatibility issues can be handled in three ways: (1) co-administration in the same intravenous catheter if compatibility has been confirmed; (2) adjustment of medication administration times to avoid co-administration if the two agents are incompatible; or (3) placement of additional intravascular catheters.

3.3.2 Renal Dosage Adjustment

Renal dysfunction is known to affect the clearance of renally eliminated medications, and it is well understood that dosage adjustment is often necessary in the setting of renal insufficiency. Pharmacists are responsible for ensuring that the ordered dose of a medication is appropriate for the patient's renal status, not only at the time the drug is initially ordered but also for the duration of therapy as renal function may change throughout the hospitalization. If a dosage change is warranted, pharmacists call the prescriber to recommend the change. However, an institution-wide protocol allowing pharmacists to automatically adjust the dosing of antibiotics according to renal function can make this process more efficient. Although changes in renal function and drug elimination are typically regarded as pharmacokinetic issues, the importance of pharmacodynamic considerations should not be overlooked when creating an institution-wide renal dosing protocol. For example, the recommended ciprofloxacin dose for patients receiving hemodialysis is 250 mg orally or 200 mg intravenously every 12 h (standard doses: 500 mg orally, 400 mg intravenously every 12 h) [26]. However, because fluoroquinolones are concentration-dependent antibiotics, the pharmacodynamics can be optimized by maintaining the dose but extending the interval (i.e., 500 mg orally or 400 mg intravenously every 24 h) rather than decreasing the dose and maintaining the interval. This type of modification may not be possible with all antibiotics due to dose-dependent toxicities.

4 Notes

1. In order to accommodate the need for additional ID-trained pharmacists beyond what is possible with currently available residency and fellowship training programs, two certificate programs have been developed. Both the Society of Infectious Diseases Pharmacists (SIDP) and the Making a Difference in Infectious Diseases Pharmacotherapy (MAD-ID) organization offer antimicrobial stewardship certification that helps to prepare pharmacists for ASP-focused practice.
2. Background should include the impact of antimicrobial resistance on patient outcomes and costs, a brief review of key antimicrobial stewardship literature, and recent, relevant policies, regulations, and/or legislation [e.g., Centers for Medicare and Medicaid Services (CMS) Readmission Reduction program or reimbursement changes for catheter-associated urinary tract infections or bloodstream infections] and how antimicrobial stewardship may help. With regard to personnel, inclusion of necessary compensation as well as future plans for additional personnel is recommended. When outlining the goals and outcomes, the period of review should be defined. For example, how often will the outcome measures be assessed? Garnering support from hospital or health-system administration early in the process is essential, and regular reporting to appropriate administrators ensures that program successes are transparent at a high level. Efforts should be made to integrate the ASP personnel into the committee infrastructure of the institution (e.g., Infection Prevention, Quality & Patient Safety, Pharmacy & Therapeutics) because this will help ensure continued enthusiasm and support for the program. As this relationship builds, and data-driven results are available, proposals for continued or additional funding for the ASP should be presented to leadership. For ASPs that encompass more than a single institution, collaborating with the health system's internal communications personnel may assist with disseminating key information to leaders across multiple campuses. The initial financial justification should strive to promote cost avoidance as opposed to direct cost savings as an acceptable method of showing the value of an ASP to hospital administration. Although length of stay (LOS) may be a useful outcome measure, a promise to reduce LOS should not be used for financial justification of developing an ASP.

3. Key questions to consider during implementation of an ASP include the following:
   (a) What are the most obtainable targets (e.g., "low-hanging fruit"), and what are the top priorities at your institution for action?
   (b) Who are the physician and hospital administrator champions who will serve as resources to assist with medical staff relationship development?
   (c) What information technology infrastructure is available? Do you have access to real-time data? What type of reports can be generated/queries can be conducted? Do you need information technology personnel support?
   (d) During what hours will ASP personnel be available? If not around the clock, what happens with antimicrobial stewardship-related issues that arise during off hours? Who will provide coverage in the absence of ASP personnel (e.g., vacation, professional meeting attendance)?
   (e) How will recommendations be communicated to providers? If communication is placed in the patient medical record, will the communication be a permanent part of the medical record? What is the course of action if the provider does not respond (i.e., a page/phone call is not returned, communication in medical record is not addressed)?
   (f) Will the ASP have any prescriptive authority, and if so in what situations?
   (g) How will interventions be documented and tracked?
   (h) What outcomes will be reported, to whom, in what format(s), and how often? Will ASP meeting minutes be provided to anyone outside of the ASP team, and if so to whom?
4. The steps involved in the development and implementation of an institution-wide dosing protocol include the following:
   (a) Gather evidence. Collect internal data to demonstrate the need for the protocol, and summarize published literature to provide supporting rationale for the protocol. Seeking insight from external institutions that have implemented a similar protocol may also be helpful.
   (b) Identify key stakeholders and collaborate to develop the protocol. Consider not only those stakeholders who will support the protocol but also those who will be affected by the protocol and/or may not be in favor of the protocol. Involvement of "naysayers" early in the process may cause a delay but ultimately is beneficial in building buy-in, anticipating problems, and overcoming barriers as early as possible.

(c) Take the protocol through the necessary committee infrastructure for approval. Consideration should be given to integrating the protocol into a decision support algorithm within the electronic medical record, which may add to the necessary committees for approval but also will likely improve adherence to the protocol.

(d) Once approved, educate the staff on the new protocol. This should include broad-based, general education, such as institution-wide newsletters or e-mails, and targeted education to those groups likely to be directly affected (e.g., pharmacists and prescribers). Development of enduring materials is helpful to allow for reeducation, if necessary, and education of new staff members as they are hired. The importance of this step should not be underestimated.

(e) Launch the protocol. Select a go-live date and include this date in the staff education. Ensure that all supporting materials (e.g., pre-programmed infusion pumps, compatibility tables, dosing reference tables, electronic orders) are in place and functioning prior to go-live.

(f) In the first weeks to months, provide active support and feedback to protocol users. Ensure that there is a contact available to help troubleshoot as all become proficient in applying the new process.

(g) Review the protocol on a regular basis and revise as necessary based on changing internal or external data or practices.

References

1. Centers for Disease Control and Prevention (2013) Antibiotic resistance threats in the United States. http://www.cdc.gov/drugresistance/threat-report-2013/. Accessed 1 Feb 2014
2. Huttner A, Harbarth S, Carlet J, Cosgrove S, Goossens H, Holmes A, Jarlier V, Voss A, Pittet D (2013) Antimicrobial resistance: a global view from the 2013 World Healthcare-Associated Infections Forum. Antimicrob Resist Infect Control 2(1):31
3. World Health Organization (2001) WHO global strategy for containment of antimicrobial resistance. World Health Organization, Geneva, WHO/CDS/CSR/DRS/2001.2
4. Dellit TH, Owens RC, McGowan JE Jr, Gerding DN, Weinstein RA, Burke JP, Huskins WC, Paterson DL, Fishman NO, Carpenter CF, Brennan PJ, Billeter M, Hooton TM (2007) Infectious Diseases Society of America and the Society for Healthcare Epidemiology of America guidelines for developing an institutional program to enhance antimicrobial stewardship. Clin Infect Dis 44(2):159–177
5. Boucher HW, Talbot GH, Bradley JS, Edwards JE, Gilbert D, Rice LB, Scheld M, Spellberg B, Bartlett J (2009) Bad bugs, no drugs: no ESKAPE! An update from the Infectious Diseases Society of America. Clin Infect Dis 48(1):1–12
6. Rice LB (2008) Federal funding for the study of antimicrobial resistance in nosocomial pathogens: no ESKAPE. J Infect Dis 197(8):1079–1081
7. Policy statement on antimicrobial stewardship by the Society for Healthcare Epidemiology of America (SHEA), the Infectious Diseases Society of America (IDSA), and the Pediatric Infectious Diseases Society (PIDS). Infect Control Hosp Epidemiol 33(4):322–327

8. Centers for Disease Control and Prevention (2014) Core elements of hospital antibiotic stewardship programs. http://www.cdc.gov/getsmart/healthcare/implementation/core-elements.html. Accessed 2 Apr 2014
9. Chung GW, Wu JE, Yeo CL, Chan D, Hsu LY (2013) Antimicrobial stewardship: a review of prospective audit and feedback systems and an objective evaluation of outcomes. Virulence 4(2):151–157
10. DiazGranados CA (2012) Prospective audit for antimicrobial stewardship in intensive care: impact on resistance and clinical outcomes. Am J Infect Control 40(6):526–529
11. Ramirez E (2013) Improving linezolid use decreases the incidence of resistance among Gram-positive microorganisms. Int J Antimicrob Agents 41:174–178
12. Fowler S, Webber A, Cooper BS, Phimister A, Price K, Carter Y, Kibbler CC, Simpson AJ, Stone SP (2007) Successful use of feedback to improve antibiotic prescribing and reduce *Clostridium difficile* infection: a controlled interrupted time series. J Antimicrob Chemother 59(5):990–995
13. Malani AN, Richards PG, Kapila S, Otto MH, Czerwinski J, Singal B (2013) Clinical and economic outcomes from a community hospital's antimicrobial stewardship program. Am J Infect Control 41(2):145–148
14. Kumar A, Roberts D, Wood KE, Light B, Parrillo JE, Sharma S, Suppes R, Feinstein D, Zanotti S, Taiberg L, Gurka D, Cheang M (2006) Duration of hypotension before initiation of effective antimicrobial therapy is the critical determinant of survival in human septic shock. Crit Care Med 34(6):1589–1596
15. Wright DH, Brown GH, Peterson ML, Rotschafer JC (2000) Application of fluoroquinolone pharmacodynamics. J Antimicrob Chemother 46(5):669–683
16. Moise-Broder PA, Forrest A, Birmingham MC, Schentag JJ (2004) Pharmacodynamics of vancomycin and other antimicrobials in patients with *Staphylococcus aureus* lower respiratory tract infections. Clin Pharmacokinet 43(13):925–942
17. Brown J, Brown K, Forrest A (2012) Vancomycin AUC24/MIC ratio in patients with complicated bacteremia and infective endocarditis due to methicillin-resistant *Staphylococcus aureus* and its association with attributable mortality during hospitalization. Antimicrob Agents Chemother 56(2):634–638
18. Kullar R, Davis SL, Levine DP, Rybak MJ (2011) Impact of vancomycin exposure on outcomes in patients with methicillin-resistant *Staphylococcus aureus* bacteremia: support for consensus guidelines suggested targets. Clin Infect Dis 52(8):975–981
19. Rybak M, Lomaestro B, Rotschafer JC, Moellering R Jr, Craig W, Billeter M, Dalovisio JR, Levine DP (2009) Therapeutic monitoring of vancomycin in adult patients: a consensus review of the American Society of Health-System Pharmacists, the Infectious Diseases Society of America, and the Society of Infectious Diseases Pharmacists. Am J Health Syst Pharm 66(1):82–98
20. Neely MN, Youn G, Jones B, Jelliffe RW, Drusano GL, Rodvold KA, Lodise TP (2014) Are vancomycin trough concentrations adequate for optimal dosing? Antimicrob Agents Chemother 58(1):309–316
21. Khatib R, Riederer K, Shemes S (2013) Correlation of methicillin-resistant *Staphylococcus aureus* vancomycin minimal inhibitory concentration results by Etest and broth microdilution methods with population analysis profile: lack of Etest overestimation of the MIC. Eur J Clin Microbiol Infect Dis 32:803–806
22. Rybak MJ, Vidaillac C, Sader HS (2013) Evaluation of vancomycin susceptibility testing for methicillin-resistant *Staphylococcus aureus*: comparison of Etest and three automated testing methods. J Clin Microbiol 51:2077–2081
23. Holmes NE, Turnidge JD, Munckhof WJ, Robinson JO, Korman TM, O'Sullivan MV, Anderson TL, Roberts SA, Warren SJ, Gao W, Howden BP, Johnson PD (2013) Vancomycin AUC/MIC ratio and 30-day mortality in patients with *Staphylococcus aureus* bacteremia. Antimicrob Agents Chemother 57(4):1654–1663
24. Nicolau DP, Freeman CD, Belliveau PP, Nightingale CH, Ross JW, Quintiliani R (1995) Experience with a once-daily aminoglycoside dosing program administered to 2184 adult patients. Antimicrob Agents Chemother 39:650–655
25. Lodise TP Jr, Lomaestro B, Drusano GL (2007) Piperacillin-tazobactam for *Pseudomonas aeruginosa* infection: clinical implications of an extended-infusion dosing strategy. Clin Infect Dis 44(3):357–363
26. Gilbert D (2013) The Sanford guide to antimicrobial therapy. 43rd edn. Antimicrobial Therapy, Inc. Sperryville, VA

Index

A

Abacavir ... 477–478
ABLC. *See* Amphotericin B lipid complex (ABLC)
Absorption, disposition, metabolism, and excretion (ADME) ... 159
ABSSSI. *See* Acute bacterial skin and skin structure infections (ABSSSI)
ABW. *See* Actual body weight (ABW)
Acinetobacter baumannii
  gram-positive bacteria ... 243
  lpx gene ... 229
  regrowth ... 238
Acquired-immunodeficiency syndrome (AIDS) ... 442
Actual body weight (ABW) ... 262
Acute bacterial pneumonia ... 64–65
Acute bacterial skin and skin structure infections (ABSSSI) ... 133
Acyclovir
  herpes labialis and genital HSV ... 443
  intravenous administration ... 444
  intravenous formulation ... 444
  in vitro cell culture analyses ... 445
  kidneys ... 446
  and penciclovir ... 443
    monophosphate ... 444
    resistance ... 447
  protein-binding capacity ... 446
  triphosphate ... 444
ADME. *See* Absorption, disposition, metabolism, and excretion (ADME)
AIDS. *See* Acquired-immunodeficiency syndrome (AIDS)
Albany Medical Center Hospital (AMCH) ... 527
Allometry ... 608, 611
AMCH. *See* Albany Medical Center Hospital (AMCH)
Amikacin (AK) ... 207, 386
Aminoglycosides ... 162–164, 641–642
  beta-lactam antibiotics ... 587
  broadening empiric spectrum ... 212
  burn patients ... 212
  cell wall active agents ... 204–205
  CF ... 211
  characteristics ... 201
  chemical structure ... 200–202
  concentration-dependent bactericidal activity ... 199
  concentration-dependent killing ... 203–204
  cystic fibrosis ... 586
  dosing regimen design ... 199
  EIAD ... 207–208
  extended-interval dosing ... 585
  febrile neutropenia ... 587
  frequent dosing and drug monitoring ... 587
  gentamicin and tobramcyin ... 585–587
  gram-positive synergism ... 212–213
  intra-abdominal infections ... 213
  meta-analysis ... 586
  MIC ratio ... 207
  monotherapy/combination therapy ... 200, 586
  nephrotoxicity and ototoxicity ... 586, 588
  nomograms ... 214
  ototoxicity and nephrotoxicity ... 587
  PAE ... 204
  P. aeruginosa ... 586
  pediatrics/neonates ... 211
  pharmacokinetics ... 202–203
  pneumonia ... 213
  and polypeptides ... 405
  pregnancy ... 211
  protein synthesis ... 203
  renal impairment ... 211
  resistance mechanisms ... 205–206
  soil microorganisms ... 199
  TDM ... 209, 210
  tobramycin ... 586
  toxicity ... 208–209
  traditional dosing ... 207
  urinary N-acetyl-D-glucosaminidase: creatinine ratio ... 588
  urinary tract infections ... 213
8-Aminoquinolines ... 428–429
Amphotericin B lipid complex (ABLC) ... 375
Animal age effect ... 61
Animal models ... 62–63, 69, 70
  acute bacterial pneumonia ... 64–65
  bacterial thigh infection ... 63–64
  chronic bacterial pneumonia ... 65–66
  description ... 397
    (*see also* Fungal infections)
  granuloma formation ... 398
  host susceptibility
    age effect ... 63
    immune suppression ... 62–63

John C. Rotschafer et al. (eds.), *Antibiotic Pharmacodynamics*, Methods in Pharmacology and Toxicology,
DOI 10.1007/978-1-4939-3323-5, © Springer Science+Business Media New York 2016

Animal models (*cont.*)
infectious endocarditis 71
intraperitoneal infection 72
Kramnic mouse 398
necrotic granulomas 398
(*see also* Pharmacokinetics (PK))
STIs (*see* Sexually transmitted infections (STIs))
UTIs (*see* Urinary tract infections (UTIs))
Antagonism 100
Antibacterial activity
erm-methylated ribosomes 348
erythromycin 348
macrocyclic ring 348
macrolides & ketolides 347
mef efflux pump 348
polypeptide site 347
Antibacterial classes 542–553
aminoglycosides 542
antibiotic effect 542
beta-lactam antibiotics
ceftazidime & cefepime 542
clinical outcome 545, 546
continuous infusion 543
gram-negative pathogens 542
PK/PD target attainment 544, 545
characteristics 541
ciprofloxacin
hydrophilic antibiotics 549
lipophilic antibiotic 549
sepsis 549
colistin
colistimethate sodium 552
hydrophilic polymyxin antibiotic 552
nephrotoxicity & neurotoxicity 552
steady-state plasma 553
daptomycin
creatinine kinase 552
hydrophilic antibiotic 550
peripheral neuropathy 552
S. aureus 551
sepsis/septic shock 551
dosing 542
fluoroquinolones 542
gentamicin
aminoglycosides 548
gram-negative infections 548
sepsis & septic shock 548
linezolid
dosing 550
epithelial lining fluid 549, 550
hydrophilic antibiotic 549
interstitial fluid 550
sepsis & septic shock 550
MIC 542
vancomycin
AUC_{0-24}/MIC 546, 547
infective endocarditis 546
meta-analysis 547
nephrotoxic drugs 547
nephrotoxicity 548
S. aureus 546, 547
Antibiotic combinations 99–105
antimicrobial properties 92
bactericidal activity 90
beta-lactams 91
community-acquired infections 92
community-acquired pneumonia 92
emerging health care 89
gram-negative bacteremia 90
innovative strategies
azithromycin 104, 105
azithromycin dosing 103
bacterial population 102
drug-induced nephrotoxicity 103
front-loaded colistin 103
infective endocarditis 103
mechanisms 102
microbiology 104
P. aeruginosa 103
plasma concentrations 103
prominently multidrug-resistant populations 103
pulse combinations 103
quorum sensing 104
renal/hepatic dysfunction 103
short-course combination therapy 103
virulence 104
in vitro and in vivo studies 97–99
meta-analyses 90
monotherapy 89
mortality benefit 90
multidrug resistance 90
multidrug-resistant pathogens 92
multiple antibiotics vs. monotherapy 90
odds ratio 90
P. aeruginosa 93
patient characteristics 92
pharmacodynamic analysis and mathematical modeling issues
analysis synergy 101, 102
antagonism 100
bactericidal activity 100
drawback 99
heterogeneous subpopulations 101
linezolid 99
log ratio area formula 101
synergy 100
Pseudomonas 91
randomized controlled trials 92

SIRS 91
Streptococcus pneumoniae 91
superinfections 90
Antibiotic drug development 624–625
Antifolates and sulfonamides
proguanil and cycloguanil 431–432
pyrimethamine 432
and sulfones 432
Antifungal PK–PD 375–379
combination therapy 380
concentration-dependent/time-dependent activity 373
drug concentrations 370
drug exposure 370
echinocandins (*see* Echinocandins)
flucytosine (*see* Flucytosine)
free non-protein bound drug 370
galactomannan 374
invasive fungal pathogens 369
in vitro drug potency 370–371
in vitro PK–PD models 371–372
laboratory animal models 372–373
Monte Carlo simulation 374
peak:MIC, AUC:MIC and T>MIC 373
pharmacodynamic index 373
polyenes (*see* Polyenes)
population pharmacokinetic models 374
serum/plasma 369
triazoles (*see* Triazoles)
Anti-infective agents 111
ADME 159
advantages and disadvantages 111, 112
aminoglycosides 162–164
amphotericin B 169–170
applications 160
azole antifungal drugs 168–169
beta-lactams 166–168
biological proteins 109
clinical safety 160
daptomycin 162
dose and biological effect 160
drug development 160
MIC 118–122
nonclinical setting 160
non-plasma drug concentrations 161
pathogen 110
PD and PK 160
pharmacodynamics activity 109, 110
pharmacokinetic techniques 159
plasma protein binding (*see* Plasma protein binding)
vancomycin and teicoplanin 161, 162
Antimalarial drugs .... 418–421, 429–430, .
See also 4-Substituted quinolines
8-aminoquinolines 428–429
antibacterials 432–433,
(*see also* Antifolates and sulfonamides)
artemisinins (*see* Artemisinins)
atovaquone 430, 431
atovaquone plus proguanil 423
biochemical mechanisms 425
drug resistance 422–423
erythrocytic forms 422
(*see also* Experimental agents)
group I, II and III drugs 422
human disease, female Anopheline mosquito 421
in vitro
growth inhibition 420
parasiticidal vs. parasitistatic activity 420
pharmacokinetic/pharmacodynamic linkage 421
speed of action and PRR 420–421
in vivo
avian malaria 418
biological and pharmacological investigations 418
humans 419–420
nonhuman primate 419
rodent malaria parasites 418
monotherapy 423
PK/PD linkage 424–425
public health campaigns/regimens 422
rational drug development 425
safety 425
SERCaP 426
sulfonamide/antifolate synergy 423
Antimicrobial
body weight 614
daptomycin 613
dosing paradigm 602, 603, 614
drug CL and weight 613
drug dosing 614
effect endpoint analysis 51–53
FDA clinical pharmacology 614
novel antibiotics 613
obese patients 615
obesity 613
PK-PD indices 604
population PK model 613
post hoc analysis 614
SSTI 614
telavancin dosing 614
therapeutic index 613
Antimicrobial resistance 633
Antimicrobial stewardship programs (ASPs) 639–644
antibiogram 635
antibiotic police 636
antibiotic utilization and expenditures 528
antimicrobial formulary restriction 637
antimicrobial resistance 644
antimicrobial therapy 636, 638

Antimicrobial stewardship programs (ASPs) (*cont.*)
- audit and feedback 637
- CDC 635, 636, 638
- clinical and economic outcomes 529
- clinical pharmacist and authorization 637
- *Clostridium difficile* infection 636
- CMS 644
- core members 634, 635
- core strategies 636
- DDD 529
- developmental procedure 639
- dose-optimized regimens 528
- hospital-acquired infections 635
- IDSA/SHEA guidelines 634, 636
- ID-trained pharmacists 644
- implementations 645
- infectious disease 634
- institution-wide dosing protocol 645, 646
- length of stay 644
- method 637
- mortality 528
- nosocomial transmission of resistant organisms 635
- patient outcomes 528
- pharmacodynamics 634 (*see* Pharmacodynamics (PD))
- piperacillin-tazobactam 529
- policy statement recommendations 638
- process and outcome metrics 528
- P&T-approved policies 637
- resources 634–635
- restriction and authorization programs 638
- SIDP 644
- superinfections 528
- supplemental strategies 638

Antimicrobial tissue concentrations
- aspiration pneumonia 608
- cefazolin 607
- cefoxitin 607
- dialysis fluid 606
- direct soft tissue evaluation 606
- dose selection 608
- drug concentration measurements 606
- end-tidal functional residual capacity 608
- ertapenem 607
- microdialysis 606, 607
- necrotic material 606
- non-skin and skin structure sites 608
- pharmacokinetics, cefazolin 607
- post cefazolin dosing 607
- protocols 606
- semipermeable membrane 606
- skin structure tissue 606
- superimposable subcutaneous cefoxitin concentration 607
- vascular and interstitial concentrations 606

Antiretroviral agents (ARV) 469
- entry inhibitor 494–495
- fusion inhibitor 493–494
- HIV (*see* Human immunodeficiency virus (HIV))
- lopinavir concentrations 472, 474
- parameters 472
- plasma drug concentrations 472
- raltegravir concentrations 472, 474

Antiviral agents 446, 447
- acyclovir and penciclovir 443, 444
- cidofovir 448
- clinical application
  - acyclovir 446, 447
  - dose–response relationship 446
  - dosing regimens 446
  - glomerular filtration and tubular secretion 446
  - hemodialysis 446
  - prophylaxis 446
  - renal tubules 447
  - side effects 446
  - valacyclovir 446
- CMV 442
- cytoplasm 443
- endocytosis 443
- foscarnet 448
- ganciclovir 448
- healthy volunteers and HIV/AIDS patients 449
- hemagglutinin binds 443
- herpesviridae viruses 441
- HSV 442
- induction therapy 451–452
- influenza 442
- intracellular viral replication 443
- maintenance therapy 452
- neuraminidase 443
- penciclovir 443
- pharmacokinetic parameters 449
- prophylactic usage 450–451
- resistance 447–448, 453–454
- sialic acid-recognizing glycoproteins 443
- toxicity 452–453
- vaccination 443
- valacyclovir and famciclovir 443
- valganciclovir 448
- viral morphologic characteristics 443
- VZV 442

Area under the concentration curve (AUC) 640

Area under the inhibitory curve (AUIC) 52

Artemisinins
- active moiety, *Artemesia annua* 429, 430
- artemether, arteether and artesunate 429
- dihydroartemisinin 429
- genetic studies 430
- hemolysis and hypersensitivity reactions 430
- long-lived endoperoxides 429

Atazanavir 487–488
Atovaquone
  antifolates and sulfonamides 430, 431
  asexual erythrocytic forms 430
  drug-resistant *P. falciparum* 431
AUC. *See* Area under the concentration curve (AUC)
AUIC. *See* Area under the inhibitory curve (AUIC)
Avian malaria 418
Azithromycin 104, 105

B

Bactec 460 TB system 393, 394
BACTEC 960 MGIT system 393, 394
Bacterial thigh infection 63–64
Bactericidal therapy 334
BAL. *See* Bronchoalveolar lavage (BAL)
Bayesian analysis 278–279
Bedaquiline 407
Beta-lactam antibiotics 518, 519
  adult data 585
  amoxicillin 582
  antibiotic resistance rates 584
  antibiotics 581
  antimicrobial agents 529
  antimicrobial therapy 582
  assessment 507–508
  aztreonam 584
  bacteremia 585
  benefits 515
  carbapenems and piperacillin-tazobactam 515
  CART 514
  cefepime 514
  ceftazidime 583
  ceftriaxone 582
  CI 515, 516
  clinical cure and microbiologic eradication 584
  clinical and pharmacokinetic outcomes 513
  computer simulations 513
  continuous and prolonged infusion programs 529, 530
  CSF 583
  cystic fibrosis 583
  dosage 582
  dose-optimized infusion strategies 529
  experimental animal models 583
  ex vivo data 511–513
  frequent dosing and extended/continuous infusions 584
  gram-negative infections 515
  immune response system 582
  meropenem and piperacillin 582–584
  Monte Carlo method 581
  multivariate model 514
  neutropenia 584
  P. aeruginosa 581
  PD targets 582
  pediatric patients 581
  pharmacoeconomic data
    carbapenems 518
    cost-benefit analyses 518
    cost-effectiveness analyses 519
    economic benefit 519
    P. aeruginosa 518
    pharmacodynamic parameters 518
    piperacillin-tazobactam 518
    QALYS 518
  pharmacokinetic and pharmacodynamic
    properties 569–577
  PI 515, 517
  piperacillin-tazobactam 515, 584
  PK-PD 508–510
  plasma antibiotic concentrations 513
  PTA 581
  ticarcillin-clavulanate 584
  time-dependent bactericidal effects 581
Body mass index (BMI) 566, 599, 601, 614
Bronchoalveolar lavage (BAL) 235
Broth microdilution (BMD) 266

C

CABP. *See* Community-acquired bacterial pneumonia (CABP)
CAPD. *See* Continuous ambulatory peritoneal dialysis (CAPD)
Capreomycin (CM) 386
CART. *See* Classification and regression tree analysis (CART)
CCR5. *See* Chemokine receptor 5 (CCR5)
CDC. *See* Centers for Disease Control and Prevention (CDC)
Cefepime 515
Centers for Disease Control
    and Prevention (CDC) 623, 635
  biofilm reactor 37
Cerebrospinal fluid (CSF) 264, 583
CF. *See* Cystic fibrosis (CF)
Chemokine receptor 4 (CXCR4) 470
Chemokine receptor 5 (CCR5) 470
Chloroquine
  dose- and age-related toxicity 427
  heme detoxification 426
  PfCRT mutations 426
Chronic bacterial pneumonia 65–66
CI. *See* Continuous-infusion (CI)
Ciprofloxacin 180
  antibacterial effects 186
  intra-pulmonary distribution 180
  and levofloxacin 181
  metabolism 179
  Monte Carlo simulations 187
  peak serum concentration 179
  plasma protein binding 180
  S. epidermidis 192
  and sparfloxacin 188

Classification and regression tree analysis (CART)..........514
Clinical Laboratory Standards Institute (CLSI)........32, 371
CM. *See* Capreomycin (CM)
CMV. *See* Cytomegalovirus (CMV)
Cockcroft–Gault equation..........277
Colistin..........222–223
Colistin methanesulfonate (CMS)..........223–224
Combination antifungal therapy..........380
Combination therapy models
antibiotics..........50
description..........38
in vitro combination PD model..........50
Community-acquired bacterial pneumonia (CABP)..........133, 624
Computerized provider order entry (CPOE)..........525
Concentration–response..........495
Continuous ambulatory peritoneal dialysis (CAPD)..........326–327
Continuous renal replacement therapy (CRRT)..........328, 329, 540
Continuous veno-venous hemodialysis (CVVHD)..........540
Continuous veno-venous hemofiltration (CVVHF)..........540
Continuous-infusion (CI)..........507
Acinetobacter baumannii..........520
administration techniques..........510
antibiograms..........520, 521
antibiotic infusion..........527
antimicrobial resistance pathogens..........521
application..........522
audience..........527
cefepime..........521, 522
clinical outcomes..........515
comorbidities and organisms..........515
cost-effectiveness analyses..........519
education..........527
hospital population..........521
hospital-wide vs. specific population use..........522–524
institution-specific needs..........519–524
microbore tubing..........527
P. aeruginosa..........520, 521
personnel and committees..........525
pharmacoeconomic data..........518–519
physical and chemical characteristics..........526
piperacillin-tazobactam..........521, 522
plasma antibiotic concentrations..........513
technology..........525–526
vancomycin and piperacillin-tazobactam..........526
Conventional amphotericin B..........375
CPOE. *See* Computerized provider order entry (CPOE)
Creatinine clearance (CrCL)..........233
CRRT. *See* Continuous renal replacement therapy (CRRT)
CSF. *See* Cerebrospinal fluid (CSF)
Cycloserine..........407
Cystic fibrosis (CF)..........211
Cystic Fibrosis Foundation..........586
Cytomegalovirus (CMV)..........441, 442

D

Dalbavancin
acute bacterial skin and skin structure infections..........298
aerobic and anaerobic gram-positive organisms..........296
animal models..........301–302
AUC/MIC..........286
C_{max} of..........296
description..........296
endocarditis and pneumonia..........286
hepatic and renal dysfunction..........296
intermittent and continuous renal replacement..........300
in vitro models..........300–301
low BSA and CrCl..........298
New Drug Application..........302
PK and exposure-response analysis..........286
PK parameters, healthy subjects..........296, 297
renal and hepatic impairment..........299–300
serum bactericidal activity..........298
single-dose and standard therapy groups..........302
and vancomycin-linezolid groups..........303
Daptomycin
animal models..........332–333
clinical trials..........335–337
concentration-dependent bactericidal activity..........317
CrCl estimation..........319, 321
critically ill patients..........324–325
CRRT..........328, 329
Cubicin®..........320
cyclic lipopeptides..........317
(*see also* Dialysis and renal replacement therapy)
disposition and penetration..........330–331
emergence of, bacterial resistance..........320
exposure and elevation creatinine phosphokinase levels..........334–335
geriatric..........323
HD..........327–328
infants and children..........322–323
in vitro models..........331–332
median terminal half-life estimation..........321
meningitis..........326
Monte Carlo simulations..........333–334
novel cyclic lipopeptide antibiotic..........317
obesity..........323–324
PK and tolerability..........321
plasma concentration–time profile..........320
protein binding..........321
renal excretion..........321
systemic exposure and elevations, CPK..........322
Darunavir..........488–489
Days of therapy (DOT)..........529
Defined daily doses (DDD)..........529
Delavirdine..........481, 482
Dialysis and renal replacement therapy
CAPD..........326–327
description..........326

Didanosine 475
Dolutegravir 492–493
Dose selection
allometry 608, 611
aminoglycoside CL 612
antifungal voriconazole 610
antimicrobial 609, 613
ATPase binding cassette 611
biomarker serum creatinine 611
body size 608
body size descriptor method 608
cefazolin 609
CLcr 611
CYP2C19 LoF alleles 610
cytochrome P450 610
daptomycin 613
drug CL 609, 610, 612
drug metabolism and body size 609
drug–drug interactions 610
empiric approach 608
empiric population average dose 609
GFR 611, 612
glomerular hyperfiltration 611
gut microbiome 609
isoenzymes systems 610
kidney biopsy data 611
kidney function 610
linezolid 612
liver function 610
modifiable 609
pharmacologic biomarkers 612
physiologic clearance mechanisms 609
PK evaluation 611
renal tubular secretion and reabsorption 611
skeletal muscle metabolism 611
SSTI 612
TDM 610, 612
voriconazole 610
weight and height 608
DOT. *See* Days of therapy (DOT)
Drug susceptibility test (DST)
agar based 7H11 media 393
Bactec 460 TB system 393
BACTEC 960 MGIT system 393
"critical" drug concentrations 393
direct and indirect methods 392
L–J media 393
molecular tools 394
Monte Carlo simulations 394
TB patients' samples 392
wild-type *Mycobacterium tuberculosis* 392
Drug targeting index (DTI) 235
Duet pump system 43, 44

E

Echinocandins
Candida parapsilosis 378
Fks mutations 379
in vitro and experimental models 378
laboratory animal models 379
paradoxical antifungal activity 378
peak:MIC/AUC:MIC 378
preclinical models 379
therapeutic index and higher dosages 379
Efavirenz 482
EIAD. *See* Extended interval aminoglycoside dosing (EIAD)
Electronic medical records (EMR) 525
ELF. *See* Epithelial lining fluid (ELF)
Elvitegravir 491–492
EMA. *See* European Medicines Agency (EMA)
E_{max} model 14
EMR. *See* Electronic medical records (EMR)
Emtricitabine 478
Epithelial lining fluid (ELF) 60, 264
Equilibrium dialysis
materials 115
methods 116
ETA. *See* Ethionamide (ETA)
Ethambutol (EMB)
description 404
GI disturbance, arthralgia and neutropenia and thrombocytopenia 404
optic neuritis 404
Ethionamide (ETA) 406
Etravirine 483
European Committee on Antifungal Susceptibility Testing (EUCAST) methodology 371
European Committee on Standardization (CEN) 6
European Federation of Pharmaceutical Industry Associations Working Group 159
European Medicines Agency (EMA) 387, 621
Experimental agents
description 434
DSM265 433
KAE609 433
KAF 156 434
OZ439 434
Exposure-response relationships 12, 13, 15, 16, 132–136, 141–150, 152, 153
antimicrobial agents 128
Bayesian approach
antimicrobial agent 141
dichotomous efficacy 144
frequentist analyses 141, 142
HABP/VABP 141

Exposure-response relationships (*cont.*)
statistical approaches ... 141
tigecycline ... 141
treatment effect ... 142–144
components ... 127
drug development process ... 128
drug exposure and safety ... 127
efficacy
antimicrobial agents ... 132
applications ... 144–146
bacterial eradication ... 133
bacteriologic response ... 133, 134
capturing effect ... 134
characterizition ... 136
clinical data ... 136
complicated intra-abdominal infections ... 133
dichotomous efficacy endpoints ... 135
drug concentration ... 132
drug regimens ... 134, 135
Enterobacteriaceae ... 133
evaluation ... 132
group assignments ... 136
hypotheses ... 132
independent and dependent variables ... 133
linear regression ... 136
mathematical model ... 136
MIC ... 132
probability ... 135
safety ... 128, 131–132
statistical approaches ... 135
treatment effect ... 133
multivariable analyses ... 137–140
safety
aminoglycosides ... 147, 149
antimicrobial agent ... 153
beta-lactam agents ... 146
characterization ... 147
clinical development ... 147
daptomycin ... 147, 152, 153
gentamicin/tobramycin ... 150
HABP/VABP ... 149
Monte Carlo simulation ... 152
multivariable model ... 152
nausea and vomiting ... 147, 148
nephrotoxicity ... 149, 150
proximal renal tubular epithelial cells ... 149
tigecycline ... 147
Extended infusion protocol
beta-lactams ... 642, 643
intravenous medications ... 643
MIC ... 642
piperacillin/tazobactam ... 642
subtherapeutic dose ... 642
Extended interval aminoglycoside dosing (EIAD) ... 207–208
vs. traditional dosing strategies ... 208
Extensively drug-resistant tuberculosis (XDR-TB) ... 386

F

Famciclovir
acyclovir ... 447
genital HSV and VZV infections ... 443
FDA. *See* Food and Drug Administration (FDA)
FiberCell systems ... 34
FIC. *See* Fractional inhibitory concentration (FIC)
First line drugs
EMB, mycobacterial cell wall synthesis ... 388
INH pro-drug ... 388
known/proposed targets ... 389
PZA pro-drug ... 388
RNA polymerase enzyme subunits ... 388
Flucytosine
Candida albicans ... 376
cryptococcal meningoencephalitis ... 376
fractionated regimens ... 377
myelosuppression ... 377
Fluoroquinolone ... 640
adult human dose ... 164
anaerobic infections ... 192–193
antibiotics ... 177
antimicrobials ... 178
arthralgia ... 166
central nervous system ... 164
ciprofloxacin ... 165
enoxacin and sparfloxacin ... 166
gram-negative pathogens ... 178
hospital and community ... 179
hospitals/health plans ... 178
LEVO and MOXI ... 404–405
Mycobacteria and *Chlamydia* ... 177
moxifloxacin ... 165
parenteral drugs ... 179
phototoxicity ... 166
prulifloxacin ... 164
QT prolongation and ventricular arrhythmias ... 165
quinolones ... 177
retinal degeneration ... 166
scientific and medical communities ... 178
seizures ... 164
sitafloxacin and levofloxacin ... 164
toxicodynamic markers ... 178
trovafloxacin ... 166
ulifloxacin ... 164
Food and Drug Administration (FDA) ... 178, 621
Food and Drug Administration Safety and Innovation Act (FDASIA) ... 623

Fosamprenavir 488
Fractional inhibitory concentration (FIC) 243
Fungal infections
 antifungal therapy 67
 CNS models, invasive candidiasis 68
 Cryptococcus sp. 68
 dermatophytes 68
 endophthalmitis 67
 filamentous fungal pathogen models 67
 pulmonary mold infection models 66
 quantitative PCR (qPCR) 67
 site-specific infections 66
 tissue homogenation, kidneys 67
 Zygomycetes 68

G

Gentamicin 207
Glomerular filtration rate (GFR) 610–611
Gram-negative organisms
 animal infection models 185–186
 antimicrobial effects 183
 human data 186–188
 in vitro simulations 183–185

H

Hematogenous *Candida* meningoencephalitis (HCME) 375
Hematopoietic stem cell transplantation (HSCT) 372
Hemodialysis (HD) 327–328
Hepatic steatosis 602
Herpes simplex viruses (HSV) 441
Heterogeneous VISA (hVISA) 101
HFS. *See* Hollow fiber system (HFS)
High-performance liquid chromatography (HPLC) 230
Hollow fiber multi-compartment PK/PD model
 advantages 33
 analysis 45
 artificial membranes, types of 33
 depiction 34, 35
 FiberCell systems 34
 materials 34, 36
 model preparation 42–43
 organism preparation 44
 PK/PD simulation 44–45
 reservoir cap with tube connections 35, 36
Hollow fiber system (HFS) 397
Hospital-acquired bacterial pneumonia (HABP)
 Bayesian principles 141
 clinical and microbiological response 137
 tigecycline-treated patients 140
HPLC. *See* High-performance liquid chromatography (HPLC)
HSCT. *See* Hematopoietic stem cell transplantation (HSCT)
HSV. *See* Herpes simplex viruses (HSV)
Human immunodeficiency virus (HIV)
 ARV therapy 471
 drug efficacy 471
 genes, proteins and functions 470
 glycoproteins 470
 lymph nodes 471
 peripheral blood 471
 RNA retrovirus 470
 sensitive assays 471
 T cells 470
 treatment, ARV drugs 472, 473
 Virologic efficacy 471
hVISA. *See* Heterogeneous VISA (hVISA)

I

ICU. *See* Intensive care unit (ICU)
IDSA. *See* Infectious Diseases Society of America (IDSA)
Indinavir 486
Infants and children 322–323
Infectious Diseases Society of America (IDSA) 507, 634
Infectious endocarditis 71
Influenza 442, 457–460
 adamantanes (M-2 Inhibitors) 454
 clinical application
  amantadine 457
  neuropsychiatric side effects 459
  oseltamivir 457, 458
  zanamivir 457, 458
 neuraminidase inhibitors 454
 resistance
  adamantanes, 459
  children and immunocompromised patients 459
  fluorimetry-based neuraminidase inhibition assay 459
  hemagglutinin receptor 459
  laninamivir 460
  neuraminidase inhibitors 459
  oseltamivir 459, 460
  peramivir 460
  virulence and transmissibility 459
  zanamivir 460
 treatment and prevention 454
Integrase strand transfer inhibitors
 dolutegravir 492–493
 elvitegravir 491–492
 raltegravir 489
 viral life cycle 489
Intensive care unit (ICU) 514
Intermittent and continuous renal replacement 300
International Conference on Harmonisation (ICH) 621
Intraperitoneal infection 72

In vitro drug potency
CLSI and EUCAST 371
dosing interval 371
MIC value 371
minimum inhibitory concentration 370
In vitro models
dilution system 396, 397
HFS 397
pathogen, host and PK factors 397
In vitro PK/PD modeling 371–372
ceftaroline with repeated dosing 39
first-order kinetic equation 38, 39
oritavancin, single 3-h infusion dose 40
pharmacodynamic analysis 38
target concentration 39
Isoniazid
catalase peroxidase enzyme (KatG) 401, 402
"pharmacokinetic mismatch" 402
post-antibiotic effect 402
TB treatment drug 401

K

Kanamycin (KM) 386
Kernicterus 568
Klebsiella pneumoniae
capsule polysaccharide gene expression 228
doripenem 245
regrowth 238
KM. *See* Kanamycin (KM)

L

Laboratory animal models
biomarkers 372
cryptococcal meningitis 373
HSCT 372
invasive aspergillosis and candidiasis 372
kidney, quantitative cultures 372
neutropenic and non-neutropenic models 372
LAmB. *See* Liposomal amphotericin B (LAmB)
Lamivudine 476–477
Length of stay (LOS) 514, 644
Levofloxacin (LEVO) 180, 386, 404–405
anaerobic infections 192
antimicrobial effect 183
bacterial eradication 190
ciprofloxacin 179
intra-pulmonary distribution 180
in vitro dynamic model 190
in vitro model 184
Monte Carlo simulations 190
moxifloxacin 179
pharmacodynamic indices 189
S. aureus 185
S. epidermidis 191
S. pneumoniae 189
Linear regression analysis 276
Linezolid 99
Lipoglycopeptides 285, 286
dalbavancin (*see* Dalbavancin)
gram-positive microorganisms 285
oritavancin (*see* Oritavancin)
PK and PD properties 285
telavancin (*see* Telavancin)
Lipopolysaccharide (LPS) 225
Liposomal amphotericin B (LAmB) 375
Lopinavir 487
LOS. *See* Length of stay (LOS)
LPS. *See* Lipopolysaccharide (LPS)
Lung penetration and intracellular activity 306

M

Macrolide-lincosamide-streptograminB (MLSB) 347
Making a Difference in Infectious Diseases Pharmacotherapy (MAD-ID) 644
Malaria
life cycle 415, 416
mitochondrial electron transport 418
mosquito-borne infectious disease 415
Plasmodium species 415, 417
simplified pharmacodynamic specificities 416, 417
MBC. *See* Minimum bactericidal concentration (MBC)
MCS. *See* Monte Carlo simulation (MCS)
MD. *See* Microdialysis (MD)
MDR. *See* Multidrug-resistant (MDR)
MDR-TB. *See* Multidrug-resistant tuberculosis (MDR-TB)
Medicines for Malaria Venture (MMV) 433
Mefloquine 428
Meningitis 326
Meropenem 582
Methicillin-resistant *Staphylococcus aureus* (MRSA) 285–288, 291–294, 301, 302, 308, 546
Methicillin-susceptible *Staphylococcus aureus* (MSSA) 177
MIBC. *See* Minimum biofilm inhibitory concentration (MIBC)
MIC. *See* Minimum inhibitory concentration (MIC)
Microbiologic & clinical outcomes
antiviral activity 578
B-lymphocytes 579
chemotherapeutic agents 579
cytotoxic activity 578
cytotoxic natural killer cells 578
deficiencies 579
humoral/antibody-mediated immunity 579
immunologic memory and cytokine production 579
immunosuppression 579
infections 578
innate and adaptive immune responses 578
lymphocyte function development 578
neonates 578

neonates & infants....579
neutrophil count....578
phagocytic cells....578
serum immunoglobulin G (IgG) antibodies....579
serum proteins....578
T-lymphocytes....579
Toxoplasma gondii and *Listeria*....579
vernix caseosa....578
Microdialysis (MD)
bioanalysis....115
materials....111, 113
plasma protein binding....114, 115
probe recovery....114
setup....113
Minimum bactericidal concentration (MBC)....5, 7
Minimum biofilm inhibitory concentration (MIBC)....241
Minimum inhibitory concentration (MIC)....5, 132, 225, 269–271, 348, 580
and antibacterial effects....509
beta-lactam....266
BMD....266, 270
broth microdilution....266
CART analysis....270, 271
Cockcroft–Gault/MDRD creatinine clearance calculation....271
creep....266
disk-diffusion susceptibility testing method....6
drug concentrations....509
Etest and automated systems....266
factors....6
gram-negative bacteria....509
IDSA MRSA treatment....266
inoculum....6
labor-intensive methods....266
macrodilution....119, 120
materials....118
measurement, antimicrobial activity....7
microdilution....6
Mueller-Hinton....6
non-visible growth....7
P. aeruginosa....521
patients....271
pharmacodynamic target....267, 268
piperacillin-tazobactam....522
plasma antibiotic concentrations....513
time kill curve determination....120, 121
toxicity
CART analysis....269
Monte Carlo simulation....269
MRSA bacteremia....269, 270
nephrotoxicity....269–271
pharmacodynamic target attainment....269, 271
and treatment outcomes....266–267
MLSB. *See* Macrolide-lincosamide-streptograminB (MLSB)
MMV. *See* Medicines for Malaria Venture (MMV)
Monte Carlo simulation (MCS)....21, 333–334, 374, 513, 580
Moxifloxacin (MOXI)....386, 404–405
bactericidal activity....190
ciprofloxacin....179
gram-negative pathogens....183
and levofloxacin....185
Monte Carlo simulation....191
Moraxella catarrhalis....185
plasma proteins....180
S. aureus and *S. epidermidis*....192
trovafloxacin....192
MRSA. *See* Methicillin-resistant *Staphylococcus aureus* (MRSA)
MSSA. *See* Methicillin-susceptible Staphylococcus aureus (MSSA)
Multidrug-resistant (MDR)....507
Multidrug-resistant tuberculosis (MDR-TB)....386

N

Nelfinavir....485–486
Nephrotoxicity....208
Neuraminidase inhibitors
cell culture assays....455
dose fractionation....456
efficacy....456
fluorescence/chemiluminescence....455
influenza....455
in vitro analyses....455
in vitro hollow-fiber infection models....456
laninamivir octanoate....455
oseltamivir....455, 456
oseltamivir carboxylate exposure data....457
peramivir....455
PK-PD parameters....456
sialic acid....455
zanamivir....455, 456
Neuromuscular toxicity....209
Neutropenic murine-thigh infection model....141
Nevirapine....480–481
Nonhuman primate....419
Non-nucleoside reverse transcriptase inhibitors (NNRTIs)
CYP enzymes....479
delavirdine....481, 482
efavirenz....482
etravirine....483
glucuronidation....479
nevirapine....480–481
rilpivirine....483–484
Nucleoside reverse transcriptase inhibitors (NRTIs)
abacavir....477–478
didanosine....475
emtricitabine....478

Nucleoside reverse transcriptase inhibitors (NRTIs) (*cont.*)
lamivudine........476–477
stavudine........476
tenofovir........478, 479
zidovudine........474, 475

O

Obesity........323–324, 606–608
adipocytes and leucocytes........601
adipokines........601
age-dependent effect........601
antimicrobial........600
(*see* Antimicrobial tissue concentrations)
antimicrobial dosing paradigm........602–603
antiviral therapy........602
BMI........599, 601
chronic Hepatitis C virus (HCV) infection........602
definition........599–600
diabesity........600
infection........600–602
inflammatory mediators........601
lymphedema........601
macrocirculation and microcirculation........601
morbid obesity........600
and pharmacodynamic bioequivalence........603–606
post-surgical skin and skin structure infections (SSTIs)........601
pro-inflammatory effects........601
sepsis-related mortality........601
super obesity........600
vascular access and respiratory intubation........601
Ohio State University Medical Center (OSUMC)........527
One-compartment PK/PD models
analysis........42
antibiotics........31
antimicrobials evaluation........29
applications and simulations........41
central reservoir system........31, 32
designs........32
human-scaled antimicrobial exposure........30
in vitro........30
materials........32, 33
media and organism preparation........41
preparation........41–42
Oritavancin
animal models........308–309
chemical structure........303
clinical trials........309–310
dialysis, clearance........306–307
drug accumulation........304
gram-positive microorganisms........286
infections........303
in vitro models........307–308
lung penetration and intracellular activity........306
patient-specific covariates and drug variability........304
pharmacokinetic parameter estimation........304, 305
plasma and skin blister fluid........305–306
second-generation semisynthetic lipoglycopeptide antimicrobial agent........303
staphylococci and enterococci with MICs........307
Staphylococcus Aureus Bacteremia........309
synergy........287
three-compartment model........286
tissues in reticuloendothelial systems........304
Oseltamivir
bloodstream........455
carboxylate........455
gastrointestinal disturbance........458
glomerular filtration and tubular secretion........458
plasma concentrations........456
randomized, control trials........457
treatment and chemoprophylaxis........457
and zanamivir........455
OSUMC. *See* Ohio State University Medical Center (OSUMC)
Ototoxicity........209

P

PAE. *See* Post-antibiotic effect (PAE)
Paenibacillus polymyxa........221
Para-amino salicyclic (PAS) acid
GI complaints........406
granule dosage form........406
N-acetyl transferase 1 (NAT1)........406
Parasite reduction ratio (PRR)........420–421
Parasiticidal vs. parasitistatic activity........420
PAS. *See* Para-amino salicyclic (PAS) acid
Pediatric Infectious Diseases Society (PIDS)........634
Pediatrics
age groups........562
antimicrobial agents........562
antimicrobial therapy........561
dosing........562
immune system........561
pharmacodynamic........562
pharmacokinetics........561
Pediatrics/neonates........211
Penciclovir........443
Pharmacodynamics (PD)........5, 7–10, 358, 359, 538–541, 543, 642–644
acute kidney injury (AKI)
dosing........540
drug molecules........540
extravascular fluid........540
fluconazole........540
glomerular filtration........540
hydrophilic drugs........540
sepsis/septic shock........539

acyclovir and penciclovir....444
aminoglycosides....642
antibacterial activity....355
antibiotic and microorganism....3, 537
antibiotic-resistant bacteria....94
antimicrobial chemotherapy....11
antimicrobials....3, 4, 94
(*see* Antiretroviral agents (ARV))
antiviral and antifungal drugs....22
AUC/MIC ratio....12, 640, 641
augmented renal clearance....541
azalides....346, 349–351, 356, 357, 361
bactericidal activity....93
bactericidal agents....94
cell lines....445
checkerboard-type experiments and time-kill curves....24
chronic bronchitis....347
chronic diseases....94
ciprofloxacin....640, 643
clindamycin....362
clinical breakpoints and drug development....21–22
Cmax and AUC....11
concentration-effect relationships
concentration-time data....9–10
drug-receptor interactions....5
MBC....7
MIC....5
microorganisms....5
time-kill curves....7–9
concentration-time curve....11
cytomegalovirus....448
dose optimization....641–642
driver & magnitudes
azithromycin....358
bacterial density....359
clarithromycin....358
erythromycin....358
ketolides....359
macrolides....358
neutropenic murine....358
telithromycin....359
drugs....3
effective concentration (EC_{50}) values....445
emergence, resistance....22–24, 94
erythromycin....345
exposure-response relationships....12, 13, 15, 16
exposures....21
factors....4
fixed concentrations....10
fluid shifts & changes
blood flow....539
hydrophilic antibiotics....539
lipophilic antibiotics....539
sepsis....539
volume distribution....539
fluoroquinolones....640, 643
formulary decision making....640
frequency....10
ganciclovir and valganciclovir....448, 449
hepatic clearance....541
heteroaryl-alkyl....346, 347
host immune status and heterogenous
viral populations....445
human cell lines....444
hypoalbuminemia....539
hypo-perfusion & sub therapeutic tissue....539
IC_{50}....445
immunomodulatory/anti-inflammatory effects....358
infection site....356
institution-wide dose optimization
beta-lactams....642–643
renal dosage adjustment....643–644
in vitro and in vivo....16–18
in vitro models and Monte Carlo
simulations....182–183
ketolides....346, 349–351, 356, 357, 361
β-lactams, aminoglycosides....93
levofloxacin....640
limited data....445
macrocyclic lactone ring....347
macrolide....345
macrolides....346, 349–351, 356, 357, 361
macrolides & azithromycin....346
metabolic pathway....94
microorganism....11
monotherapy....93
multidrug-resistant bacteria....93
orofacial, genital, and perirectal lesions....445
parameter estimates....12
patient populations....18–20
penicillin allergic patient....345
pharmacokinetics
dosing....538, 543
hydrophilicity....538
post antibiotic effect....357–358
PRA....445
protein binding....15–16
renal replacement therapy
antibiotics....541
drug dosing....541
hemodynamic intolerance....540
intermittent hemodialysis....540
sensitive control strain....445
sepsis....537
septic shock....537
and serum drug concentrations....445
steady-state C_{max} concentrations....444, 445
superinfection....93
synergistic activity....93
(*see* Vancomycin)

Pharmacodynamics (PD) (*cont.*)
telithromycin ... 346, 347
translation ... 20–21
triphosphate ... 448
vancomycin and aminoglycosides ... 93, 641–642
white blood cells ... 356–357
Pharmacokinetics (PK)
absorption and oral bioavailability ... 179–180
advantage ... 129, 131
albumin binds ... 568
allometric method ... 565
alveolar macrophages (AM) ... 354
aminoglycosides & linezolid ... 202, 568
animal age effect ... 61
animal species, effect of ... 60
antibiotics ... 129
anti-infective agent ... 59
benefits ... 128
body composition measures ... 566, 567
chloramphenicol ... 568
clarithromycin ... 353
clinical usage ... 129
concentration-dependent bactericidal activity ... 203
creatinine clearance ... 264
cystic fibrosis ... 562
definition ... 129
distribution and tissue penetration ... 180–181
dosing interval calculation ... 265
dried blood spot technique ... 590
drug accumulation and nephrotoxicity ... 202
drug concentration measurements ... 59
drug concentrations ... 130
drug exposure ... 131
effect sites ... 129
ELF and CSF ... 264
elimination ... 181
erythromycin ... 353
extracellular fluid ... 354
flexibility ... 130
gentamicin ... 568
gestational & postnatal age ... 565
glomerular filtration rate ... 202
hepatic clearance pathways ... 565
hepatic encephalopathy/intestinal parasites ... 202
hepatic metabolism ... 568
hydrophilic drugs ... 566
infection sites ... 60
infection, effect of ... 61
inhaled (aerosolized) therapy ... 202
kernicterus ... 568
ketolides & macrolides ... 353
kidneys ... 131
liver and kidneys ... 568
maturation and organ function ... 562
mechanism ... 179
methyltransferase and sulfotransferase ... 565
microsomal cytochrome ... 568
mimic human PK ... 61–62
neonates and infants ... 566
neonates and young infants ... 566
nephrogenesis ... 565
non-absorbable antibiotics ... 202
obesity ... 566
opportunistic study design ... 590
optimal PK estimation ... 59
optimal sampling theory ... 131
oral doses ... 354
parameters ... 130
patient-specific factors ... 130
pediatric age groups ... 566
physiologic changes ... 562–564
physiologic-based parameters ... 566
plasma protein binding ... 568
properties ... 129
sparse sampling ... 590
sulfonamides & ceftriaxone ... 568
supplemental doses ... 203
tissue penetration ... 264
traditional intensive approach ... 590
two-stage approach ... 130
vancomycin ... 264
Pharmacokinetics-pharmacodynamics (PK-PD) ... 624, 625
animal models ... 626
antibacterial agents ... 624
antibiotic-resistant bacteria ... 625
antibiotics reflect ... 622
anti-infective drug development programs ... 622
antimicrobial agents ... 360, 361, 627
antimicrobial drug development ... 625, 627
bacteriostatic effect ... 360
beta-lactams ... 508–510
administration techniques ... 510–511
breakthrough therapy ... 623
CABP ... 624
chronic bronchitis ... 361
clinical data ... 136
drug development phases ... 627–628
drug-resistant bacteria ... 623
efficacy ... 135
ex vivo modeling systems ... 360
EMA ... 624
FDA ... 621, 622
FDASIA ... 623
four-tiered -approach
animal rule ... 625
infection/disease-focused approach ... 624
pathogen-focused approach ... 625
risks and limitations ... 625
health authority guidance documents ... 621–622
in vivo infection models ... 626, 629

life-threatening diseases....623
limitation....145
logistic regression/Hill-type models....135
macrolides....359
MIC, microorganism....629
multivariable analyses....137
PD marker....626
pharmacometric approaches....624, 629
preclinical infection models....628
principles....624
probability....144
QIDP....623
regulatory approval and probability of preclinical....626
translational pharmacology....624
PI. *See* Prolonged-infusion (PI)
PK-PD biofilm models
analysis....48–49
antimicrobial efficacy evaluation....37
CDC biofilm model....45, 46
CDC biofilm reactor....37
CDC model preparation....47–48
commercial assays....37
media and organism preparation....46–47
PK-PD indices
anti-infective drugs....395
beta-lactams....395
limitations....395
protein binding....395
Plaque reduction assay (PRA)....445
Plasma and skin blister fluid....305–306
Plasma protein binding
in vitro equilibrium dialysis....115, 116
in vitro microdialysis....111, 113–115
in vitro ultrafiltration....117–121
Polyenes
amphotericin B....375, 376
clinical implications....376
Polymyxin....241, 243–248
aminoglycosides....222
animals....231–233
antibacterial activity....240–241
antimicrobial agents....222
antimicrobial peptides....221
BAL....235
CMS....223–224
colistin and polymyxin B....222–223, 234
combination therapy
A. baumannii....243
amplification....241
antibiotics....241
antimicrobial agents....244
carbapenems....244
clinical investigations....246–248
colistin....243
FIC....243
gram-negative organisms....246
gram-positive bacteria....243
heteroresistant strains....243
imipenem/doripenem....244–246
immunocompetent host....246
plasma concentrations....243
resistance....241
rifampicin....244
static/dynamic time-kill methods....244
subpopulation synergy....243
synergy....244
CrCL....233
cystic fibrosis....222
DTI....235
influence....232, 236
in vitro pharmacodynamics....236–240
kidneys....235
mechanisms of resistance....228–229
microbiological and pharmacological knowledge....222
microbiological assay....230
mode of action....225–228
multidrug-resistant....222
polymyxin B....222–223
polymyxin E....221
prodrug....236
renal impairment....233
renal replacement therapy....235
safety....222
spectrum....224–225
susceptibility testing....236
toxicity....229–230
urinary tract infections....236
Population pharmacokinetic models....374
Post-antibiotic effect (PAE)....204, 239, 588
PRA. *See* Plaque reduction assay (PRA)
Preclinical toxicology....160
Priori dosing method....276
Probability of target attainment (PTA)....508, 581
Proguanil and cycloguanil....431–432
Prolonged-infusion (PI)....507
administration techniques....510
cefepime....514, 521
clinical and economic outcomes....529
clinical benefits....508
Hawthorne effect....510
mortality benefit....510
pharmacoeconomic data....518–519
piperacillin-tazobactam....515, 527
Protease inhibitors
atazanavir....487–488
darunavir....488–489
fosamprenavir....488
indinavir....486
lopinavir....487
nelfinavir....485–486

Protease inhibitors (*cont.*)
ritonavir/cobicistat 484
saquinavir 484–485
tipranavir 488
PRR. *See* Parasite reduction ratio (PRR)
Pseudomonas aeruginosa 104, 206, 514, 581
colistin 237
cystic fibrosis 222
heteroresistance 229
imipenem/doripenem 244
PTA. *See* Probability of target attainment (PTA)
Pyrazinamide (PZA)
acidic environment 403
bacterial pyrazinamidase enzyme 402
dose-dependent 403
hepatotoxicity 403
PK/PD parameter 403
Pyrimethamine 432
PZA. *See* Pyrazinamide (PZA)

Q

Qualified infectious disease product (QIDP) 623
Quality-adjusted life years (QALYS) 518
Quinine 427–428
Quinolones 177

R

Raltegravir
ANRS 139 TRIO trial 490
atazanavir 491
CD4 cell 490
efficacy 490
HIV-infected adults 489
lopinavir/ritonavir 491
nucleoside-sparing regimens 491
rifampin 490
tenofovir and emtricitabine 489
viral suppression and immune restoration 490
Reactive oxygen species (ROS) 228
Receiver operating characteristic (ROC) 145
Renal and hepatic impairment 299–300
Renal dysfunction 643
Resistance development
bactericidal effects 390
chromosomal mutations 390
drug exposure among patients 392
gene and product correlation 390, 391
patient adherence to treatment 390
spontaneous mutations and cross-resistance 390
Resistance mechanisms
active efflux 206
amino/hydroxyl functions 205
aminoglycosides 205
anaerobic bacteria 205
antimicrobials 205
broad spectrum 205
genetic elements 205
P. aeruginosa 206
phenotypes 205
plazomicin 206
sisomicin 206
target modification 206
Rifabutin 400
Rifampin 399–400
Rifamycins
clinical utility, anti-TB drugs 399
concentration-dependent killers 399
monotherapy 399
TB treatment 399
Rifapentine
culture conversion, groups 400
cyclo-pentyl derivative, rifampin 400
Guinea pig model 401
isoniazid 401
Rilpivirine 483–484
ROC. *See* Receiver operating characteristic (ROC)
Rodent malaria parasites 418
ROS. *See* Reactive oxygen species (ROS)

S

Saquinavir 484–485
SCVs. *See* Small-colony variants (SCVs)
Second line drugs
aminoglycosides 389
DNA gyrase 389
PAS mechanism 390
peptidoglycan synthesis and d-alanine metabolism 390
SERCaP. *See* Single exposure radical cure and prophylaxis (SERCaP)
Sexually transmitted infections (STIs)
Chlamydia trachomatis 70
congenital syphilis 70
description 69
genital tract disease 70
genitourinary tract disease models 69
localized infection 69
SHEA. *See* Society for Healthcare Epidemiology of America (SHEA)
Single exposure radical cure and prophylaxis (SERCaP) 426
SIRS. *See* Systemic inflammatory response syndrome (SIRS)
SLED/SLED-*f*. *See* Sustained low-efficiency daily dialysis/diafiltration (SLED/SLED-*f*)
Small-colony variants (SCVs) 306
Society for Healthcare Epidemiology of America (SHEA) 507, 634

Society of Infectious Diseases Pharmacists (SIDP)..........644
Spectrum & potency
  clarithromycin..........348
  erm genes..........352
  erythromycin..........348
  Haemophilus influenzae..........348
  ketolides..........348
  macrolides..........348
  pharmacokinetic & pharmacodynamic..........348
  S. pyogenes..........352
  streptococci..........348, 352
  telithromycin..........352
Staphylococcus aureus..........103, 141, 152, 191–192, 309
Stavudine..........476
STIs. *See* Sexually transmitted infections (STIs)
Streptococcus pneumoniae..........91
  chronic bronchitis..........188
  ciprofloxacin and sparfloxacin..........188
  levofloxacin..........188, 189
  microbiologic eradication..........188
  Monte Carlo simulations..........188
  moxifloxacin..........189
4-Substituted quinolines
  amodiaquine..........428
  chloroquine..........426–427
  lumefantrine..........428
  mefloquine..........428
  piperaquine..........428
  quinine..........427–428
  and structurally related compounds..........426, 427
Sulfones..........432
Sustained low-efficiency daily dialysis/diafiltration (SLED/SLED-*f*)..........540
Synergy
  antagonism..........100
  azithromycin..........104
  Bliss independence..........97
  microbiology..........104
  β-lactams, aminoglycosides..........93
  oewe additivity..........95–97
Systemic inflammatory response syndrome (SIRS)..........91

T

T-cell proliferation..........601
TDM. *See* Therapeutic drug monitoring (TDM)
Telavancin
  animal models..........293–294
  ATLAS I and II studies..........295
  ATTAIN trials..........295
  covariates..........289
  disposition and penetration..........291–292
  European Medicines Agency..........287
  FAST 1 and 2 trials..........294
  in vitro models..........292–293
  lipophilic side chain..........287
  maximum and minimum plasma concentrations..........287
  methicillin-resistant *S. aureus* (MRSA)..........285
  PK at steady state..........288
  population PK estimated parameters..........289
  post hoc analysis..........295
  primary urinary excretion..........286
  special populations..........290–291
  VanA VRE against VanB VRE..........287
Tenofovir..........478, 479
Therapeutic drug monitoring (TDM)
  characteristics..........495
  clinical and virologic outcomes..........495
  drug serum concentrations..........210
  intra-patient and inter-patient..........496
  NRTIs..........496
  populations..........497
  ritonavir..........496
  toxicity monitoring..........210
Thymidine kinase (TK)..........444, 447, 448
Time-kill curves..........396
  determination..........120, 121
Tipranavir..........488
Tobramycin..........207
Toxicity
  hematological side effects..........209
  hypersensitivity reactions..........209
  linezolid..........279
  nephrotoxicity..........208, 279
  neuromuscular..........209
  optimal dosing..........280
  ototoxicity..........209, 280
  oxidative stressor..........279
  renal dysfunction..........279, 280
Toxicokinetics (TK)
  clinical safety issues..........159
  drug development..........160
  guinea pig model..........163
  in vivo kinetics..........159
  preclinical toxicology..........160
Triazoles
  antifungal therapy, humans..........377
  dose fractionation studies..........377
  fluconazole..........377
  invasive candidiasis..........377
  itraconazole and posaconazole..........378
  oropharyngeal candidiasis..........378
Tuberculosis (TB) drugs..........392, 402–404
  aminoglycosides and polypeptides..........405
  animal models..........397–398
  bedaquiline..........407
  cycloserine..........407
  dose optimization tools..........398
  DST (*see* Drug susceptibility test (DST))

Tuberculosis (TB) drugs (*cont.*)
ELF 398
EMB 386
(*see* Ethambutol (EMB))
ETA 406
first line drugs 388–389
fluoroquinolones 404–405
HIV, sole infectious agent 385
INH, RIF and PZA 386
isoniazid 401–402
in vitro models 396–397
MDR-TB 386
Mycobacterium tuberculosis 385
PAS acid 406
PK/PD indices 395
PZA (*see* Pyrazinamide (PZA))
resistance development 390–392
rifabutin 400
rifampin 399–400
rifamycins 399
rifapentine 400–401
second line drugs 389–390
sputum samples 399
streptomycin treatment 385
TDM 407–408
time-kill curves 396
treatment drugs, chemical structure 386, 387
Two-compartment models. *See also* Hollow fiber multi-compartment PK/PD model

U

Ultrafiltration
materials 117
methods 117, 118
Urinary creatinine clearance 540
Urinary tract infections (UTIs)
antimicrobial efficacy assessment 70
antimicrobial therapy 71
bacterial pathogens 71
pathogenic microorganisms 71

V

Valacyclovir
dose–response relationship 446
high serum levels 445
oral formulations 443
Vancomycin 641–642
ABW and creatinine clearance estimation 262, 277
AUC/MIC 589
augmented renal clearance 274–275
Bayesian analysis 278–279
Bayesian estimation and Monte Carlo simulations 588
beta-lactam antibiotics 588
broth microdilution and E-test methods 588
Cockcroft–Gault equation 277
continuous infusion 274
developmental and renal maturation 588
dosing chart 276
efficacy 261
feasibility 589
linear regression analysis 276
loading doses 273–274
Matzke and Moellering nomograms 277
MDRD 277
MIC 262
(*see* Minimum inhibitory concentration (MIC))
monitoring guidelines 262–264
monitoring serum and pre-dose trough concentrations 262
MRSA infections 261
nephrotoxicity 261, 589
nomograms 276
obesity 272–273
optimal therapy 262
PAE 588
pathogens 262
patients 277
peak and trough concentrations 590
pediatrics 272
pharmacokinetics 264–265
preterm and full-term neonates 589
priori dosing method 276
serum creatinine and post-menstrual age 589
skin infections 262
therapeutic drug monitoring 275–276
toxic exposure 589
toxicity and adverse reactions 279–280
Varicella-zoster virus (VZV) 441, 442
Ventilator-associated bacterial pneumonia (VABP)
clinical and microbiological response 137
microbiological 140
VZV. *See* Varicella-zoster virus (VZV)

X

XDR-TB. *See* Extensively drug-resistant tuberculosis (XDR-TB)

Z

Zanamivir
influenza 457
intravenous formulations 460
oral inhalation 455
and oseltamivir 455
parenteral formulation 455
treatment and prophylaxis 457
Zidovudine 474, 475